WC
100

2008

D1433821

WC
100

2008

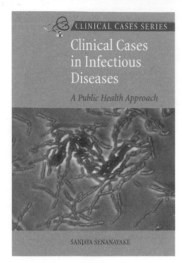

Clinical Cases in Infectious Diseases
Sanjaya Senanayake

ISBN 9780074716625

Effective management of most communicable diseases involves not only a clinical response, but a public health response. Clinical Cases in Infectious Diseases: A Public Health Approach, by Sanjaya Senanayake, increases our understanding of the synergy generated by these groups when they work closely together to fight notifiable infections. 22 clinical cases comprehensively discuss 23 infections in a problem-based format. Each chapter is modelled on an interactive scenario with characters and dialogue, incorporating clinical, laboratory and public health aspects.

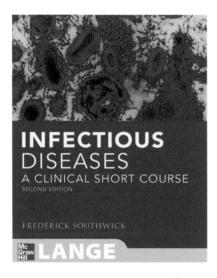

Infectious Diseases: A Clinical Short Course 2e
Frederick Southwick

ISBN 9780071477222

Infectious Diseases: A Clinical Short Course 2e, by Frederick Southwick, is a self-instruction tool organised by body systems/regions as opposed to pathogens, simulating how common pathogens and disorders would be encountered by clinicans in rounds or in practice. Key features include case examples, key point summaries, questions to aid comprehension, and 24 colour plates depicting key pathogens.

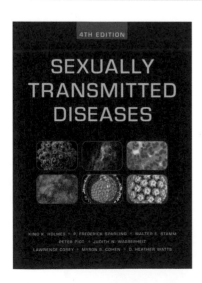

Sexually Transmitted Diseases 4e
King K. Holmes, Frederick P. Sparling, Walter E. Stamm, Peter Piot, Judith N. Wasserheit, Lawrence Corey, Myron Cohen

ISBN 9780071417488

Sexually Transmitted Diseases 4e, by King Holmes et al, covers all aspects of STDs, from epidemiology to diagnosis and public health measures. Featuring an exciting new full-colour format, the fourth edition of Sexually Transmitted Diseases delivers the most encyclopaedic overview of the clinical, microbiological and public health aspects of STDs, including HIV.

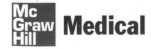

INFECTIOUS DISEASES

ATLAS • CASES • TEXT

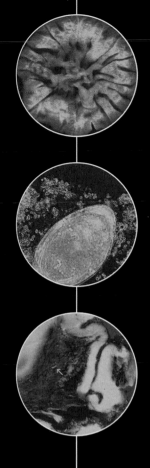

INFECTIOUS

DISEASES

ATLAS • CASES • TEXT

NORTH HAMPSHIRE HOSPITAL HEALTHCARE LIBRARY

The **McGraw·Hill** Companies

Sydney New York San Francisco Auckland
Bangkok Bogotá Caracas Hong Kong
Kuala Lumpur Lisbon London Madrid
Mexico City Milan New Delhi San Juan
Seoul Singapore Taipei Toronto

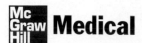

Notice

Medicine is an ever-changing science. As new research and clinical experience broaden our knowledge, changes in treatment and drug therapy are required. The editors and the publisher of this work have checked with sources believed to be reliable in their efforts to provide information that is complete and generally in accord with the standards accepted at the time of publication. However, in view of the possibility of human error or changes in medical sciences, neither the editors, nor the publisher, nor any other party who has been involved in the preparation or publication of this work warrants that the information contained herein is in every respect accurate or complete. Readers are encouraged to confirm the information contained herein with other sources. For example, and in particular, readers are advised to check the product information sheet included in the package of each drug they plan to administer to be certain that the information contained in this book is accurate and that changes have not been made in the recommended dose or in the contraindications for administration. This recommendation is of particular importance in connection with new or infrequently used drugs.

Photographs © 2008 Robin A. Cooke

Text and illustrations © 2008 McGraw-Hill Australia Pty Ltd

Every effort has been made to trace and acknowledge copyrighted material. The authors and publishers tender their apologies should any infringement have occurred.

Reproduction and communication for educational purposes

The Australian *Copyright Act 1968* (the Act) allows a maximum of one chapter or 10% of the pages of this work, whichever is the greater, to be reproduced and/or communicated by any educational institution for its educational purposes provided that the institution (or the body that administers it) has sent a Statutory Educational notice to Copyright Agency Limited (CAL) and been granted a licence. For details of statutory educational and other copyright licences contact: Copyright Agency Limited, Level 15, 233 Castlereagh Street, Sydney NSW 2000. Telephone: (02) 9394 7600. Website: www.copyright.com.au

Reproduction and communication for other purposes

Apart from any fair dealing for the purposes of study, research, criticism or review, as permitted under the Act, no part of this publication may be reproduced, distributed or transmitted in any form or by any means, or stored in a database or retrieval system, without the written permission of McGraw-Hill Australia including, but not limited to, any network or other electronic storage.

Enquiries should be made to the publisher via www.mcgraw-hill.com.au or at the address below.

National Library of Australia Cataloguing-in-Publication Data

Author:	Cooke, Robin A.
Title:	Infectious diseases: atlas, cases, text/Robin A. Cooke.
ISBN:	9780070159068 (hbk.)
Notes:	Includes index.
Subjects:	Communicable diseases—Atlases.
	Communicable diseases—Case studies.
Dewey Number:	616.9

Published in Australia by

McGraw-Hill Australia Pty Ltd

Level 2, 82 Waterloo Road, North Ryde NSW 2113

Publisher: Elizabeth Walton
Managing Editor: Kathryn Fairfax
Associate Editor: Hollie Zondanos
Production Editor: Kim Ross
Copy Editor: Connie de Silva
Cover design: Patricia McCallum
Typesetter: Midland Typesetters, Australia
Proofreader: Pamela Dunne
Indexer: Max McMaster
Printed in China on 105 gsm matt art by CTPS

Foreword

For the visually-oriented medical student or physician, a wealth of highly relevant knowledge is transmitted in Robin A Cooke's lifetime's work of collecting outstanding quality images: clinical photographs, gross pathology specimens, radiographs, and photomicrographs of pathologic lesions. For those to whom the real disease alterations carry more meaning and lasting impression on the memory, these illustrations reveal the reality that words alone cannot convey. From the novice student who sees a lumbar puncture procedure and the appearance of pathologic cerebrospinal fluid for the first time, to the expert subspecialist who has never personally diagnosed yaws, *Mycobacterium marinum* infection, or donovanosis, there is valuable knowledge to be obtained from these pages.

Infectious diseases clearly have not disappeared from the earth. Understanding their nature has never been more important as both treatment and epidemiologic control require a timely and accurate diagnosis. Tropical diseases, such as those so well-represented from Papua-New Guinea in this atlas, remain important components of the global burden of infections. These clinical, usually cutaneous, manifestations demand our attention and comprehension.

Most of the chapters represent a group of etiologic agents in a taxonomic category such as bacteria, viruses, fungi, protozoa or helminths. Moreover, the greatest threat of infectious diseases is presented in separate chapters on pandemic diseases and emerging viral infections. Contained therein are some jewels of contemporary pathology, including HIV immune reconstitution syndrome, a wonderfully illustrated case of SARS (severe acute respiratory syndrome), human monkeypox, and two spectacular demonstrations of Hendra virus infection. The readers will be unlikely to miss these diagnoses when they reappear in their pathology department.

Throughout the book, Dr. Cooke has provided appropriate interesting historical vignettes, photographs of key persons and places, and numerous clinical cases to enhance one's desire to know more about the diseases and the medical science that has illuminated them. It is amazing and intriguing, both to those from 'down under' and to persons from the other continents alike, how many important discoveries in medical sciences have originated in Australia. Liberal doses of pride and appreciation await the Aussies and non-Aussies who absorb this beautifully illustrated view of infectious diseases from an Australian perspective. The general clinician will find the work as attractive and useful as the medical student, registrar, practicing pathologist, and dermatologist. It would take a lifetime to gain the experience that is acquired by a just few hours of perusing the atlas.

David H. Walker, MD
The Carmage and Martha Walls Distinguished University Chair in Tropical Diseases
Professor and Chairman, Department of Pathology
Executive Director, Center for Biodefense and Emerging Infectious Diseases
University of Texas Medical Branch

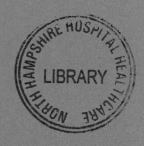

Brief Contents

Detailed Contents

Preface

I decided to produce this atlas to attempt to meet a perceived lack of published, high quality illustrations of tropical and other infectious diseases. It is difficult for a single author to collect such illustrations, but I was fortunate to work in a tertiary referral centre in which personal contact between clinicians, patients, nurses and laboratory staff was still maintained. Before that I had worked in Papua New Guinea where tropical diseases abound, and I maintained close contact with practitioners in Papua New Guinea. I established cordial relationships with infectious disease pathologists throughout the world. As a result of this it was possible to gather clinical and other information on most of the patients, and to maintain a fairly uniform standard in the quality of the recording.

Emphasis is placed on the clinical presentation and laboratory diagnosis of the diseases considered. Treatment is rarely mentioned because it changes as new therapies are introduced. It is hoped that the information provided is accurate, but in-depth scientific information is not a feature of the text. Such information can be obtained in comprehensive text books. Few references are given because it is meant to be mainly an atlas, and up to date references can be obtained from the internet.

Not all infectious diseases present with clinical signs that can be photographed. For this reason, some common diseases have been omitted. Some rare diseases have been included in the hope that they illustrate some general principles rather than being just 'so what' cases.

The text is presented in a somewhat conversational style, and, as far as possible, in the form of case histories, so that it is easy to read and in a format that may be useful for teachers. In an attempt to add further interest to the text some historical anecdotes are included with some current photographs of the places where these original observations were made.

Diseases such as leprosy, syphilis, smallpox and yaws could be regarded as being diseases that have been controlled, and descriptions of them are of historical value only. However, it is hard to find concise illustrations of the clinical and pathological features of these conditions, and some of them are showing signs of resurgence.

Diseases such as tuberculosis and malaria are now rarely encountered in economically affluent societies, but they are very important tropical diseases and travel medicine doctors, in particular, need to know how to diagnose and treat them. Due to the speed and availability of modern means of travel, the world has become a much smaller place, and doctors everywhere need to have some knowledge of the clinical manifestations of most of the diseases illustrated in this atlas.

Some diseases that may be caused by a number of different organisms, such as meningitis and infective endocarditis, are presented as a disease entity rather than in the more traditional manner of presentation by organism type.

Mention is made of 'emerging infections' partly to illustrate their features, and partly to illustrate how their causes were identified. Organisms mutate quite quickly so it will always be necessary for all categories of health workers to maintain their vigilance. By doing this they will ensure that any new disease will be recognised as a clinical entity and its cause identified, so that it can be controlled as quickly as possible.

Mention is also made of bio-terrorism since this is set to become an unfortunate fact of life.

The disciplines of immunology and molecular biology are advancing very rapidly, and increasingly laboratory diagnoses in many fields are being made by immunological tests. Some of these are mentioned in the text, but the rate of introduction of new tests would make a detailed listing obsolete before it was printed. Older methods of diagnosis are emphasised because many countries in which tropical and other infectious diseases are most prevalent cannot afford the new immunological tests.

The author hopes that this atlas will be of use to students in all fields of biological study, to clinical and laboratory health workers, to travel medicine doctors and perhaps even to specialist infectious disease physicians who may only need to 'borrow' some of the images for their lecture presentations.

Robin A. Cooke,
Brisbane, Australia.
June 2008

The Author

Professor ROBIN A. COOKE
OBE, OAM, MD, DCP, FRCPA, FRCPath, FACTM, FAICD
Brisbane, Australia

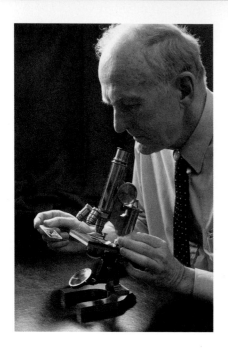

Professor Cooke graduated from the University of Queensland Medical School in Brisbane, Australia, in 1959. He trained in pathology in Brisbane and at the Royal Postgraduate Medical School, London, and in the 1960s he established the pathology services in Papua New Guinea. Stationed in Port Moresby, he had the fascinating opportunity to study the pathology of 3 million Stone Age people as they came into contact with western medicine for the first time. This study continued for the next 40 years and in 2003 he was awarded an Order of the British Empire by the PNG Government for his contribution to medicine in that country.

For 23 years Professor Cooke was Director of Anatomical Pathology at the Royal Brisbane Hospital, one of the largest teaching hospitals in Australia. During this time he built on his New Guinea experience and became an expert in Tropical Diseases.

Together with Brian Stewart he published *A Colour Atlas of Anatomical Pathology* (Churchill Livingstone). The 3rd edition was released in 2003 and editions were published in Spanish, Japanese, Greek and Russian.

Since 1995 Professor Cooke has been editor and producer of *International Pathology*, the news bulletin of the International Academy of Pathology (circulation 23 000 worldwide) and in this capacity was invited to be the editor and main contributor to a commemorative publication to mark the 100th anniversary of the IAP.

In 2001 Professsor Cooke received the Distinguished Pathologist award from the Australasian Division of the IAP, and in 2006 the rare distinction of a gold medal from the International body of the IAP.

Brian Stewart is a photographer/illustrator who has enjoyed a 40 year career in applied photography. For 20 years he was photographer in the pathology department and later, photographer in charge of the medical illustration department of the Royal Brisbane Hospital. This was followed by a 6 year period as medical photographer at the Wesley Hospital Brisbane.

He was a foundation member of the Australian Institute of Medical and Biological Illustration (AIMBI).

In later years he has ably assisted Professor Cooke in the preparation of illustrative material for ongoing education programs and for numerous publications.

Acknowledgments

Brian Stewart was the image manipulator for the images in this book. We have worked closely together since 1968, and without his assistance much of the material that I have published would never have seen the light of day. His wife, Dot has patiently put up with us both spending many hours in photographic endeavours.

Editorial advice was kindly provided by **Joan Faoagali**, Director of Microbiology, Royal Brisbane, Royal Women's and Royal Children's hospitals, Pathology Queensland, Herston Campus, Brisbane, Australia, and **Ian Wilkey**, formerly Director General of Health, Queensland, Australia,

The chapters in the book were very kindly reviewed by the following experts in the relevant subjects:

Graeme Nimmo, Director of Microbiology, Pathology Queensland, Princess Alexandra Hospital, Brisbane

Chris Coulter, Director of Microbiology and Infectious Diseases Departments, Pathology Queensland, The Prince Charles Hospital, Brisbane, and Head of the WHO Western Pacific Region Mycobacterial Reference Laboratory

Grace Warren, reconstructive surgeon and senior consultant in leprosy to the World Leprosy Mission

Ken Clezy, former Professor of Surgery and Dean of the Faculty of Medicine, University of Papua New Guinea, and senior consultant in leprosy and senior surgeon, Health Department, Papua New Guinea

Joan Faoagali, Director of Microbiology, Royal Brisbane, Royal Women's and Royal Children's hospitals, Pathology Queensland, Herston Campus, Brisbane

John Patten, Director, Sexual Health Unit, Queensland Health, Brisbane, Australia

David Ellis, Head, Mycology Unit, Women's and Children's Hospital, Adelaide and Head of the Mycology reference centre for Australia

David Siebert, Director, Virology, Royal Brisbane, Royal Women's and Royal Children's hospital, Pathology Queensland, Herston Campus, Brisbane, Australia

Jenny Robson, Head, Microbiology Department, and Infectious Disease Physician, Sullivan Nicolaides Pathology, Brisbane

Joe McCormack, Professor and Director of Infectious Diseases, Mater Hospital, Brisbane.

Special topics were contributed by the following:

HIV/AIDS: cases and commentary courtesy of **Ann Marie Nelson**, Chief, Division of AIDS Pathology, Armed Forces Institute of Pathology, Washington, USA

SARS: case and commentary courtesy of **Jiang Gu**, Professor and Chair, Department of Pathology, and Dean (in association with staff member, Xueying Shi), School of Basic Medical Sciences, Peking University, Beijing, China

Monkeypox virus: case and commentary courtesy of **Sherif R Zaki**, Chief, Infectious Disease Pathology Activity, Division of Viral and Rickettsial Diseases, National

Center for Infectious Diseases, Centers for Disease Control and Prevention, Atlanta, USA

'Basidiobolus': case and commentary courtesy of **Michel Huerre**, Chief, Histopathology Unit, Pasteur Institute, Paris, France

Hendra virus pneumonitis: courtesy of **Anthony J Ansford**, Director of Forensic Pathology, Pathology Queensland, Brisbane, and **Joseph G. McCormack**, Professor and Director of Infectious Diseases Mater Hospital, Brisbane

Hendra virus Encephalitis: courtesy of **Ian Brown**, Sullivan and Nicolaides Pathology, and **John O'Sullivan**, Neurologist, Brisbane

Hendra virus Equine cases: Courtesy of **Roger Kelly**, Head, Veterinary Pathology Department, University of Queensland, Brisbane

Lyssa virus: courtesy of **Tom Robertson**, Director of Anatomical Pathology, Royal Brisbane, Royal Women's and Royal Children's hospitals, Queensland Health, Herston Campus, Brisbane

Melioidosis: courtesy of **Norain Karim**, Consultant pathologist and Head of Pathology Department, Ipoh Hospital, Ipoh, Perak, Malaysia

Rickettsia australis: case, photographs and commentary courtesy of **Bernie Hudson**, Head of Microbiology and Infectious Diseases Departments, Royal North Shore Hospital, Sydney.

Those photographs not taken by Brian Stewart or myself were contributed by numerous colleagues from around the world. These are acknowledged individually. Some of the photographs came from the pre-1990 photograph collection of the Pathology Department, Royal Brisbane Hospital. These are reproduced with permission of Michael Whiley, Director of Pathology Queensland, Brisbane.

A number of photographs are reproduced from Cooke, R.A. and Stewart, B: *Colour Atlas of Anatomical Pathology*. Edinburgh, Churchill Livingstone, 2004. They are reproduced with permission of the authors and the publisher, Churchill Livingstone.

The author wishes to thank his colleagues in the Pathology Department, (staff pathologists, trainee pathologists, scientists and secretaries) of the Royal Brisbane Hospital, and the other major pathology laboratories in Brisbane; the staff of the Pathology Department, University of Queensland; clinical colleagues, nursing and allied health colleagues and administrators in all departments of the Royal Brisbane, Royal Women's and Royal Children's hospitals; clinical colleagues in private practice in Brisbane and elsewhere; laboratory and clinical colleagues in Papua New Guinea; colleagues from many different countries around the world; and the patients who kindly allowed us to photograph themselves in the interest of medical teaching.

Kathy Bevin typed most of the original drafts of the book and I am grateful to her for this. I am also grateful for the care and expertise with which the editors and proof readers at McGraw-Hill treated the manuscript which was greatly improved as a result of their efforts.

My wife, Roma has been a constant and patient friend and companion for the past 50 years during the collection of the material that is included in this book.

Robin A. Cooke
Brisbane, Australia
June 2008

Historical overview

Infectious diseases have been a significant cause of morbidity and mortality throughout the whole of human existence. Human beings throughout the centuries have wrestled with the problems of how to explain their occurrence, and how to prevent and treat them. Religious and metaphysical explanations were popular, particularly when trying to explain the cause of epidemic and pandemic infections.

The French microbiologist Louis Pasteur (1822–1895) (depicted in Fig. 1.1) introduced the 'germ theory of disease' and, in doing so, became the 'father of microbiology'. He began his observations with studies on fermentation, which he published in 1857. The formal introduction in 1880 of the germ theory of disease was received with mixed reactions of belief and disbelief.

In Berlin, Robert Koch (1843–1910), the German physician and Nobel laureate, also supported the germ theory of disease. He identified the causative organisms for tuberculosis, anthrax, cholera and many other diseases. Between them, Pasteur and Koch began the specialty of microbiology. Shortly after Koch identified the anthrax bacillus, Pasteur successfully developed a vaccine to the organism, having found that by repeated subcultures of the organism it lost its virulence. This 'attenuated strain' of the organism injected into an animal made it immune to infection with the unattenuated (wild or natural) organism.

Farmers in a town in the south of France offered Pasteur 60 sheep on which to demonstrate the efficacy of his vaccine. Of these, 25 were vaccinated and 25 were not. Both of these groups were then infected with live anthrax organisms. The remaining 10 had no injections and served as controls. On 5 May 1881, the trial began amid considerable press publicity and much public interest. By the end of a month, all 25 unvaccinated sheep had died or were on the point of death. All 25 vaccinated sheep were alive and well, as were the 10 controls. The farmers believed in Pasteur's vaccine, but some of the academicians of the medical establishment in Paris did not. As a result of this experiment, Pasteur became famous.

On 6 July 1885, Pasteur was presented with a shepherd boy, Joseph Meister, who had been bitten 2 days before by a dog infected with rabies (depicted in Fig. 1.2). This infection was regarded as almost a sentence of death because it was known that rabies had a very high mortality. Pasteur, who had been experimenting with a vaccine for rabies, gave the boy a course of vaccination. The boy survived and stayed on as a servant to Pasteur.

Pasteur was already world famous at this point and after the success with Joseph Meister, people came from all over Europe to be vaccinated against rabies. He was not a medical doctor and thus could not give the injections himself, but was always in attendance.

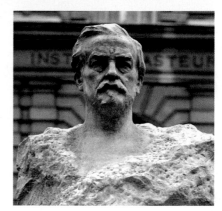

▲ **Fig. 1.1** Bust of Louis Pasteur in the front garden at the entrance to the Institut Pasteur in Paris. This building was constructed for Pasteur as a laboratory and a home by the French government in 1888.

▼ **Fig. 1.2** The story of Joseph Meister being bitten by a rabid dog is commemorated by this statue at the entrance to the Institut Pasteur in Paris.

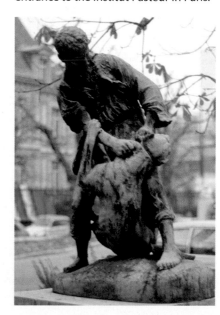

Descriptions of discoveries made by doctors, scientists and other researchers in the field if infectious diseases are provided in this book. Many of the summaries and facts were drawn from this source: Simmons, J. G., *Doctors and Discoveries: Lives that Created Today's Medicine*, Houghton Mifflin Company, Boston, 2002.

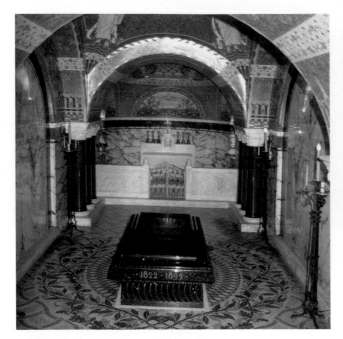

▲ **Fig. 1.3** Tomb of Louis Pasteur in the memorial chapel in the Institut Pasteur, Paris.

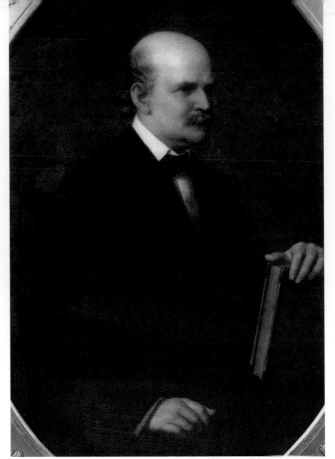

▲ **Fig. 1.4** Ignaz Semmelweis (1818–1865).

Following Pasteur's death in 1895, a memorial chapel was built that year in the Institut Pasteur and his body placed in a black basalt coffin in front of the altar (see Fig. 1.3). With donations from grateful patients, the ceiling of the chapel was decorated with ceramics that commemorate the various experiments that made him famous.

Following on from the work of Pasteur, it is not surprising that his successors at the Pasteur Institute were pioneers in immunology and vaccine production. The Institute remains one of the premier centers of medical research in the world, and is still a leader in the fields of immunology and vaccine production.

Quite soon after its opening, the Institute began to establish branch laboratories throughout the world. It took a keen interest in tropical diseases, which included every type of infectious disease. It continues this interest to the present day, not only in the headquarters laboratory in Paris but also in its branch laboratories in countries around the world.

Empirical observations that preceded the germ theory of disease

Ignaz Semmelweis and washing hands

Before the germ theory of disease was established, many empirical observations about the organismal cause of disease were made. Perhaps the most famous person in this regard was Ignaz Semmelweis (1818–1865), the Hungarian physician and obstetrician (see Fig. 1.4).

Semmelweis graduated in medicine from the Vienna Medical School, then the most famous school in Europe. He specialized in obstetrics. The fame of the Vienna Medical School derives from the advances to medical knowledge based on careful correlation between the clinical features of diseases compared with the pathologic changes seen at post mortem.

As well as his clinical duties, Semmelweis was appointed in charge of all post mortems on obstetrical cases from the hospital. At that time, the hospital was the biggest in Europe with in excess of 3000 deliveries per year.

Most of the clinics in the hospital were divided into two units. The first maternity clinic was staffed by doctors and the second clinic by midwives. In 1846, the maternal mortality in the first clinic was 13 per cent and in the second it was 2 per cent. Women in labor begged not to be admitted into the first clinic.

In puzzling over this discrepancy in outcomes, Semmelweis wondered whether the students and doctors were taking something from the post-mortem room into the delivery rooms. His suspicions were confirmed when a pathologist colleague died after cutting himself while performing a post mortem. At the post mortem on the pathologist, it was noticed that the changes seen in his organs were similar to those seen in women who had died of 'child bed fever'. In May 1847, Semmelweis insisted that all students and doctors must wash their hands in bowls of chlorinated lime water, and must clean under their finger-nails before going to the delivery rooms. The mortality in the first clinic in June 1847 decreased to 3 per cent. Soon it dropped further. In spite of this resounding vindication of his observations, he fell out with the hospital authorities and, disappointed, he returned to his home city of Budapest, Hungary, where he spent the rest of his life.

John Snow's research on cholera

The British physician John Snow (1813–1858) working in London, England, investigated an outbreak of cholera in August 1854, that in 10 days caused 500 deaths. Those who died had been living in houses around Golden Square in central London (see Fig. 1.5). Snow carefully compiled a record of 83 of the victims. From his work with a previous epidemic of cholera in 1848, he suspected drinking water as the cause of the disease. He found that all of the deceased had drunk water from a common water pump situated in the nearby Broad Street. He persuaded the authorities to remove the handle from the pump (shown in Figs 1.6 and 1.7). The death rate in the area dropped at once. Snow's

empirical observation was confirmed in 1883, when Robert Koch working with patients in Egypt and India identified the causative organism of cholera—the *Vibrio cholerae*.

Snow followed up with further studies on the waters of the River Thames. His research showed that discharge of raw sewage into drinking water was the cause of the cholera outbreak, but the politicians did not believe him. It was not until the terrible stench of sewage effluent stopped the proceedings in Parliament in 1858 that a major engineering enterprise was commissioned to build a sewerage system to pipe the sewage from the city, well down to near the mouth of the River Thames. Snow died before the sewers were constructed.

Clinical observations on cholera

Clinically, cholera presents with severe diarrhea. Fluid loss is massive and death occurs from dehydration and electrolyte imbalance. Epidemics occur frequently, and there are always new strains of the organism appearing. Cholera continues to be a common infection in Kolkata (formerly Calcutta) India (see Fig. 1.8 overleaf). The National Institute of Cholera and Enteric Diseases (NICED), a reference center for monitoring epidemics and identifying new mutations of the *Vibrio cholerae* organism, established there in the early twentieth century, is still functioning.

Antisepsis

Another important empiricist was the British surgeon Joseph Lister (1827–1912), a contemporary of Pasteur, who worked mainly in Scotland. Lister read Pasteur's observations on fermentation and putrefaction and he applied them to a common surgical problem—infection in compound fractures of bones (that is, fractures in which the bone protrudes through the skin).

From 1865, after treatment of a fracture, Lister applied dressings soaked in carbolic acid—a substance that had

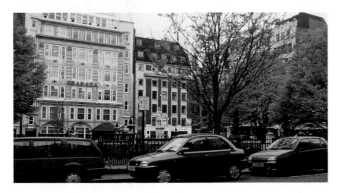

▲ **Fig. 1.5** Golden Square in London, England, where a fatal outbreak of cholera occurred in 1854.

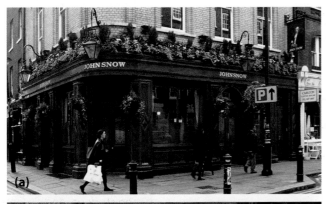

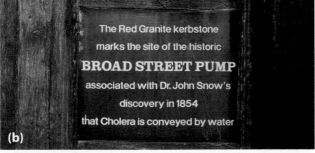

▲ **Fig. 1.6(a)** The John Snow pub built on the site of the Broad Street Pump. **(b)** Plaque on the wall at the entrance to the pub.

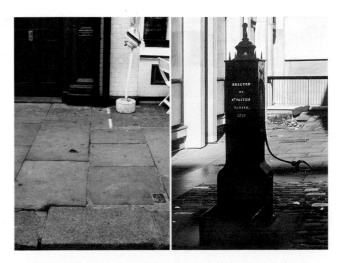

▲ **Fig. 1.7** The red stone in the footpath that marks the site where the common pump once stood. Beside it is a pump similar to the original one.

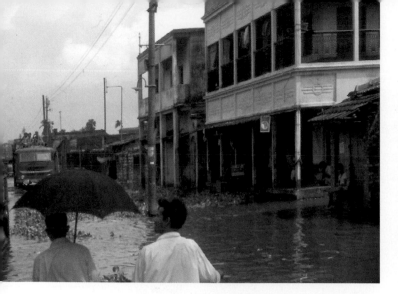

▲ **Fig. 1.8** From a tourist bus passing through the flooded streets of Kolkata today, one may observe the sewage being mixed with the drinking water, as it has been for centuries.

been used effectively in the treatment of sewage. This method of antisepsis was successful in reducing the rate of infection in the wounds he treated. In 1870 he introduced a device that sprayed carbolic acid over the operating site, which came to be called 'the Lister spray' (shown in Fig. 1.9). It was cumbersome to operate and was abandoned by 1887; however, the concept of antisepsis was well established by this time.

Then, compound fractures of the limbs were notorious for becoming infected, as they still are today. Before Lister, an untreated compound fracture was almost uniformly fatal as a result of the infection. The treatment of such fractures was amputation of the limb—a daunting operation (see Figs 1.10 and 1.11). It was done without anesthetic and with a mortality of about 50 per cent.

Such amputations were the main operation performed for centuries by military surgeons. The surgeon's operating area below deck on naval ships was painted red so as to obscure the appearance of the large amounts of blood that spilled during surgery.

The history of penicillin

Alexander Fleming's discovery

In 1928, the Scottish microbiologist Alexander Fleming (1881–1955), working at St Mary's Hospital in London (see Fig. 1.12), noticed that cultures of the fungus *Penicillium notatum* inhibited the growth of colonies of *Staphylococcus aureus* inoculated onto the same culture plate. He examined a culture of *S. aureus* under a dissecting microscope. This involved having the lid off the Petri dish for some time. The lid was replaced, and the plate was left on the laboratory bench for about 2 days (Fig. 1.13). When he came back to examine it again, he noticed that a mold had grown on the plate; the colonies around the mold had decreased in size and many of them had disappeared. He rightly concluded that something was being produced by the mold that diffused into the surrounding medium, causing the death of the organisms.

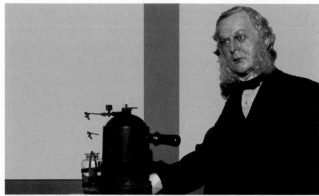

▲ **Fig. 1.9** Display in the Museum of the Royal College of Surgeons of Edinburgh, Scotland, showing Lister with his 'Lister spray'.

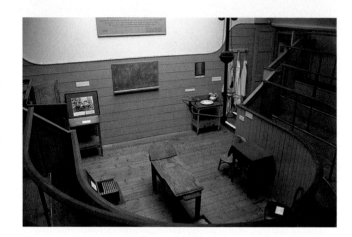

▲ **Fig. 1.10** St Thomas's Hospital, London. The old operating theatre has been preserved intact since closure in 1862. The photo shows the operating table on which the patient was laid. The extension to the table was drawn out and the leg to be amputated placed upon it. The surgeon operated in street clothes, without gloves. A box of sawdust (seen in the bottom of the photo) was positioned under the operating site to soak up the blood. The surgeon would kick the box to the required strategic position. No ligatures were used. The leg stump was dipped into boiling oil to staunch the bleeding. If the patient survived, chronic osteomyelitis was the normal consequence.

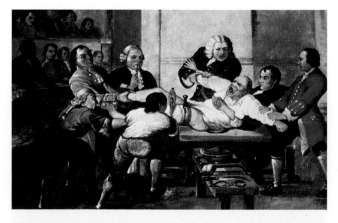

▲ **Fig. 1.11** The painting on the wall of the operating theatre shows the scene. The patient was blindfolded and held down to minimize movement.

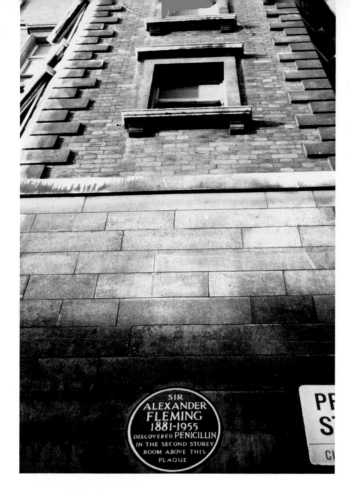

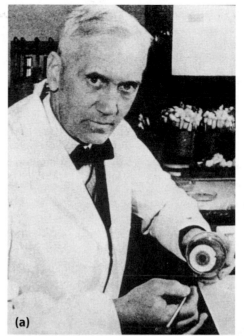

(a)

▲ **Fig. 1.12** St Mary's Hospital, London, where Alexander Fleming worked as a microbiologist.

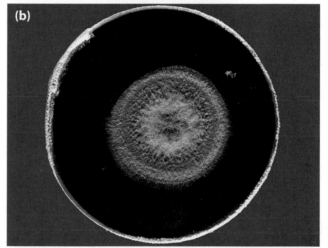

(b)

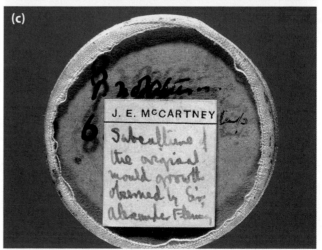

(c)

Fleming had been investigating substances called 'antibiotics' for some time. Such substances had been known since 1889. He noticed that mucus from his nasal secretions contained an enzyme—which he called lysozyme—that inhibited the growth of nonpathogenic organisms. Thus, while his observation was a flash of genius, his mind had been prepared for such a chance happening.

He then proceeded to grow the mold in a broth. He filtered this and used the filtrate to test against a number of common organisms. He made a trench across an agar plate and placed agar mixed with the filtrate into the trench. The active substance in the filtrate diffused into the adjacent medium. Test organisms were then streaked up to the trough, and their sensitivity to the filtrate could be assessed. Organisms such as *Staphylococci*, *Streptococci* and *Pneumococci* were sensitive, while organisms such as *Escherichia coli* and *Bacillus subtilis* were resistant.

He further tested some of the properties of the substance and showed that the dilute broth was effective in inhibiting growth of organisms up to a dilution of 1/1000—that is, three times the dilution at which phenol (an antiseptic agent) became inactive. The substance was quite unstable; its activity fell off on standing; it was sensitive to pH, to freezing and to heating. He could not do any more with these observations because he had neither the chemical know-how nor the equipment to further concentrate and purify his substance.

▲ **Fig. 1.13(a)** Fleming, after he became famous, used to make small culture plates of *P. notatum*, which he gave as souvenirs to his friends. Here in his laboratory, he is holding such a plate. **(b) and (c)** One of these plates Fleming gave to James McCartney, later Professor of Bacteriology at the University of Adelaide, Australia.

The work of Howard Florey and Ernst Chain

In 1938, the medical scientist Howard Florey (1898–1968) (Figs 1.14 and 1.15) originally from Adelaide, Australia, and the biochemist Ernst Chain (1906–1979) from Berlin, Germany, working together in Oxford, England, completed a series of experiments on the enzyme lysozyme, which Chain was able to crystallize. They then decided to investigate the properties of antibiotic substances. They examined the literature and, after reading Fleming's papers, decided that penicillin was worth studying. They concentrated the substance and produced it in pure powder form.

As a powder, it was quite stable and it was effective at a dilution of 1/1 000 000. It was not effective if taken by mouth, but worked well when given by injection. They tested mice infected with different organisms and reported their results in 1940.

In February 1941, Florey and Chain reported the first human trial of penicillin. The patient was a 43-year-old policeman, who had developed a massive mixed streptococcal and staphylococcal septicemia following a small cut on his face, acquired while he was working in his rose garden. By 24 hours he had improved, and by day five he was afebrile and eating. Believing that he was on the way to recovery, Florey and Chain used the remainder of their penicillin to treat a 15-year-old boy with osteomyelitis following a hip operation which involved the insertion of a pin. The boy made an initial recovery, but when the penicillin ran out and the pin was removed, the infection recurred. He had a stormy relapse but eventually recovered. The policeman remained stable for 10 days but then he relapsed and died, as there was no penicillin left for treatment.

At the time of Florey and Chain's research, which occurred during the years of World War Two, Britain was fighting for its life, and it was not possible to develop an industrial process to manufacture this new antibiotic product. So, Florey was impelled to take a dangerous flight to the USA, carrying with him some of the purified penicillin and the culture of *P. notatum*. He visited a US Government Research Laboratory in Peoria, Illinois, which soon afterwards started work on developing a technique for manufacturing commercial amounts of penicillin. They used deep broth cultures in 10 000–15 000 gallon tanks. The culture medium was corn steep liquor, a by-product of the manufacture of starch from corn (maize). The vast cultures were kept aerated by thin jets of air constantly blown into the tanks. The chief mycologist was Charles Thorn (1872–1956).

The staff at Peoria tested molds from all over the world. The yields from these were variable but they got the best yield from *Penicillium chrysogenum*, grown from a cantaloupe bought in the local market. Various American pharmaceutical companies—Merck, Squibb, Pfizer, Abbott and Winthrop—joined a crash program to develop penicillin. Preliminary clinical tests showed that penicillin was effective against a wide range of organisms.

In 1944, when the Allied armies landed in Normandy, France, the US manufacturers had produced enough penicillin for it to be used prophylactically on all soldiers suffering severe injuries. There was a dramatic reduction in infected war wounds sustained in that battle, as compared with the campaigns of the preceding years.

After this dramatic initial success, the drug was tested in a variety of clinical situations; and its indications, dosage and toxicity were established. Clearly, it heralded a new era in medicine. Fleming, Florey and Chain shared a Nobel Prize in 1945 for their contribution to this achievement.

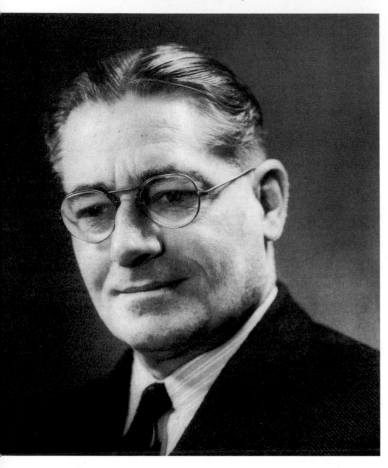

▲ **Fig. 1.14** Howard Florey (1898–1968).

▼ **Fig. 1.15** The Sir William Dunn School of Pathology in Oxford where Florey worked.

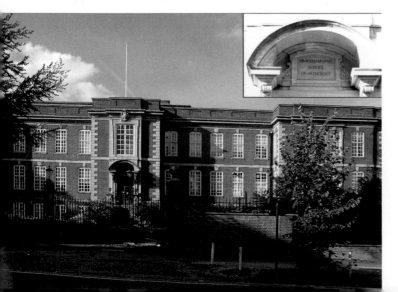

Subsequent advances in antibiotic research

After the cessation of World War Two, the hunt for new antibiotics was on in earnest. Molds from all over the world were tested for their antibiotic properties. By the mid 1950s, a number of new antibiotics were in routine use in medicine. The first of these after penicillin was streptomycin, which was very effective in treating tuberculosis as well as other infections.

It is hard to capture the excitement of laboratory workers in those heady days. The enduring memories of two Australian scientists—a biochemist and a microbiologist—may illustrate the mood.

In 1966, a then recently retired biochemist still vividly recalled the excitement in Florey's laboratory in the late 1940s, where she had been sent from the fledgling Commonwealth Serum Laboratories in Melbourne, Australia, to learn how to make penicillin for manufacture in Australia.

In 2000, a professor of microbiology in his retirement speech from the University of Queensland, spoke with lively recall about his time as a Fulbright Scholar at the University of Wisconsin in the early 1950s. Then, the hunt for new antibiotics was in full cry and the entire staff was swept up by 'the excitement of the chase'.

Vaccines

The first effective vaccine was introduced by Edward Jenner in 1796. This prevented the recipient of the cowpox vaccination from contracting smallpox, and resulted in the saving of numerous lives. Since then, many different types of vaccine have been introduced, and they have been responsible for changing the incidence of many common infectious diseases.

Jenner's vaccine was a simple use of a pure organism (cowpox), which caused a minor disease: the immunity produced protected against infection by a more virulent organism (smallpox).

The vaccines that followed this were also simple preparations of organisms that were attenuated in various ways so that a mild infection caused by them rendered the recipient immune to infection by a virulent organism.

In recent years, scientists have developed many different methods of producing vaccines that use only a small part of the organism or even artificial antigens to produce immunity in recipients of the vaccine.

Some vaccines that are currently available

- Anthrax
- Cholera
- Diphtheria
- Hepatitis A and hepatitis B
- Haemophylus influenzae type b (Hib)
- Human papilloma virus (HPV)
- Influenza
- Lyme disease
- Measles
- Meningococcal infection
- Monkeypox
- Mumps
- Pertussis (whooping cough)
- Pneumococcal infection
- Poliomyelitis
- Q fever
- Rabies
- Rotavirus

Many more vaccines are being developed and are undergoing field trials. One of the better known vaccines under trial is a vaccine for malaria.

Acknowledgments

- Fig. 1.3 Photographed with permission of the Curator of the Pasteur Museum, Pasteur Institute, Paris, France.
- Fig. 1.4 Courtesy of Anna Kadar, Semmelweis University, Budapest, Hungary.
- Fig. 1.9 Photographed with permission of the Curator of the Museum of the Royal College of Surgeons in Edinburgh, Scotland.
- Fig. 1.10 Photographed with permission of the Curator of the Garret Museum, London.
- Fig. 1.13(b) and (c) Photographed with permission of Mrs Peggy McCartney, Adelaide, Australia.

2

Bacterial infections

Bacterial infections are presented here in the context of the bacteria that more commonly cause disease in humans, rather than as the complete spectrum of bacterial infections. Some have been controlled by preventive and therapeutic measures, and a few are specifically important in certain areas of the world.

Meningitis

By definition, meningitis is an inflammation of the membranes that cover the nervous system. Meningitis can occur at all ages but is more common in children. The presenting symptoms are fever, headache, drowsiness and neck stiffness. Convulsions may occur. Untreated, the patient becomes unconscious and mortality is high. Antibiotic treatment is highly effective in treating most cases of meningitis.

More often than not, a specific organism causing meningitis is not isolated. The types of organisms isolated from cases of meningitis vary in different environmental situations.

Organisms that most commonly cause meningitis

Under 'ordinary community practice conditions' the ones most commonly isolated are:

- *Haemophilus influenzae*
- *Neisseria meningitidis*
- *Streptococcus pneumoniae*.

Less common organisms that cause meningitis

Less common organisms that cause meningitis are:

- *Mycobacterium tuberculosis*
- *Staphylococcus aureus*
- *Cryptococcus neoformans*
- free-living amebas (*Naegleria*).

Organisms that cause meningitis found particularly in neonates

Some organisms that cause meningitis are found particularly in neonates. These are:

- *Coliform organisms*
- *Listeria monocytogenes*
- Group B Streptococci.

Pathology

The inflammation of meningitis causes raised intracranial pressure. This can be seen in infants as a tense or bulging anterior fontanelle (shown in Fig. 2.1). Specifically, the acute inflammation of the meninges causes neck stiffness. In advanced cases of meningitis, the irritation of the meninges may cause severe spasm of back muscles (opisthotonos) (see Fig. 2.2).

Diagnosis

The diagnosis of meningitis is confirmed by lumbar puncture. For this procedure to be performed with the least trauma and the best results, the patient must be placed so that the spine is parallel to the bed. Children must be held firmly so that the operator can put the needle cleanly into the subarachnoid space, where the cerebrospinal fluid (CSF) is found (see Figs 2.3 and 2.4). Normal CSF is a clear fluid. In meningitis, it is turbid; and if the lumbar puncture is traumatic, it is blood stained (Fig. 2.5 overleaf).

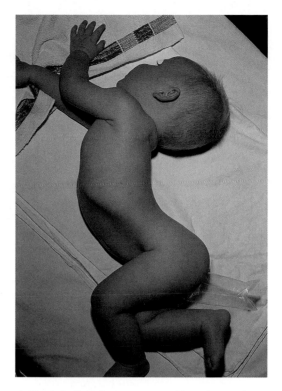

▲ **Fig. 2.2** Opisthotonos caused by advanced meningitis.

▼ **Fig. 2.1** Bulging fontanelle from raised intracranial pressure resulting from meningitis.

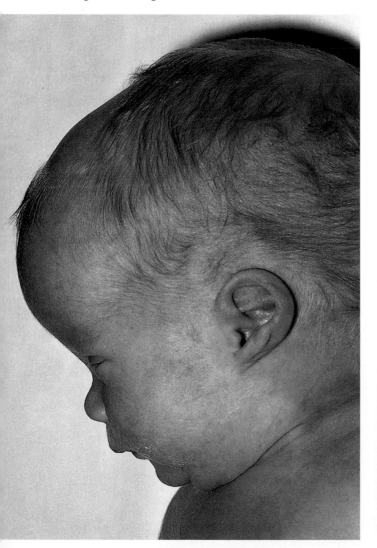

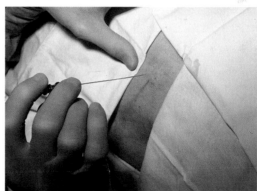

▲ **Fig. 2.3** Lumbar puncture being performed. After skin preparation, local anesthetic is injected and the needle is inserted.

▼ **Fig. 2.4** The stillette is removed and CSF drains from the needle. It is noted whether the CSF is under increased pressure and whether it is a clear color, turbid or purulent.

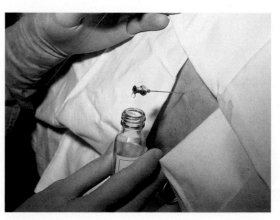

Figure 2.6 shows a segment of spinal cord removed at post mortem on a child who died from meningitis. The dura mater (the thick, tough membrane that covers the brain and spinal cord) has been opened to show the leptomeninges (pia arachnoid), the soft covering of the spinal cord. The lumbar puncture needle encounters resistance as it passes through the dura mater. When this is penetrated, the operator enters the subarachnoid space, where the CSF is found. At this stage of the procedure, the CSF begins to flow through the needle (as shown in Fig. 2.4 on page 9).

The pia arachnoid covers the whole of the brain and spinal cord, and the CSF circulates through this space. In meningitis, pus is found throughout the space. The images in Fig. 2.7 show pus in the subarachnoid space on the upper and inferior surfaces of the brain.

Fig. 2.8 is a microscopic section showing the pus (neutrophils) in the subarachnoid space and extending into the underlying brain via the perivascular space (the Virchow Robin space), which surrounds the blood vessels that leave the meninges to enter the substance of the brain.

In neonates who die from meningitis, the pus in the subarachnoid space is usually much thicker than it is in older children and adults (illustrated in Fig. 2.9).

▼ **Fig. 2.5** These three samples of CSF are—(from left) blood stained, clear, turbid.

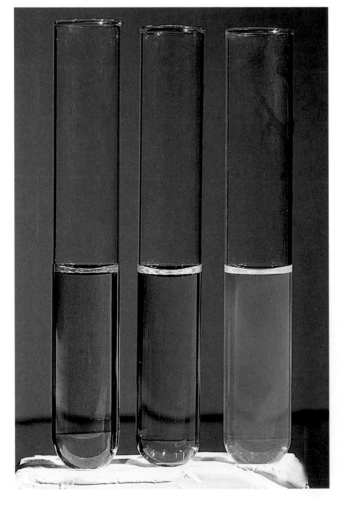

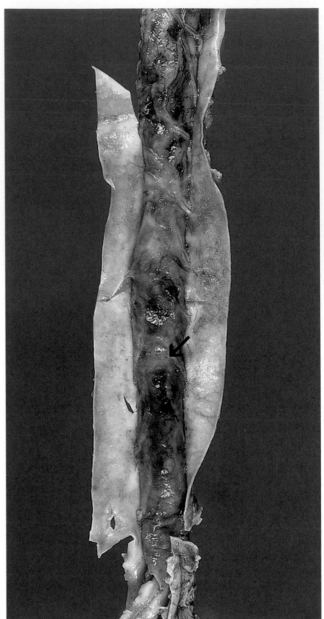

▲ **Fig. 2.6** Spinal cord from a child who died from meningitis. The dura mater has been opened to show the leptomeninges covering the spinal cord. The subarachnoid space is filled with pus. It is into this space that the doctor inserts a needle to aspirate CSF for testing.

▼ ▶ **Fig. 2.7(a) and (b)** The brain from the same patient as in Fig. 2.6 shows the white pus in the subarachnoid space over the surface of the brain. **(c)** Pus in the interpeduncular cistern can be seen on the basal surface of the brain. Thick pus along the base of the brain may impede the flow of CSF causing obstruction and raised intracranial pressure.

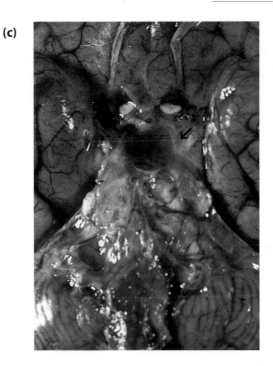

(c)

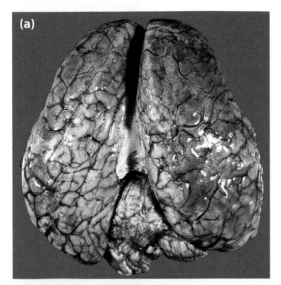

(a)

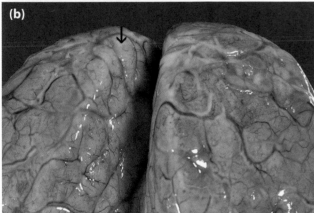

(b)

▼ **Fig. 2.8** Microscopic examination shows the purulent infiltration in the subarachnoid space over the surface of the brain. Almost all the cells are neutrophils.

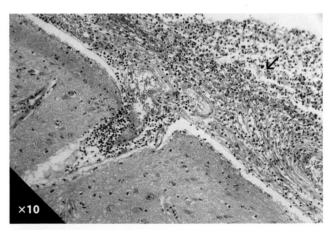

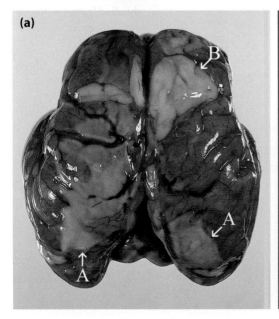

(a)

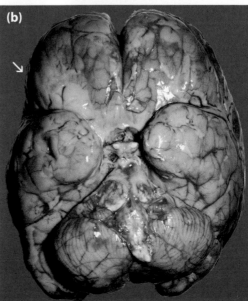

(b)

◀ **Fig. 2.9(a) and (b)** These two brains came from neonates who died from meningitis. Both infections were caused by *E. coli*. Note the very thick pus in the subarachnoid space. In **(a)** the arrows labeled A show pus and the arrow labeled B shows normal cerebral cortex from which the meninges have been accidentally torn.

Biochemical and microbiological tests performed on the CSF

Biochemical tests are performed on the aspirated cerebrospinal fluid (CSF). In meningitis, the results are as follows:

- protein—usually increased
- sugar—usually decreased.

A cell count is performed on a white-cell counting chamber (see Figs 2.10 and 2.11).

- In bacterial meningitis, there is an increased cell count, mostly neutrophils.
- In tuberculous meningitis, cryptococcal meningitis and viral meningitis, there is an increased cell count (mostly lymphocytes).

While these are the usual results, opposite results may be encountered.

Gram stain and culture are performed on the CSF (see Figs 2.12–2.19, continued overleaf). As a rule of thumb, any CSF in which there is a lymphocytosis is worth testing for *C. neoformans* and *M. tuberculosis*. An India Ink stain for Cryptococci is less sensitive than a Cryptococcal antigen test, which is the one recommended.

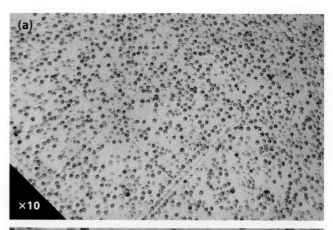

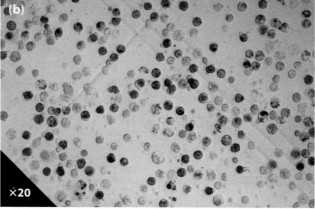

▲ **Fig. 2.11(a) and (b)** Sample of CSF in a counting chamber. There is a very high cell count, mostly neutrophils.

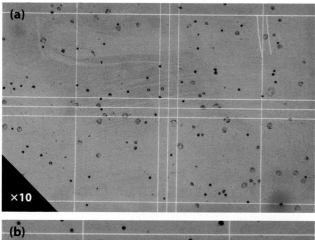

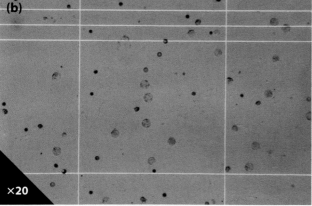

▲ **Fig. 2.10(a) and (b)** Sample of CSF in a counting chamber. There is a modestly increased cell count, mostly neutrophils.

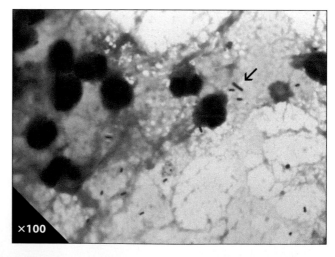

▲ **Fig. 2.12** Gram stain showing the pleomorphic (where some organisms are longer than others) Gram-negative bacilli of *H. influenzae*.

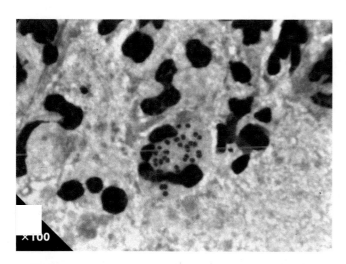

▲ **Fig. 2.13** Gram stain showing the Gram-negative intracellular diplococci of *N. meningitidis*.

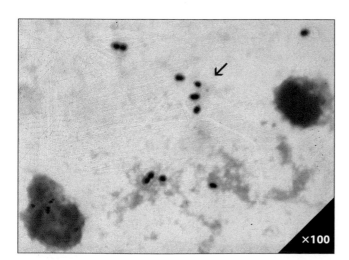

▲ **Fig. 2.14** Colonies of *N. meningitidis* growing on a chocolate agar plate.

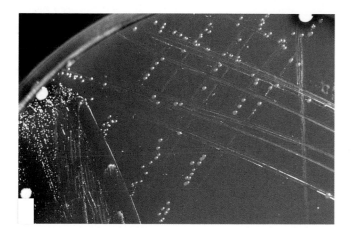

▲ **Fig. 2.15** Gram stain showing the diplococci of *S. pneumoniae*. Note the unstained halo around each pair of cocci. This is the capsule from which pneumococcal vaccine is made. This vaccine has been shown to reduce the incidence of childhood deaths from pneumococcal pneumonia.

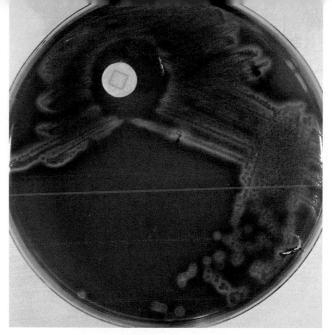

▲ **Fig. 2.16** Blood agar culture plate showing Optochin inhibition typical of *S. pneumoniae*. An Optochin disc is placed on the agar plate that has been inoculated with the test organism before the plate is incubated.

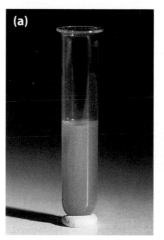 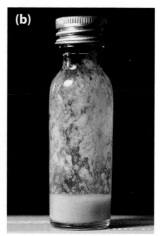

▲ **Fig. 2.17(a)** The CSF here is blood stained and purulent. **(b)** This CSF came from a 40-year-old diabetic man. It was so purulent and viscous that it would barely pass through the needle. Gram stain and culture showed *S. aureus*. In spite of the seriousness of the infection, the patient recovered.

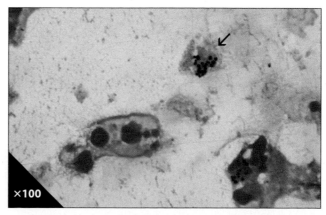

▲ **Fig. 2.18** Gram stain from the CSF shown in Figure 2.17(b). It shows the clumped Gram-positive cocci of *S. aureus*.

Cryptococcal meningitis is illustrated in Figures 2.20–2.26, continued overleaf. To exclude tuberculosis, culture of a large volume of CSF is recommended. This may involve a number of serial lumbar punctures. A single Ziehl Neelsen (ZN) stain for acid-fast bacilli (AFB) is much less sensitive (see Fig. 2.27, overleaf).

Rarely, meningitis can be caused by free-living amebas. One such organism is *Naegleria fowleri* (illustrated in Fig. 2.28, overleaf).

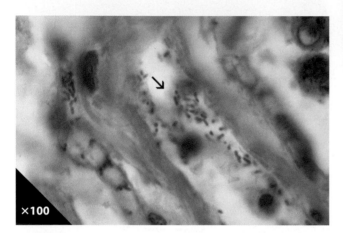

▲ **Fig. 2.19** Gram stain showing Gram-negative bacilli consistent with coliforms. *E. coli* was cultured.

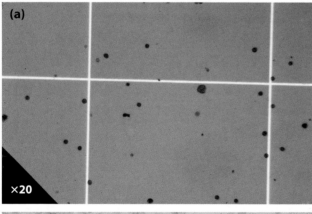

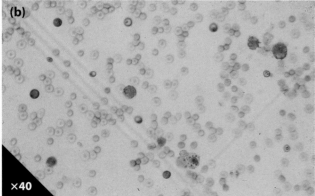

▲ **Fig 2.20(a) and (b)** In this CSF count, there is an increase in mononuclear cells. Some of these cells are lymphocytes and some are not.

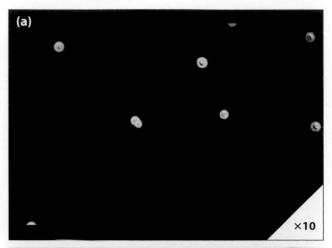

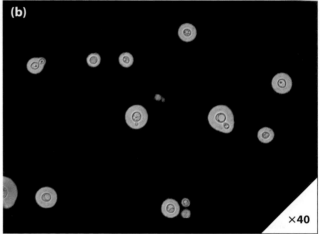

▲ **Fig. 2.21(a) and (b)** In these two images, an India Ink stain has been performed on the CSF shown in Fig. 2.20(a) and (b). One drop of CSF was mixed with a drop of India Ink. This accentuated the thick capsule of the organism *Cryptococcus neoformans*.

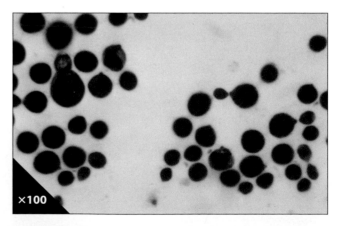

▲ **Fig. 2.22** The budding yeasts can also be seen in the Gram stain, which is a routine test on purulent CSF.

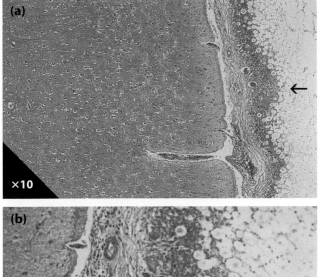

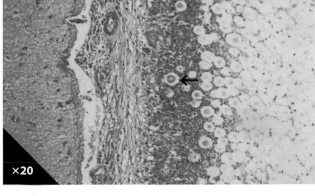

▲ **Fig. 2.23(a) and (b)** Subarachnoid space in a patient who died from cryptococcal meningitis. It shows the characteristic inflammatory reaction elicited by this organism. There is a minimal amount of cellular reaction with large amounts of mucoid material. Within this, one sees the round yeasts surrounded by an unstained halo, which represents the capsule of the yeast.

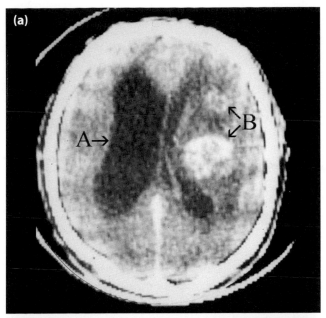

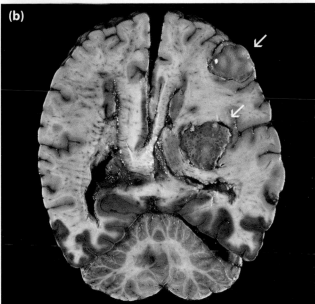

▲ **Fig. 2.25(a)** Brain scan of an adult patient with cryptococcal meningitis shows dilated ventricles (A) and the presence of two radio-opaque areas (B) that represent cryptococcomas (or, by the older name for the organism, torulomas)—inflammatory masses that resemble neoplasms. **(b)** Brain at post mortem confirms the presence of the two cryptococcomas.

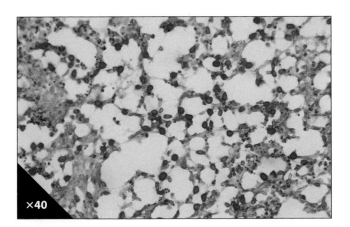

▲ **Fig. 2.24** With a Periodic Acid Schiff (PAS) stain, the yeasts stain pink and the capsule remains unstained.

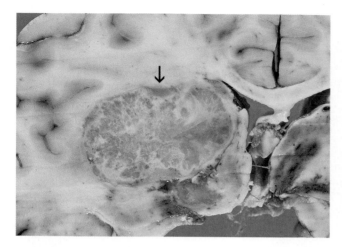

▲ **Fig. 2.26** Brain from a male, aged 50 years, who died from cryptococcal meningitis. A cryptococcoma in the thalamic region shows the typical multiloculated mucoid appearance of this condition.

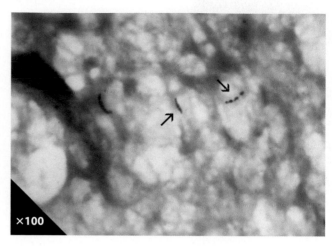

▲ **Fig. 2.27** ZN stain on the CSF of a patient with tuberculous meningitis showing the presence of acid-fast bacilli.

▼ **Fig. 2.28(a) and (b)** Amebic meningitis. Microscopic sections from the brain of a male, aged 6 years, who died from amebic meningitis. The small amebas of *Naegleria fowleri* can be seen in the perivascular space. There is also a perivascular infiltration of lymphocytes giving the appearance of an encephalitic reaction.

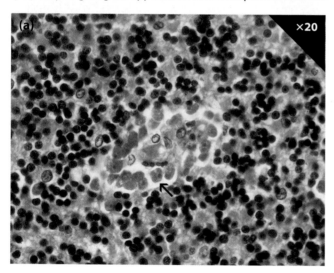

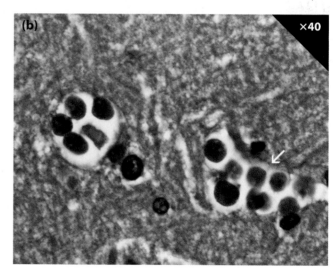

Complications of meningitis

Waterhouse-Friderichsen syndrome

Waterhouse-Friderichsen syndrome most often occurs as a complication of *N. meningitidis* infection, but other bacteria may cause the syndrome.

Clinical features

A female, 6 months of age, was well in the morning; became febrile at mid-day; developed a red, hemorrhagic rash soon afterwards (shown in Fig. 2.29); and died in the late afternoon. This sequence of events can occur at any age, but it is most common in children.

A common complication of Waterhouse-Friderichsen syndrome is bilateral adrenal hemorrhage with adrenal failure (see Fig. 2.30). There is still a significant mortality from this condition, but with early diagnosis and treatment of the adrenal failure, deaths are much less frequent than they used to be.

Septicemia

Meningitis may be complicated by septicemia, a disease caused by toxic microorganisms circulating in the blood-stream, which may cause abscesses in other organs, for example in bone (see Fig. 2.31).

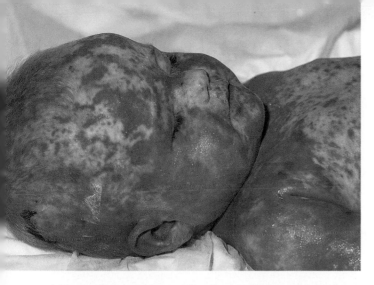

▲ **Fig. 2.29** Female, 6 months of age, with the rash of Waterhouse-Friderichsen syndrome.

Cortical infarction following neonatal meningitis

Meningitis may be complicated by a cortical infarction. Pediatricians carefully measure the head circumference in children with meningitis. If the head is getting bigger, this may indicate the presence of hydrocephalus. If it is getting smaller, it may mean that there has been a cerebral infarction (see Fig. 2.32).

Obstructive hydrocephalus

Meningitis may be complicated by obstructive hydrocephalus. A normal cerebellum, as seen in Figure 2.33, exhibits transparent meninges covering the outlets of the fourth ventricle into the cisterna magna.

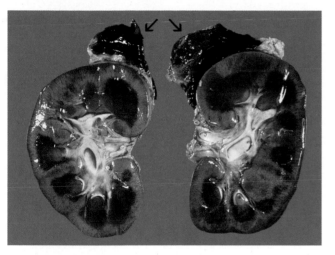

▲ **Fig. 2.30** Waterhouse-Friderichsen syndrome. This post-mortem specimen shows bilateral adrenal hemorrhage, a common complication of this syndrome.

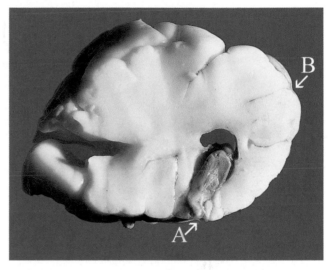

▲ **Fig. 2.32** Neonatal meningitis complicated by a cortical infarction (A). Neonatal brains do not have well-demarcated grey matter (B).

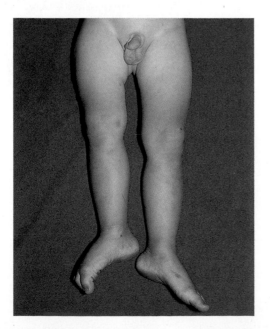

▲ **Fig. 2.31** Male, aged 30 months, developed septicemia following meningitis. This resulted in acute osteomyelitis in the head of the right femur and shortening of the leg.

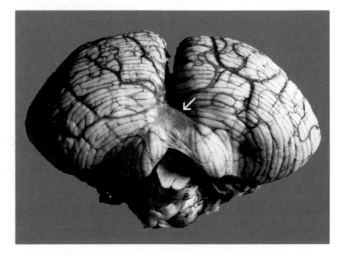

▲ **Fig. 2.33** Normal cerebellum, showing transparent meninges covering the outlets of the fourth ventricle into the cisterna magna.

Two causes of obstructive hydrocephalus are illustrated here.

- Obstruction to the outflow tracts of the fourth ventricle, as shown in Figures 2.34–2.37.
- Obstruction to the cerebral aqueduct, as indicated in Figures 2.38, 2.39 and 2.40.

Obstruction to the outflow tracts of the fourth ventricle

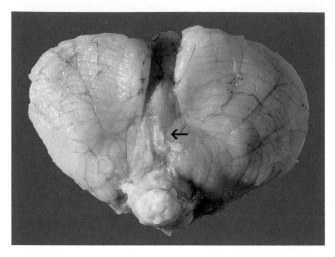

▲ **Fig. 2.34** Obliteration of the cisterna magna by the purulent exudate of acute neonatal meningitis in a female aged 3 months.

▼ **Fig. 2.35** Dilatation of the fourth ventricle.

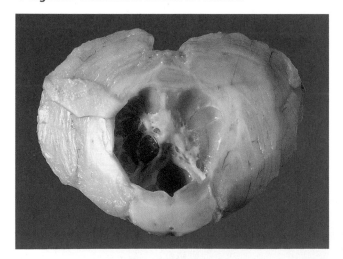

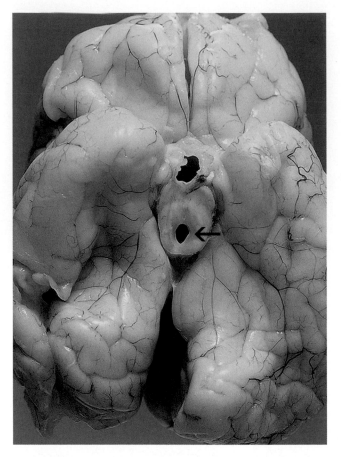

▲ **Fig. 2.36** Dilatation of the cerebral aqueduct.

▼ **Fig. 2.37** Dilatation of the third ventricle and both lateral ventricles.

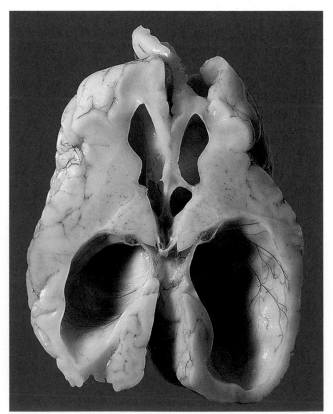

Obstruction to the cerebral aqueduct

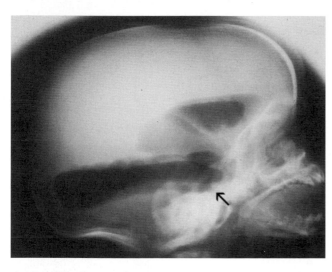

▲ **Fig. 2.38** Plain X-ray of the skull showed raised intracranial pressure causing widening (springing) of the suture lines of the skull.

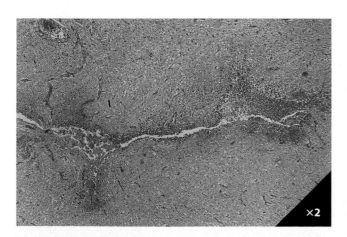

▲ **Fig. 2.39** Air encephalogram showed the obstruction to be in the region of the cerebral aqueduct. (This investigation has been superseded by magnetic resonance imaging (MRI) technology.)

×2

▲ **Fig. 2.40** Microscopic examination of the aqueduct after death confirmed the site of the inflammatory obstruction.

Cerebral abscess

Meningitis may be complicated by the formation of an abscess in the cerebrum (illustrated in Fig. 2.41).

Subdural hematoma

The features of a chronic subdural hematoma—a complication of meningitis—are illustrated in Figure 2.42.

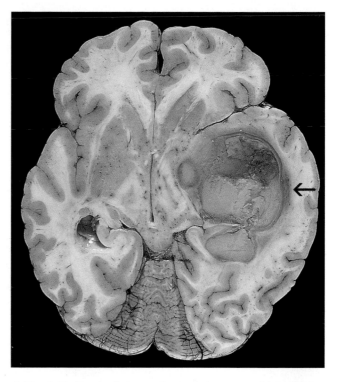

▲ **Fig. 2.41** Cerebral abscess in the right temporal lobe of the brain of a male aged 9 years.

▼ **Fig. 2.42** A 9-year-old male had had many aspirations of a subdural hematoma. At the time of his death there was a chronic hematoma with multiple layers of fibrous tissue.

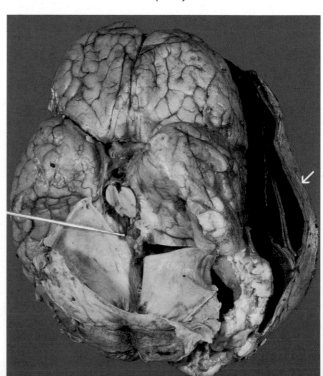

Beta hemolytic streptococcal (*Streptococcus pyogenes*) infections

Streptococcus pyogenes organisms occur in the normal flora of the nasopharynx. They are the usual cause of acute tonsillitis. A syndrome called scarlet fever, caused by the erythrogenic toxin of the *S. pyogenes* used to be fairly common. It had a considerable mortality, but it has become a rare disease since the introduction of penicillin.

The clinical features of scarlet fever are fever, a bright red skin rash (shown in Fig. 2.43), an area of pallor around the mouth (Fig. 2.44) and a red tongue (Fig. 2.45).

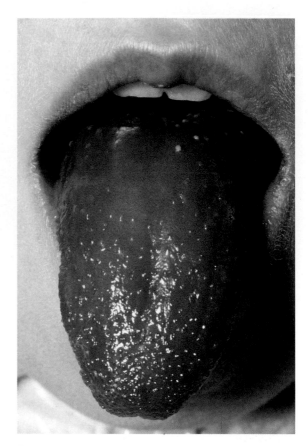

▲ **Fig. 2.45** Scarlet fever—bright red tongue.

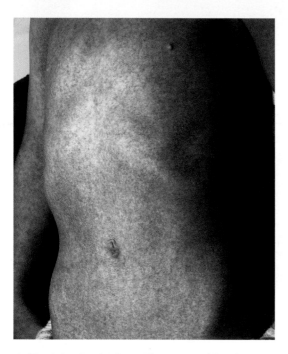

▲ **Fig. 2.43** Scarlet fever. This 6-year-old male shows the skin rash of this disease.

▼ **Fig. 2.44** Circum oral pallor—an area of pallor around the mouth—is a feature of this disease.

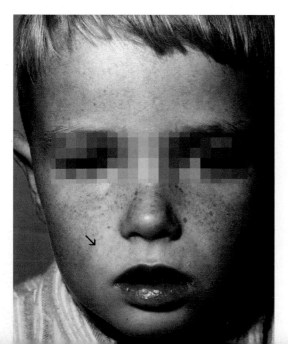

Complications of *S. pyogenes* infections

Two diseases that may follow in 1 to 3 weeks after *S. pyogenes* infections are acute nephritis and rheumatic fever. They are thought to be immunologically induced. A streptolysin O toxin has been identified in rheumatic fever.

Acute nephritis

Acute nephritis occurs in children. It presents with a mixture of symptoms including fever, periorbital edema, oliguria, hematuria and complications of hypertension (heart failure or cerebral edema with fitting). The underlying pathology consists in enlargement and hypercellularity of glomeruli throughout both kidneys (Fig. 2.46).

Rheumatic fever

Rheumatic fever is characterized by fever, transient pain and stiffness in large joints, and symptoms and signs of cardiac dysfunction.

Death is uncommon. When death does occur, the myocardium shows multiple focal areas of inflammation in the interstitial tissue. These foci of inflammation are called Aschoff nodules, after Ludwig Aschoff (1866–1942), the German pathologist from Freiburg. They consist of focal necrosis of myocardial fibres, with a mononuclear inflammatory cell infiltration that includes mononuclear histiocytes with prominent nucleoli. These nucleoli are called Anitschkow myocytes, after Nikolai Anitschkow, the twentieth-century Russian pathologist from St Petersburg.

Aschoff nodules and Anitschkow myocytes are shown in Figure 2.47.

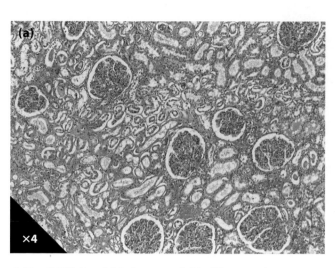

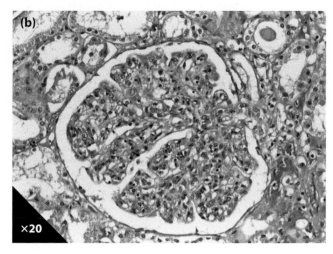

▲ **Fig. 2.46(a) and (b)** Acute nephritis. Microscopic appearances of a kidney examined at low and high magnifications. They show enlargement and hypercellularity of glomeruli throughout the kidney.

▼ **Fig. 2.47(a) and (b)** Aschoff nodules with Anitschkow myocytes in the myocardium of a child who died from acute rheumatic fever.

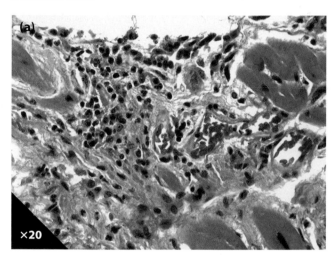

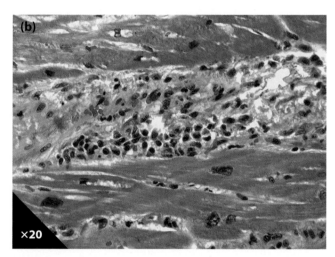

Long-term cardiac complications of rheumatic fever

The complications of *S. pyogenes* infections described here are now uncommon in countries where modern medical facilities are readily available, but they are still quite often seen in less well medically endowed countries, and they manifest in some indigenous groups within the better medically endowed countries.

Valve stenosis/incompetence

A late complication of rheumatic fever is fibrous thickening (often with calcification) of the mitral and aortic valves (shown in Figs 2.48 and 2.49, continued overleaf). This results in stenosis/incompetence of the valves. Mitral stenosis may present without any clear history of previous rheumatic fever. This manifests itself, for example, as heart failure in early pregnancy.

▼ **Fig. 2.48** Stenotic and incompetent mitral valve viewed from the dilated left atrium. Because of the fibrosis, the valve is stiff and immobile. The left atrium shows compensatory dilatation resulting from the stenotic effect of the valve.

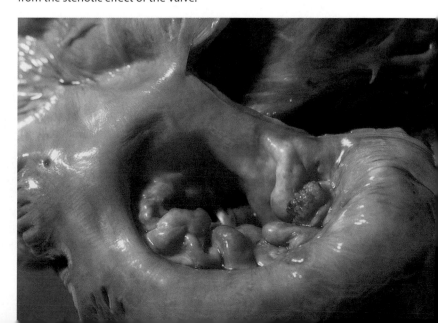

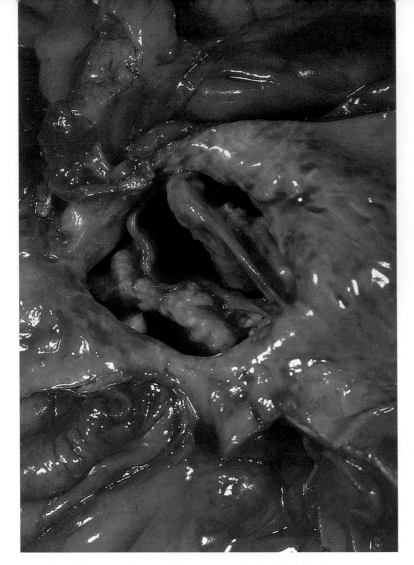

▲ Fig. 2.49 Stenotic and incompetent aortic valve. Surgical replacement of these damaged valves results in alleviation of the impairment in their function.

Infective endocarditis

Another late complication of rheumatic fever is infective endocarditis (previously called bacterial endocarditis). Organisms circulating in the bloodstream colonize the damaged valves. Vegetations consisting of fibrin, inflammatory cells and organisms form on the valves (shown in Fig. 2.50).

When the disease is caused by an organism of relatively low virulence (e.g. *Streptococcus viridans*), the organisms usually invade already damaged valves, and tiny fragments of the vegetations break off and circulate in the bloodstream as emboli. These emboli may lodge in vessels in other organs and cause infarcts (illustrated in Figs 2.51, 2.52 and 2.53). The symptoms and signs of infarctions in internal organs depend on the organ and on the size of the embolus.

On the other hand, when the organism is more virulent, for example *S. aureus*, the organisms attack normal valves and often damage them with, for example, perforation of the valve causing a sudden, serious incompetence. The emboli from these organisms are more likely to cause septic infarcts in internal organs, with the formation of abscesses.

Clinical features of *S. viridans* infective endocarditis include low-grade fever accompanied by symptoms and signs caused by emboli, which occlude small blood vessels throughout the body.

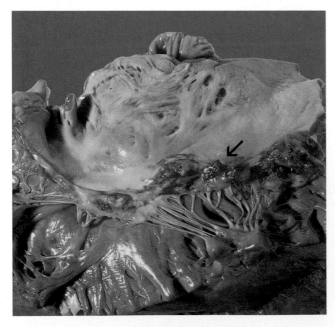

▲ Fig. 2.50 *S. viridans* infective endocarditis. The mitral valve leaflets have numerous small vegetations attached to their free edges.

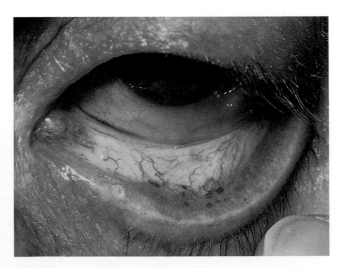

▲ Fig. 2.51 *S. viridans* infective endocarditis. In the conjunctiva, there are 'splinter' hemorrhages resulting from occlusion of capillaries by emboli. (Similar hemorrhages may be seen in the nail beds of the fingers and toes.)

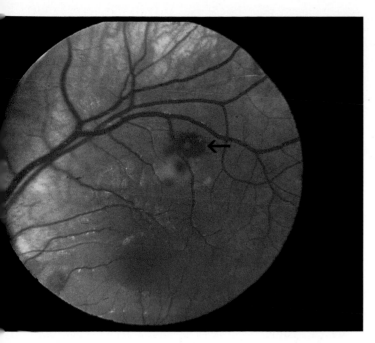

▲ **Fig. 2.52** *S. viridans* infective endocarditis. Micro-infarcts in the retina caused by tiny emboli.

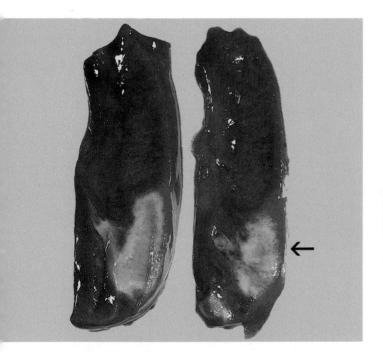

▲ **Fig. 2.53** *S. viridans* infective endocarditis. Renal infarct. Emboli lodge in the small arteries of internal organs causing infarctions. This specimen of kidney shows an embolic infarction.

Erysipelas

The toxins of *S. pyogenes* may affect the skin and result in the clinical condition called erysipelas. The patient has a rapid onset of fever with septicemia and skin rash with marked subcutaneous edema. The head and neck are the sites most often involved. Before the introduction of penicillin, this was a very serious infection (illustrated in Fig. 2.54).

▼ **Fig. 2.54** Wax model in the Department of Pathology in the University of Bologna, Italy, shows the clinical features of erysipelas.

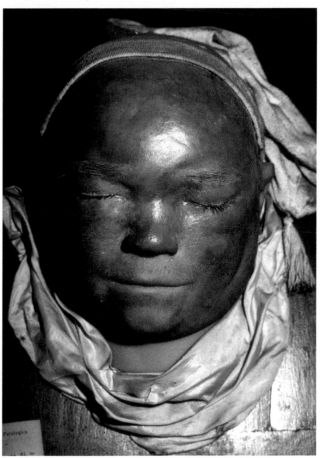

Streptococcus pneumoniae

Streptococcus pneumoniae organism is a part of the normal flora of the upper respiratory tract. When infection of the lungs occurs, it results in what is called pneumonia. This may be seen in two morphological forms: involvement of a single lobe—lobar pneumonia (see Fig. 2.55, overleaf), or involvement of multiple lobules throughout both lungs—bronchopneumonia.

Bronchopneumonia is the most commonly encountered form. Before the introduction of penicillin, lobar pneumonia was a common and serious infection with a high mortality. Nowadays, it is regarded as a relatively trivial infection. Occasionally, it still causes death, with a rapid onset of illness leading to death in a day or two in spite of vigorous antibiotic treatment.

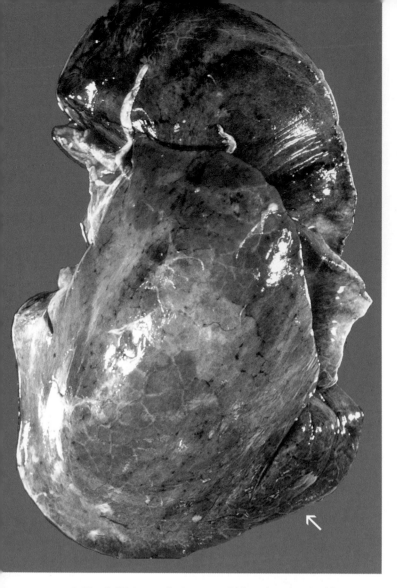

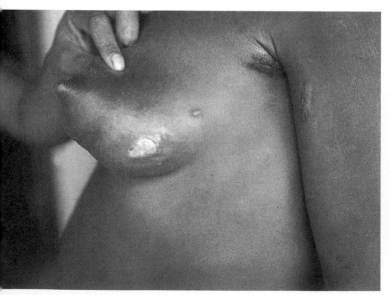

▲ Fig. 2.55 Lung of a 38-year-old female, who died from lobar pneumonia. One lobe is full of purulent exudate. The pleural surface shows a fibrinous pleurisy. This patient would have complained of fever, dyspnea and pleuritic pain.

▼ Fig. 2.56 Female, aged 19 years, has a breast abscess that is ulcerating through the skin.

While *S. pneumoniae* is probably the most common cause of pneumonia, many other organisms may cause the clinical and pathologic features of pneumonia, and it is important to perform sputum cultures and other investigations to establish an etiological diagnosis in each case. A vaccine has been made against *S. pneumoniae* and its use has reduced the number of infections from this organism.

Staphylococcus aureus

Staphylococcus aureus organism is a member of the normal flora of the nose and skin. The carriage rate decreases with age. The overall carriage rate is 20–30 per cent. *S. aureus* causes a great variety of conditions, only a few of which will be considered here. Its biological properties have been extensively investigated because it quickly developed resistance to penicillin. Now, infections by resistant strains are a serious problem.

Abscesses

S. aureus is a common cause of abscesses in all sites. Before penicillin, breast abscesses in lactating women were common. Organisms entered through cracks in the nipple and grew rapidly in the rich culture medium of the milk (see Fig. 2.56).

Osteomyelitis

Staphylococcal infection of bone results in acute osteomyelitis (see Fig. 2.57). This is associated with septicemia and the pus trapped in the bone marrow cavity causes local pain. Before penicillin, this was often a fatal disease. Even with modern antibiotic treatment, infection may continue, causing chronic osteomyelitis with sinuses that continue to discharge pus.

▼ Fig. 2.57 Acute osteomyelitis. A 21-year-old female died from acute leukemia. The marrow cavity is filled with pus, which may need to be drained via drill holes in the bone.

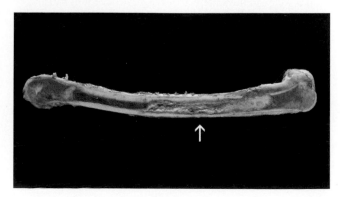

Pneumonia

Staphylococcal pneumonia is a serious form of pneumonia. It causes multiple abscesses throughout both lungs. Abscesses frequently rupture into the pleural space causing empyema (illustrated in Fig. 2.58). Metastatic abscesses occur in other organs as a result of colonization by organisms which circulate in the blood as a result of the septicemia.

The boy whose lung is demonstrated in Figure 2.58 was among a number of cases that occurred during a period of a few months at the Royal Children's Hospital in Brisbane, Australia. This necrotizing pneumonia is caused by S. aureus, *which is associated with a strain of the organism that carries Panton-Valentine leukocidin, a cellular toxin transmitted between different strains of* S. aureus *by bacteriophage.*

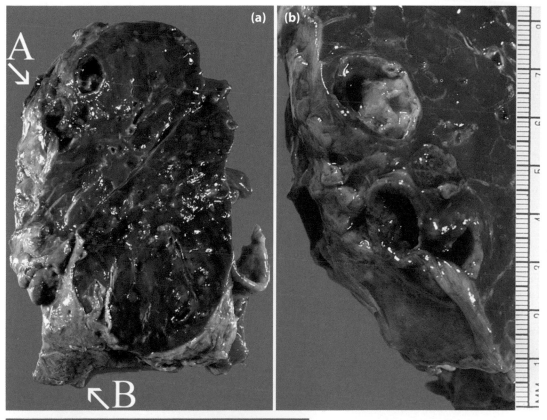

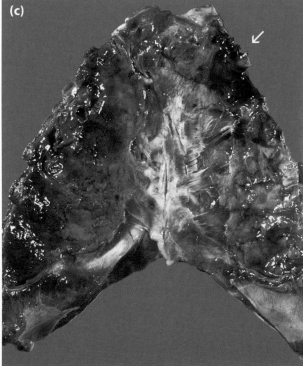

▲ ◄ **Fig. 2.58** Lung of 11-year-old male, who died 1 month after the onset of pneumonia. **(a)** Note the many abscesses and purulent exudate (empyema) in the pleural cavity (A). The pleural surfaces are greatly thickened as a result of inflammation (B). These are the typical appearances of staphylococcal pneumonia. **(b)** A close-up view of the abscesses. **(c)** View of the posterior surface of the rib cage shows the pus of the empyema adherent to the pleural surface.

Toxic epidermal necrolysis (scalded skin syndrome)

As with *S. pyogenes*, *S. aureus* produces a toxin that can cause toxic necrosis of the skin. The condition is called toxic epidermal necrolysis (scalded skin syndrome) (see Fig. 2.59).

Disseminated intravascular coagulation

An uncommon complication of septicemia, disseminated intravascular coagulation is caused by a number of different organisms. It results in occlusion of small arteries in the peripheries of the body—fingers, ears, toes. This results in infarction and gangrene of these extremities, which may require amputation of the affected parts for cure (see Fig. 2.60).

▶ **Fig. 2.59(a)** Legs of a 2-year-old female, who developed toxic epidermal necrolysis 'scalded skin syndrome' as a complication of staphylococcal pneumonia following thoracic surgery. **(b)** Left arm of the same 2 year old.

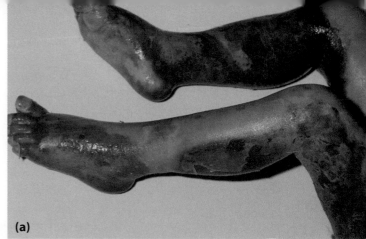

(a)

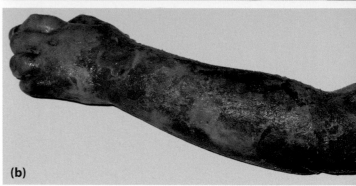

(b)

▼ **Fig. 2.60** A 5-year-old male had staphylococcal pneumonia, and then developed the complication of disseminated intravascular coagulation. This resulted in thrombotic obstruction of the small arteries in peripheral tissues; and necrosis of the tips of his ears, lips, fingers, hand and nose.

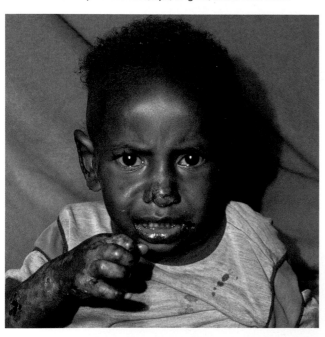

Enterobacteriaceae

The Enterobacteriaceae group of organisms includes the species *Escherischia*, *Shigella* and *Salmonella*. They cause acute enterocolitis. Infection is acquired from contaminated food or water. Other organisms such as pathogenic coliforms and viruses can cause a similar pathology (see Fig. 2.61).

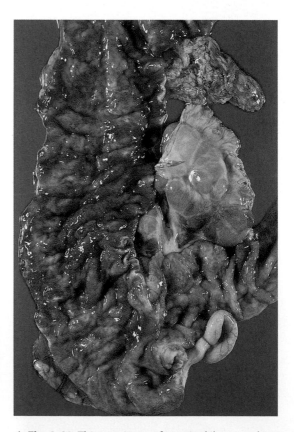

▲ **Fig. 2.61** This specimen of terminal ileum and ascending colon shows redness of the mucosal surface of the colon and terminal ileum—a mild acute enterocolitis. The specimen was obtained at post-mortem examination on a female aged 19 months. She died from acute dehydration before treatment could be started. A *Shigella* organism was isolated from the feces collected before death.

Typhoid fever

Typhoid fever is caused by the organism *Salmonella typhi*. Infection is acquired by drinking contaminated water. Clinical features are quite varied. There is fever with a relatively slow pulse rate and a low white cell count.

> *Physicians who see numerous typhoid cases at a clinic claim that typhoid patients may be identified by their facial appearance—the 'typhoid facies' (see Fig. 2.62), an appearance described by physicians some 100 years ago.*
>
> *The author, having been at a typhoid clinic and having seen some 'typhoid facies' cases proven by positive blood culture of the* Salmonella typhi *organism, observed that the claim may be true.*

Some patients develop a red spotty skin rash—the so-called 'rose red spots' (Fig. 2.63). Some patients have diarrhea. Some have abdominal pain suggestive of a bowel obstruction. Some have rectal bleeding, and some have peritonitis from perforation of the small intestine (Fig. 2.64).

There is a typhoid vaccination available for travelers to regions of high prevalence of typhoid fever, and it is strongly recommended as a prophylactic measure.

Other species of Salmonella cause food poisoning. This presents about 48 hours after eating the contaminated food, with a sudden onset of fever, nausea, vomiting, abdominal pain and a profuse, watery diarrhea. Symptoms usually last for a few days and subside with symptomatic treatment.

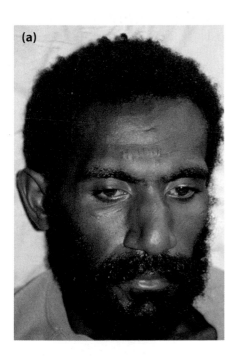
(a)

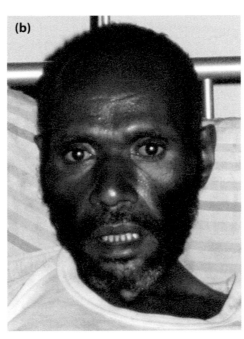
(b)

◀ **Fig. 2.62(a) and (b)** Typhoid facies.

▼ **Fig. 2.63** 'Rose red spots' of typhoid fever on the abdomen.

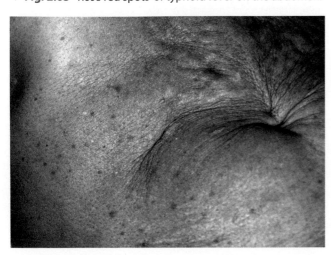

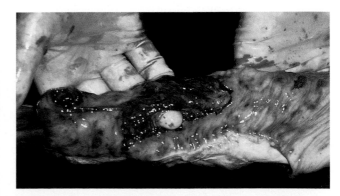

▲ **Fig. 2.64** A 23-year-old male patient, who had typhoid fever, died from perforation of a Peyer's patch, inflamed as a result of the infection. In typhoid fever, the small bowel shows inflammation, ulceration and hemorrhage—particularly affecting the Peyer's patches.

Helicobacter

Helicobacter pylori is a curve-shaped bacillary organism found in the stomach in excess of 90 per cent of cases of acute and chronic gastritis, and of peptic and duodenal ulcers. In 1982, two Australians, Robin Warren pathologist, and Barry Marshall gastroenterologist (pictured in Fig. 2.65) indicated that this organism was the cause of acute gastritis and peptic ulcers. They showed that by treating the infection and eradicating the organism, acute gastritis and peptic ulcers could be cured. For this discovery, they were awarded the Nobel Prize in 2005.

The bacilli are seen in the mucus on the surface epithelium of the gastric mucosal cells and in the gastric crypts. They are easily seen in routine hematoxylin and eosin (H&E) sections (shown in Figs 2.66 and 2.67), but may be more easily seen in sections stained with Giemsa or Warthin Starry silver stain.

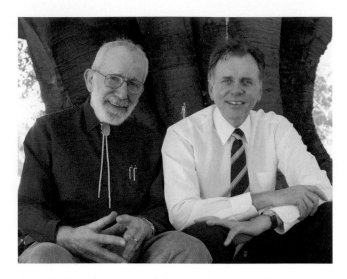

▲ **Fig 2.65** Robin Warren (*left*), pathologist, and Barry Marshall, gastroenterologist, shared the Nobel Prize in 2005 for showing that acute gastritis and peptic ulcers were caused by *H. pylori* infection and that these conditions could be cured by treatment with antibiotics.

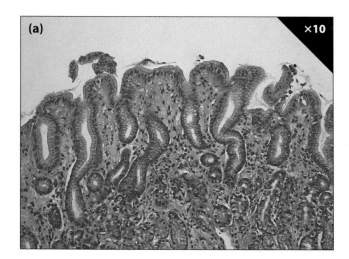

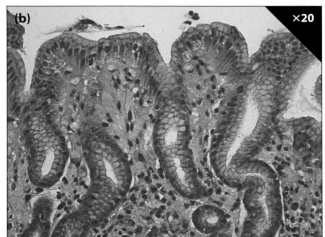

▲ **Fig. 2.66(a) and (b)** Section of a gastric biopsy from a 40-year-old male, who complained of indigestion. The gastric mucosa shows an excess of cells in the lamina propria. The cells consist of a mixture of mononuclear cells and neutrophils. These appearances are consistent with acute on chronic gastritis.

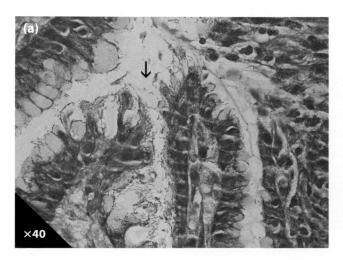

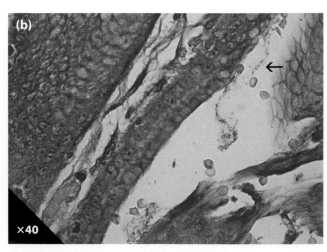

▲ **Fig. 2.67(a) and (b)** Curved bacilli of *H. pylori* can be seen in the surface mucus and in the gastric crypts.

Diphtheria

Diphtheria is caused by the Gram-positive bacillus *Coryne-bacterium diphtheriae*. On Gram stain, metachromatic granules can be seen in the bacilli. The organism grows best on tellurite agar medium. It is a normal inhabitant of the upper respiratory tract.

Much of the early work on *C. diphtheriae* was done by Emile Roux (1853–1933), who followed Louis Pasteur as Director of the Pasteur Institute in Paris. Roux demonstrated that the pathologic effects of this organism were caused by an exotoxin that it secreted. The production of an antitoxin led to the development of an inactive toxoid which, when injected prophylactically, resulted in protection against diphtheria.

Diphtheria presents clinically as an acute tonsillitis, with fever and sore throat. The tonsils are enlarged, and they are usually covered by an adherent, grey membrane. Before the days of prophylactic immunization and antibiotics, it was a very serious infection with significant mortality.

The disease occurred mainly in children, and tonsillar enlargement and accumulation of purulent exudate in the trachea caused respiratory obstruction (see Fig. 2.68). In many cases, by this stage of the disease, the exotoxin was causing neuritis, resulting especially in paralysis of the palate, which added to the respiratory difficulty; and was also causing toxic myocarditis, resulting in cardiac irregularity and the complications of this.

Family doctors, and doctors in children's hospitals were very aware of the respiratory complications of diphtheria. If the airway was becoming obstructed, as shown by the presence of stridor, they knew this to be a medical emergency that required urgent tracheostomy to save the child's life. At the time when diphtheria was prevalent, family doctors were often required to perform tracheostomies in the patients' homes because transportation to a hospital was slow and difficult.

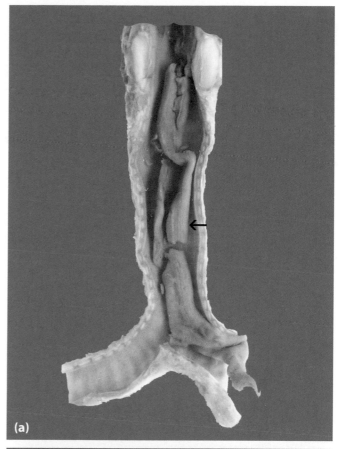

(a)

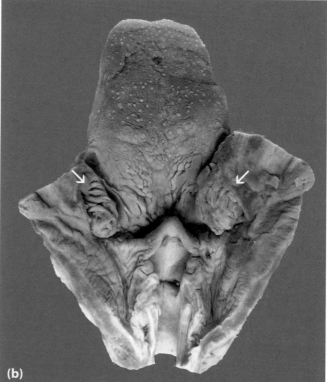

(b)

▲ **Fig. 2.68** Specimens from children 5 years of age, who died from asphyxiation during an epidemic of diphtheria in Brisbane, Australia. **(a)** Trachea filled with thick, purulent exudate. **(b)** Much enlarged tonsils with purulent exudate on their surfaces. The tonsils occluded the airway.

In some children's hospitals, bells would be rung when a child with stridor was admitted to the emergency ward. When the bells rang, doctors would rush to emergency to perform the tracheostomy. This was done by making an incision through the skin in the suprasternal notch and removing a small piece of cartilage from the trachea just below the larynx. An elderly ear, nose and throat surgeon remembered the drama associated with these tracheostomies in the late 1930s when he was a junior doctor. Removal of the piece of trachea resulted in an immediate in-drawing of air followed by an exhalation or a cough that expelled blood and pus with considerable force. The operator had to quickly move out of the 'firing line' to avoid being splashed by it.

The patient pictured in Figure 2.69 shows a scar in her suprasternal notch. This scar resulted from a tracheostomy performed in the winter of 1954 by a family doctor at her home in Auckland, New Zealand. That winter, there was an epidemic of diphtheria in which a number of children died.

Diphtheria toxoid for immunization against diphtheria only became readily available for widespread use in the late 1940s. At that time, diphtheria was so common and the effects so dramatic that parents were eager to comply with the recommendation of the public health authorities that all children be immunized (see Fig. 2.70). As a result, diphtheria 'disappeared' as a serious infection.

▼ **Fig. 2.69** A 55-year-old female with a scar in the suprasternal notch area of the neck, photographed in 2005. This scar was the result of a tracheostomy performed by a family doctor called to her home when she was aged 4 years, and in danger of dying from laryngeal obstruction caused by diphtheria. She was one of the children who had not yet been immunized. When she recovered, a photograph of herself and the doctor who performed the tracheostomy was published in a local newspaper in an effort to encourage parents to have their children immunized.

In recent years, for various reasons, some parents have not had their children immunized. Consequently, sporadic cases of diphtheria are occurring once again. Such an attitude of parents, who have no knowledge of the possible severity of diphtheria, may lead to a drop in the 'herd' immunity and expose the community to new epidemics.

Rhinoscleroma

Rhinoscleroma is a rather rare, chronic inflammatory condition affecting the nose and nasopharynx. It occurs in most countries, with pockets of increased incidence in some. It is caused by the organism *Klebsiella rhinoscleromatis*.

Patients present with symptoms of nasal obstruction. The inflammatory mass grows slowly over many months, causing increasing obstruction. Ultimately, it protrudes from one or both nostrils. The surface may become ulcerated and may then bleed (shown in Fig. 2.71).

Rhinoscleroma diagnosis is made by examination of biopsy specimens (see Fig. 2.72). Sections show an inflammatory mass with a cell population of lymphocytes, plasma cells and variable numbers of histiocytes with foamy cytoplasm, in which the characteristic bacillary organisms can be demonstrated with a Warthin Starry silver stain (see Fig. 2.73).

Culture of biopsy material allows the organism to be grown on blood agar or MacConkey's agar. It does not respond well to antibiotic treatment, and surgical removal is the preferred treatment.

▼ **Fig. 2.70** Immunization clinic in Brisbane, Australia, 1941. Anxious mothers bring their children for immunization after a report that two non-immunized children had died of diphtheria. There were rumors that an epidemic was imminent.

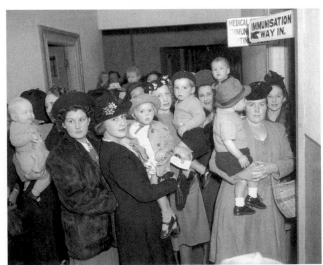

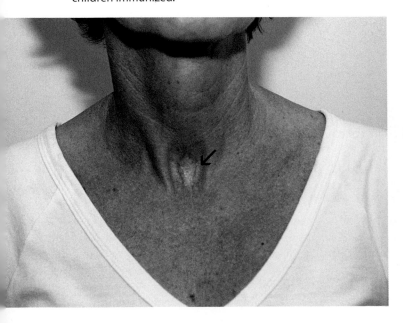

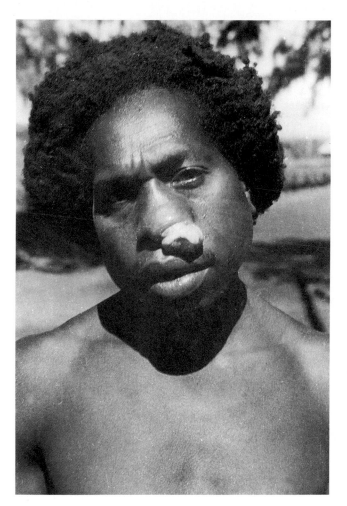

▲ **Fig. 2.71** Rhinoscleroma. Male, aged about 18 years, from the Western Highlands region of Papua New Guinea (where the disease is endemic) has enlargement of his nose, with a polypoid, ulcerated tumor protruding from his left nostril.

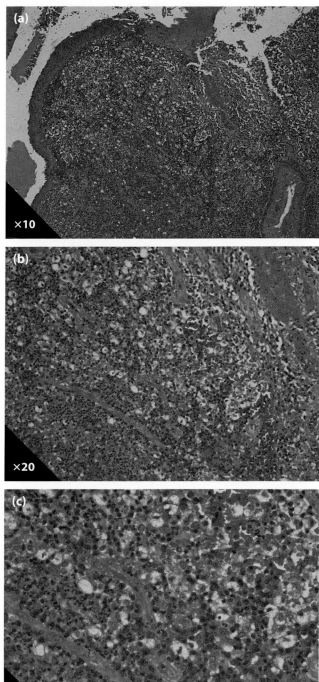

▲ **Fig. 2.72(a), (b) and (c)** Views of the biopsy show an inflammatory cell infiltration consisting mainly of lymphocytes, plasma cells and numerous large histiocytes with foamy cytoplasm.

◀ **Fig. 2.73** Warthin Starry stain shows the presence of bacillary organisms in the cytoplasm of the histiocytes.

Clostridial infections

The organisms that cause clostridial infections are large Gram-positive anaerobic rods containing spores. They secrete exotoxins. The main members of this group are:

- *Clostridium tetani*
- *Clostridium difficile*
- *Clostridium perfringens*.

C. tetani—the cause of tetanus

Tetanus infection results in muscle spasm (depicted in Fig. 2.74). Generalized painful muscle spasms are induced by noise and jolting of the patient. The muscle spasm usually begins in the facial muscles causing 'lock jaw', which prevents eating.

The organisms live as commensals in the gut of humans and of animals. The spores are found in soil. Soil contamination of wounds is the source of infection. In warfare and severe civilian injuries, infection used to be common.

In countries with poor health services, contamination of the umbilical cord occurs when babies are delivered on the earth floors of village houses. As a result, neonatal tetanus is common, and it is a cause of infant deaths. Tetanus can be prevented by vaccination with tetanus toxoid.

C. difficile—the cause of membranous colitis

In *C. difficile*, diarrhea occurs in patients who are taking broad-spectrum antibiotics, especially ampicillin. The broad-spectrum antibiotic inhibits the normal flora, allowing an overgrowth of *C. difficile*. If this is not corrected, death may occur from the effects of the toxemia and fluid loss from the diarrhea. Now that this complication of broad-spectrum antibiotics is better understood, the condition is rarely seen.

Grossly, the mucosal surface of the colon shows the presence of multiple, rounded, yellowish areas (shown in Fig. 2.75). This can be seen easily during colonoscopic examinations. On microscopic examination, these deposits consist of accumulations of purulent exudate that have formed over an area of mucosal ulceration. The pus appears to be rising from the ulcer in the shape of a mushroom, like the cloud caused by an atomic bomb explosion.

▼ **Fig. 2.74** The characteristic flexor spasm of the muscles caused by tetanus is seen in a soldier of the Battle of Waterloo (1815), depicted in a famous painting by Charles Bell, housed in the Museum of the Royal College of Surgeons of Edinburgh, Scotland.

▼ **Fig. 2.75** Membranous colitis in a female aged 68 years. She had been taking ampicillin (a broad-spectrum antibiotic). She had an overgrowth of *C. difficile* in her colon. The characteristic rounded deposits of purulent exudate can be seen on the mucosal surface of the colon.

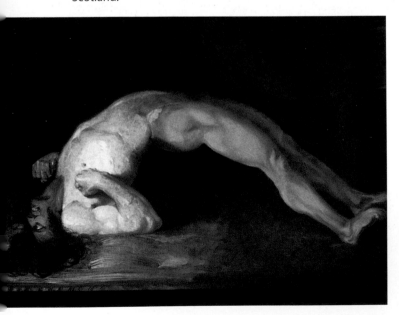

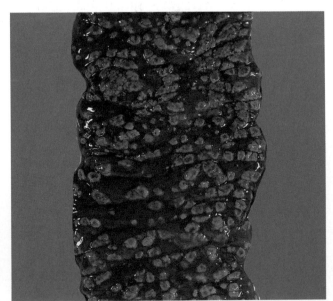

C. perfringens—the cause of gas gangrene, food poisoning and puerperal infection

C. perfringens is a cause of gas gangrene and food poisoning (particularly from reheated meat). It is a rare cause of puerperal infection.

Gas gangrene is a condition where a wound is contaminated by spores of *C. perfringens*, which is normally found in soil. The spores germinate and the organisms produce exotoxins (see Fig. 2.76) that cause muscle necrosis and gas production (see Fig. 2.77). This type of wound contamination occurs particularly after severe trauma (for example, traffic accidents and war wounds). During World War Two, the use of the newly found penicillin dramatically reduced the incidence of death from battle injuries in the Allied forces during the 1944 Normandy landing in France.

Clinical presentations of *C. perfringens*

Bubbles of gas begin to form within hours of the wound contamination. The gas travels quickly along the muscle planes. This gives the sign of crepitus (crackling) in the muscle. The dead muscle soon becomes black. If the spread of the gas gangrene is not controlled, death results from the effects of the toxemia.

To prevent gas gangrene occurring, soil contaminated wounds are 'debrided'. They are scrubbed to remove the soil and other contamination, and any dead tissue is excised. They are then left open and 'drained', rather than sutured at once.

The microscopic features of gas gangrene are muscle necrosis; the presence of gas bubbles; multiple, large, Gram-positive bacilli; and very little inflammatory cell reaction (see Fig. 2.77).

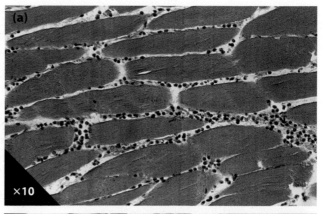

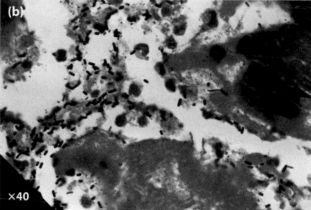

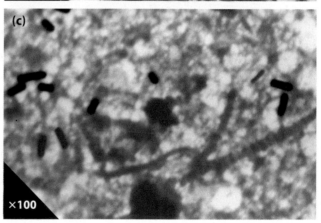

▲ **Fig. 2.77(a)** Post-mortem section of the quadriceps femoris muscle shows necrosis, hemorrhage, and little inflammatory reaction. **(b) and (c)** Gram stain shows the presence of multiple large, Gram-positive bacilli consistent with *C. perfringens*.

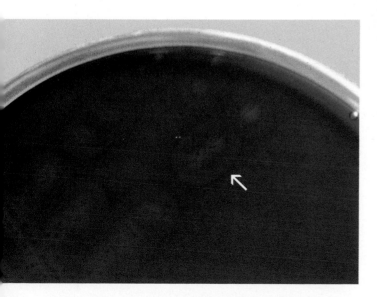

▲ **Fig. 2.76** Culture of *C. perfringens* on a blood agar plate shows the characteristic double ring of hemolysis caused by two of the exotoxins secreted by the organism.

Case 2.1

A 20-year-old female was admitted to the emergency ward of a hospital in Papua New Guinea after having recently delivered a baby. She was 'in extremis' with a barely recordable blood pressure and a hemoglobin that was also barely recordable. She died soon after being examined.

Post mortem was performed within a few hours of death. The myometrium of the uterus showed necrosis and numerous gas spaces characteristic of gas gangrene caused by *C. perfringens* (see Fig. 2.78).

The intimal lining of the aorta was stained red as a result of hemolysis. *C. perfringens* causes hemolytic anemia, which would have been the cause of this woman's low hemoglobin and also the red staining of the aorta (see Fig. 2.79).

▼ **Fig. 2.78** Uterus of a female, aged 20 years, who died soon after delivery. The myometrium contained numerous gas spaces characteristic of gas gangrene caused by *C. perfringens*.

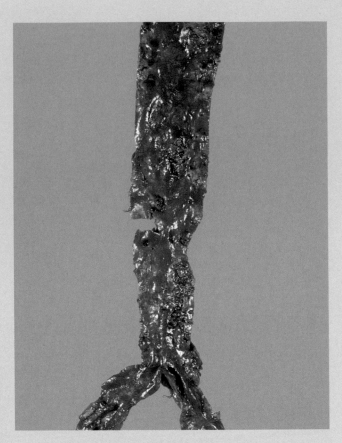

▲ **Fig. 2.79** Intimal lining of the aorta is stained red from hemolysis. This is frequently seen in death from *C. perfringens* infection.

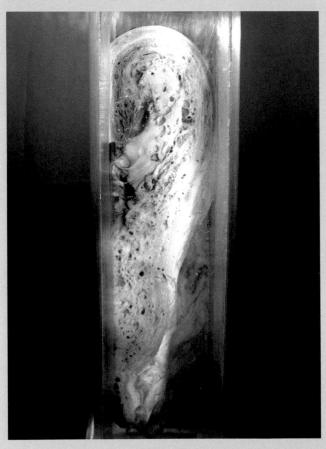

Case 2.2

A male, aged 10 years, had a compound fracture of both ulna and radius of the right forearm. Bubbles of gas were observed accumulating in the muscle from infection with *C. perfringens* (shown in Fig. 2.80).

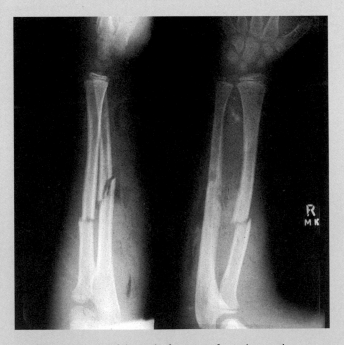

▲ **Fig. 2.80** X-ray of the right forearm of a male, aged 10 years. Compound fracture of radius and ulna with gas gangrene.

Case 2.3

A male, aged 20 years, had a motorcycle accident on the road just outside the entrance to the accident and emergency department of a hospital. He sustained head injuries and a compound fracture of his left femur.

He received immediate and optimum treatment, but gas gangrene developed quite quickly, and he died the next day. Muscle crepitus was present and the tissue was edematous and necrotic (see Fig. 2.81).

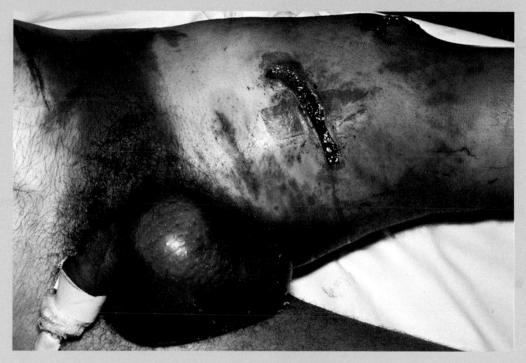

▲ **Fig. 2.81** Male, aged 20 years, with a compound fracture of the left femur complicated by gas gangrene.

Anthrax

Anthrax is a disease caused by the *Bacillus anthracis*, which is a large, aerobic, Gram-positive, spore-bearing bacillus.

It is a disease primarily of herbivorous animals. Spores from dead animals contaminate pastures. Animals grazing on the contaminated pastures become infected with the spores.

Humans become infected either by contact with sick animals; or with spore-contaminated animal products, skins and bristles; or with fertilizers that contain contaminated animal protein.

Necrotizing hemorrhagic skin lesions occur on fingers and hands. Systemic lesions are very rare, but pathologically they are characterized by hemorrhage, very little inflammatory reaction, and large numbers of Gram-positive bacilli.

Melioidosis

Melioidosis is a disease caused by *Burkholderia (Pseudomonas) pseudomallei*, which is a Gram-negative, motile bacillus.

It can be cultured on modified MacConkey's agar. Serologic tests are available, but are not entirely reliable in diagnosis.

The disease is fairly common in South-East Asia, northern Australia and in the tropical zones of India, Africa and the United States. It lives in the soil just below the surface during dry seasons and it comes to the surface in wet seasons. Infection occurs in animals, as well as in humans. Most cases occur in the wet seasons. The organism seems to gain access to the body via skin abrasions.

Infection is more commonly seen in farmers. There is no transmission from animal to human, nor from human to human. A significant proportion of patients have diabetes. Lung infection is the most common form of the disease, but other organs may be affected.

Case 2.4

Four weeks before being admitted in a moribund state, a 38-year-old Chinese fisherman in Malaysia had had an abscess in his right lower chest drained, and he had been treated with antibiotics. His chest X-ray on admission showed multiple, bilateral, miliary nodules (see Fig. 2.82).

Post-mortem examination showed multiple, well-circumscribed, yellowish nodules throughout both lungs (shown in Fig. 2.83). Similar nodules were present in the liver, the spleen, both kidneys and the right adrenal. Microscopic examination showed the nodules to be abscesses in which Gram-negative bacilli could be demonstrated (shown in Figs 2.84, 2.85 and 2.86).

B. pseudomallei was cultured from a number of organs.

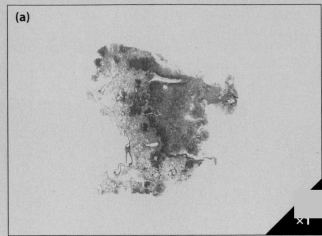

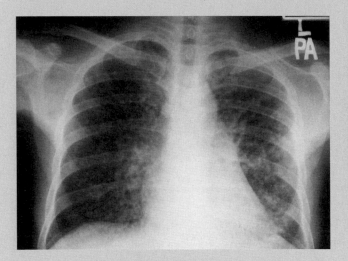

▲ **Fig. 2.82** Chest X-ray of a male, aged 38 years, showing multiple, bilateral, miliary nodules.

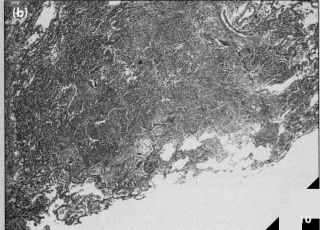

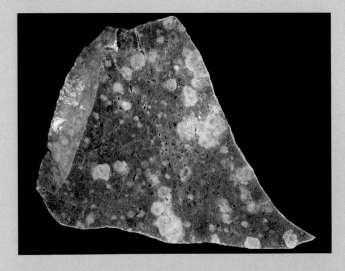

▲ **Fig. 2.83** Lung showing multiple, well-circumscribed, yellowish nodules.

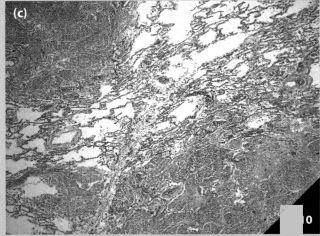

▲ **Fig. 2.84(a), (b) and (c)** Low magnification views of the nodules.

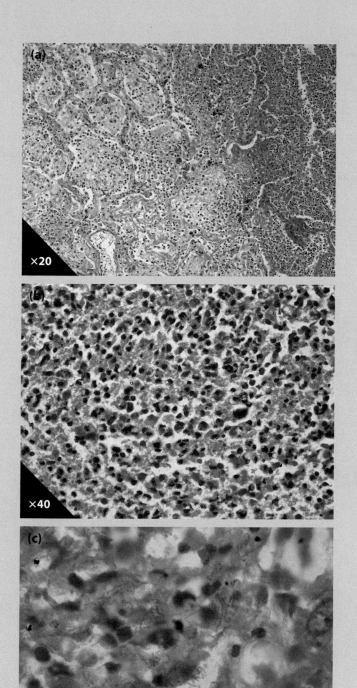

▶ **Fig. 2.85(a), (b) and (c)** Higher magnification views showed the nodules to be abscesses.

▼ **Fig. 2.86** Gram stain showing the presence of Gram-negative bacilli in the abscesses.

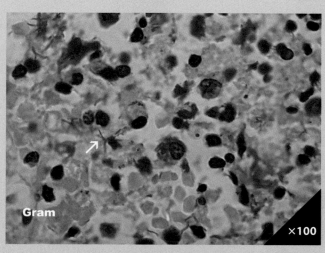

Acknowledgments

- Fig. 2.1 From Cooke, R.A. and Stewart, B., *Colour Atlas of Anatomical Pathology*, third edn, Churchill Livingstone, Edinburgh, 2004.
- Fig. 2.2 From Cooke, R.A. and Stewart, B., *Colour Atlas of Anatomical Pathology*, third edn, Churchill Livingstone, Edinburgh, 2004.
- Fig. 2.6 From Cooke, R.A. and Stewart, B., *Colour Atlas of Anatomical Pathology*, third edn, Churchill Livingstone, Edinburgh, 2004.
- Fig. 2.7 From Cooke, R.A. and Stewart, B., *Colour Atlas of Anatomical Pathology*, third edn, Churchill Livingstone, Edinburgh, 2004.
- Fig. 2.26 From Cooke, R.A. and Stewart, B., *Colour Atlas of Anatomical Pathology*, third edn, Churchill Livingstone, Edinburgh, 2004.
- Fig. 2.29 From Cooke, R.A. and Stewart, B., *Colour Atlas of Anatomical Pathology*, third edn, Churchill Livingstone, Edinburgh, 2004.
- Fig. 2.31 From Cooke, R.A. and Stewart, B., *Colour Atlas of Anatomical Pathology*, third edn, Churchill Livingstone, Edinburgh, 2004.
- Fig. 2.32 From Cooke, R.A. and Stewart, B., *Colour Atlas of Anatomical Pathology*, third edn, Churchill Livingstone, Edinburgh, 2004.
- Figs 2.34 –2.37 From Cooke, R.A. and Stewart, B., *Colour Atlas of Anatomical Pathology*, third edn, Churchill Livingstone, Edinburgh, 2004.
- Fig. 2.41 From Cooke, R.A. and Stewart, B., *Colour Atlas of Anatomical Pathology*, third edn, Churchill Livingstone, Edinburgh, 2004.
- Fig. 2.48 From Cooke, R.A. and Stewart, B., *Colour Atlas of Anatomical Pathology*, third edn, Churchill Livingstone, Edinburgh, 2004.
- Fig. 2.49 From Cooke, R.A. and Stewart, B., *Colour Atlas of Anatomical Pathology*, third edn, Churchill Livingstone, Edinburgh, 2004.
- Fig. 2.50 From Cooke, R.A. and Stewart, B., *Colour Atlas of Anatomical Pathology*, third edn, Churchill Livingstone, Edinburgh, 2004.
- Fig. 2.51 Courtesy of John Tyrer, Brisbane, Australia.
- Fig. 2.52 Courtesy of John Tyrer, Brisbane, Australia.
- Fig. 2.53 From Cooke, R.A. and Stewart, B., *Colour Atlas of Anatomical Pathology*, third edn, Churchill Livingstone, Edinburgh, 2004.
- Fig. 2.54 Courtesy of Vincenzo Eusebi, Bologna, Italy.
- Fig. 2.55 From Cooke, R.A. and Stewart, B., *Colour Atlas of Anatomical Pathology*, third edn, Churchill Livingstone, Edinburgh, 2004.
- Fig. 2.57 From Cooke, R.A. and Stewart, B., *Colour Atlas of Anatomical Pathology*, third edn, Churchill Livingstone, Edinburgh, 2004.
- Fig. 2.58(a) and (b) From Cooke, R.A. and Stewart, B., *Colour Atlas of Anatomical Pathology*, third edn, Churchill Livingstone, Edinburgh, 2004.
- Fig. 2.61 From Cooke, R.A. and Stewart, B., *Colour Atlas of Anatomical Pathology*, third edn, Churchill Livingstone, Edinburgh, 2004.
- Figs 2.62 and 2.63 Courtesy of Robert Ayres, Toowoomba, Australia.
- Fig. 2.64 Courtesy of John Richens, Papua New Guinea and London, England; and from Cooke, R.A. and Stewart, B., *Colour Atlas of Anatomical Pathology*, third edn, Churchill Livingstone, Edinburgh, 2004.
- Fig. 2.65 Courtesy of Frances Andrijick, photographer, Perth, Australia.
- Fig. 2.69 Courtesy of the person in the photograph.
- Fig. 2.70 Courtesy of Neil Wiseman and the *Courier Mail*, Brisbane, Australia.
- Fig. 2.71 Courtesy of Charles Haszler, Papua New Guinea and Sydney, Australia.
- Fig. 2.74 Courtesy of the Museum of the Royal College of Surgeons in Edinburgh, Scotland.
- Fig. 2.75 From Cooke, R.A. and Stewart, B., *Colour Atlas of Anatomical Pathology*, third edn, Churchill Livingstone, Edinburgh, 2004.
- Fig. 2.86 Case courtesy of Norain Karim, Ipoh, Malaysia.

Tuberculosis

Tuberculosis (TB) has been an important disease throughout the world for centuries. It is a disease caused by the bacterium *Mycobacterium tuberculosis*. Transmitted mainly by respiratory droplet infection, in some cases it may be spread by drinking infected milk. It has been largely controlled in countries with well-funded public health programs that aim to diagnose patients with the disease, and to treat and isolate them from the uninfected population until cured. Programs such as these are expensive in terms of money and human resources. In countries with small health budgets, tuberculosis is now raging almost unchecked.

This great resurgence of tuberculosis has been compounded by the large number of AIDS patients who contract it, and by the emergence of multiple, drug-resistant strains of *M. tuberculosis*. It is important for health workers to be able to recognize the many ways in which tuberculosis may present, particularly in poorer countries with small health budgets. It is also important in the wealthier countries, because now that it is less common there, it has become harder to diagnose, since health workers have had little experience with it—either during their training or since—making it a 'forgotten' disease.

Some manifestations of tuberculosis

Lymphadenopathy

In countries where TB is endemic, cervical lymphadenopathy is one of the most common modes of presentation, as illustrated in Figures 3.1–3.6, continued overleaf. A Ziehl Neelsen (ZN) stain for acid-fast bacilli (AFB) should be performed whenever granulomas—such as those in Figure 3.4, overleaf—are seen in biopsy tissue. In TB lymph nodes, however, AFBs are not always found.

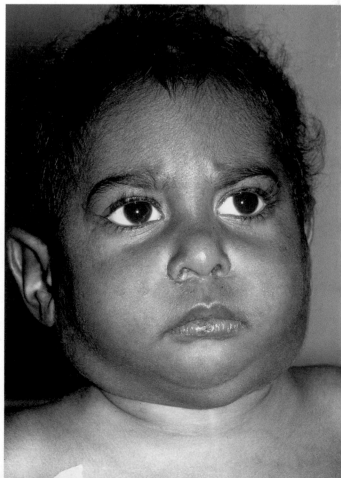

▶ **Fig. 3.1** This child was referred to a children's hospital in Brisbane, Australia, with bilateral cervical lymphadenopathy. The provisional diagnosis was malignant lymphoma. A lymph node biopsy was performed.

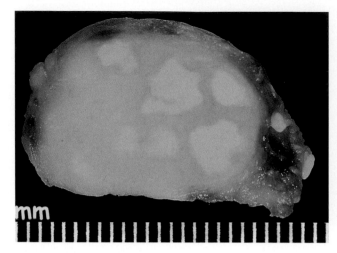

▲ **Fig. 3.2** Gross examination of the cut surface of the lymph node from the child in Figure 3.1 shows that it is replaced by rubbery white tissue with a number of areas of caseation.

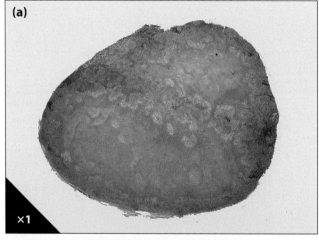

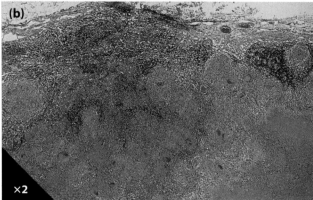

▲ **Fig. 3.3(a) and (b)** At low magnification, it can be seen that the lymph node, shown in Figure 3.2, is replaced by multiple granulomas with extensive caseation.

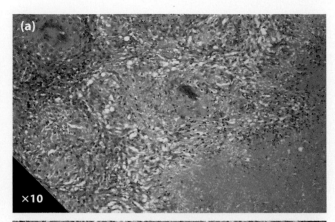

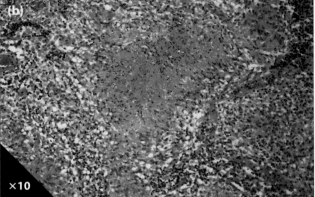

▲ **Fig. 3.4(a) and (b)** Higher magnification views of the lymph node, shown in Figure 3.2, show the detail of the granulomas. They consist of collections of epithelioid cells with central areas of caseous necrosis. At the edges of the granulomas, there are a few multinucleated giant cells. These appearances are typical of the granulomatous inflammation that occurs as a response to infection with *M. tuberculosis*.

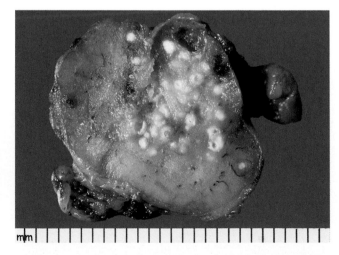

▲ **Fig. 3.5** Cut surface of a lymph node that is less completely infiltrated by 'tubercles'.

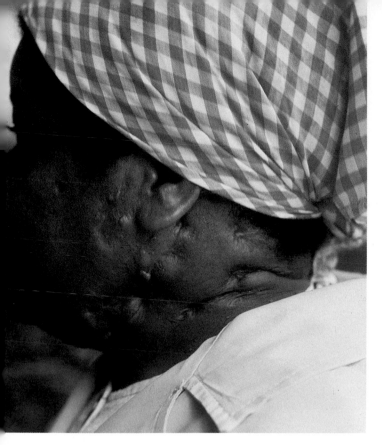

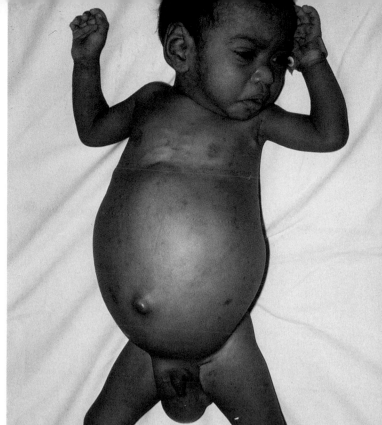

▲ **Fig. 3.6** This woman from Melanesia (an island group in the western Pacific Ocean) was treated for acute tuberculous lymphadenitis with multiple discharging sinuses. Healing has resulted in extensive scarring in the neck.

▲ **Fig. 3.7** This child presented with ascites (fluid in the abdomen). Ascites is a fairly common presentation of tuberculosis in endemic areas.

When a lymph node biopsy is taken for a possible diagnosis of TB, it should be sent to the laboratory in a sterile container without any fixative. A culture for *M. tuberculosis* can then be performed.

If it is not possible to get the specimen to the laboratory in less than an hour, the node should be sliced down the middle, and placed in a container of 10 per cent formalin for transport to a laboratory for histologic examination. In many places where TB is prevalent, laboratory facilities will not be readily available and culture will not be possible, but a diagnosis can nevertheless be made by histologic examination.

Gastrointestinal tract

Another relatively common presentation of tuberculosis is with gastrointestinal involvement, which may present as ascites (excessive fluid in the abdominal cavity) (see Figs 3.7 and 3.8). In such cases, the serosal surfaces in the abdomen are studded with multiple, small nodules which are tuberculous granulomas. Surgeons who open the abdomen of a person with abdominal tuberculous often mistake these nodules for secondary deposits of malignant tumors. Indeed, the granulomatous inflammation may produce thickenings in the bowel that mimic the appearance of tumors (see Figs 3.9, 3.10 and 3.11, overleaf). Mucosal inflammation causes ulceration (as shown in Fig. 3.12, overleaf), which in turn results in diarrhea.

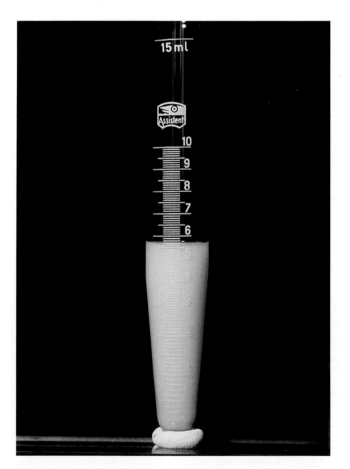

▲ **Fig. 3.8** Ascitic fluid showing the features of chyle. TB ascites is sometimes chylous due to damage to the large lymphatic ducts.

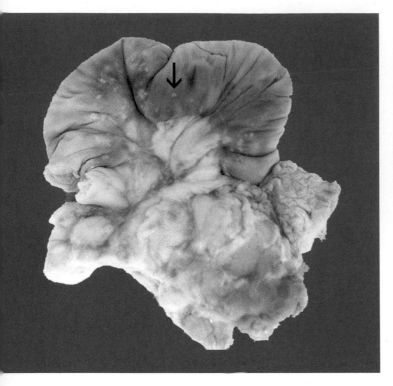

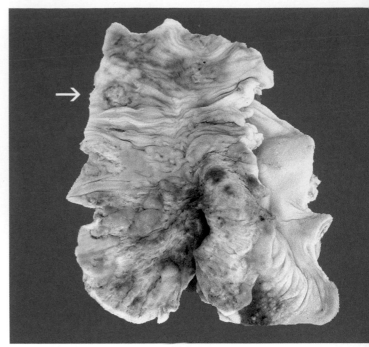

▲ **Fig. 3.9** Gross appearance of the small intestine, seen in a child who died from disseminated tuberculosis. The serosal surface of the bowel is studded with multiple, small nodules. The peritoneum shows similar nodules (tubercles), and the mesenteric lymph nodes are enlarged. Surgeons who are not aware of this pathology may mistake it for disseminated malignancy.

▲ **Fig. 3.11** Gross appearance of the ileo cecal region in the post mortem illustrated in Figure 3.9. There is mucosal ulceration and marked thickening of the area. This inflammatory thickening may sometimes cause the symptoms of intestinal obstruction leading, in an adult, to an erroneous diagnosis of carcinoma of the cecum.

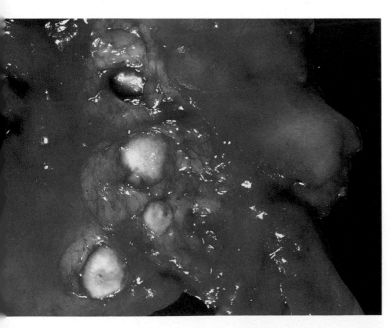

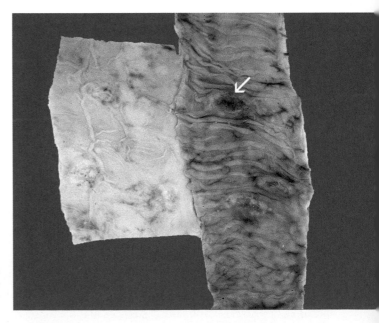

▲ **Fig. 3.10** Fresh specimen of tuberculous mesenteric lymph nodes.

▲ **Fig. 3.12** Gross appearance of the opened transverse colon on the left and the small intestine on the right. In the small intestine, the ulcers are typically transverse. In this case, there were mucosal ulcers throughout the length of the colon as well.

Lungs

Pulmonary involvement is common in tuberculosis. The X-rays in Figures 3.13 and 3.14 show two of the most common patterns seen in this condition—miliary and cavitating.

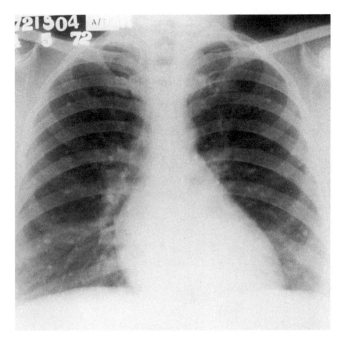

▲ **Fig. 3.13** Chest X-ray showing the typical features of miliary tuberculosis. There are small, round opacities scattered throughout both lungs.

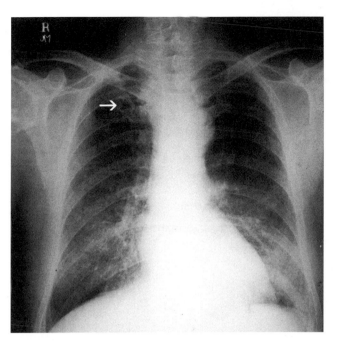

▲ **Fig. 3.14** Chest X-ray showing the usual features of tuberculosis with pneumonic infiltrates and multiple cavities, particularly in the apices of the lungs.

Case 3.1

A 4-year-old female was referred to a children's hospital in Brisbane, Australia, after being sick with a high fever for some days. No localizing signs could be detected. A chest X-ray was reported as showing widening of the mediastinum, with some nonspecific changes in the lungs. The widening of the mediastinum was thought to be due to a thymus gland (see Fig. 3.15).

Soon after admission, she became drowsy and then became comatose. An air encephalogram showed marked hydrocephalus with dilatation of all the ventricles (shown in Fig. 3.16 overleaf). A day later she died, and a post-mortem examination was performed.

The post mortem revealed that the child had tuberculous meningitis and miliary tuberculosis. In this condition, as illustrated in Figures 3.17–3.28 (see pages 44–47), organisms spread throughout the body via the bloodstream and lodge in the various organs, producing microscopic foci of infection—miliary tubercles.

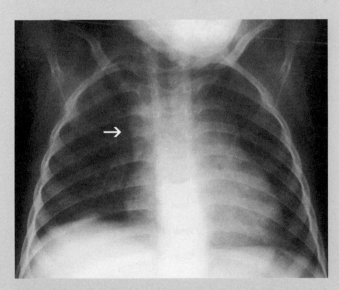

▲ **Fig. 3.15** Chest X-ray of the 4-year-old female was reported as showing widening of the mediastinum, with some nonspecific changes in the lungs. The widening of the mediastinum was thought to be due to a thymus gland.

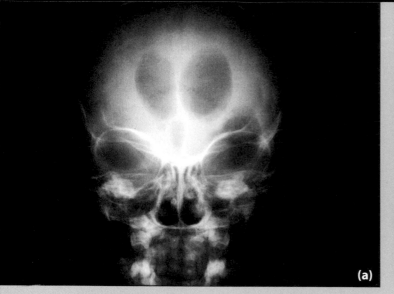
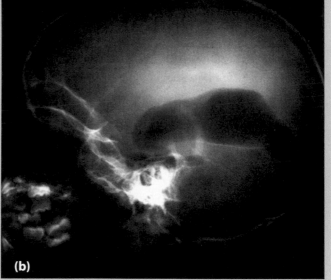

▲ **Fig. 3.16(a) and (b)** An air encephalogram showed marked hydrocephalus with dilatation of all the ventricles. (This technique is no longer used.)

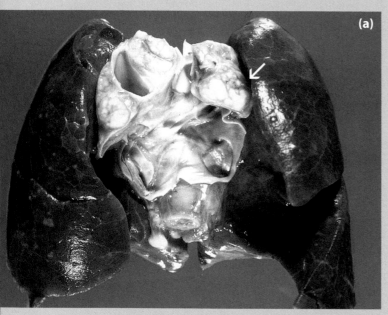

(a)

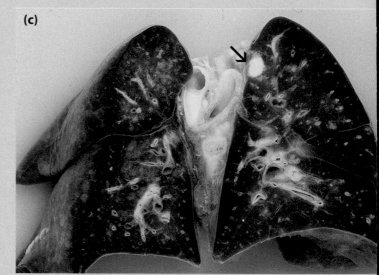

(c)

▲ **Fig. 3.17(c)** A further slice through the lungs showed the presence of a rounded area of white caseous material just beneath the pleural surface of the medial aspect of the upper lobe of the left lung. This appearance has been called a Gohn focus. It is more frequently seen in children than in adults. Miliary tubercles can be seen throughout the lungs.

▲ **Fig. 3.17(a)** Post-mortem examination showed that the widening of the mediastinum was not due to a thymus, but to enlargement of the mediastinal lymph nodes by tuberculous granulation tissue. Miliary tubercles can be seen beneath the pleura of the lungs.

▼ **Fig. 3.17(b)** Miliary tubercles are more clearly seen in this close-up view.

▼ **Fig. 3.18** Another example of a Gohn focus with involvement of the mediastinal lymph nodes. This appearance used to be called 'primary tuberculosis'.

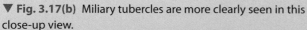

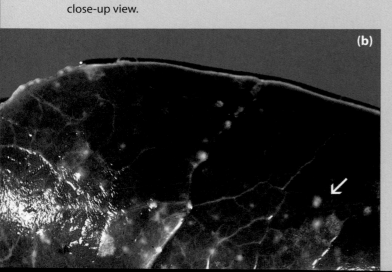

(b)

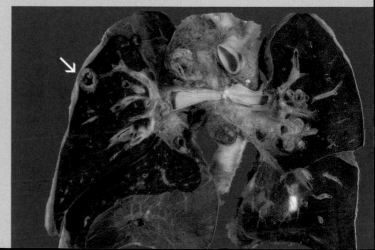

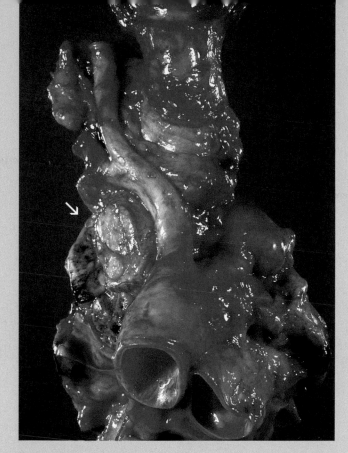

▲ **Fig. 3.19** Fresh specimen of tuberculous involvement of mediastinal lymph nodes.

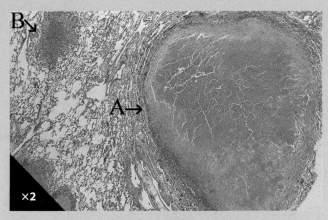

▲ **Fig. 3.20** Low-magnification view of the Gohn focus (A) and miliary tubercles (B) in the lung.

▼ **Fig. 3.21(a), (b), (c) and (d)** Higher magnification views of the miliary tubercles. Note that the inflammatory response in acute tuberculous infection as seen in this case is a neutrophilic one, and not a granulomatous one. Quite often in acute tuberculous inflammation, the cellular infiltrate is neutrophilic without any granulomas or multinucleated giant cells. There are usually numerous acid-fast bacilli in the inflammatory infiltrate, as seen in **(d)**. This feature of acute tuberculous inflammation may sometimes lead to an incorrect diagnosis if the pathologist is not aware of this possibility.

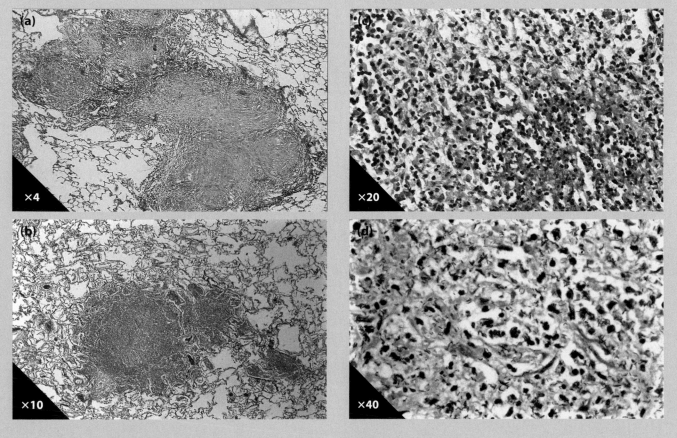

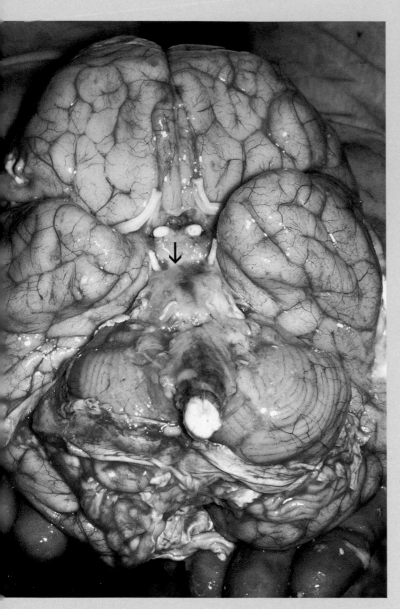

▲ **Fig. 3.22** Examination of the brain showed that the hydrocephalus was due to tuberculous meningitis. The brain is viewed from its under surface. It shows the characteristic features of tuberculous meningitis with pus accumulation along the base obstructing the outflow tracts of the fourth ventricle resulting in hydrocephalus.

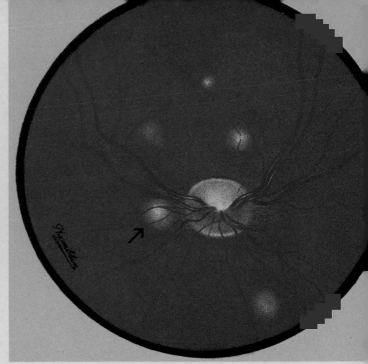

▲ **Fig. 3.23** Drawing of miliary tubercles in the retina seen through an ophthalmoscope.

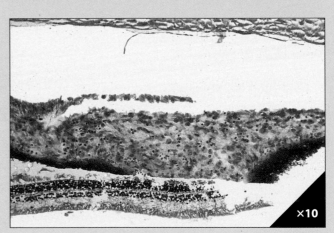

▲ **Fig. 3.24** Microscopic section of a miliary tubercle in the retina.

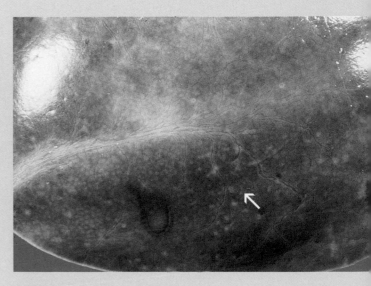

▲ **Fig. 3.25** Miliary tubercles in the liver.

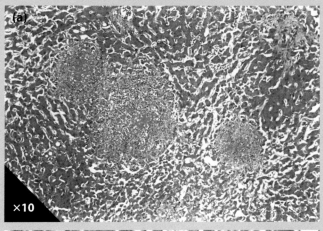

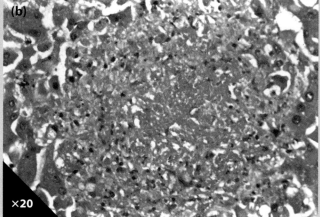

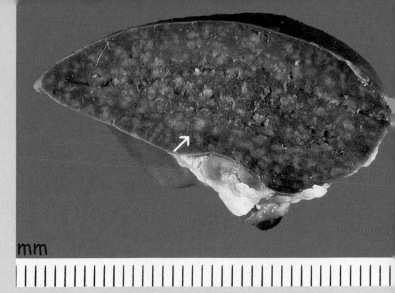

▲ **Fig. 3.27** Miliary tubercles in the spleen.

▲ **Fig. 3.26(a) and (b)** Higher magnification views of miliary tubercles in the liver.

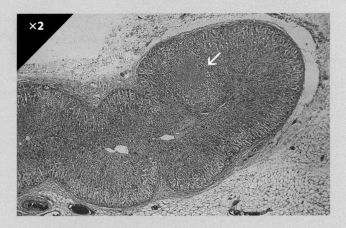

▲ **Fig. 3.28** Miliary tubercles in the adrenal gland.

Case 3.2

In 1965, a teenage male, who had been sick with fever and wasting for some weeks, presented to the hospital in Port Moresby, the capital of Papua New Guinea (PNG), for treatment (see Fig. 3.29, overleaf). He had a cough, hemoptysis and discharging sinuses in the neck and axilla; and he was having night sweats. He had clinical evidence of pneumonic involvement of both lungs.

His chest X-ray showed cavitating pneumonia typical of tuberculosis (illustrated in Fig. 3.30, overleaf). His sputum was cultured by inoculation of a Lowenstein Jensen culture slope. A ZN stain on the sputum revealed the presence of acid-fast bacilli.

He was diagnosed as having tuberculosis and he was treated with streptomycin, isoniazid and pas—the antibiotic regime of the time.

He responded quickly to this treatment, and a week later he was almost unrecognizable. His energy had returned; he was putting on weight, and his signs of disease were abating. This was a common response in the early days after the first introduction of streptomycin.

▼ **Fig. 3.29(a)** This teenage male, who had been sick with fever and wasting for some weeks, presented to the hospital in Port Moresby, the capital of PNG, for treatment of his rampant tuberculosis.

(a)

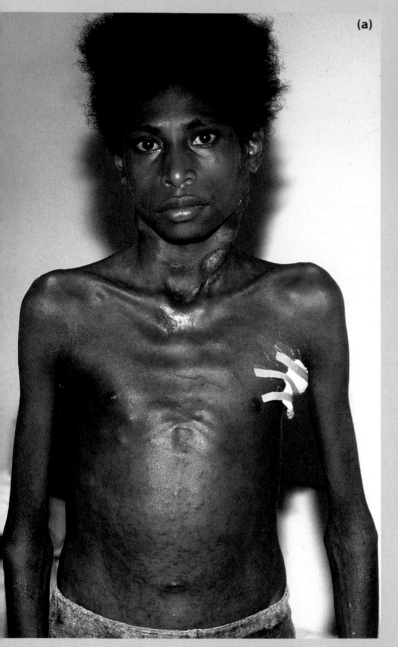

(b)

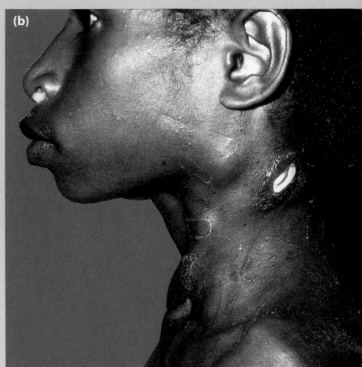

▲ **Fig. 3.29(b)** Close-up view of the sinuses in the neck, resulting from tuberculous inflammation of the cervical lymph nodes.

▼ **Fig. 3.30** Chest X-ray of the teenage patient showed cavitating pneumonia typical of tuberculosis.

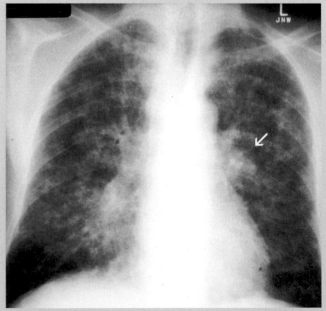

Frequently, tuberculosis affects the apices of the lungs (see Figs 3.31, and 3.32 overleaf). Before the introduction of antibiotic treatment, there were many adults in the community who had pulmonary tuberculosis that caused them ill health, but it would grumble on for many years without causing severe incapacity. Their sputum contained acid-fast bacilli and it was sometimes blood stained. These people were a constant source of infection, particularly to children. From time to time, they would have a recrudescence of their disease, and ultimately they would develop an acute recrudescence of infection that would be fatal. Examination of the lungs at post mortem would show old cavities and areas of calcification in the apices with acute pneumonia in the adjacent lung (shown in Fig. 3.33 overleaf).

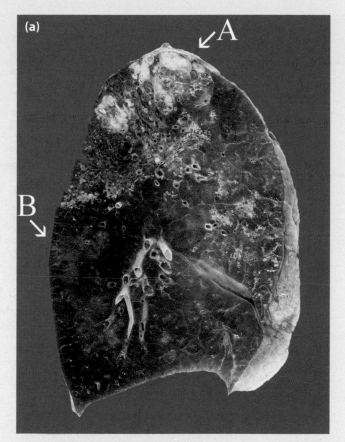

▶ **Fig. 3.31(a)** Lung of a coalminer from a mining city near Brisbane, Australia, who died from a recrudescence of tuberculosis. The lung shows a minor degree of coalminers' pneumoconiosis with deposition of moderate amounts of carbon, some fibrosis and some emphysema. Cavitating lesions of tuberculosis are affecting the apex of the lung (A), and an acute pneumonia is extending beyond this to the surrounding areas of the lung (B).

▶ **Fig. 3.31(b)** Closer view of the acute pneumonia.

▼ **Fig. 3.31(c)** Closer view of the emphysema and cavitating pneumonia in the apex of the lung.

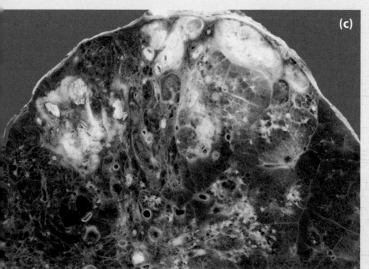

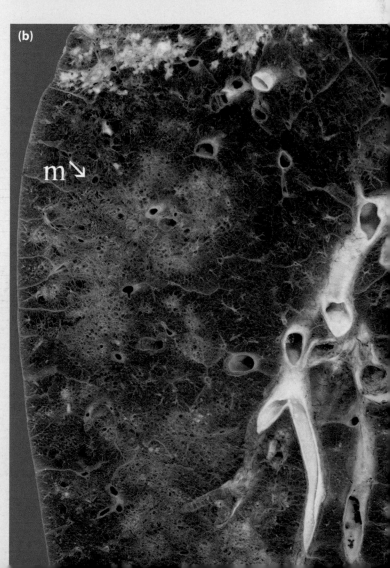

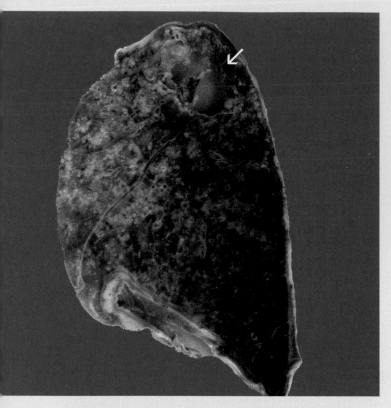

▲ **Fig. 3.32** For comparison to the condition illustrated in Fig. 3.31, this lung from a patient from Papua New Guinea shows the features of an acute tuberculous pneumonia. There is an acute abscess cavity in the apex.

Tuberculosis used to be a common complication of coalminers' lung, a condition characterized by the deposition of black carbon dust causing fibrosis and emphysema of the lung. Tuberculosis was a secondary infection.

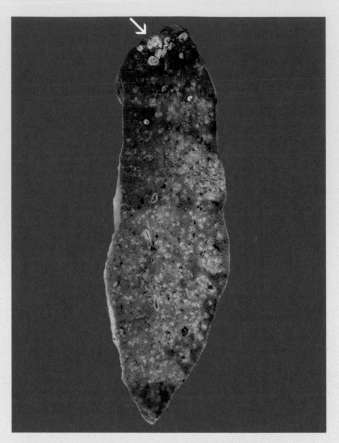

▲ **Fig. 3.33** Lung from a patient, who died before the introduction of streptomycin, shows the features of longstanding tuberculosis. The disease in the apex has undergone healing with calcification. Death occurred because there was a recrudescence of the disease.

▶ **Fig. 3.34** This severely fibrotic lung was one of those removed during the vogue for pneumonectomy or lobectomy for the treatment of severely damaged lungs that resulted from cure of the tuberculous infection.

In the 1950s and 1960s, patients were cured of longstanding tuberculosis as a result of antibiotic treatment. This left them with severely fibrotic, poorly functioning lungs. In an effort to improve the function of the remaining lung substance, thoracic surgeons excised either the most severely affected segment or the whole lung (see Fig. 3.34).

This treatment was ultimately abandoned when it was found that it did not significantly improve lung function. Another reason for its abandonment was that antibiotic treatment was given early in the course of the disease and such severely damaged lungs were no longer seen, thus this pathology disappeared.

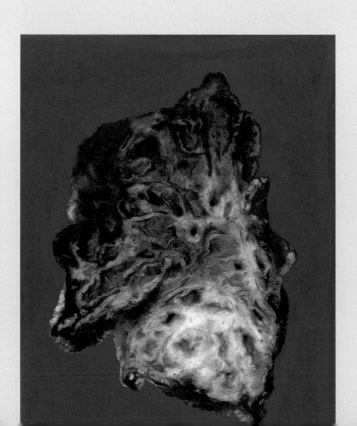

Bones

Tuberculosis particularly affects the spine (see Figs 3.35 and 3.36) and the large joints—hips, knees and ankles. The most characteristic presentation that results from tuberculous involvement of bone is the collapse of vertebral bodies giving rise to a deformity called 'Pott's disease of the spine', named after Percival Pott (1713–1788), depicted in Figure 3.37, overleaf. One of Pott's specimens is housed in St Bartholomew's Hospital, London (see Fig. 3.38, overleaf).

A more recent specimen of Pott's disease of the spine is shown in Figure 3.39, overleaf. Paravertebral abscess from tuberculosis of the lower lumbar spine is shown in Figure 3.40, overleaf.

▼ **Fig. 3.35** Vietnamese boy with Pott's disease of the spine.

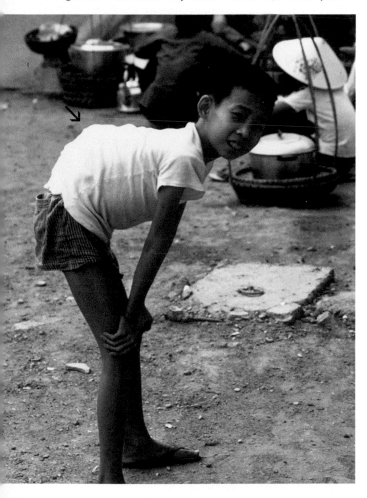

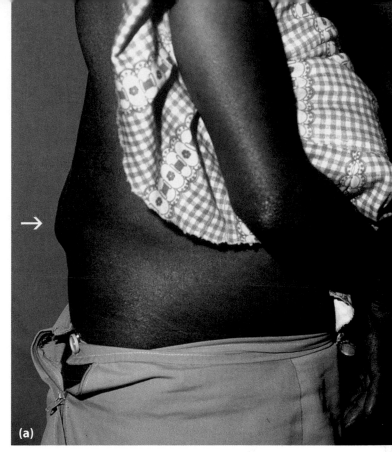

(a)

▲ **Fig. 3.36(a)** Papua New Guinean woman with Pott's disease of the spine.

▼ **Fig. 3.36(b)** X-ray of the woman's spine shows the collapsed lower lumbar vertebrae that caused the deformity.

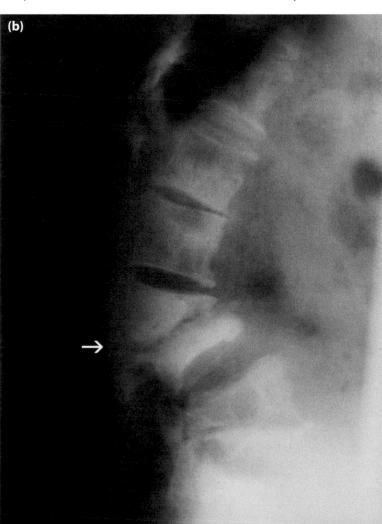

(b)

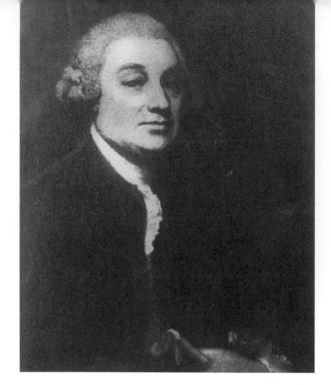

▲ **Fig. 3.37** Percival Pott (1713–1788), after whom the fracture of the vertebrae is named, worked at St Bartholomew's Hospital in London.

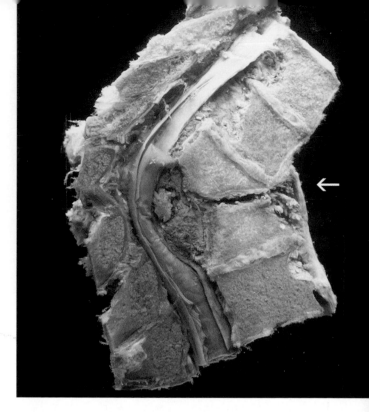

▲ **Fig. 3.38** One of Percival Pott's specimens, *c.*1777, that is still housed in the St Bartholomew's Hospital Pathology Museum, London.

▼ ▶ **Fig. 3.39(a) and (b)** A more recent specimen shows the collapsed vertebrae and the pus that tracks into the psoas muscle.

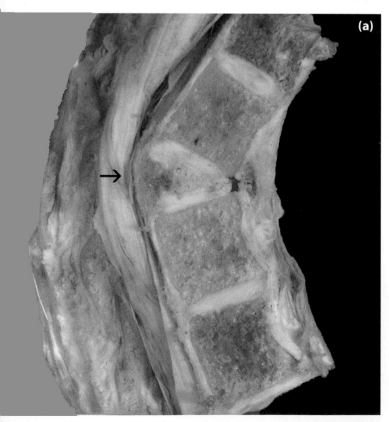

(a)

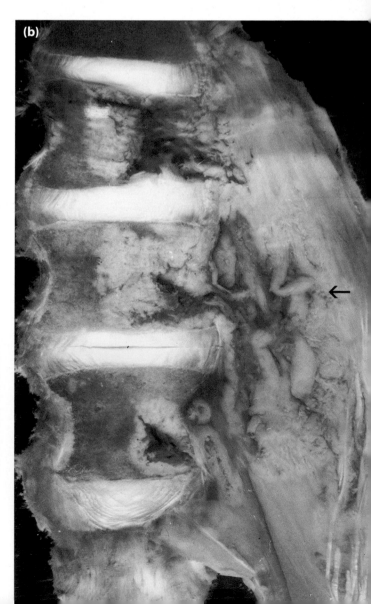

(b)

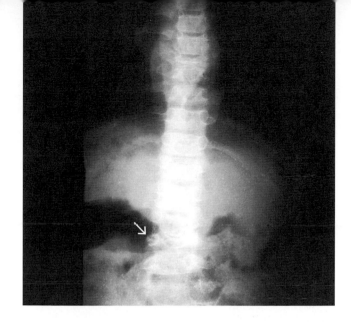

▶ **Fig. 3.40** X-ray from a young Papua New Guinean man, who developed a sudden pain in his back and paralysis of his legs. He has a paravertebral abscess from tuberculosis of the lower lumbar spine.

Central nervous system

Case 3.3

A 30-year-old Sri Lankan immigrant to Australia had been in the country for 6 months, and he had been sick with fever for a few weeks. He accompanied his family for a week-long drive from Melbourne in the south, to Brisbane in the north. During the journey, he became more sick, and by the time they reached Toowoomba, a city 80 miles (129 km) west of Brisbane, he was becoming drowsy.

He was admitted to a Toowoomba hospital and investigations showed that he had meningitis and hydrocephalus with no localizing signs (see Fig. 3.41). He became unconscious and was sent by ambulance to a neurosurgical unit of a hospital in Brisbane. He died shortly after admission.

Post-mortem examination confirmed the presence of meningitis, which had the typical gross features of being caused by tuberculosis (see Figs 3.42–3.45, overleaf).

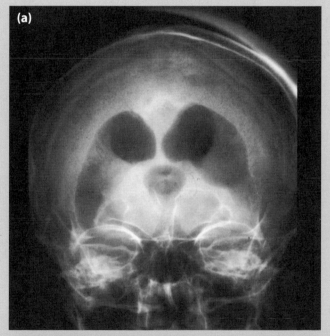

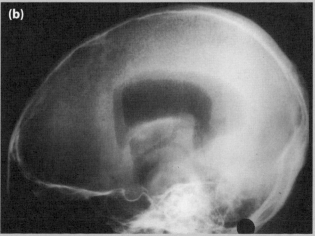

▶ **Fig. 3.41(a) and (b)** An air encephalogram showed marked hydrocephalus.

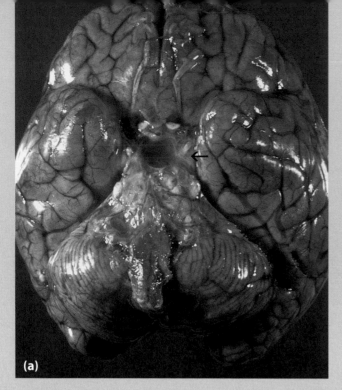

(a)

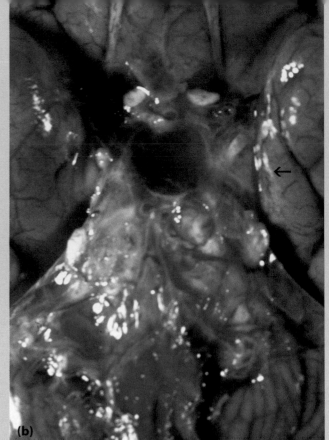

(b)

▲ ▶ **Fig. 3.42(a) and (b)** The brain viewed from its under surface showed an accumulation of pus along its base, with opacity of the subarachnoid space in the interpeduncular cistern.

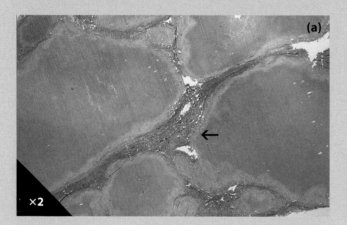

(a)

×2

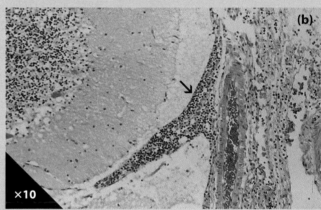

(b)

×10

▲ **Fig. 3.43(a) and (b)** Microscopic examination shows pus in the subarachnoid space—the hallmark of meningitis. At the high magnification, it can be seen that the predominant inflammatory cell is the lymphocyte.

▼ **Fig. 3.44** Occasional acid-fast bacilli are present in the inflammatory infiltrate (ZN stain).

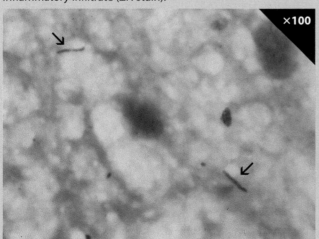

×100

▼ **Fig. 3.45** In this section, the inflammatory reaction extends into the brain substance (B), rather than remaining in the subarachnoid space (A), as it seems to do in cases of meningitis caused by other organisms. This may explain why treatment of tuberculous meningitis results in more complications than does treatment of the more commonly occurring bacterial meningitides.

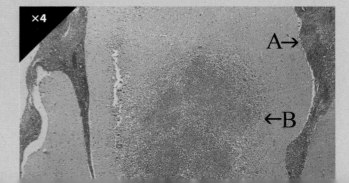

×4

A→

←B

Other intracerebral complications of tuberculosis

Case 3.4

A young man from Papua New Guinea with a left hemiplegia and a space-occupying lesion in his right frontal hemisphere was referred to the neurosurgical unit of a hospital in Queensland, Australia. He died soon after admission. Post-mortem examination showed the presence of an abscess in the right frontal lobe. As shown in Figure 3.46, there are also two localized, firm, white areas: one in the right frontal lobe and the other in the cerebellum. These are tuberculomas. Tuberculomas may present with the symptoms and signs of an intracerebral space-occupying lesion (see Fig. 3.47, overleaf). In an endemic area of tuberculosis, one should be wary of such a lesion in a patient with a fever. It could be due to tuberculosis and not to a neoplasm. Treatment is not very satisfactory.

▼ **Fig. 3.46(a)** Post-mortem examination showed the presence of an abscess in the right frontal lobe (A). There are also two localized, firm white areas: one in the right frontal lobe (B), and the other in the cerebellum (C). These are tuberculomas—solid areas of tuberculous granulation tissue.

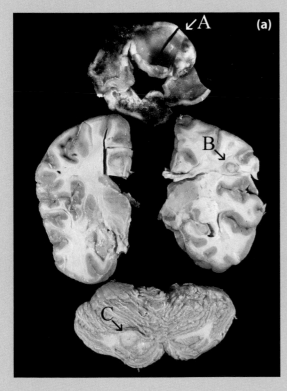

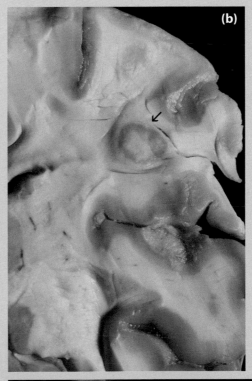

◀ **Fig. 3.46(b)** Closer view of the tuberculoma in the right frontal lobe.

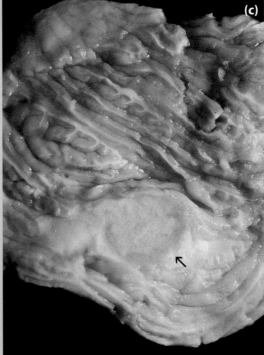

◀ **Fig. 3.46(c)** Closer view of the tuberculoma in the cerebellum.

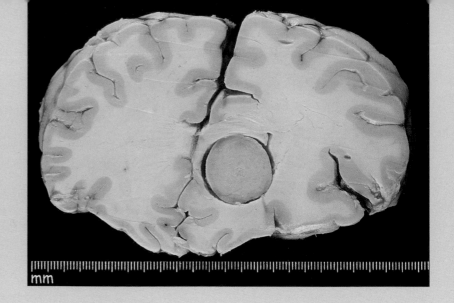

▶ Fig. 3.47 When examined at post mortem, this tuberculoma shelled out like a pea from a pod, but clearly there was more pathology there than was apparent to gross examination.

Kidneys

Case 3.5

A 25-year-old Australian-born* man presented with renal colic and hematuria. An intravenous pyelogram showed right-sided hydronephrosis, with what appeared to be a stricture at the lower end of the right ureter (see Fig. 3.48). The surgeon intended to excise the segment of damaged ureter near the pelvic brim and to re-anastomose the ends. When he viewed the pathology at operation, he realized that he could not do this because the whole length of the ureter was thickened, so he performed a right nephro-ureterectomy (as illustrated in Figs 3.49 and 3.50).

TB was virtually eliminated from the Australian population by about 1970 and it was seen only in immigrants or travelers.

In the routine follow-up of contacts, the patient's father was found to have pulmonary tuberculosis. Father and son were both successfully treated with appropriate chemotherapy.

▼ Fig. 3.48 An intravenous pyelogram showed right-sided hydronephrosis (A), with what appeared to be a stricture at the lower end of the right ureter (B).

▼ Fig. 3.49 The gross specimen showed marked thickening of the ureter and the pelvis (A), with pyoureter and pyonephrosis (B).

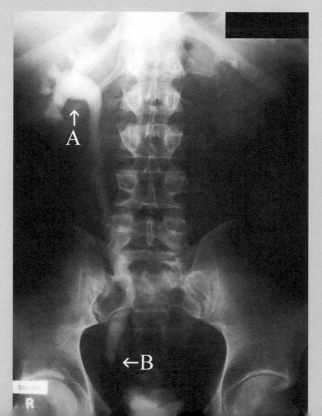

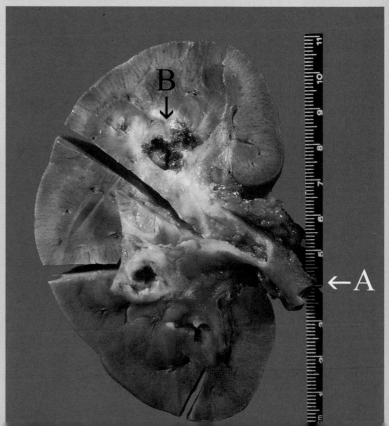

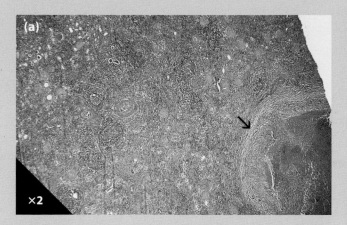
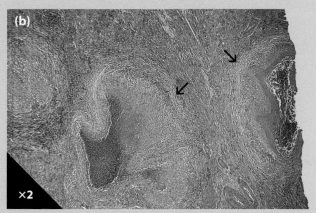

▲ **Fig. 3.50(a) and (b)** Microscopic examination shows granulomas with central caseation in the renal parenchyma. These gross and microscopic features are typical of those seen in renal tuberculosis.

Gastrointestinal tract

Case 3.6

A 25-year-old man from Papua New Guinea (PNG) was referred to Brisbane, Australia, to have a colonoscopy. He had severe colitis, present for about 6 months.

Acute generalized colitis was seen, and random biopsies of the colon were taken (see Fig. 3.51). These biopsies were reported as showing acute nonspecific colitis (see Fig. 3.52, overleaf) by a pathologist, who had been given no history apart from the fact that this was a colonic biopsy.

The gastroenterologist asked for another opinion on the biopsy, and provided the following more complete history.

History: This man had been in the United States 6 months previously on a postgraduate scholarship. While in the US, he had complained of abdominal pain, and an appendectomy was performed. Granulomas were seen and a provisional diagnosis of Crohn's disease was made. He was still very sick when he returned home to PNG, and his family took him to see a specialist there. The man was referred to Brisbane for further management.

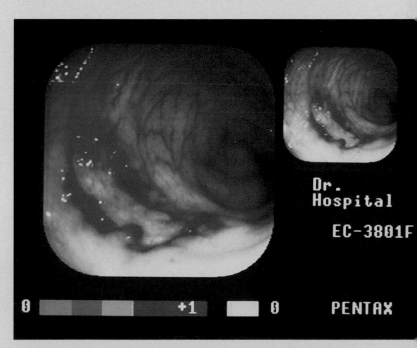

▲ **Fig. 3.51** Endoscopic examination showed a generalized acute colitis.

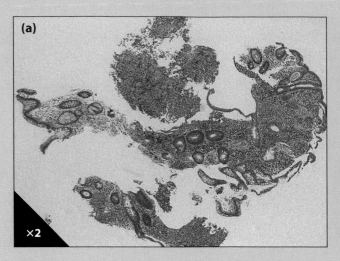

(a)

×2

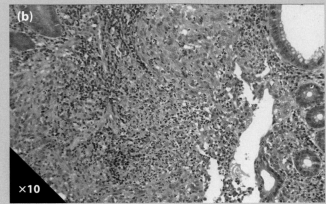

(b)

×10

▲ **Fig. 3.52(a) and (b)** Views of the colonic biopsy show an acute colitis. The inflammation consists of neutrophils.

Diagnosis: The diagnosis is clearly acute tuberculous colitis (see Fig. 3.53, in which a ZN stain was performed). Once a proper history was available, the diagnosis was easy. An acute inflammatory reaction is quite commonly seen in acute tuberculosis. A ZN stain in such circumstances often shows the biopsy to be teeming with acid-fast bacilli, as it was here.

The patient was transferred to an infectious diseases ward. He responded quickly to effective anti-tuberculosis treatment. A week later, he was feeling much better, was eating voraciously and beginning to put on weight.

▶ **Fig. 3.53** ZN stain showed the biopsy to be teeming with acid-fast bacilli.

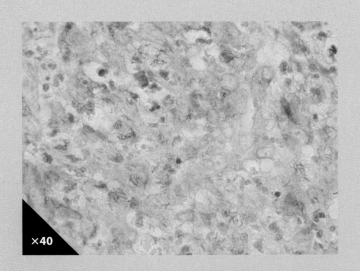

×40

The hallmark of TB infection is the presence of granulomas and this is why pathologists may miss TB when it causes a tissue response that is unusual—even though it is commonly seen in countries where TB is common. So, there are two reasons why the pathologist in Case 3.6 missed the diagnosis: one is that he was given no history and the second is that he was not aware that TB can present with a tissue reaction that is more characteristic of an acute infection caused by some of the other organisms.

The lesson for the pathologist is that TB can present with an acute inflammatory reaction, as well as with granulomas. Diagnosis is always easier when the history is adequate.

Male genital tract

Tuberculosis involves the testis and epididymis and it may produce a discharging sinus that opens posteriorly through the scrotum (see Fig. 3.54).

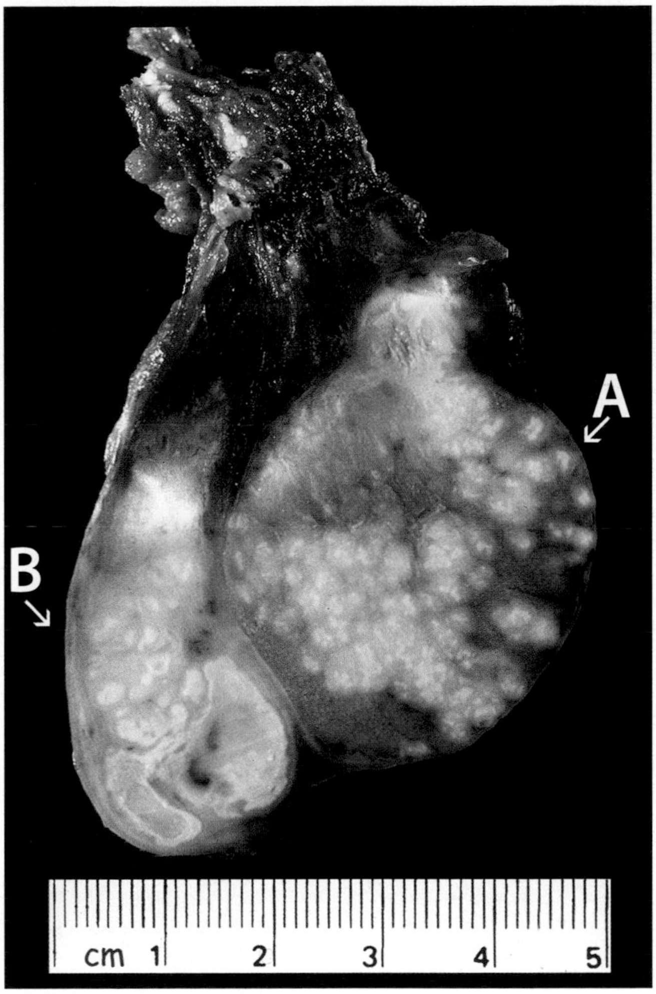

▶ **Fig. 3.54** Testis and epididymis from a male, aged 42 years, from Papua New Guinea. He had a mass in the scrotum, which was thought to be a tumor. The body of the testis (A) is extensively replaced with a cream-colored mass of tissue. The epididymis (B) is extensively replaced by a similar type of infiltrate. This is tuberculous granulation tissue.

Female genital tract and breast

Tuberculosis involves the female genital tract in two main ways.

- Endometrial involvement causes menorrhagia. Granulomas can be seen in secretory phase endometrium. If tuberculosis is suspected, a curettage should be performed late in the secretory phase of the cycle, so as to allow the granulomas time to form. The cyclical shedding of the endometrium means that the granulomas are being continually shed with the endometrium.
- The second site for tuberculosis of the female genital tract to occur is the Fallopian tubes. The Fallopian tubes become obstructed by granulation tissue and this results in sterility. Multiple, small nodules (granulomas) can be seen on the serosal surfaces of the tubes.

The breast may be affected, usually as part of a more widespread infection (illustrated in Fig. 3.55).

▼ **Fig. 3.55** This young woman from Papua New Guinea has pulmonary and disseminated tuberculosis with involvement of the left breast. The tissue wasting is an effect of the TB.

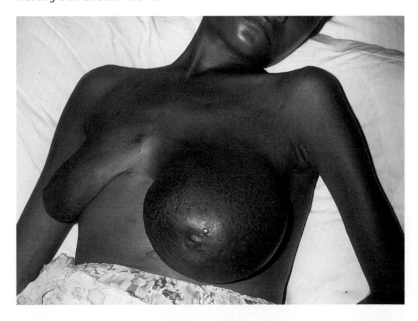

Adrenal gland

Tuberculous granulation tissue may replace virtually the whole of the adrenal gland (see Figs 3.56 and 3.57). This results in Addison's disease—named after Thomas Addison (1793–1860), the British physician. As the adrenal hormonal secretions are reduced by this infiltration, the patient's skin becomes a dark brown to black color.

Some of Thomas Addison's original cases were caused by tuberculous replacement of the adrenal gland. These cases can be seen in the Gordon Museum in Guy's Hospital, London. They look just like the case illustrated here, where a male aged 49 years presented a month before death with an acute onset of adrenal insufficiency.

▶ **Fig. 3.56(a) and (b)** The tuberculous cause of this case was not diagnosed prior to death. Both adrenal glands are extensively replaced with white material, which on microscopic examination is tuberculous granulation tissue.

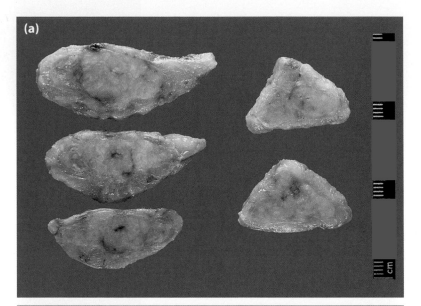

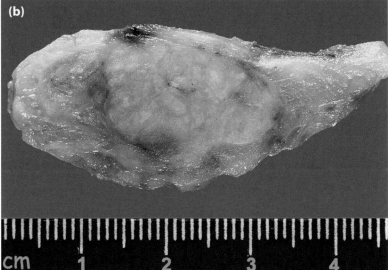

▼ **Fig. 3.57** Whole mount of the microscopic section of the adrenal gland, which confirms the replacement of the adrenal tissue with tuberculous granulation tissue.

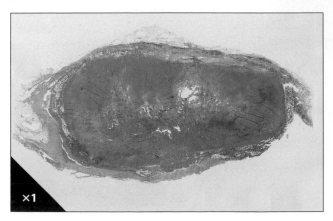

Heart

The myocardium may be involved in cases of miliary tuberculosis, and then one sees miliary tubercles in the myocardium. Involvement of the serosal surface of the heart results in a pericardial effusion (see Fig. 3.58). Longstanding infection of the pericardium results in adhesion between the two layers of pericardium and, ultimately, fibrosis. As occurs with longstanding tuberculosis in the lungs and elsewhere, calcification occurs in the pericardium. The clinical consequence of this is constrictive pericarditis (shown in Fig. 3.59).

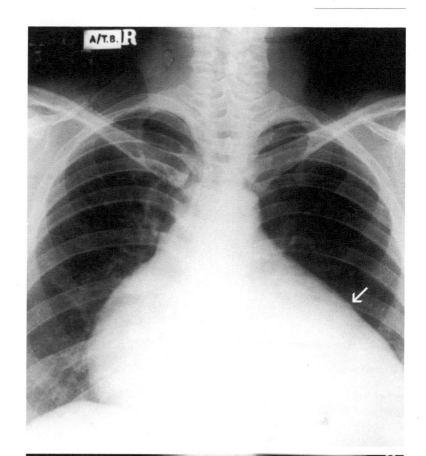

▶ **Fig. 3.58** Chest X-ray of a patient with tuberculous pericarditis causing a pericardial effusion and cardiac tamponade.

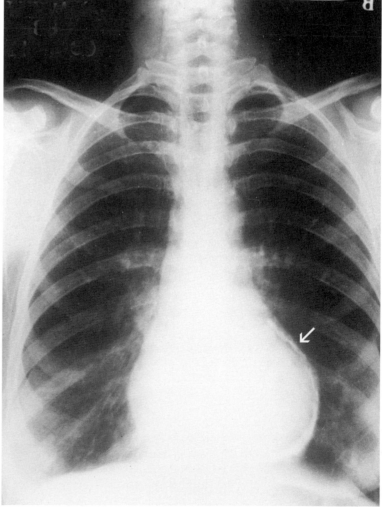

▶ **Fig. 3.59** Chest X-ray showing constrictive pericarditis with calcification caused by tuberculosis. Pericardiectomy in patients like this is effective in relieving the symptoms of constriction.

Skin—lupus vulgaris

Tuberculosis may involve the skin—lupus vulgaris, as illustrated in Figures 3.60 and 3.61.

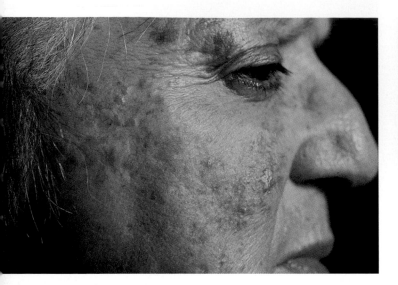

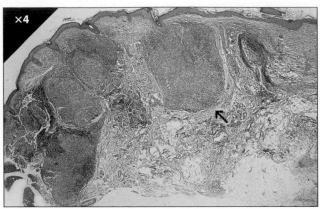

▲ **Fig. 3.61** Skin biopsy showing granulomas in the dermis.

▲ **Fig. 3.60** This 64-year-old female had a rash on the right side of her face. Biopsy showed a granulomatous reaction in the dermis, and culture of the biopsy was positive for tuberculosis.

Historical overview

Robert Koch (1843–1910) (depicted in Fig. 3.62) was the microbiologist who identified the acid-fast bacillus *Mycobacterium tuberculosis*. A small museum in the Institute of Bacteriology, University of Berlin, Germany, commemorates his work (see Figs 3.63, 3.64 and 3.65).

The anatomic pathologist Rudolph Virchow (1821–1902) worked at the Charité Hospital, Berlin, at the same time as Robert Koch. There are a number of specimens of tuberculosis affecting various organs displayed in the Virchow Museum in the Institute of Pathology at the University of Berlin (see Fig. 3.66).

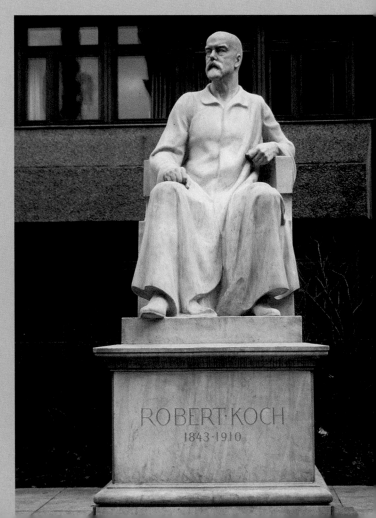

▶ **Fig. 3.62** Monument at the entrance to the Charité Hospital in Berlin, commemorating Robert Koch (1843–1910), the microbiologist who identified the acid-fast bacillus *M. tuberculosis*. He worked in the Charité Hospital in Berlin at the same time as the anatomic pathologist Rudolph Virchow.

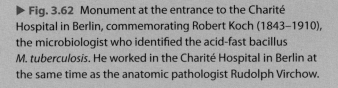

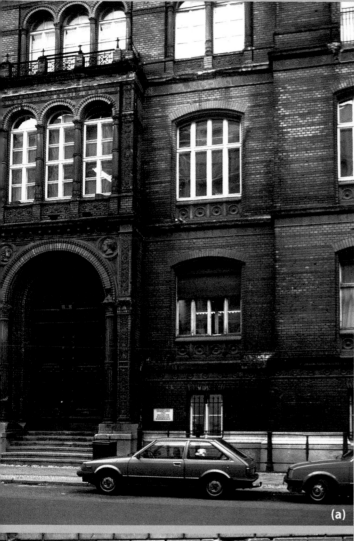

▼ **Fig. 3.63(a) and (b)** Entrance to the Institute of Bacteriology, University of Berlin, where Koch worked.

(a)

(b)

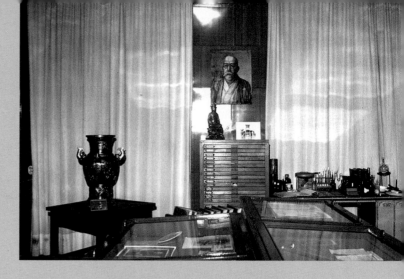

▲ **Fig. 3.64** Institute of Bacteriology, University of Berlin. A small museum commemorates the work of Robert Koch. The museum contains some of the awards given to him by heads of state in a number of countries, including China and Japan. It also contains some of the instruments he used.

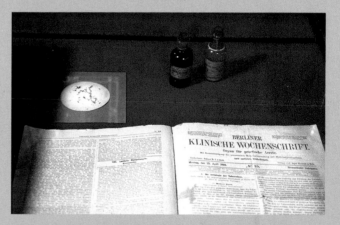

▲ **Fig. 3.65** Robert Koch's first report of the finding of the acid-fast bacillus of *M. tuberculosis,* bottles of stain, and a micro photograph of the acid-fast bacilli.

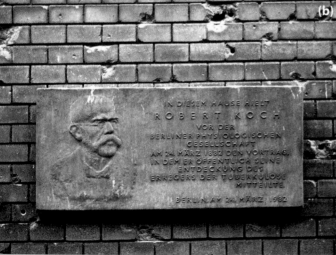

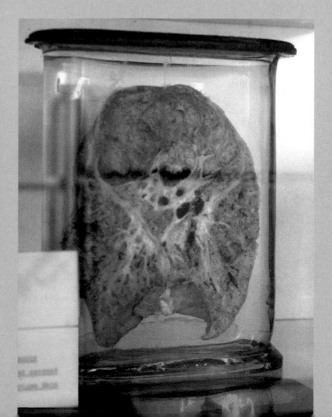

▶ **Fig. 3.66** Specimen of pulmonary tuberculosis in the Virchow Museum, dating from the time when Robert Koch was making his discoveries.

Acknowledgments

- Fig. 3.2 From Cooke, R.A. and Stewart, B., *Colour Atlas of Anatomical Pathology*, third edn, Churchill Livingstone, Edinburgh, 2004.
- Fig. 3.7 From Cooke, R.A. and Stewart, B., *Colour Atlas of Anatomical Pathology*, third edn, Churchill Livingstone, Edinburgh, 2004.
- Fig. 3.18 Photograph provided courtesy of Victor Harrison, London, England.
- Fig. 3.23 Courtesy of John Rendle Short, Brisbane, Australia.
- Fig 3.29(b) Cooke, R.A. and Stewart, B., *Colour Atlas of Anatomical Pathology*, third edn, Churchill Livingstone, Edinburgh, 2004.
- Fig. 3.33 Photograph provided courtesy of Victor Harrison, London, England.
- Fig. 3.35 Courtesy of Geoffrey Bourke, Brisbane, Australia.
- Fig. 3.38 Photograph provided courtesy of the Curator, St Bartholomew's Hospital, London.
- Fig. 3.39(b) Cooke, R.A. and Stewart, B., *Colour Atlas of Anatomical Pathology*, third edn, Churchill Livingstone, Edinburgh, 2004.
- Fig. 3.42 Cooke, R.A. and Stewart, B., *Colour Atlas of Anatomical Pathology*, third edn, Churchill Livingstone, Edinburgh, 2004.
- Fig. 3.47 Cooke, R.A. and Stewart, B., *Colour Atlas of Anatomical Pathology*, third edn, Churchill Livingstone, Edinburgh, 2004.
- Fig. 3.54 From Cooke, R.A. and Stewart, B., *Colour Atlas of Anatomical Pathology*, third edn, Churchill Livingstone, Edinburgh, 2004.
- Fig. 3.55 Courtesy of Kamal SenGupta, Adelaide, Australia.
- Fig. 3.58 Courtesy of Stan Wigley, Papua New Guinea and Sydney, Australia.
- Fig. 3.59 Courtesy of Stan Wigley, Papua New Guinea and Sydney, Australia.
- Fig. 3.60 Courtesy of Graeme Beardmore, Brisbane, Australia.
- Fig. 3.65 Photographs provided courtesy of the Curator, Robert Koch Museum, Berlin, Germany.
- Fig. 3.66 Photograph provided courtesy of the Curator, Virchow Museum, Berlin, Germany.

Leprosy

Leprosy is a disease caused by infection with the acid-fast bacillus *Mycobacterium leprae*. The *M. leprae* is genetically so similar to the *M. tuberculosis* that it is suggested they may be derived from a common ancestor organism. A person with multibacillary disease may transmit the organisms to a genetically and immunologically susceptible person by droplet aerosol dissemination or by contact.

The organism first attacks nerves, and the most prominent clinical features are skin lesions (changes in texture and color) and enlargement of nerves, particularly the greater auriculars, the ulnars and the lateral popliteals (see Fig. 4.1). The nerves are thickened because they have been infiltrated by inflammatory cells. This causes destruction of the nerve fibers and replacement by fibrous tissue (shown in Figs 4.2 and 4.3, overleaf).

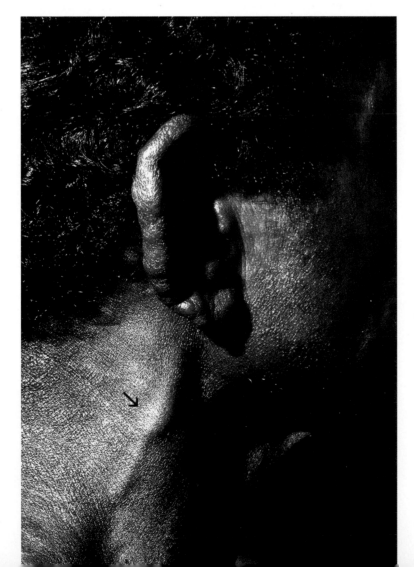

◄ **Fig. 4.1** Advanced lepromatous leprosy. This patient has multiple nodules in his ear and the greater auricular nerve is markedly thickened.

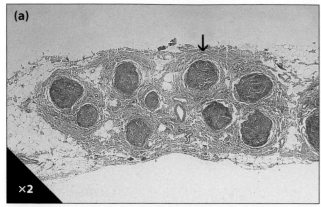

×2

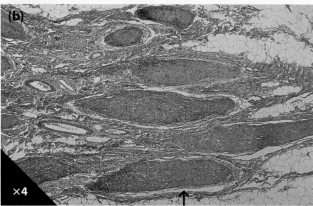

×4

▲ **Fig. 4.2(a) and (b)** Transverse and longitudinal sections of a thickened nerve. The nerve fibers have been destroyed and replaced by fibrous tissue.

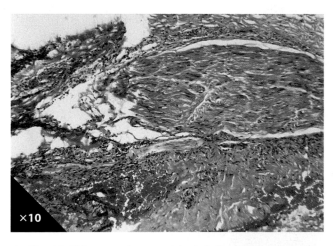

×10

▲ **Fig. 4.3** This nerve shows a chronic inflammatory cell infiltration as well as fibrosis.

There is usually a rash, which affects any or all parts of the body. It is usually erythematous, a feature that is not easily seen in black skins. There are depigmented areas, too, and these are more easily seen in black skins. The depigmented areas in particular are usually insensitive to light touch. Intradermal nodules are a feature of lepromatous leprosy. They are most easily palpated along the supraorbital ridges, on the face and in the ear (especially in the ear lobes).

Clinical examination of a patient suspected of having leprosy

Experienced leprosy physicians examine patients from the front. The examination procedure is as follows.

- Look for a skin rash and for depigmented areas.
- Look for loss of eyebrows.
- Feel for nodules along the supraorbital ridges and in the ear lobes.
- Test for any weakness of the facial nerves.
- Feel with both hands for the presence of thickened nerves—greater auriculars, ulnars and lateral popliteals.
- Turn the patient around and examine the back, especially the buttocks, because any rash may be more visible on the buttocks.
- Test suspect areas for loss of sensation with a piece of cotton wool.
- Test for motor function of the hands and feet.

Laboratory investigations

Some leprologists use a smear test for looking for acid-fast bacilli. This is done by making a small, superficial incision in the skin at the site of a suspect lesion and smearing the fluid from this onto a glass microscope slide and then staining this with a Wade Fite stain (a modified Ziehl Neelsen (ZN) stain).

The main laboratory test in the diagnosis of leprosy is a skin biopsy. If placed in formalin, a biopsy from the edge of a lesion (to include lesion and normal skin) can be mailed to a pathology laboratory anywhere in the world for a report by a qualified pathologist.

A polymerase chain reaction (PCR) test is now available as well.

Historical overview

The polyneuritis caused by inflammatory reaction results in loss of all modalities of nerve function—importantly in the hands and feet. There is loss of pain sensation, loss of motor function and loss of autonomic function. Claw hands commonly result (see Fig. 4.4).

Hand function then becomes awkward. The fingers grip more strongly than a normal hand would, causing trauma to the insensitive skin, resulting in ulceration (shown in Figs 4.5 and 4.6). Infection follows, with extension to bone. The low-grade osteomyelitis results in loss of the bone, and the digits are slowly absorbed and 'disappear' (or, in lay terms, 'fall off'). A similar mechanism results in ulceration of the toes and feet with, ultimately, loss of the feet. This is seen especially in people who do not wear protective footwear. See Figures 4.7 and 4.8 overleaf.

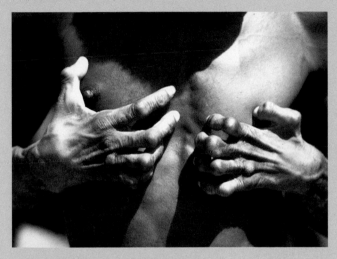

▲ **Fig. 4.4** Both hands show the features of 'claw hand'. Note the wasting of the interosseous muscles.

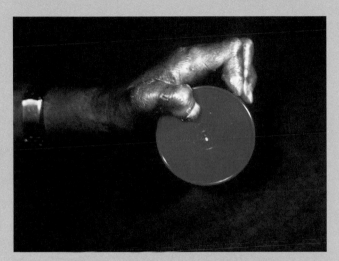

▲ **Fig. 4.5** Damaged hand of a patient with leprosy, illustrating the abnormal grip that causes damage to the tips of anesthetic fingers.

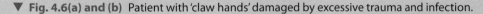

▼ **Fig. 4.6(a) and (b)** Patient with 'claw hands' damaged by excessive trauma and infection.

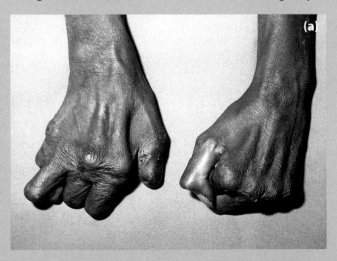

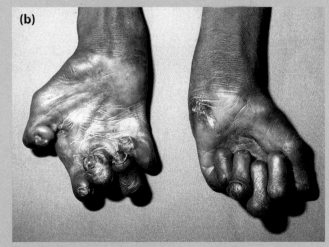

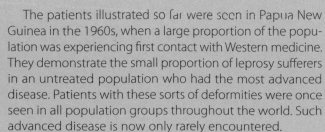

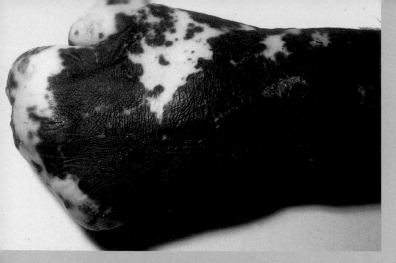

▲ **Fig. 4.7** Hand of a patient who had leprosy before effective drug treatment became available. All of the fingers have disappeared.

The patients illustrated so far were seen in Papua New Guinea in the 1960s, when a large proportion of the population was experiencing first contact with Western medicine. They demonstrate the small proportion of leprosy sufferers in an untreated population who had the most advanced disease. Patients with these sorts of deformities were once seen in all population groups throughout the world. Such advanced disease is now only rarely encountered.

Understanding the underlying pathology of the disease has allowed health professionals to educate patients in the proper care of anesthetic hands and feet. Relatively simple measures can result in improvement of established deformities, and prevention of further damage (as shown in Fig. 4.9).

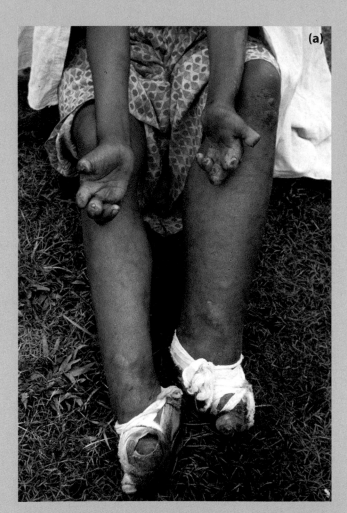

(a)

◄ ▼ **Fig. 4.8(a) and (b)** These patients, who had advanced leprosy before the introduction of effective treatment, show the results of trauma to anesthetic hands and feet.

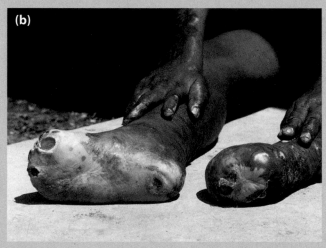

(b)

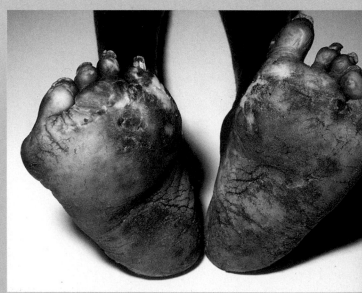

▶ **Fig. 4.9** The ulcers on this patient's anesthetic feet have been healed by a combination of specific therapy for the leprosy, daily treatment of the ulcers, and prevention of further trauma by the wearing of protective footwear.

Contribution by D.C. Danielssen and Armauer Hansen to leprosy research

The Norwegian physician D.C. Danielssen (1815–1894) described the clinical features of leprosy in 1848. His son-in-law Armauer Hansen (1841–1912), reported finding acid-fast organisms in the nodular lesions of leprosy in 1874, and correctly postulated that it was an infectious disease.

Danielssen and Hansen worked in the busy port city of Bergen in Norway. Sailors had a significant incidence of leprosy and the disease was also fairly common among the farmers, whose tiny farms still cling to the steep cliffs of the Norwegian fiords. The old port buildings in Bergen are preserved, and the leprosy hospital where Hansen worked is in a nearby street (see Figs 4.10–4.14, continued overleaf).

▼ **Fig. 4.10** Old port buildings in Bergen, Norway. The Norwegian physician Danielssen, who described the clinical features of leprosy in 1848, worked in Bergen with Armauer Hansen.

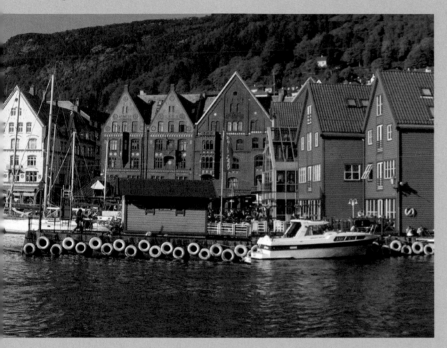

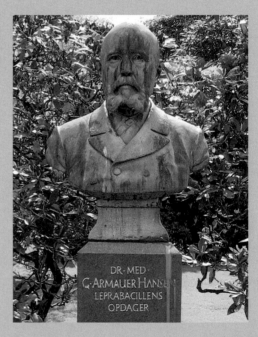

▲ **Fig. 4.11** Bust of Armauer Hansen (1841–1912), on his grave in Bergen, Norway.

◀ **Fig. 4.12** The hospital in which Hansen worked has been renovated and is situated to the right behind this church in Bergen, Norway.

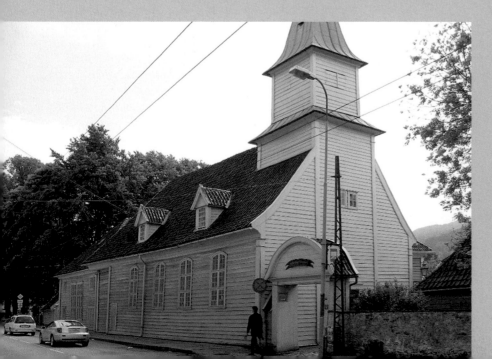

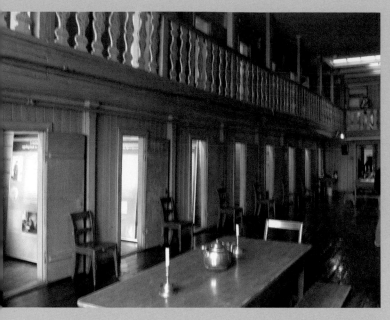

▲ **Fig. 4.13** Interior of the hospital in which Hansen worked.

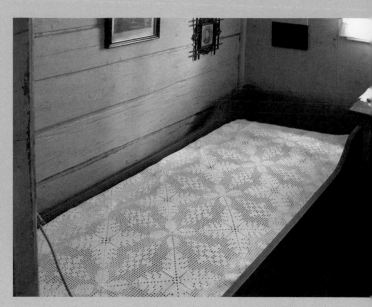

▲ **Fig. 4.14** Cubicle in the ward in which Hansen worked. Often there were three patients in each cubicle.

The diagnosis of leprosy depends on a clinicopathologic correlation. In the 150 years since Danielssen's first description of the disease, its clinicopathologic correlations have been refined, standardized and agreed upon internationally.

Classification of leprosy

There are two polar types of leprosy—lepromatous leprosy and tuberculoid leprosy. The clinical features of these two types are fairly distinct. Immunologically, they appear to be distinct, and the microscopic appearances of skin biopsies are distinct for each polar type.

- In lepromatous leprosy, there are numerous acid-fast bacilli (multibacillary disease), and the body has a poor or nonexistent T-cell immune response. Hence, the inflammatory reaction consists of numerous histiocytes filled with acid-fast bacilli and few lymphocytes.
- In tuberculoid leprosy, there are few or no acid-fast bacilli (pauci bacillary disease), and the body mounts a strong, granulomatous inflammatory response to the infection. There are epithelioid cell granulomas (lepromas), with multinucleated giant cells and large numbers of lymphocytes.

The majority of patients fall between these two extremes, and show a mixture of clinical and pathologic features of both polar types. These patients are classified as having borderline leprosy. They are further classified as having borderline tending toward lepromatous or tuberculoid types of leprosy.

The short forms for these classification terms are: LL (lepromatous leprosy), BL (borderline lepromatous leprosy), BB (borderline borderline), BT (borderline tuberculoid), TT (tuberculoid).

Lepromatous leprosy

Clinical features

Patients with well-established disease have an erythematous rash. There are intradermal nodules and thickened nerves. The outer halves of the eyebrows are lost. The nasal septum may collapse. Clinical appearances differ slightly depending on the amount of racial pigmentation present (illustrated in Figs 4.15, 4.16 and 4.17).

▼ ▶ **Figs 4.15, 4.16 and 4.17** Lepromatous leprosy in three patients of different racial origins with different amounts of skin pigmentation. The patient shown in Figure 4.17 has a collapsed nasal septum.

◀ **Fig. 4.15**

▼ **Fig. 4.16(a) and (b)**

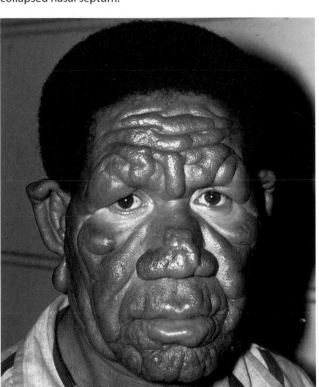

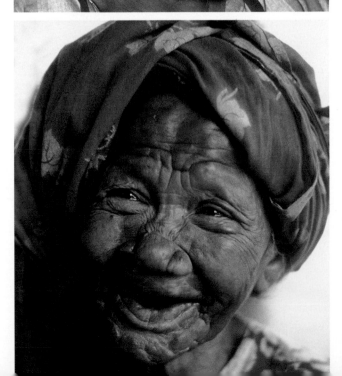

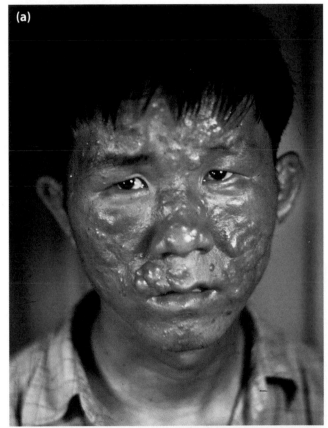

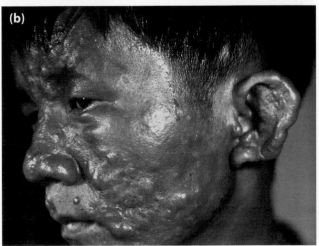

◀ **Fig. 4.17**

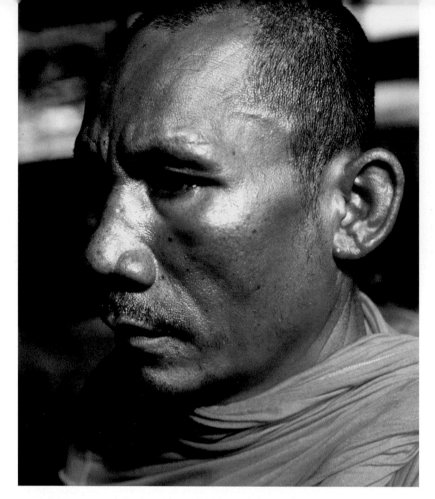

A medically interesting and sometimes confusing presentation is the diffuse type of rash that may be seen in lepromatous leprosy. Again, note the difference in appearance in the two different skin tones (shown in Figs 4.18 and 4.19).

▲ **Fig. 4.18** Lepromatous leprosy. A reddish, diffuse type of rash in an Asian patient.

▼ **Fig. 4.19(a) and (b)** Lepromatous leprosy. A reddish diffuse type of rash in a white Caucasian.

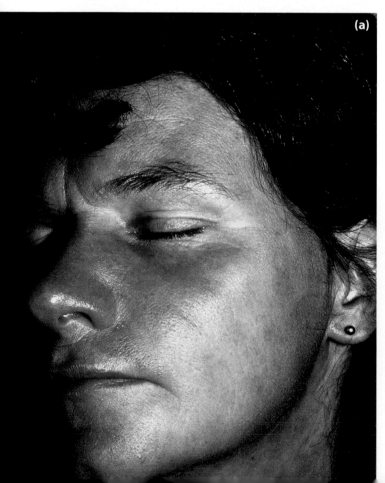

(a)

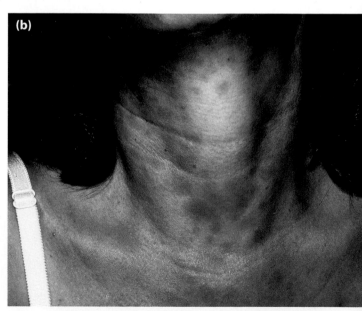

(b)

Histologic features in a skin biopsy—lepromatous leprosy

Scanning magnification examination shows an inflammatory infiltrate throughout the dermis. The reaction consists of pale-staining histiocytes, with no multinucleated giant cells. There are variable numbers of lymphocytes in the inflammatory infiltrate, but they are rather sparse. There is a clear, uninvolved zone in the upper dermis between the basal layer of the epidermis and the inflammatory infiltrate. Cutaneous nerves associated with the skin appendages are not destroyed. Large numbers of acid fast bacilli can be seen in the cytoplasm of the histiocytes. Sometimes, there are solid clusters of bacilli in the intercellular connective tissue. These clusters are sometimes called globi (see Figs 4.20–4.24, continued overleaf).

▼ **Fig. 4.20(a), (b) and (c)** Lepromatous leprosy. There is an inflammatory infiltrate throughout the dermis.

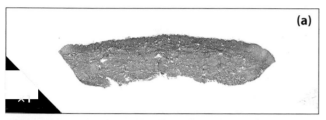

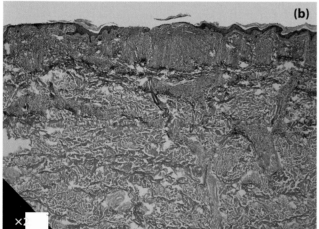

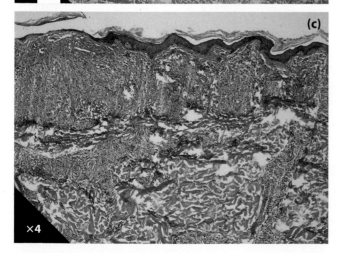

▼ **Fig. 4.21(a) and (b)** There is a clear, uninvolved zone (a gren zone) between the basal layer of the epidermis and the inflammatory infiltrate.

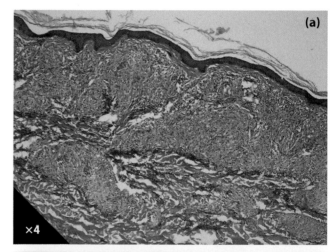

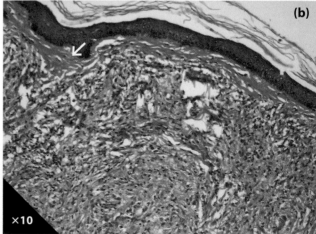

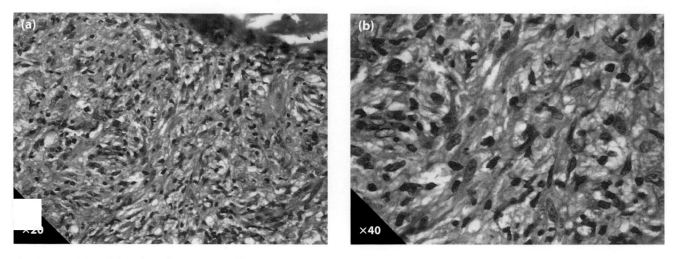

▲ **Fig. 4.22(a) and (b)** The inflammatory infiltrate consists of histiocytes with foamy cytoplasm, and variable numbers of lymphocytes and plasma cells.

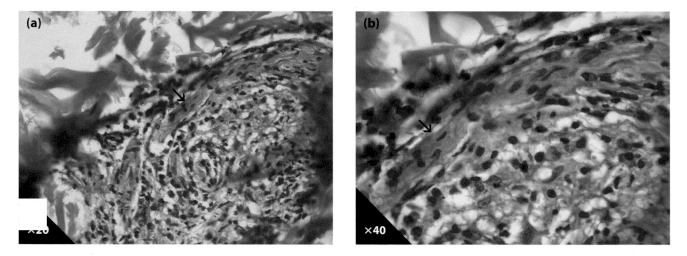

▲ **Fig. 4.23(a) and (b)** Cutaneous nerves associated with skin appendages are not destroyed.

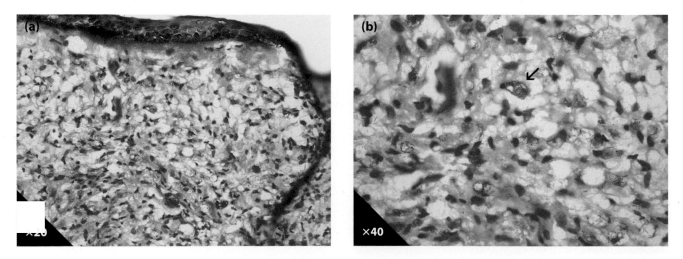

▲ **Fig. 4.24(a) and (b)** Wade Fite stain (a ZN stain modified to stain *M. leprae* organisms) showing the presence of large numbers of acid-fast bacilli in the cytoplasm of the histiocytes. In **(b)** there are a few solid clusters of bacilli (globi).

Tuberculoid leprosy

Clinical features

In pure tuberculoid leprosy, there is only one large area of depigmented skin, but the current World Health Organization (WHO) classification allows up to five lesions before calling it borderline tuberculoid. The depigmented area is anesthetic to light touch. Often, a thick cutaneous nerve can be seen, or felt, supplying the area. Other nerves—particularly the greater auriculars, ulnars and lateral popliteals—are also enlarged. This condition is demonstrated in Figures 4.25–4.28.

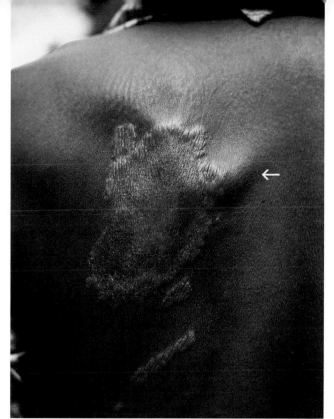

▲ **Fig. 4.27** Tuberculoid leprosy. A thickened cutaneous nerve is clearly visible going towards the area of depigmentation.

▼ **Fig. 4.28** Predominantly tuberculoid leprosy. This young woman has a number of depigmented areas on her face, with a large one on her left cheek and another on her left upper arm. Smaller lesions are present on her chest.

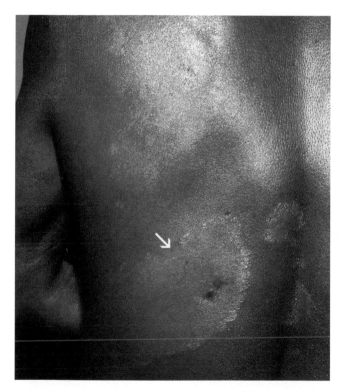

▲ **Fig. 4.25** Predominantly tuberculoid leprosy. A large depigmented, anesthetic area of skin in the left loin. A few smaller lesions are also visible.

▼ **Fig. 4.26** Biopsy has been taken from near the center of this lesion. It has not been taken from the best place. The best site from which to take a biopsy of any skin lesion is from the growing edge to include normal and abnormal skin. Healing has usually started in the center and the diagnostic features have been lost.

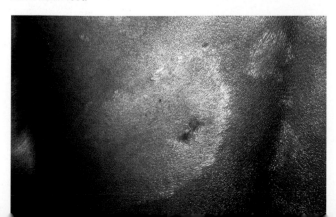

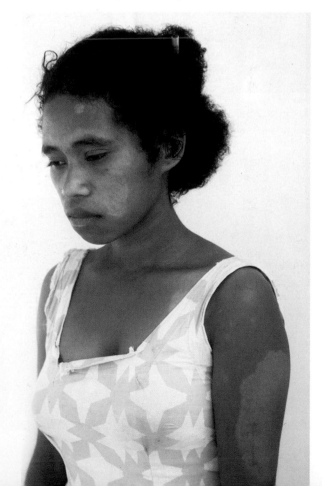

Histologic features in a skin biopsy—tuberculoid leprosy

Scanning magnification examination shows granulomatous inflammatory infiltrates throughout the dermis. In the inflammatory reaction, epithelioid cells and multinucleated giant cells are prominent. The reaction extends right to the base of the epidermis. The inflammatory reaction occurs around skin appendages and the cutaneous nerves are destroyed. There are variable numbers of lymphocytes in the inflammatory reaction and no acid-fast bacilli can be seen (as illustrated in Figs 4.29–4.33).

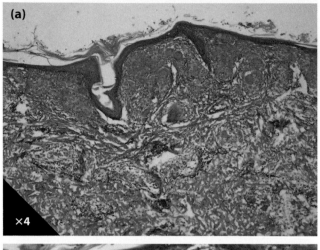

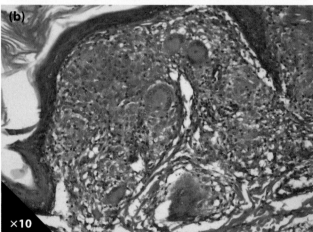

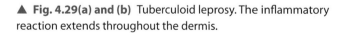
▲ **Fig. 4.29(a) and (b)** Tuberculoid leprosy. The inflammatory reaction extends throughout the dermis.

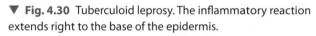
▼ **Fig. 4.30** Tuberculoid leprosy. The inflammatory reaction extends right to the base of the epidermis.

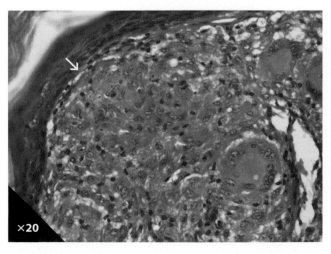

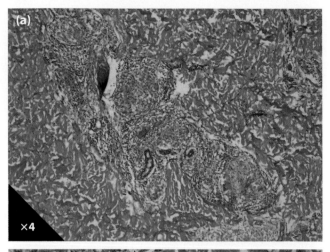

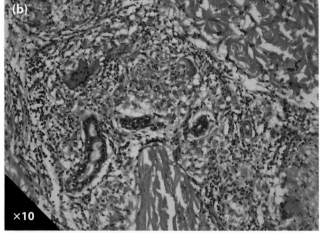

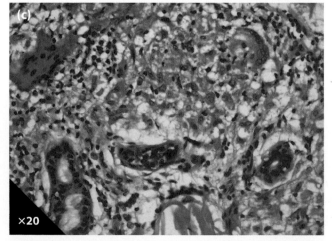

▲ **Fig. 4.31(a), (b) and (c)** The inflammatory reaction around skin appendages in the dermis destroys the cutaneous nerves.

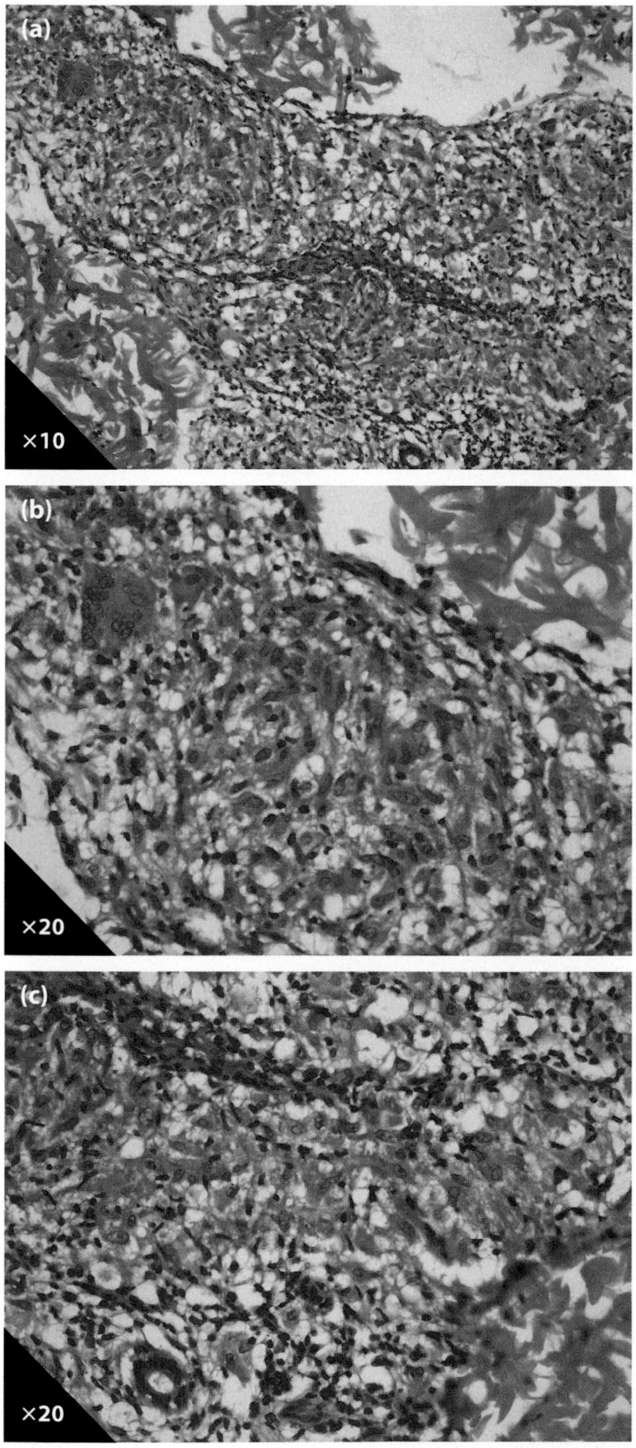

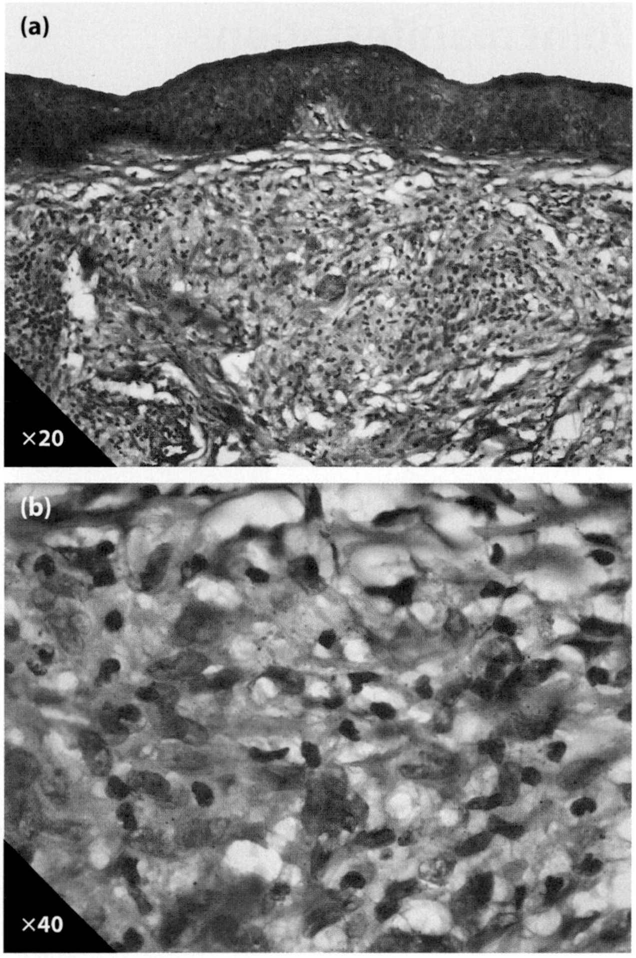

▲ **Fig. 4.33(a) and (b)** No acid-fast bacilli can be seen in a Wade Fite stain.

▲ **Fig. 4.32(a), (b) and (c)** Further illustrations of the inflammatory reaction with destruction of cutaneous nerves.

Joint manifestations

Joint manifestations are illustrated here in two patients: a teenage, male immigrant to Australia; and a 10-year-old Papua New Guinean schoolboy.

- A teenage male, who was a recent immigrant, presented at a hospital in Brisbane, Australia, with acute dactylitis (see Fig. 4.34). His left ulnar nerve was markedly enlarged. This condition is illustrated in another patient shown in Figure 4.35.
- A 10-year-old Papua New Guinean schoolboy had been diagnosed as having borderline lepromatous leprosy. He was suffering a reaction in which his rash had become edematous. He had periorbital edema, and he had developed a painful dactylitis (see Fig. 4.36).

▶ **Fig. 4.34** Acute dactylitis involving the left little finger of a teenage male.

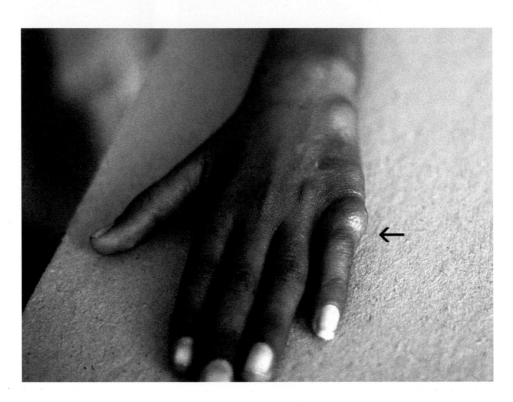

▼ **Fig. 4.35 (a) and (b)** Acute dactylitis. This patient had marked enlargement of his left ulnar nerve.

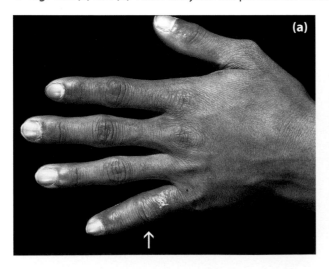

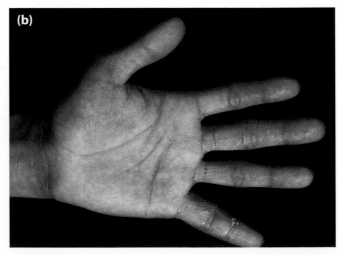

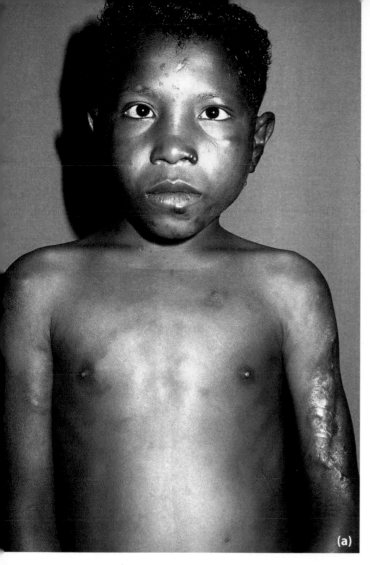

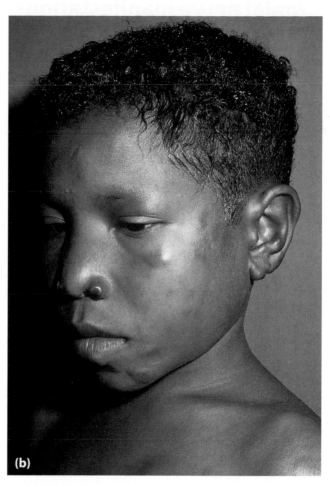

▲ Fig. 4.36(a) and (b) Typical features of lepromatous leprosy. This 10-year-old boy has lost the outer half of each eyebrow. He has a number of nodules on his face. His ears, particularly his ear lobes, show the presence of a number of nodules.

▼ Fig. 4.36(c) Both hands are swollen and all the interphalangeal joints are swollen, stiff and painful.

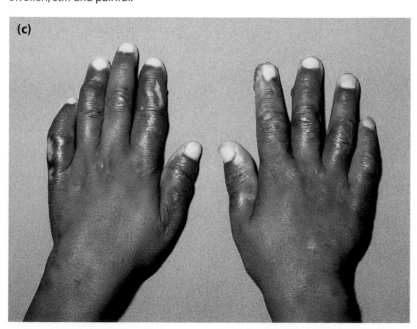

Cranial nerve manifestations

Cranial nerve manifestations present as ptosis of the eyelids from facial nerve palsy. This condition is often bilateral (see Fig. 4.37).

Eye manifestations

Eye manifestations present as iritis, cataract and scleritis. These conditions are illustrated in Figures 4.38, 4.39 and 4.40.

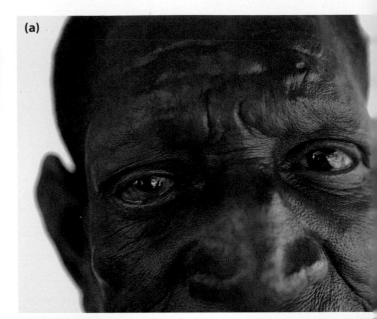

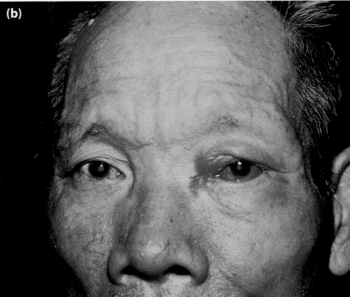

▲ **Fig. 4.38(a) and (b)** Acute iritis.

▲ **Fig. 4.37** Bilateral ptosis. The facial nerve is the cranial nerve most frequently involved and this is often bilateral.

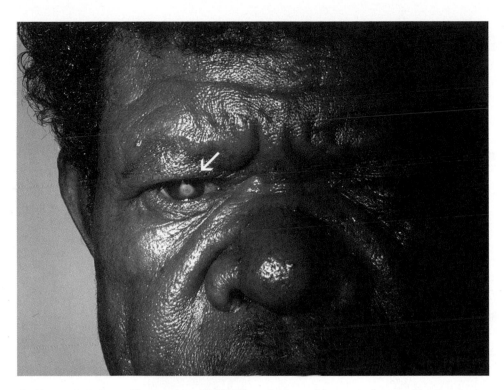

▲ **Fig. 4.39** Cataract. The pupil is white because the lens of the eye is damaged by the inflammatory reaction and has become opaque.

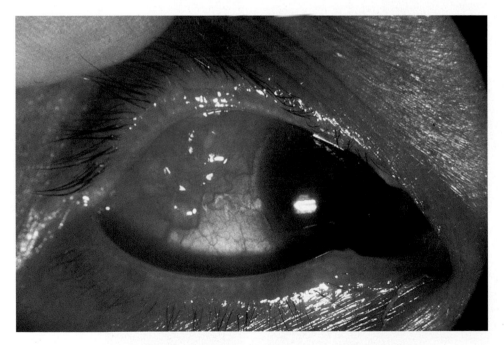

▲ **Fig. 4.40** Granulomas (lepromas) full of organisms may form on the sclerotic.

Pathologic changes in nerves

In tuberculoid leprosy, there is a granulomatous infiltration, sometimes with areas of necrosis. No organisms are seen (see Figs 4.41 and 4.42).

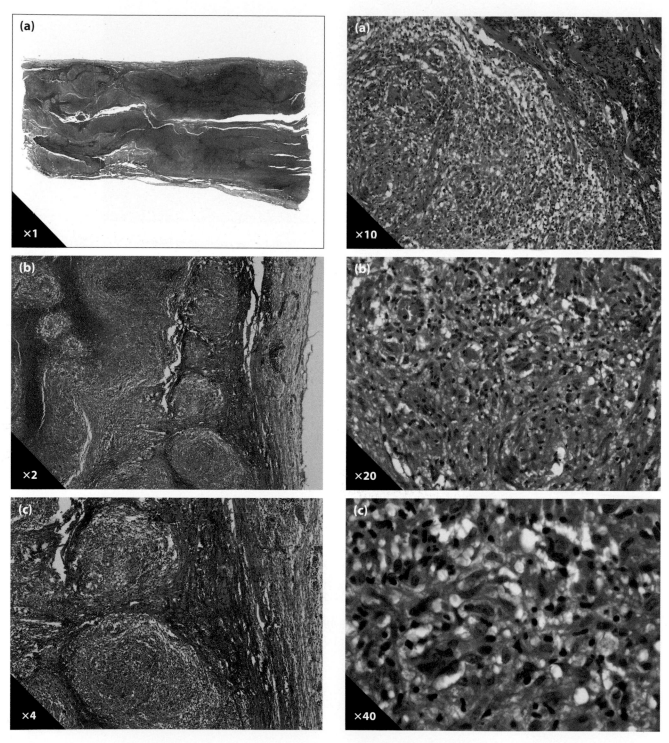

▲ **Fig. 4.41(a), (b) and (c)** Tuberculoid leprosy. A longitudinal section of an ulnar nerve, greatly enlarged by a granulomatous-type inflammatory reaction. Areas of necrosis can be seen. The nerve fibers have almost all been destroyed.

▲ **Fig. 4.42(a), (b) and (c)** Tuberculoid leprosy. Ulnar nerve at higher magnifications. The epithelioid cells, multinucleated giant cells and lymphocytes of the inflammatory reaction can be seen. No acid-fast bacilli were present.

In lepromatous leprosy, the inflammatory infiltrate consists of histiocytes filled with acid-fast bacilli (see Fig. 4.43).

In both forms of leprosy, the inflammatory reaction in the nerves ultimately subsides and a fibrosed nerve is all that remains (shown in Figs 4.44, 4.45 and 4.46, continued overleaf).

Acute painful enlargement of nerves may occur during leprosy reactions. This needs to be treated with steroids to prevent permanent damage to the nerve. In rare cases in which the nerve pain is not relieved by steroids, and the nerve appears to be 'compressed', it may be moved surgically in an attempt to relieve the pain (see Figs 4.47 and 4.48, overleaf).

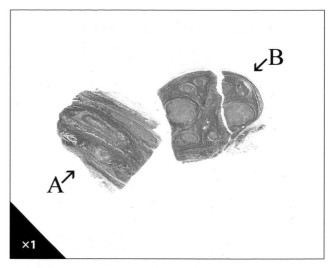

▲ **Fig. 4.44** Longitudinal (A) and transverse (B) section through an enlarged nerve in a patient with longstanding leprosy.

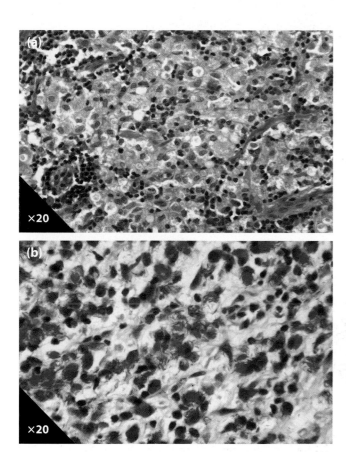

▲ **Fig. 4.43** Lepromatous leprosy. **(a)** The nerve is infiltrated by histiocytes with clear cytoplasm. **(b)** Wade Fite stain shows that the cytoplasm of the cells is filled with acid-fast bacilli. Variable numbers of lymphocytes are present as well.

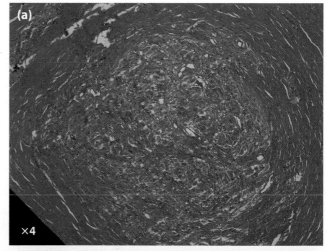

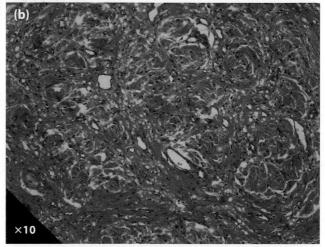

▲ **Fig. 4.45(a) and (b)** In the late stages of both forms of leprosy, the nerves are extensively destroyed and replaced by fibrous tissue.

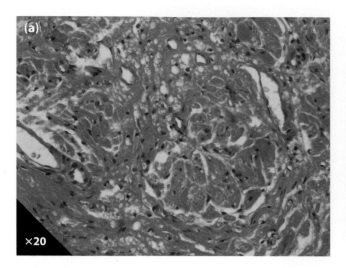
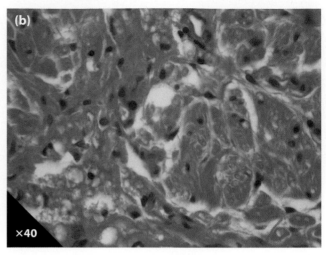

▲ **Fig. 4.46(a) and (b)** Acute painful enlargement of nerves. A few nerve fibers survive after inflammatory reaction in the nerves subsides. This represents 'end stage' disease with virtually no inflammatory cells and no acid-fast bacilli.

▶ **Fig. 4.47** Acute painful enlargement of nerves. 'Nerve abscess' in the left ulnar nerve.

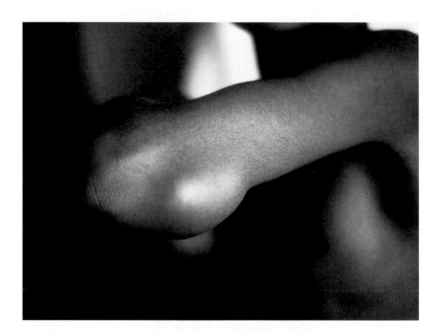

▼ **Fig. 4.48(a) and (b)** Acute painful enlargement of nerves. In this case, the left ulnar nerve has been moved anterior to the medial epicondyle of the humerus in an attempt to relieve the pain.

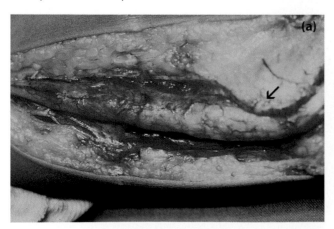
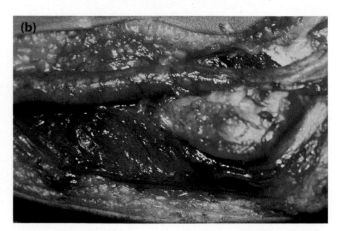

Systemic involvement in leprosy

In lepromatous leprosy, all the organs in the body may be affected. The pathologic changes of this are most easily seen in some organs (for example lymph nodes, spleen and liver).

- Lymph nodes may be enlarged because of an infiltration of pale-staining histiocytes through the sinusoids of the nodes. These histiocytes are full of acid-fast bacilli (see Figs 4.49, 4.50 and 4.51, continued overleaf).
- The spleen may be similarly affected (see Fig. 4.52, overleaf).
- In the liver, collections of foamy histiocytes containing acid-fast bacilli accumulate in the portal tracts (see Figs 4.53, 4.54 and 4.55, overleaf).

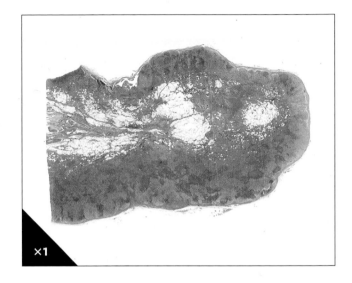

▶ **Fig. 4.49** Lepromatous leprosy. Section of an enlarged lymph node.

▼ **Fig. 4.50(a), (b), (c) and (d)** Lepromatous leprosy. The architecture of the lymph node is retained and there is an extensive infiltration of histiocytes through the sinusoids of the node.

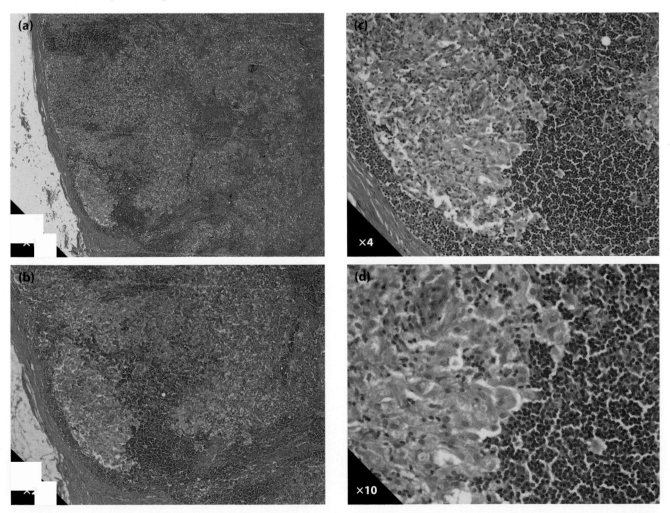

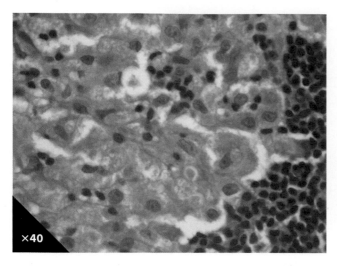

▲ **Fig. 4.51** Lepromatous leprosy. At high magnification the organisms are almost visible in the hematoxylin and eosin (H&E) section. Wade Fite stain was positive.

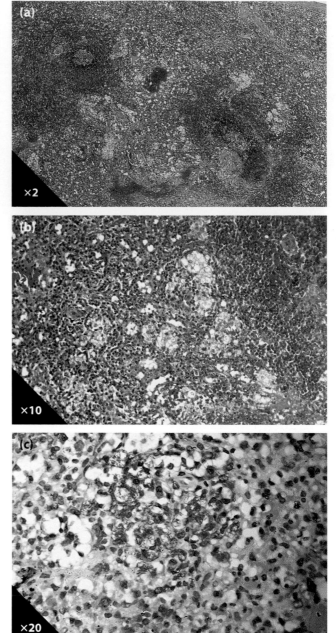

▲ **Fig. 4.52(a), (b) and (c)** Lepromatous leprosy. The spleen shows an infiltration of its sinusoids by histiocytes filled with acid-fast bacilli.

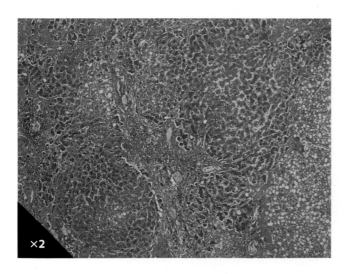

◀ **Fig. 4.53** Lepromatous leprosy. A section of liver showing the presence of cirrhosis. The cirrhosis is not caused by the leprosy.

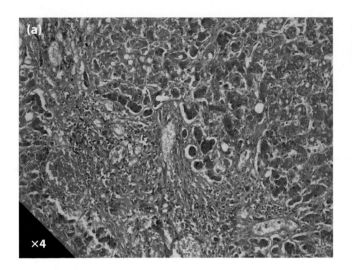

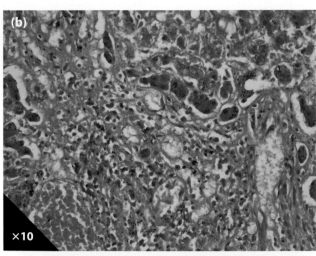

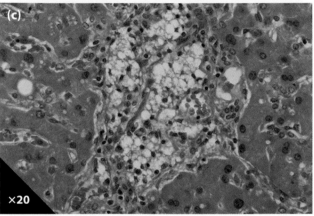

▲ ▶ **Fig. 4.54(a), (b) and (c)** The liver shows portal tracts with accumulations of histiocytes with pale staining cytoplasm.

▶ **Fig. 4.55** Lepromatous leprosy. Wade Fite stain shows the presence of acid-fast bacilli in the histiocytes.

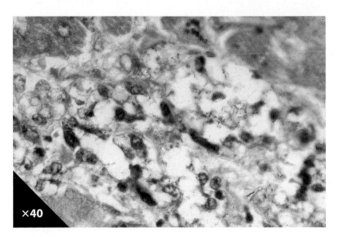

Amyloidosis in leprosy

Lepromatous leprosy can be complicated by disseminated secondary amyloidosis. The prevalence of this complication seems to vary in different population groups. It is very common in Papua New Guinean people, but uncommon in the Chinese. Amyloid can be seen in most organs, but the kidney is particularly affected (see Figs 4.56 and 4.57). Rectal biopsy shows amyloid deposited in the walls of the small blood vessels and this is sometimes used to diagnose the presence of amyloidosis in leprosy patients. This test is easier to perform, but perhaps not so reliable as a renal biopsy.

▼ **Fig. 4.56** Amyloidosis. Almost every glomerulus in this kidney is replaced by amyloid.

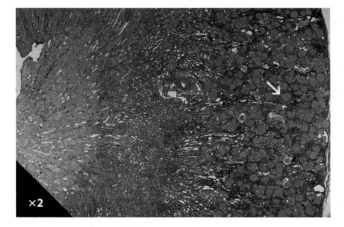

×2

▼ **Fig. 4.57** The amyloid glows with a green birefringence when a congo red stain is examined under polarized light.

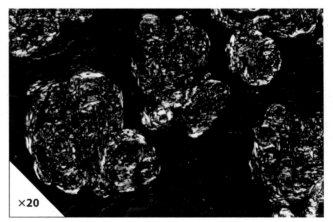

×20

Illustrative case histories

Case 4.1

A 23-year-old postgraduate student from South-East Asia presented to a university medical clinic in Australia for advice about a rash on his face. The clinic doctor noticed some rounded lesions on both cheeks and on the forehead. She noted that the lesions were anesthetic to cotton-wool touch and made a clinical diagnosis of leprosy. She took a skin biopsy, which showed the features of borderline lepromatous leprosy (see Fig. 4.58).

Leprosy is a notifiable disease in Australia. Upon notification, the authorities decided that the student should be repatriated to his home country. 'Not on our airplanes', declared the various airline companies—echoing a widely held community fear of this disease, dating from the Middle Ages. So, the student had 2 years of treatment, finished his course of studies, and cured of his disease, he made his way home without incident.

▼ ▶ **Fig. 4.58(a), (b), (c) and (d)** Borderline lepromatous leprosy in a 23-year-old male from South-East Asia.

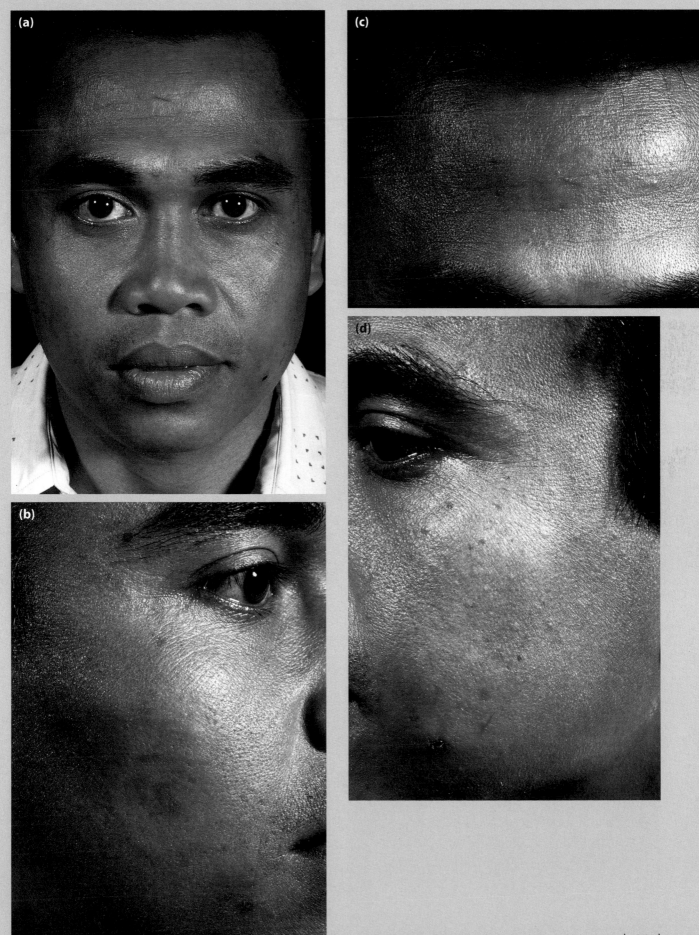

Case 4.2

A 32-year-old woman from India, living temporarily in Brisbane, Australia, presented with a discharging sinus from a lump on the right side of the neck (shown in Fig. 4.59). The clinical diagnosis was 'discharging tuberculous lymph node': this node was excised.

Microscopic examination showed the presence of a nerve abscess in tuberculoid leprosy (see Fig. 4.60). Closer inspection after the pathology report was made showed the presence of a round, anesthetic, depigmented area just below and anterior to her right ear. The patient was treated successfully before she returned home.

▼ **Fig. 4.59(a) and (b)** Tuberculoid leprosy. A 32-year-old woman with a nerve abscess in her right, greater auricular nerve. There was a round, anesthetic, depigmented area just below and anterior to her right ear.

▼ **Fig. 4.60(a), (b) and (c)** Microscopic section of the nerve abscess. No organisms were detected.

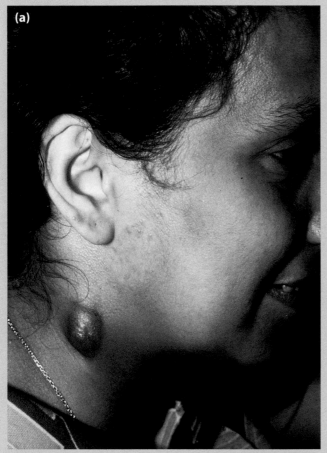

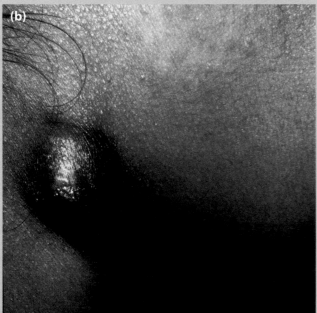

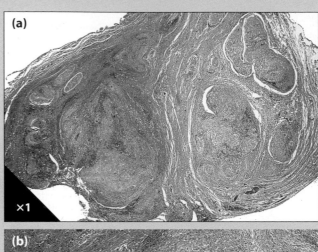

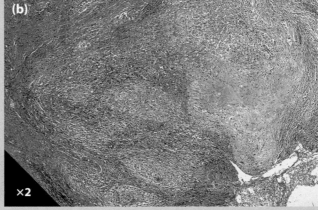

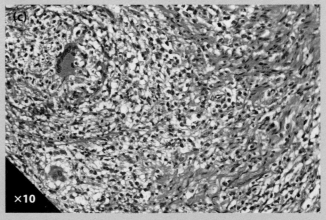

Case 4.3

A 15-year-old Papua New Guinean schoolboy had a rash on his face with a round, red, firm nodule on his chin. This was insensitive to cotton-wool touch. Palpation of his forehead and ear lobes revealed the presence of a number of nodules. He had a round, anesthetic lesion on his left buttock. A diagnosis of leprosy was made and a biopsy of the nodule on his chin showed the features of borderline lepromatous leprosy (see Fig. 4.61).

▼ **Fig. 4.61(a)** Borderline lepromatous leprosy in a 15-year-old male.

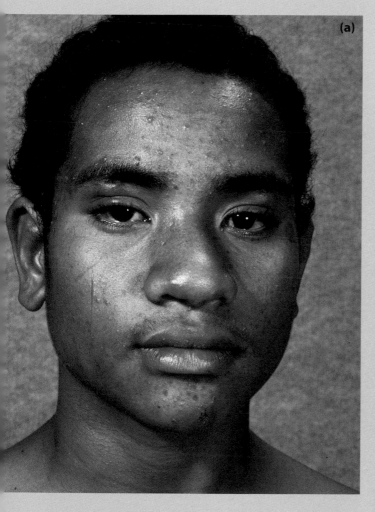

▼ **Fig. 4.61(b)** Examination of the patient's buttocks showed an anesthetic, depigmented area on the left buttock.

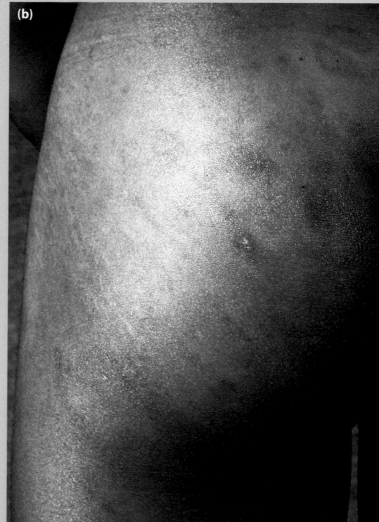

Lepromatous leprosy may present with an inflammatory mass that mimics the clinical features of a neoplasm. Anatomical sites in which this phenomenon occurs with some regularity are the testis and the nasopharynx.

Case 4.4

An orchidectomy was performed on a Papua New Guinean man, aged 25 years, for a clinical diagnosis of testicular neoplasm. The testis was enlarged and felt rubbery.

Microscopic examination showed the presence of a fibrotic mass with many collections of histiocytes containing acid-fast bacilli distributed through it. A diagnosis of leprosy involvement of the testis was made (see Fig. 4.62).

▼ ▶ **Fig. 4.62(a), (b), (c), (d) and (e)** Lepromatous leprosy. Section through a mass in the epididymis. The mass is fibrotic, and through it there are many collections of foamy histiocytes that contain acid-fast bacilli.

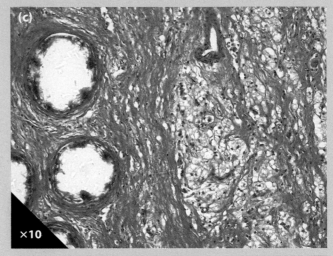

×10

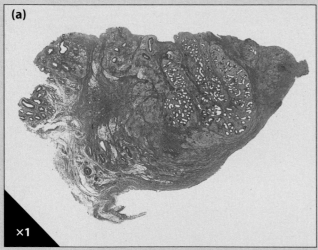

×1

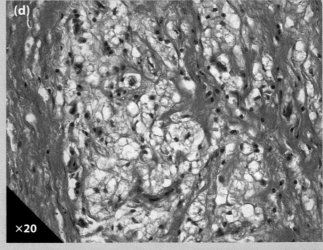

×20

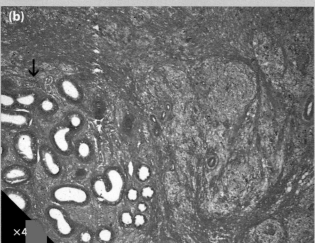

×4

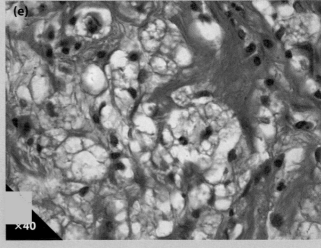

×40

Case 4.5

A 45-year-old man complained of nasal obstruction. He had 'snuffles' for about 2 years. A tumor seen in the left nostril was biopsied.

Microscopically, there was no tumor but an infiltration of histiocytes filled with acid-fast bacilli. A diagnosis of lepromatous leprosy causing a localized tumor was made (see Figs 4.63, 4.64 and 4.65).

A more critical clinical examination (post biopsy) revealed that the patient had lost the outer half of both his eyebrows, and he had a few subcutaneous nodules on his face. His greater auricular, ulnar and lateral popliteal nerves were enlarged. There were pressure-induced ulcers on the tips of all of the fingers of both hands (shown in Figs 4.66 and 4.67, overleaf).

The patient was born in Australia and lived in south-east Queensland. He had never traveled outside the country and had no known contact with another person with leprosy.

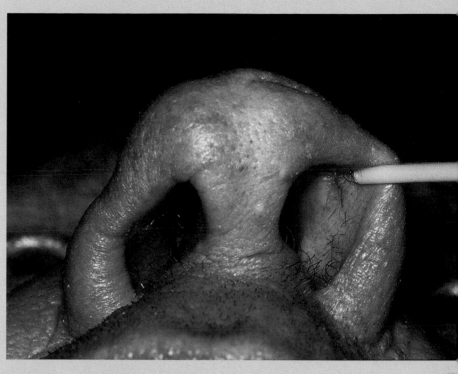

▲ **Fig. 4.63** Lepromatous leprosy. Tumor obstructing the left nostril.

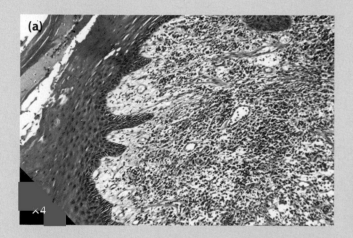
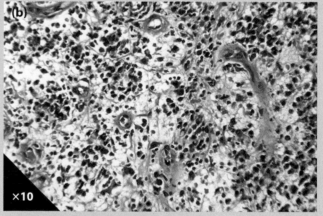

▲ **Fig. 4.64(a) and (b)** Biopsy of the nasal tumor showed an inflammatory mass consisting of lymphocytes, plasma cells and histiocytes.

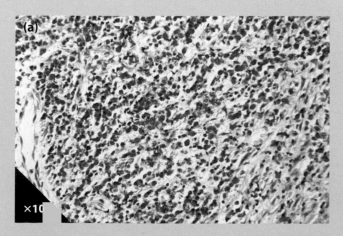
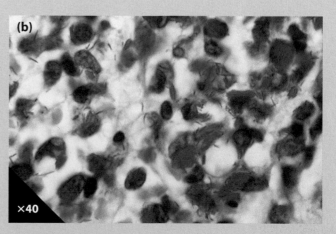

▲ **Fig. 4.65(a) and (b)** Wade Fite stain showed that the histiocytes were full of acid-fast bacilli.

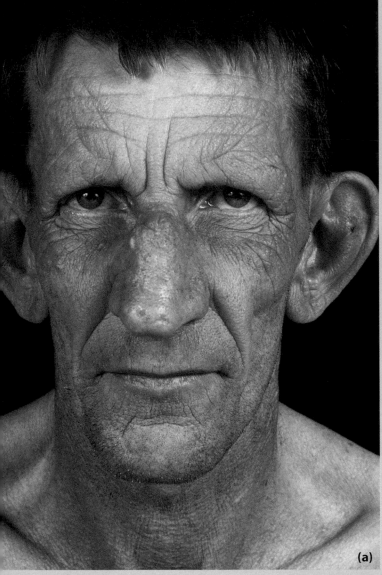

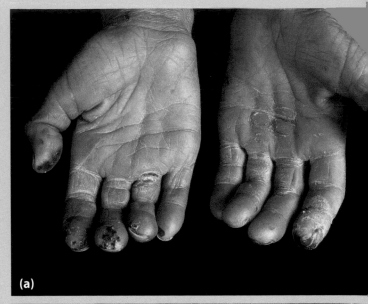

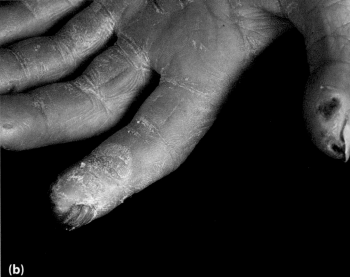

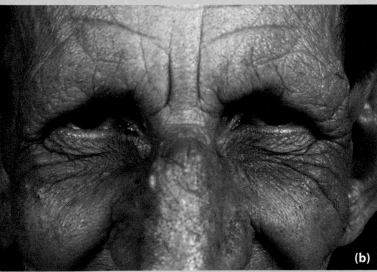

▲ **Fig. 4.66(a) and (b)** Lepromatous leprosy. The patient has lost the outer half of both his eyebrows, and he has a few subcutaneous nodules on his face.

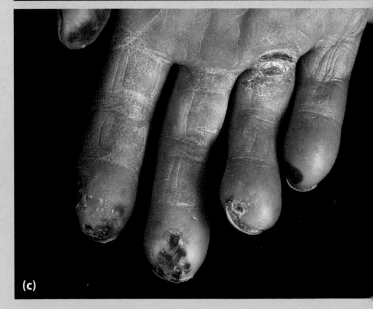

▲ **Fig. 4.67(a), (b) and (c)** Pressure-induced ulcers on the tips of all of the fingers of both of his hands.

Case 4.6

A 40-year-old man, who had immigrated to Australia from Yugoslavia 15 years previously, presented with a right-sided foot drop. He had the signs of a peripheral neuritis and enlargement of the right lateral popliteal nerve. There was an irregular, reddish rash on his back (see Fig. 4.68). The central portions of this rash were insensitive to light touch.

This patient worked as a laborer on a sugar cane farm. He often worked in his bare feet and he had noticed that the dirt did not stick to the affected foot. Presumably, this was because his autonomic nerves were involved and he was not sweating on this side.

Leprosy is one of the causes of a mononeuritis, but the clinical signs that suggest the diagnosis of leprosy are very subtle. Signs of a skin lesion must be looked for and, if found, must be biopsied. Any enlarged nerve may be biopsied, but if no such nerve can be found, a sural nerve biopsy is the investigation of choice. It will frequently reveal the typical changes of leprosy.

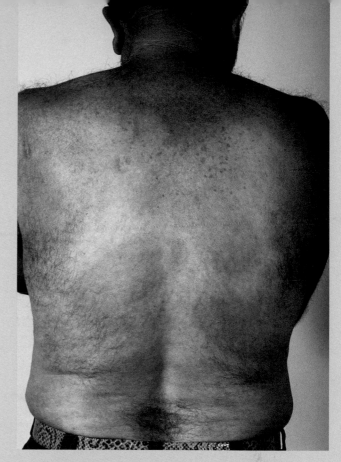

▲ **Fig. 4.68** Tuberculoid leprosy. This 40-year-old man presented with a mononeuritis of his right lateral popliteal nerve. He had an irregular, reddish rash on his back. The central portions of this rash were insensitive to light touch.

Reactions in leprosy

Acute reaction (Type 1 reaction)

Acute reaction (Type 1 reaction) is also called reversal or upgrading reaction.

The biological progression of leprosy is characterized by recurrent periods of acute activity, which are called reactions. They are seen most frequently in multibacillary (borderline lepromatous) leprosy. They appear to be a feature of the normal progression of the disease as the T-cell response begins to move the disease (upgrade it) toward the tuberculoid end of the spectrum; but they may be triggered by intercurrent infection, pregnancy or psychological stress. Occasionally, this type of reaction occurs soon after the commencement of drug therapy.

Case 4.7

An 8-year-old female, who came to Australia as a refugee, had been living in Australia for 6 months. Three weeks before her clinical presentation, she developed a rash. In the week prior to clinical presentation, it had become considerably worse—with swelling and scaling.

Clinical examination revealed an elevated, edematous, scaly, red rash all over her body (as shown in Fig. 4.69). Her

▼ ▶ **Fig. 4.69(a), (b), (c), (d), (e) and (f)** An 8-year-old female with a Type 1 lepra reaction.

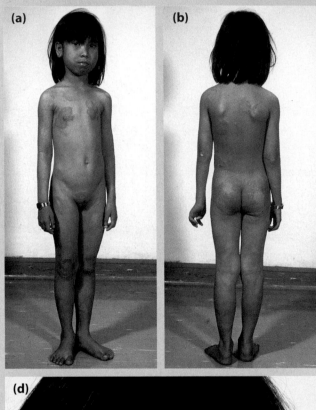

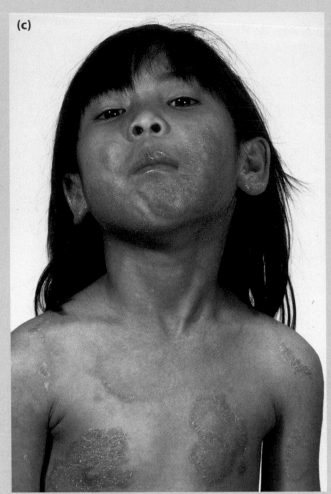

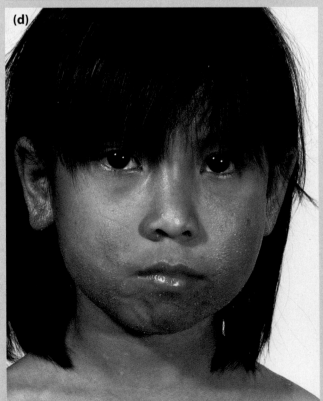

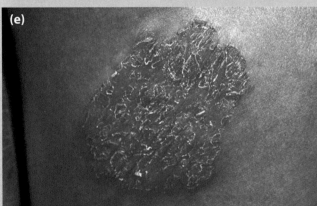

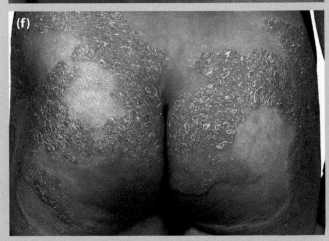

ear lobes were red, swollen and nodular, and her lateral popliteal nerves were somewhat enlarged. Some areas of the rash were insensitive to light touch with cotton wool.

A skin biopsy showed the features of borderline lepromatous leprosy.

The patient responded well to antileprosy therapy. At her review appointment 12 months later, she showed minimal sequelae (see Fig. 4.70).

This patient shows the typical features of a Type 1 reaction in borderline leprosy. She probably had the disease while she was in her home country. The immigration medical examination did not show any signs of leprosy, so presumably it was quiescent at this time. She would have undergone severe psychological stress in leaving her home and settling in a new country. Her nutritional state would have improved since coming to Australia, and all these factors probably triggered the reaction.

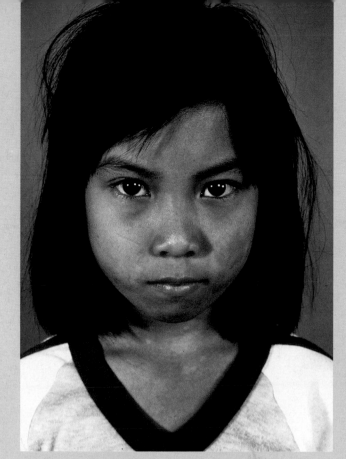

▲ **Fig. 4.70** The patient responded well to antileprosy therapy. At her review appointment 12 months later, she showed minimal sequelae.

Erythema nodosum leprosum (Type 2 reaction)

Erythema nodosum leprosum (Type 2 reaction), a reaction in lepromatous leprosy, is thought to be a result of an immune complex reaction initiated by the release of dead bacteria.

Case 4.8

A 33-year-old female presented because she felt extremely ill, having developed a fever of 104°F (40°C) and multiple red lumps all over the body 1 week before admission to hospital (see Fig. 4.71 overleaf).

She had had a similar but less severe episode 8 months prior to this one. The first episode had settled without treatment in 2–3 weeks.

A clinical diagnosis of erythema nodosum was made and a skin biopsy performed. It showed the features of erythema nodosum leprosum (see Fig. 4.72 overleaf).

After the results of the skin biopsy were known, further examination was performed. The lumps were tender, but not anesthetic. There was a band of anesthesia over the left calf. This area was burned by a cigarette 2 years previously and she did not feel it. There was no known contact with another case of leprosy.

She was treated with antileprosy drugs plus prednisone, and had many periods of quiescence interspersed with acute reactions. Two years after first diagnosis, she was still very ill (as shown in Figs 4.73 overleaf and 4.74 on page 100), so she was started on thalidomide and continued on a maintenance dose of clofazimine.

At follow-up 7 years after this treatment was started, she remained well (see Fig. 4.75 on page 100).

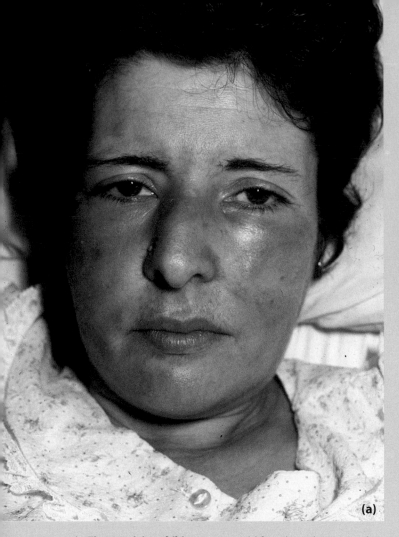

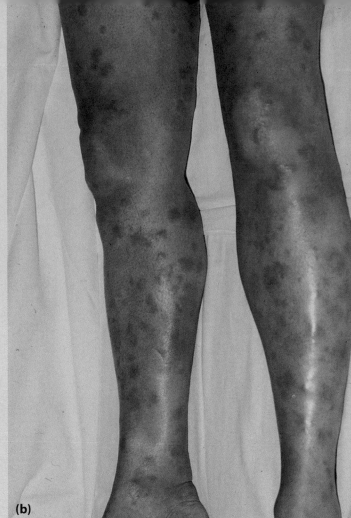

(a)

(b)

▲ **Fig. 4.71(a) and (b)** A 33-year-old female with a Type 2 lepra reaction.

▼ ▶ **Fig. 4.72(a) and (b)** Skin biopsy showed marked edema in the superficial dermis and a mixed inflammatory cell infiltrate (which included many neutrophils) throughout the dermis. Admixed with the inflammatory cells, there were many foamy histiocytes. **(c)** These contained numerous acid-fast bacilli.

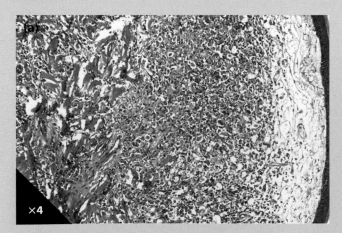

(a)

×4

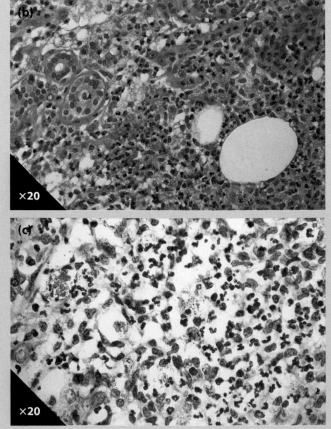

(b)

×20

(c)

×20

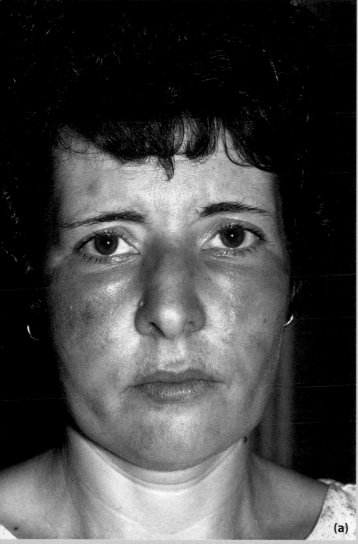

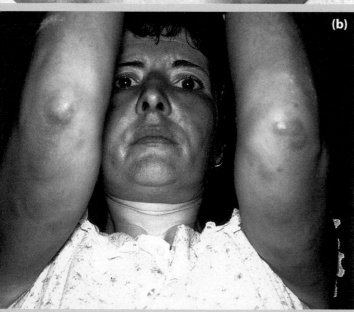

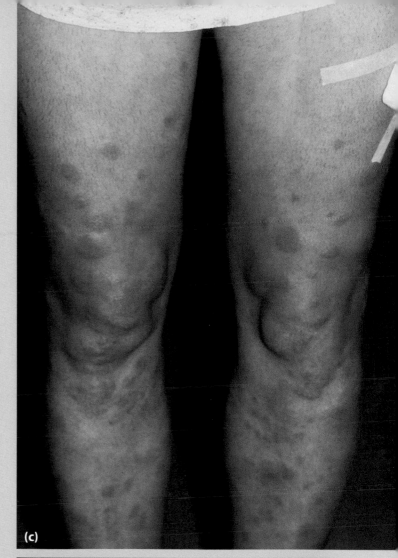

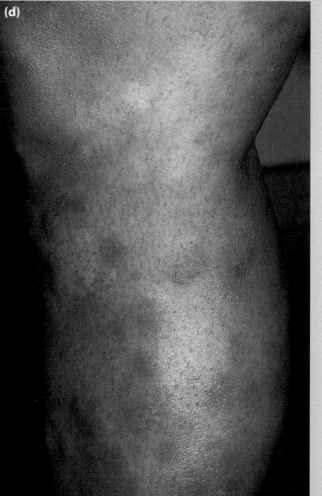

▼ ▶ **Fig. 4.73(a), (b), (c) and (d)** Clinical features shown in one of the patient's recurrent acute reactions.

(a)

(b)

(c)

(d)

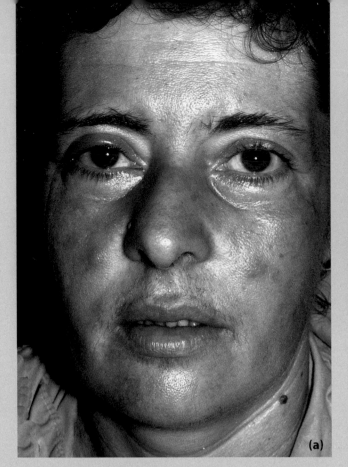

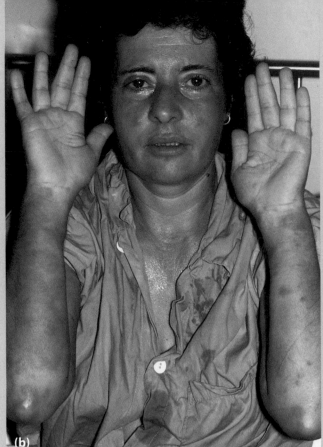

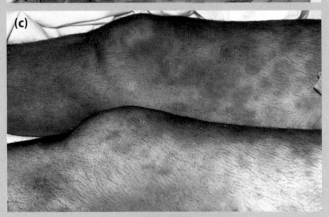

▲ ▶ **Fig. 4.74(a), (b) and (c)** Two years after first diagnosis, this patient was still very ill, so she was started on thalidomide and continued on a maintenance dose of clofazimine.

▼ ▶ **Fig. 4.75(a) and (b)** At follow-up 7 years after this treatment was started, the patient remained well.

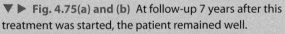

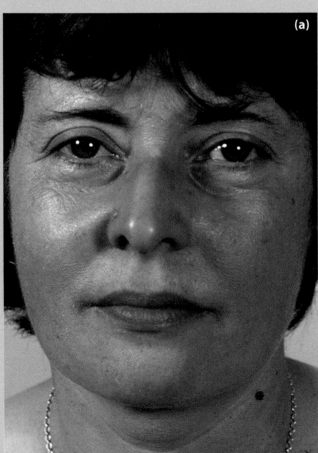

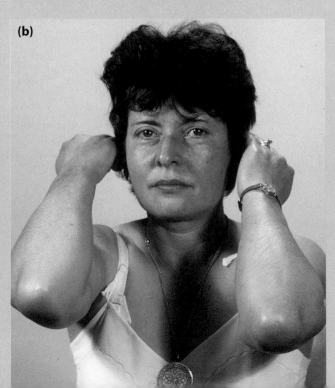

Social attitudes to leprosy

For centuries, patients with leprosy have undergone social stigmatization. They have been regarded as being 'unclean' and have been social outcasts.

The young man whose right arm is shown in Figure 4.76 had tried to hide his leprosy lesion with a tattoo. The biopsy was interesting: there were two types of granuloma in the dermis—one from the leprosy and one from the tattoo. The tattoo granuloma can be recognized by the presence of black carbon pigment. The leprosy granuloma has no pigment (see Figs 4.77, 4.78 and 4.79, continued overleaf).

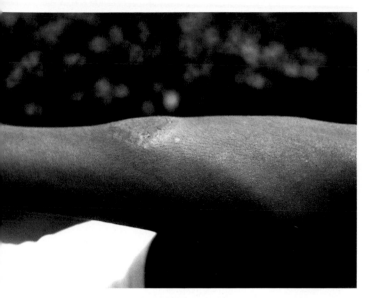

▲ **Fig. 4.76** This young man has a tattoo on his right arm to disguise the presence of a skin lesion of leprosy.

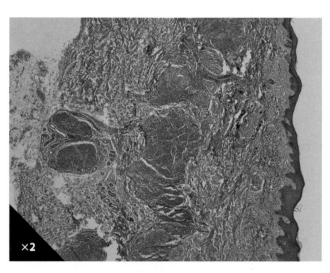

▲ **Fig. 4.77** Low-magnification view of the skin biopsy shows an inflammatory infiltration involving all levels of the dermis.

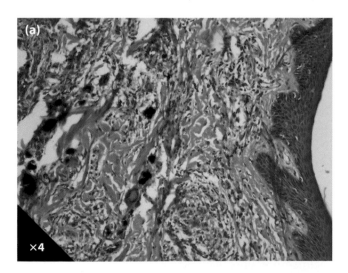

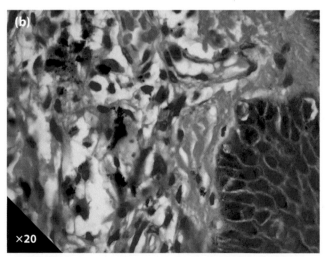

▲ **Fig. 4.78(a) and (b)** The granulomatous reaction in the upper dermis contains black carbon pigment—a tattoo granuloma.

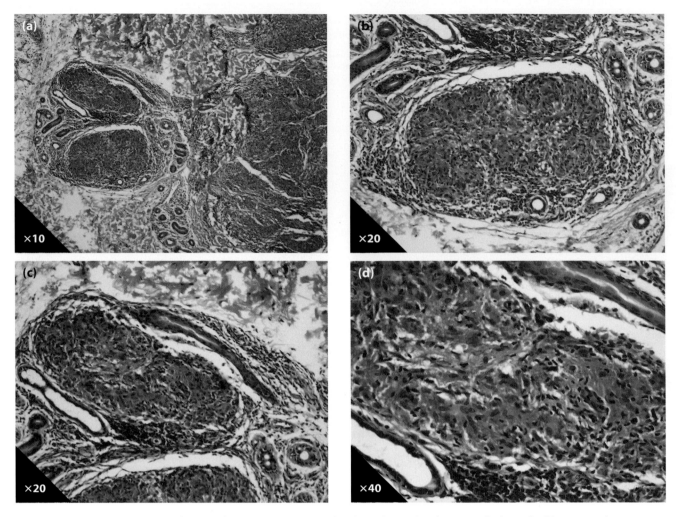

▲ **Fig. 4.79(a), (b), (c) and (d)** The granulomatous reaction in the deep dermis has features of tuberculoid leprosy with destruction of cutaneous nerves associated with skin appendages.

Reconstructive surgery in leprosy

Since the early 1950s, surgeons have been attempting to repair the damage done by leprosy in patients who have been cured of their disease by the drugs that are now available for treatment. Perhaps the best-known operative procedures are the transfer of tendons, particularly in hands and feet, so that muscles that are still innervated can be transferred to replace the function of the ones that have become paralyzed. These muscles can be trained to restore lost hand function. The man shown in Figure 4.80 has had plastic surgery to replace his lost eyebrows.

▼ **Fig. 4.80(a) and (b)** This man had lost his eyebrows. They were restored by plastic surgery, much to his satisfaction.

In chronic diseases, such as leprosy, the patient has to cooperate with the therapist to get results. Lack of patient cooperation may be a significant contributing factor to prolonged hospitalization. The Fijian man shown in Figure 4.81 had been an inmate of a well-run leprosy hospital for many years. Despite the many years of hospitalization, he still had chronic ulcers on his anesthetic hands and feet.

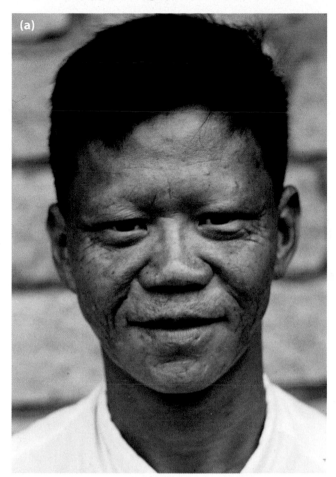

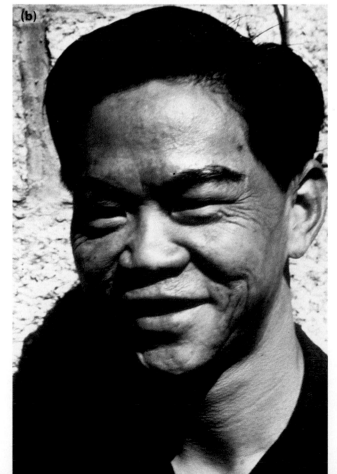

▼ **Fig. 4.81(a) and (b)** This Fijian man was an inmate of a leprosy hospital in Fiji for many years. Despite the many years of hospitalization, he still had chronic ulcers on his anesthetic hands and feet. Was he just happy to stay on in the hospital?

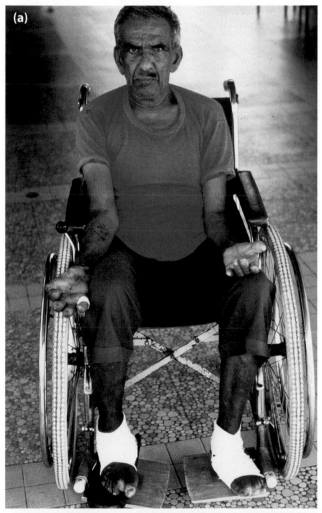

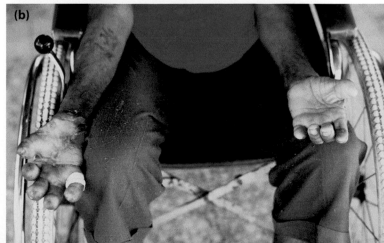

Research in leprosy

In the 1960s, the eight-banded armadillo, shown in Figure 4.82, that lives in some desert areas of the USA was found to harbor naturally large numbers of *M. leprae* organisms. This property led to its becoming an important source of organisms for research on leprosy. Prior to this, research was hampered by the fact that the organism could not be cultured in artificial media.

▼ **Fig. 4.82** The eight-banded Armadillo naturally harbors large numbers of *M. leprae* organisms.

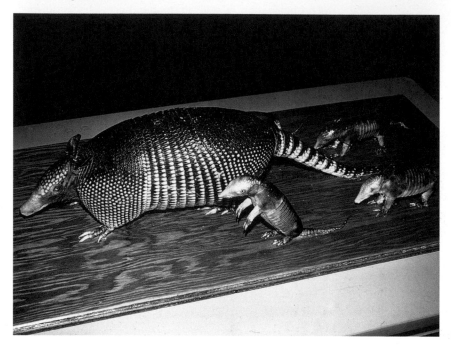

Acknowledgments

- The author thanks the following people for their generosity in sharing with him their knowledge and their patients' stories and photographs and knowledge over many years: Ken Clezy, Douglas Russell and Grace Warren; all international consultants on leprosy; and fellow physicians on the staff of the Royal Brisbane Hospital, Brisbane, Australia.
- Fig. 4.10 Courtesy of Roy Pugh, Brisbane, Australia.
- Figs 4.11–4.14 Courtesy of Roy Axelsen, Brisbane, Australia.

5

Sexually transmitted infections (STIs)

Many sexually transmitted infections (STIs) are caused by organisms that are difficult to culture on artificial media, are slowly growing and require special conditions, for example added carbon dioxide (Neisseria) or special cells (such as Chlamydia). The fastidious nature of the causative agents makes laboratory testing difficult, but the difficulties are magnified when poor or low-quality samples are collected by the requesting clinicians.

Various techniques have been employed over the years to improve the diagnostic yield. Gram stain is still a useful technique for detection of some bacteria (for example *Neisseria gonorrhoeae*) because of their distinctive shape and intracellular location. However, this requires the use of stains and a microscope with a light source, and this may not be available in all environments.

Treponemas cannot be cultured. Alternative methods, such as serology, have been traditionally used to detect the specific and nonspecific antibodies found in the serum of patients infected with these organisms.

Fluorescent antibody techniques—where the organism sought is stained with an antibody linked to a fluorescing dye—have been used for difficult-to-culture organisms, such as *Chlamydia trachomatis* and *Trichomonas vaginalis*. These techniques also require the use of trained staff and expensive microscopes and reagents, so they are not readily available in the field or at the bedside.

The discovery of the technique called polymerase chain reaction (PCR), with its ability to amplify specific microbial DNA, has revolutionized the detection of many difficult-to-diagnose microbes. Because DNA is robust, samples can be collected in the field and sent to a central processing laboratory, where the technique can be automated to maximize sensitivity, decrease costs and minimize the result turnaround time. Organisms such as those causing syphilis, herpes genitalis, chlamydial infections, trichomoniasis and granuloma venereum may be detected (or excluded) in a single sample that can be tested in a laboratory far from the collection point.

While these techniques are not universally available, and are still expensive, work is ongoing to develop robust field tests that can provide data at the bedside. This will ensure that specific diagnoses are made, and that all patients receive appropriate treatment for their condition.

Causative organisms

The following list names diseases that are recognized by various medical professionals—who have written knowledgably about this area—as belonging to the category of sexually transmitted infections (STIs).

Gonorrhea, NSU (nonspecific urethritis), syphilis, donovanosis (granuloma inguinale), pubic lice, scabies and mobiluncus are described in this chapter.

- Gonorrhea (see below)
- NSU (nonspecific urethritis) (see page 107)
- Syphilis (see page 108)
- Donovanosis (*granuloma inguinale*) (see page 133)
- Pubic lice (see page 141)
- Scabies (see page 141)
- Mobiluncus (see page 145)
- Amebiasis (see page 344)
- Candida (see page 187)
- Hepatitis B and hepatitis C (see pages 266 and 269)
- HIV (human immunodeficiency virus) (see page 466)
- HPV (human papilloma virus) (see page 259)
- HSV (herpes simplex virus) (see page 252)
- Lymphogranuloma venereum (LGV) (see page 265)
- Molluscum contagiosum (see page 262)
- Trichomoniasis (see page 352)

Gonorrhea

Gonorrhea is the commonest cause of sexually transmitted infection (STI). It is caused by the Gram-negative intracellular bacillus *N. gonorrhoeae*. It presents with a painful acute urethritis that causes a purulent discharge from the urethra (shown in Fig. 5.1). This is more obvious in males than in females. In fact, infection may not be noticed by the female and acute salpingitis may develop: this condition may progress to chronic salpingitis and may cause infertility.

Patients with gonorrhea may develop an acute arthritis of large joints (such as the knees), due to a systemic bacteremia, or the arthritis may result from an autoimmune reaction.

Babies delivered through a vagina infected with the gonococcus often get an acute ophthalmitis—gonococcal ophthalmitis (see Fig. 5.2).

Gram stain of the purulent exudate shows the Gram-negative diplococci of *N. gonorrhoeae* (see Fig. 5.3). Culture on chocolate agar confirms the presence of the organism, as illustrated in Figures 5.4 and 5.5.

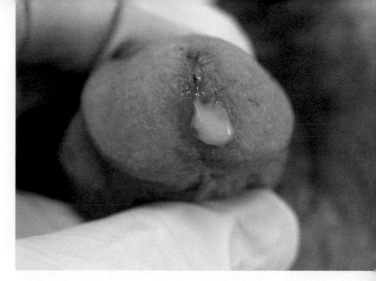

▲ **Fig. 5.1** Gonorrhea. A painful purulent urethral discharge.

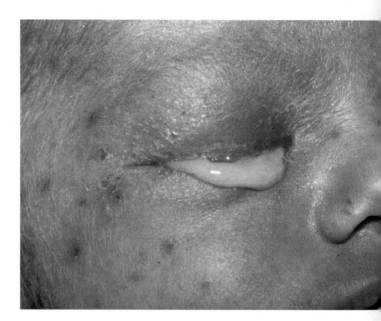

▲ **Fig. 5.2** Neonatal gonococcal ophthalmitis.

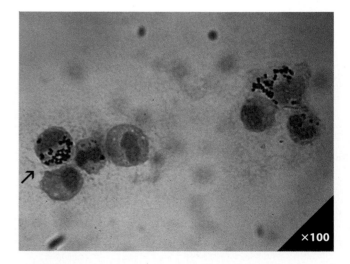

×100

▲ **Fig. 5.3** Gram stain on the purulent exudate shows the Gram-negative intracellular diplococci of *N. gonorrhoeae*.

▲ **Fig. 5.4** Chocolate agar culture plate showing the colonies of *N. gonorrhoeae*.

▼ **Fig. 5.5** Chocolate agar culture plate. A drop of oxidase solution has been dropped onto some of the *N. gonorrhoeae* colonies and the colonies have turned blue. Adjacent colonies have not been treated so as to provide a control appearance. This test is specific for *N. gonorrhoeae*.

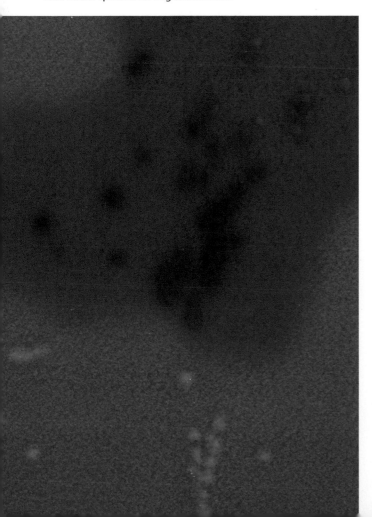

Nonspecific urethritis (NSU)

By definition, nonspecific urethritis is a urethritis in which no specific organism can be identified—it is a nongonococcal urethritis. The same clinical features are caused by infection with Chlamydia —chlamydial urethritis. The only way to detect the difference is to find no organismal cause in the former, and to have a positive test for Chlamydia in the latter. The test for Chlamydia used to be a serologic one but it has now been superseded by a very accurate PCR test.

Patients with NSU present with a urethral discharge of clear, mucoid fluid (shown in Fig. 5.6). The urethritis may be painless; more often it is painful, but less painful than gonorrhea.

▼ **Fig. 5.6** Nonspecific urethritis. A urethral discharge of clear, mucoid fluid. Marked acute inflammation of the urethral meatus is present as well, which is a little unusual.

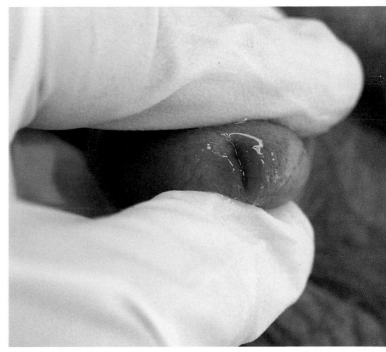

▼ **Figs 5.7, 5.8 and 5.9** Examples of primary chancres on the penis.

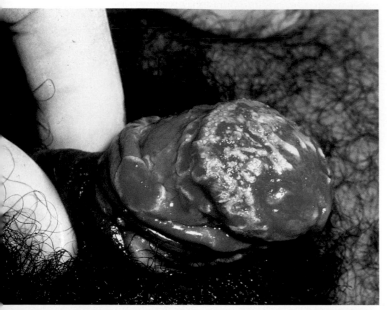

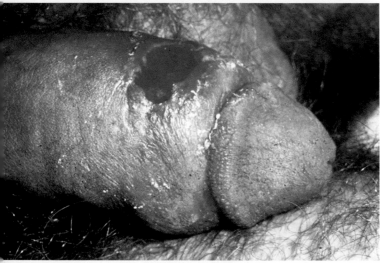

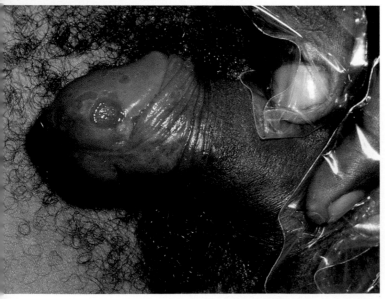

Syphilis

Syphilis is a sexually transmitted infection caused by the spirochetal organism *Treponema pallidum*. It is transmitted by sexual intercourse or transplacentally. HIV patients may contract syphilis concomitantly with their HIV infection.

Since the introduction of penicillin and other antibiotics, it has become a much less serious disease than it used to be. Long-term complications are now very rare. The last cases of long-term complications that were seen in Brisbane, Australia, were in the early 1960s, in elderly patients who had acquired their primary infection many years before the introduction of penicillin.

Syphilis occurs in all countries. Primary infections are still common.

Clinical presentation of syphilis

The first presentation of syphilis is with a painless ulcer on the penis or on the vulva. This lesion is called a chancre (illustrated in Figs 5.7–5.10).

Laboratory diagnosis

The process of laboratory diagnosis is as follows.

1. Dark ground examination of a smear from the lesion looking for motile spirochetes.
2. Serology.
3. Fluorescent antibody test.
4. Biopsy.

▼ **Fig. 5.10** Primary chancre at the introitus of the vagina.

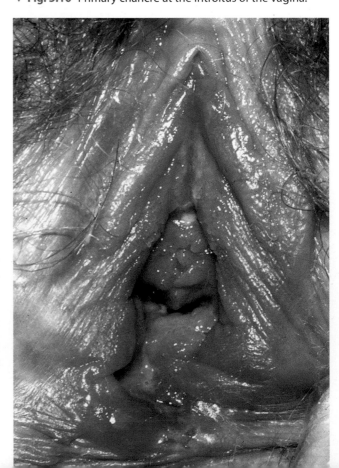

Case 5.1

A 22-year-old female presented with a generalized rash which she thought was due to an allergy. The rash involved the whole body, and the palms of both hands and the soles of both feet (shown in Fig. 5.11). She also had a chancre on the perineum (see Fig. 5.12 overleaf). Testing showed a few motile spirochetes in a smear from her perineal lesion (see Fig. 5.13 overleaf) and serologic tests for syphilis were positive. She was given a course of penicillin and her symptoms subsided.

Note: Had this patient presented in 2006 and later, she would not have had the serologic tests that were introduced in the 1940s but a fluorescent antibody test instead (see Fig. 5.14 overleaf).

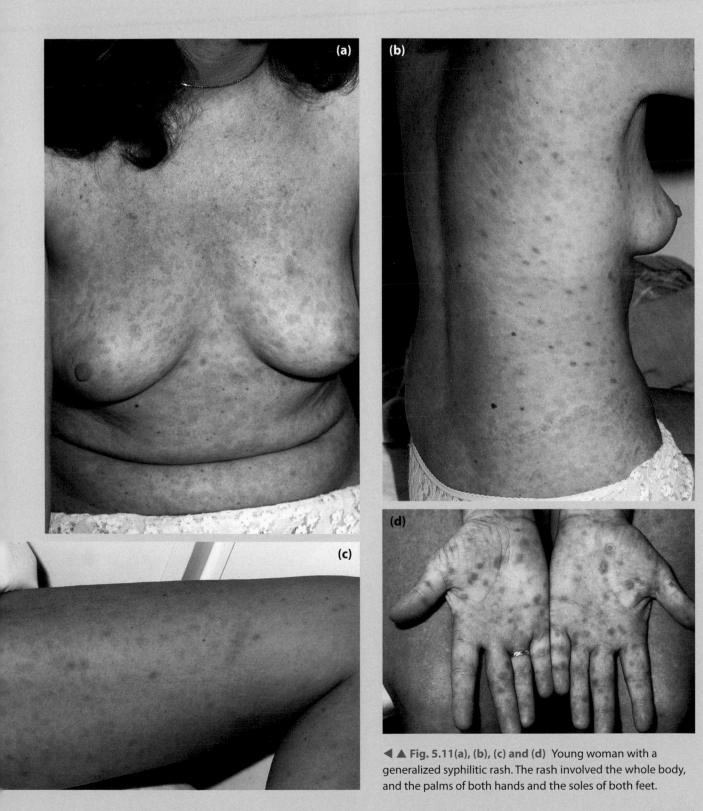

◀ ▲ **Fig. 5.11(a), (b), (c) and (d)** Young woman with a generalized syphilitic rash. The rash involved the whole body, and the palms of both hands and the soles of both feet.

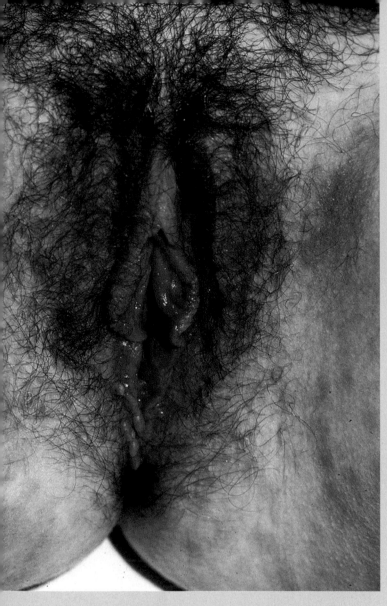

▲ **Fig. 5.12** Chancre and a few small condylomata on the vulva near the perineum.

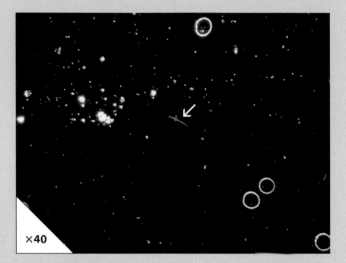

▲ **Fig. 5.13** A spirochete can be seen with dark ground illumination of a wet preparation from a smear from the surface of a chancre. In 'real time' the organism was motile.

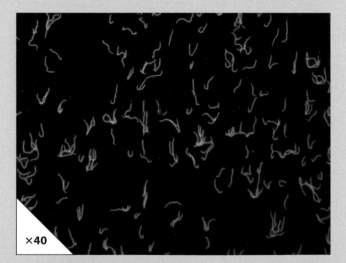

▲ **Fig. 5.14** Positive fluorescent antibody test. A culture of spirochetes is used for the test. The serum to be tested is added to the culture; a green marker dye is added; and a smear of the mixture is examined using a fluorescent microscope.

Case 5.2

A 62-year-old male presented with a typical syphilitic rash on his body and on the palms of both hands and the soles of both feet (see Fig. 5.15). He responded to a course of penicillin.

(a)

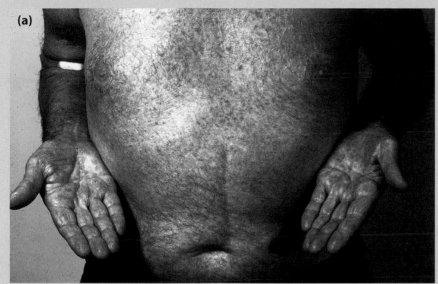

◀ ▼ **Fig. 5.15(a), (b) and (c)** Male, aged 62 years, with a typical syphilitic rash on his trunk and on the palms of his hands and the soles of his feet.

(b)

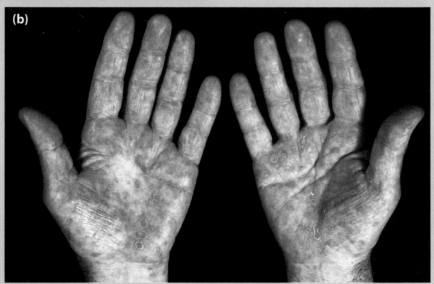

(c)

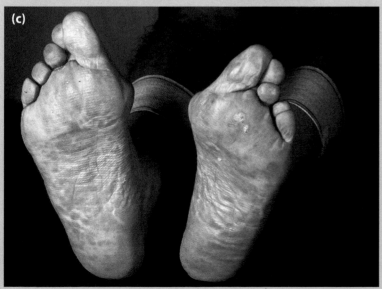

Microscopic appearance of a biopsy from a penile ulcer—a chancre

The microscopic appearance of a biopsy from a penile ulcer is seen in Figure 5.16. The biopsy shows an area of ulceration in the epidermis and an inflammatory infiltration in the upper and mid dermis. The inflammatory cells are lymphocytes and plasma cells, and there is marked swelling of the endothelial cells of the capillaries in the dermis. This tissue response is very suggestive of a spirochetal infection. Warthin Starry stain showed the presence of spirochetes in the thickened stratum corneum (shown in Fig. 5.16).

▼ **Fig. 5.16(a) and (b)** Skin biopsy shows ulceration and pseudoepitheliomatous hyperplasia of the epidermis adjacent to the ulcer.

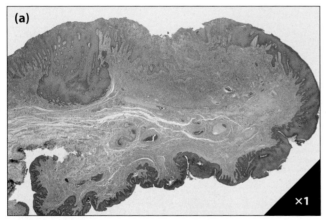

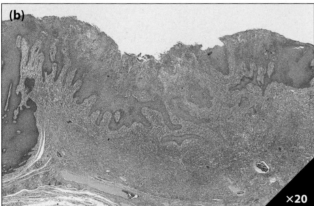

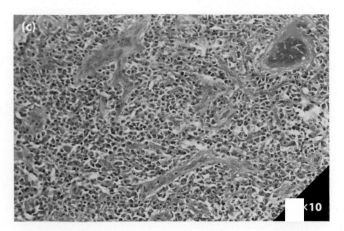

▲ **Fig. 5.16(c)** There is swelling of the endothelial cells of the capillaries in the dermis, and there is an infiltration of lymphocytes and plasma cells in the dermis. This pattern of inflammatory infiltration is typical of a spirochetal infection.

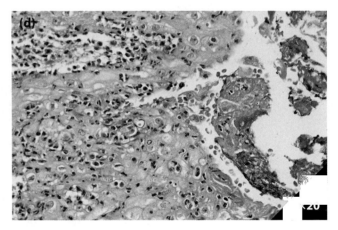

▲ **Fig. 5.16(d)** This section shows thickened keratin and debris in the base of the ulcer.

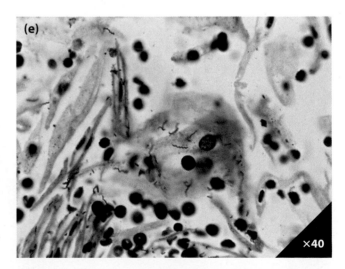

▲ **Fig. 5.16(e)** Spirochetes are seen in a Warthin Starry stain in the thickened keratin layer (not in the dermis).

Condylomata

Condylomata are localized hyperkeratotic lesions that occur:

- in the anogenital region, as shown in Figure 5.17(a) and (b)
- in the axillae, as shown in Figure 5.17(c) and (d), and
- at the base of the nostrils (but only sometimes), as shown in Figure 5.17(e).

Histologically, condylomata have a similar appearance to that illustrated in the biopsy of the chancre shown earlier in Figure 5.16.

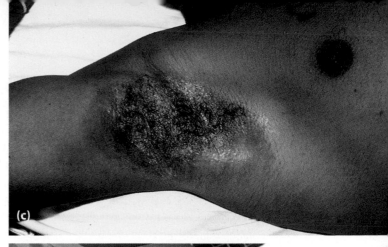

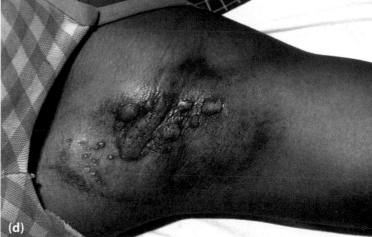

▼ **Fig. 5.17(a) and (b)** Condylomata. Localized hyperkeratotic lesions may be seen in the anogenital region.

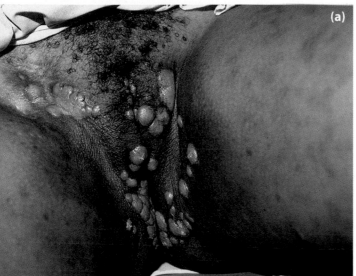

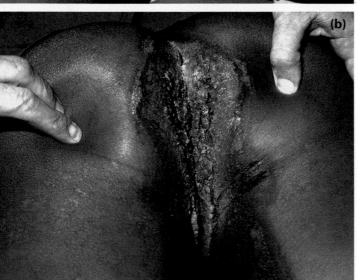

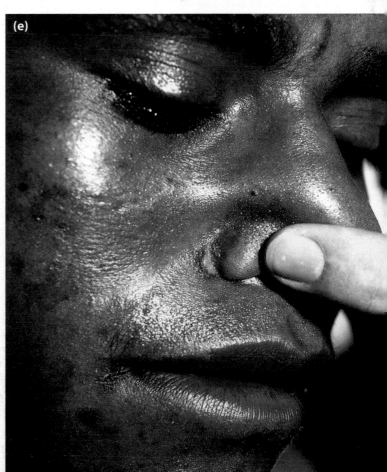

▲ **Fig. 5.17(c) and (d)** Condylomata. Localized hyperkeratotic lesions may be seen in the axillae.

▼ **Fig. 5.17(e)** Sometimes, one sees a fairly characteristic 'crack' in the skin at the base of the nostrils.

Later manifestations of syphilis

Oral lesions

Mucosal ulcers

Mucosal ulcers follow oral sex. It is anecdotally reported that some STI clinics are beginning to see increasing numbers of homosexual men who have acquired infection in this way because they think that oral sex is 'safe' (see Figs 5.18 and 5.19).

Perforation of the hard palate

Perforation of the hard palate is a late manifestation of syphilis and is now of historical interest (shown in Fig. 5.20).

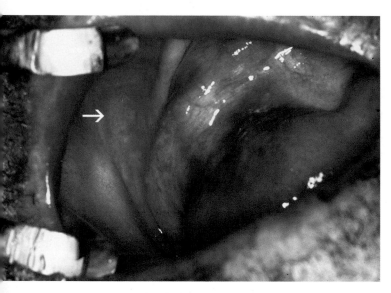

▲ **Fig. 5.18** Male, aged 59 years, with a mucosal lesion on the buccal mucosa following oral sex.

▼ **Fig. 5.19** Female, aged 16 years, with a mucosal lesion on the hard palate following oral sex. Serologic tests for syphilis were strongly positive. No organisms could be identified, but a biopsy showed a histologic appearance consistent with syphilis.

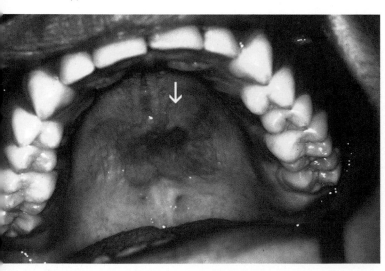

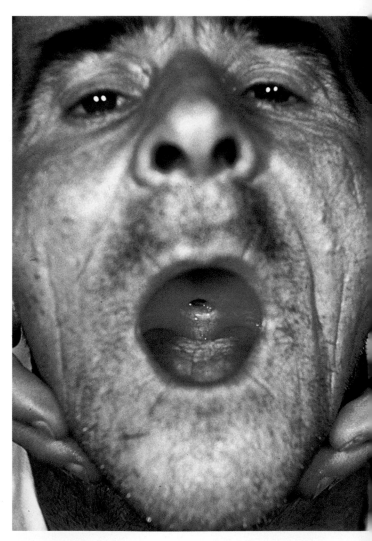

▲ **Fig. 5.20** Male, aged 46 years, with perforated hard palate. He also had Argyll Robertson pupils, which is one of the clinical signs of neurosyphilis. The pupils are small and do not react to light, but convergence is retained.

Squamous cell carcinoma of the tongue

Squamous cell carcinoma (SCC) of the tongue is a late manifestation of syphilis. The patient illustrated here, a male aged 75 years, had positive serologic tests for syphilis (see Fig. 5.21). These SCCs almost always occur in the middle of the upper surface of the tongue. This is a different location from the usual SCC of the tongue, which is the lateral border of the tongue. When one sees what appears to be an SCC in this location, one must consider syphilis or that it is a nonmalignant lesion associated with the presence of a benign tumor of the tongue—a granular cell tumor, which causes a pseudoepitheliomatous hyperplasia in the squamous epithelium.

A histologic section from the squamous cell carcinoma is shown in Figure 5.22.

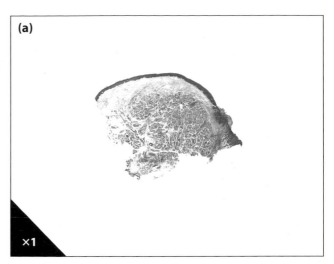

(a) ×1

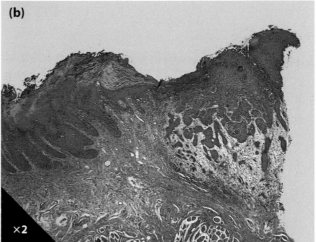

(b) ×2

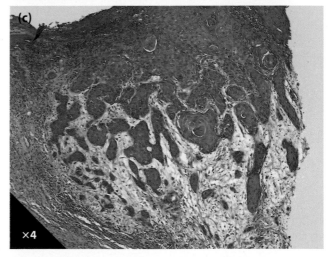

(c) ×4

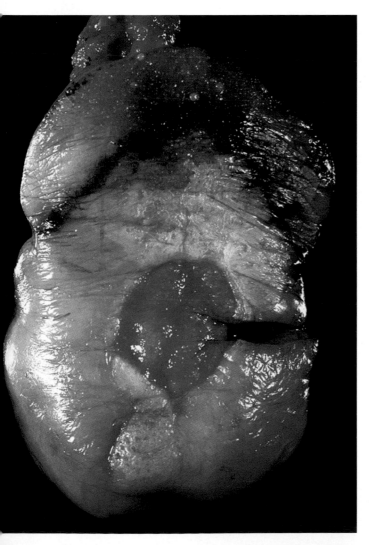

▲ **Fig. 5.21** Squamous cell carcinoma of the upper surface of the tongue in a male, aged 75 years, who had positive serologic tests for syphilis.

▲ **Fig. 5.22(a), (b) and (c)** Histologic section from the squamous cell carcinoma.

Cardiovascular lesions

The most common forms of cardiovascular syphilis are aneurysm of the aorta and aortic stenosis/incompetence.

Aneurysm of the aorta

Aneurysm of the aorta usually affects the arch of the aorta. Before the days of modern medicine, it sometimes presented clinically as a pulsating tumor bulging through the anterior chest wall, gradually enlarging and then rupturing (illustrated in Figs 5.23–5.28).

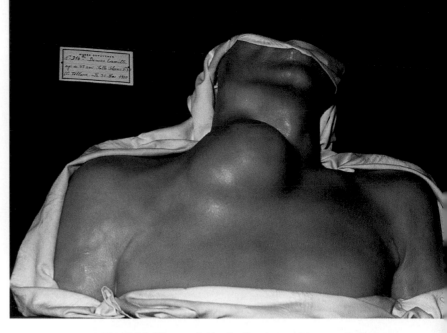

▼ **Fig. 5.23** This specimen of an aneurysm of the ascending thoracic aorta was one of the Scottish surgeon John Hunter's cases from the late 1770s. The patient was a 55-year-old British soldier in the Indian Army: he returned to London with a pulsating tumor bulging through his chest. It grew larger over a period of a year and then ruptured. The arrow labeled A shows a rib.

▲ **Fig. 5.24** Wax model in the Dupuytren Museum in Paris, France, depicts an aortic aneurysm bulging through the chest of a patient who was seen at about the same time as the John Hunter case illustrated in Figure 5.23.

▼ **Fig. 5.25** Wax model in the Dupuytren Museum in Paris, France, of a post-mortem specimen of a syphilitic aneurysm of the ascending thoracic aorta bulging through the anterior chest wall. Death was due to rupture of the aneurysm.

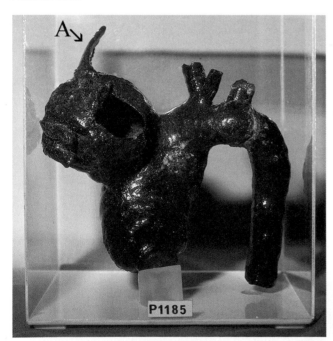

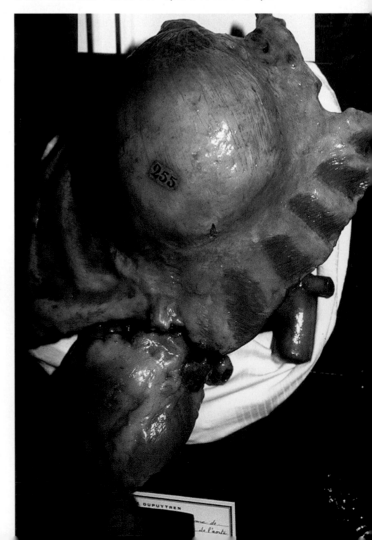

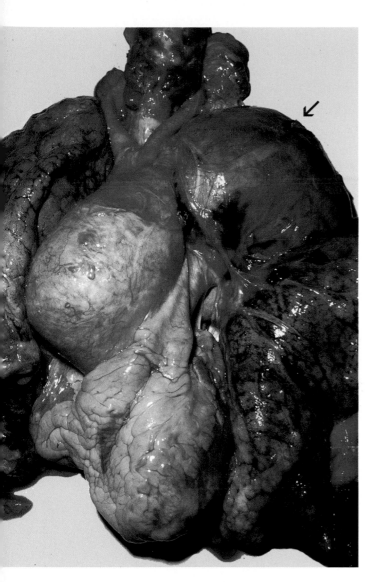

◄ **Fig. 5.26** An unfixed specimen of a syphilitic aneurysm in the arch of the aorta from a female aged 73 years. She had strongly positive serologic tests for syphilis. She died in Brisbane, Australia, in 1969.

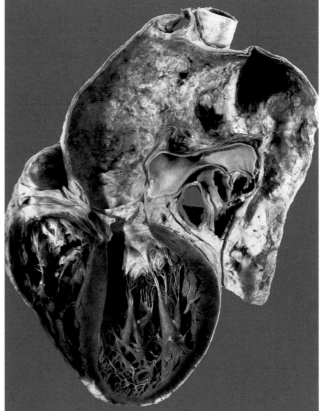

▼ **Fig. 5.27** In the opened specimen shown in Figure 5.26, note the appearance of marked thickening of all layers of the wall of the aorta, and the white, wrinkled plaques on the intimal surface. Atherosclerosis is present as well. These are the characteristic gross appearances of syphilitic aortitis.

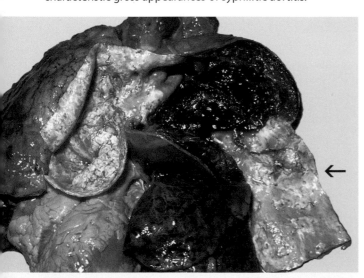

▲ **Fig. 5.28** Specimen of a syphilitic aneurysm, from the late 1960s. Note again the thickening of all layers of the wall of the aorta, and the crinkled, white plaques on its intimal surface. The free margins of the aortic valve cusps appear to be a little thickened.

Microscopic appearances of syphilitic aortitis

The microscopic appearances of syphilitic aortitis are as follows.

- Disruption and thickening of the wall of the aorta by an inflammatory infiltration (mainly of lymphocytes and plasma cells), through all layers of the wall of the aorta, and destruction of the elastic laminae of the aortic wall.
- The walls of the vasa vasora in the adventitial layer of the aorta are thickened and undergo endarteritis. There is an infiltration of lymphocytes and plasma cells in the thickened walls of the vasa vasora. This change is similar to that seen in the blood vessels in the periosteum in tertiary syphilis.

This destruction of the wall of the aorta by the inflammatory cell infiltrate and the destruction of the elastic laminae weakens the wall of the aorta, and an aneurysmal dilatation occurs.

These changes to the wall of the aorta are illustrated in Figures 5.29–5.32. The hematoxylin and eosin (H&E) stains show the cellular reaction, and the elastic stains show the destruction of the elastic laminae. Figures 5.29, 5.30 and 5.31 show increasing magnifications: the (a) images are an H&E stain and the (b) images are an elastic stain (VVG). The changes seen in the vasa vasora are similar to those shown in Figure 5.56 on page 133.

▼ **Figs 5.29, 5.30 and 5.31** Section of a syphilitic aorta showing destruction of the wall of the aorta. **(a)** Stained with H&E. **(b)** Stained with an elastic stain (VVG).

(a)

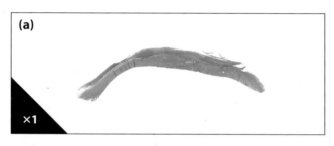

(b)

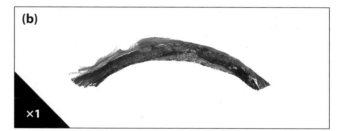

▼ **Fig. 5.30**

(a)

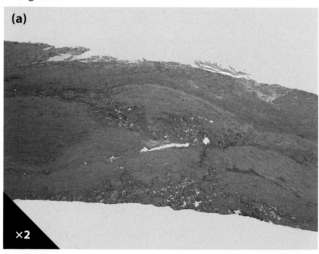

(b)

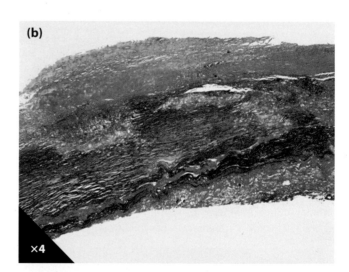

▼ **Fig. 5.31**

(a)

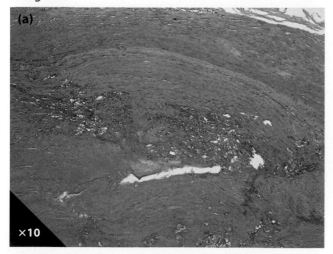

(b)

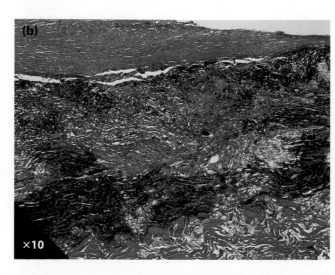

▼ **Fig. 5.32(a), (b) and (c)** Inflammatory infiltration in the wall of the aorta consists mainly of lymphocytes and plasma cells.

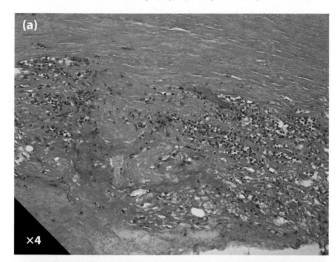

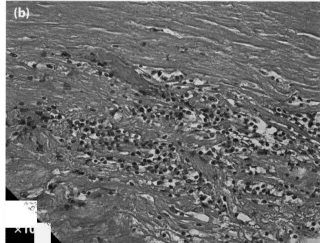

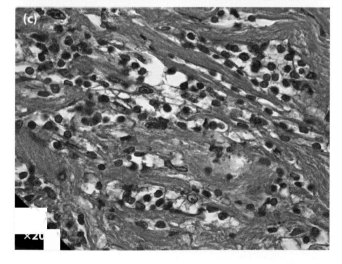

Aortic stenosis/incompetence

The inflammatory reaction in syphilis involves the cusps of the aortic valve. This causes thickening of the valves and fibrosis, which results in shortening of the cusps. This in turn leads to inability of the cusps to close completely and to aortic incompetence. The inflammatory infiltration in the intima may also cause occlusion of the ostia of the coronary arteries and myocardial ischemia (see Fig. 5.33).

▼ **Fig. 5.33** This heart has been opened to demonstrate the presence of syphilitic aortitis, thickening of the aortic cusps and the compensatory left ventricular hypertrophy.

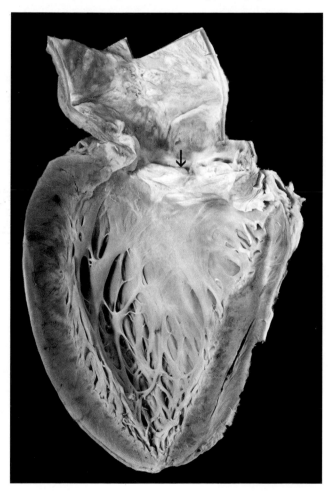

Hepatic lesions

Hepar lobatum—irregular lobation of the liver due to scarring caused by syphilitic inflammation—is shown in Figure 5.34.

Microscopically, the scarring fibrosis is seen and the vessels show endarteritis obliterans of the small arteries (see Fig. 5.35).

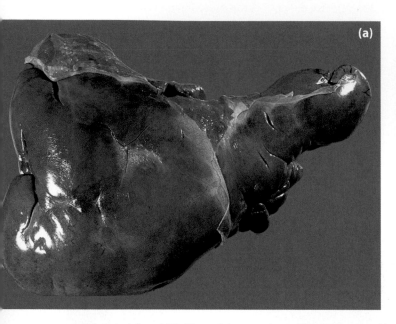

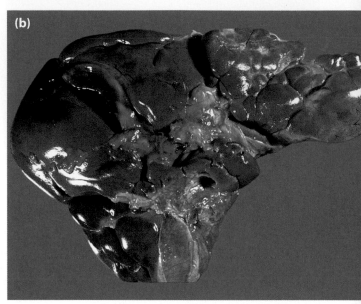

▲ **Fig. 5.34(a) and (b)** Hepar lobatum viewed from above and below. This was an incidental finding in a post mortem performed in Brisbane, Australia, in 1974, on a male aged 61 years.

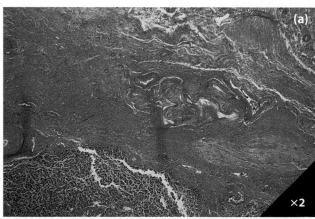

◀ ▼ **Fig. 5.35(a), (b) and (c)** Section of a hepar lobatum shows the presence of wide bands of fibrous tissue dissecting the normal liver parenchyma and endarteritis obliterans of small arteries. This is best seen in **(c)**.

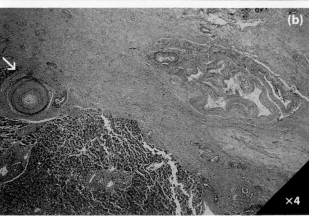

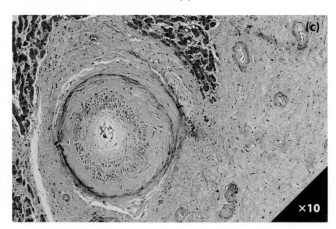

Mid face deformities

Mid face deformities are the result of inflammation and scarring of the facial cartilage and bone. The cartilage disintegrates and the nose 'collapses' (see Fig. 5.36). Similar lesions appear in yaws.

▼ **Fig. 5.36** Mid face deformity of syphilis. This man had positive serology for syphilis.

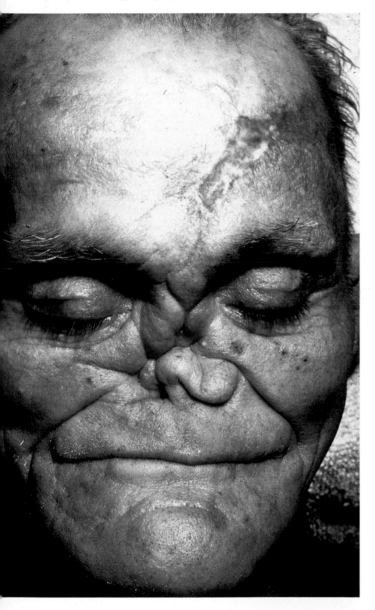

Central nervous system pathology

The spinal cord and the cerebrum are the parts of the central nervous system most commonly affected by syphilis. The inflammation in the spinal cord causes damage to the posterior columns, resulting in the clinical condition called tabes dorsalis.

The inflammatory reaction in the brain causes the clinical condition called 'general paralysis of the insane' (GPI).

Tabes dorsalis

Atrophy of the posterior columns of the spinal cord (see Fig. 5.37) results in sensory loss, and loss of proprioception, which produces a characteristic gait. The feet are placed well apart; they are lifted higher than is necessary; and then they are 'stamped' on the ground. This is the so-called 'high stepping gait'.

Other causes of atrophy of the posterior columns of the spinal cord are:

- vitamin B12 deficiency—this may be seen in chronic alcoholics, as well as in patients with pernicious anemia
- Freidreich's ataxia.

▼ **Fig. 5.37** Tabes dorsalis. This specimen of spinal cord shows atrophy of the posterior columns.

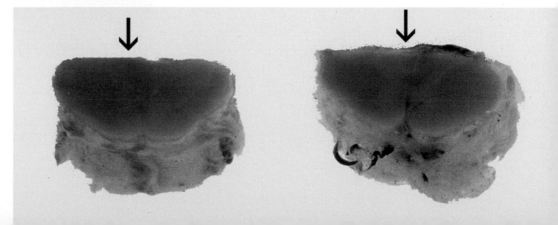

Microscopic changes in the nervous system

The inflammatory reaction in syphilis results in a meningitic type of reaction, with thickening of the meninges by an infiltration of lymphocytes and plasma cells. The illustrative images here are from a case of congenital syphilis in which the changes are similar to those seen in tertiary syphilis in adults (see Fig. 5.38).

▼ ▶ **Fig. 5.38(a), (b), (c), (d) and (e)** Section of cerebellum in a baby who died from congenital syphilis. The leptomeninges are thickened, and there is an infiltration of plasma cells and lymphocytes.

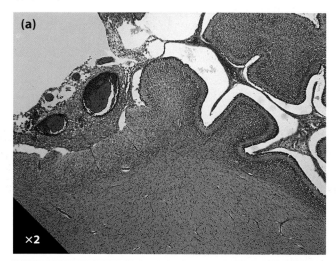

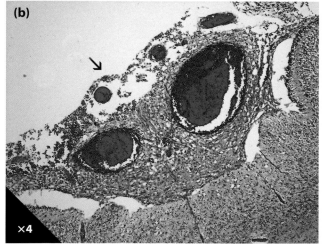

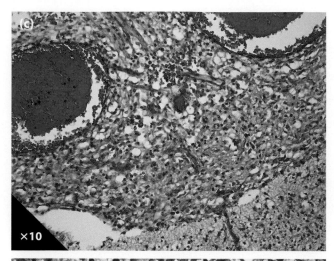

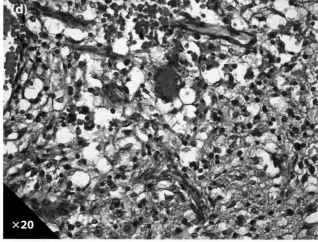

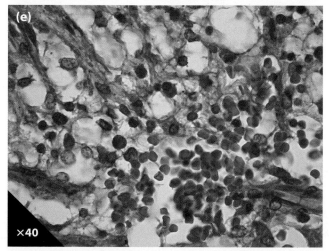

Joint pathology

The loss of proprioception that occurs in tabes dorsalis results in disorganization of hip, knee and ankle joints. This deformity is called a Charcot's joint, after the famous Parisian neurologist Jean Charcot (1825–1893), who worked at the Hopital Salpetriere in Paris (see Figs 5.39, 5.40 and 5.41).

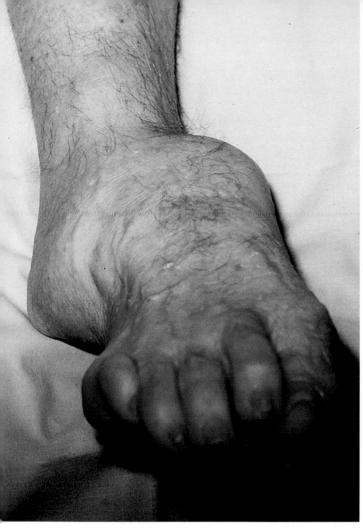 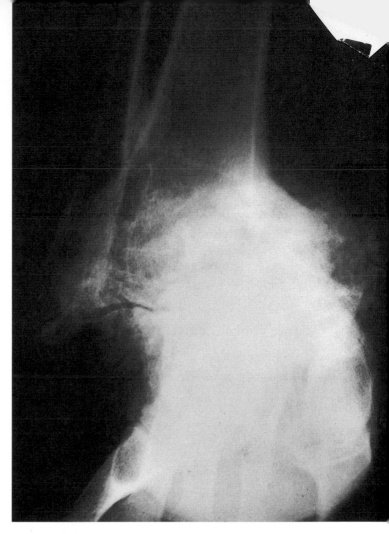

▲ **Fig. 5.39** Charcot's deformity of the ankle. A 70-year-old male patient of a hospital in Brisbane, Australia, 1960. He has gross deformity of his right ankle. His syphilis serology was strongly positive.

▲ **Fig. 5.40** X-ray of the ankle of the 70-year-old male patient in Figure 5.39.

▼ **Fig. 5.41** Charcot's deformity of the left hip. X-ray of the pelvis shows gross deformity of the left hip in a 71-year-old female patient in a hospital in Brisbane, Australia, 1960. Her syphilis serology was strongly positive.

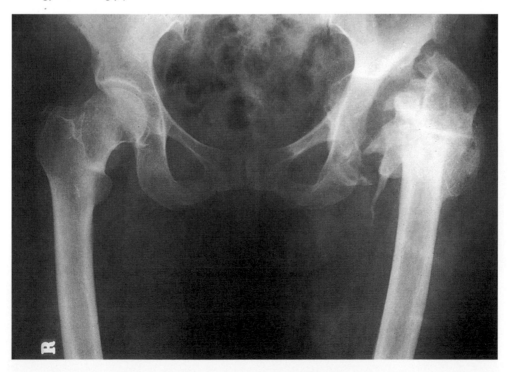

Bone pathology

Pitting of the skull in late-stage disease in adults is shown in Figure 5.42.

Disorganization of the cartilage columns in the meta-physis in long bones in congenital syphilis is discussed on pages 130–134, as is periostitis.

Congenital syphilis

Congenital syphilis occurs in the baby when a mother acquires a primary infection with the organism *Treponema pallidum* during pregnancy. Some of the pathologic changes resemble those seen in late-stage syphilis—the so-called 'tertiary syphilis' in adults.

Features of congenital syphilis

Most of the babies with congenital syphilis die before birth, at birth or soon after birth and they suffer from varying combinations of the following abnormalities.

- Fetal maceration
- Generalized rash
- Redness of palms of hands and soles of feet
- Large placenta, with the baby showing features of hydrops fetalis
- Enlargement of liver and spleen
- Multiple purpuric spots on the serosal surfaces lining the body cavities
- Excessive extramedullary hematopoiesis in the liver for the age of gestation, together with the presence of some multinucleated hepatocytes
- Excessive hair on the head and face—the so-called 'syphilitic wig'
- Bone changes consist in irregularity in the formation of the columns of cartilage in the metaphysis of long bones, and periostitis resulting in thickening of the periosteum
- Changes in the brain consist in thickening of the meninges from a meningitic, inflammatory cell infiltration
- Thymic atrophy
- Adrenal atrophy
- Spirochetes may be found in the organs at post mortem, especially in the liver. Organisms are most numerous in macerated fetuses.
- Most of these changes in babies with congenital syphilis will be demonstrated in the following four cases: Cases 5.3–5.6.

▼ **Fig. 5.42** Skull of an adult exhumed during an archeological excavation. It shows the pitting that is characteristic of advanced syphilis.

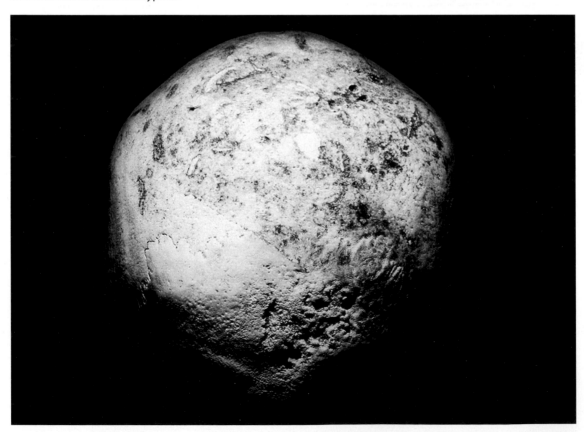

Case 5.3

A macerated fetus born at term (see Fig. 5.43), showed the presence of numerous spirochetes in the necrotic liver and spleen (see Fig. 5.44).

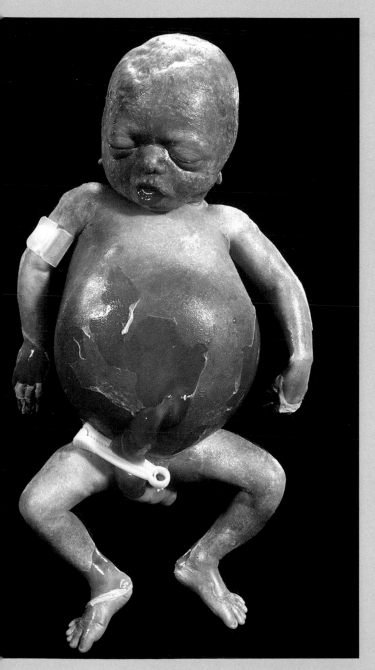

▲ **Fig. 5.43** Macerated fetus with congenital syphilis.

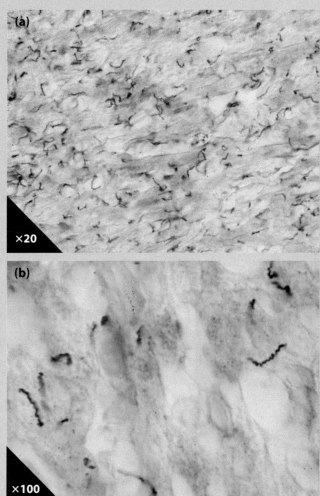

▲ **Fig. 5.44(a) and (b)** All the organs of the macerated fetus were necrotic, but numerous spirochetes were demonstrated in the liver and the spleen.

Case 5.4

A female born at 30 weeks gestation breathed for 15 minutes and then died. She had a blotchy rash all over her body, and the palms of both hands and of the soles of both feet were red, as shown in Figure 5.45.

Laboratory tests were as follows:

- Mother: Serologic tests for syphilis strongly positive.
- Baby: Serologic tests for syphilis positive.
- Motile treponemes seen in cord blood with dark ground illumination.

The pathologic changes seen at post mortem are illustrated in the various images presented here.

The placenta was enlarged, as illustrated below in Figure 5.46.

The liver and spleen were enlarged and there were multiple purpuric spots on the serosal surfaces lining the body cavities (see Fig. 5.47).

In the liver, there was excessive extramedullary hematopoiesis for the age of gestation; there were a few multinucleated hepatocytes present; and a few spirochetes were present (as illustrated in Fig. 5.48 overleaf).

Also present were thymic atrophy with fibrosis; and adrenal atrophy with loss of the X zone and a moderate degree of giant cell transformation in the cells of the adrenal cortex.

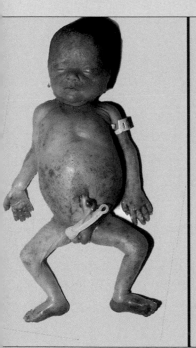
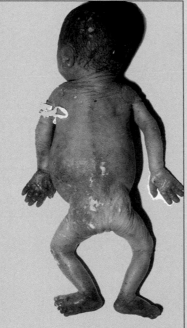
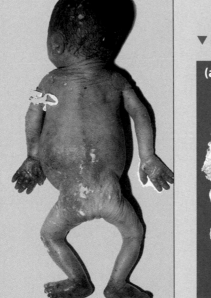

▲ **Fig. 5.45** Congenital syphilis. Female born at 30 weeks gestation. This baby had a generalized rash and there was redness of the palms of both hands and of the soles of both feet.

▼ **Fig. 5.46(a) and (b)** This baby had an enlarged placenta.

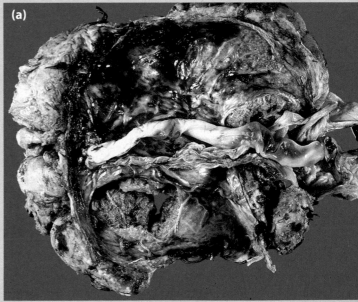

(a)

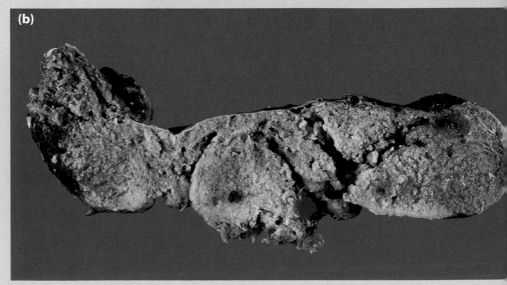

(b)

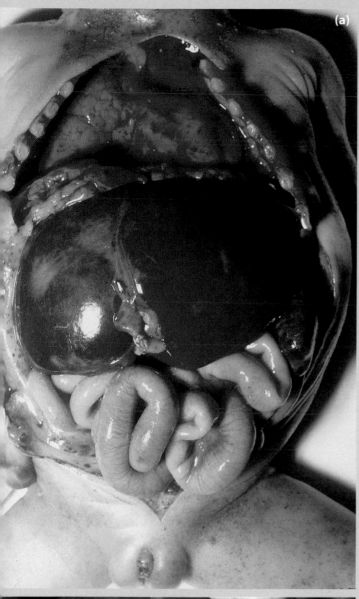

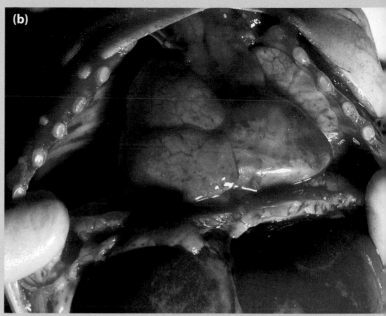

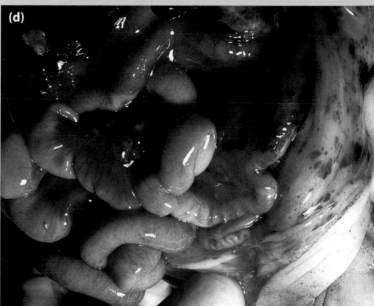

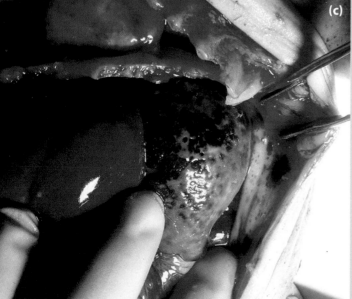

◀ ▲ **Fig. 5.47(a), (b), (c) and (d)** The liver and spleen of the baby were enlarged and there were multiple purpuric spots on the serosal surfaces lining the body cavities.

▼ ▶ **Fig. 5.48(a), (b) and (c)** There was excessive extramedullary hematopoiesis in the liver for the age of gestation (A). **(d)** Some hepatic giant cells were present (B). **(e)** A few spirochetes were present.

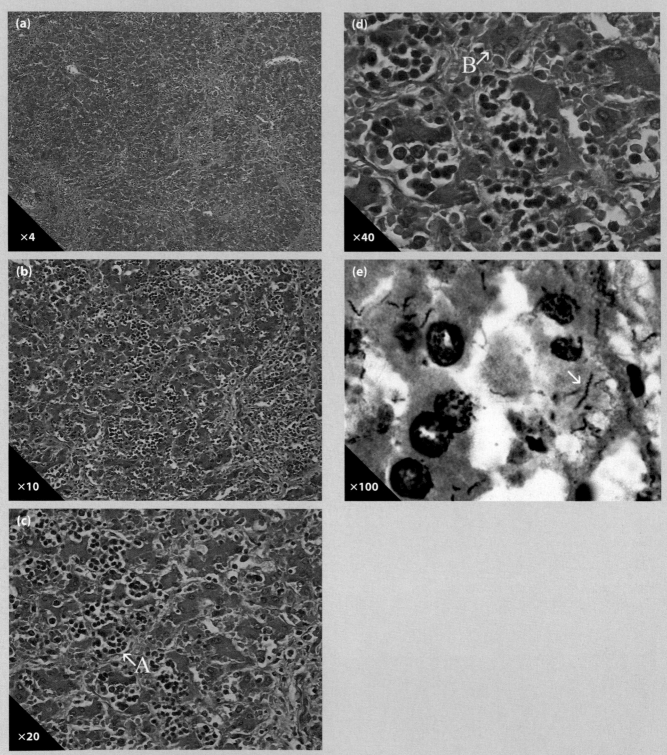

Case 5.5

A female was born at term and died 5 hours later. Both baby and mother had positive syphilis serology. The baby had excessive amounts of hair on the head and face that is sometimes referred to as the 'syphilitic wig' (see Fig. 5.49).

At post-mortem examination, the liver was enlarged and there were a number of greyish areas beneath the capsule. On histologic sections, these areas showed inflammatory changes that resembled 'gummas'. This condition is illustrated in Figure 5.50

▶ **Fig. 5.49** This female baby born at term died 5 hours later. She demonstrated excessive growth of hair—the 'syphilitic wig'.

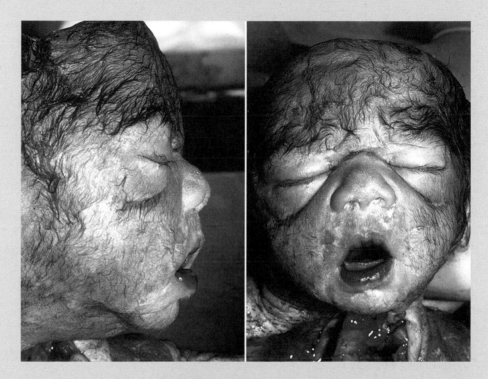

▶ **Fig. 5.50** At post-mortem examination, the baby's liver was enlarged. There were a few grey-white areas beneath the capsule. On section, these showed inflammatory changes that resembled 'gummas'—the granulomatous inflammatory reaction seen in tertiary syphilis in adults.

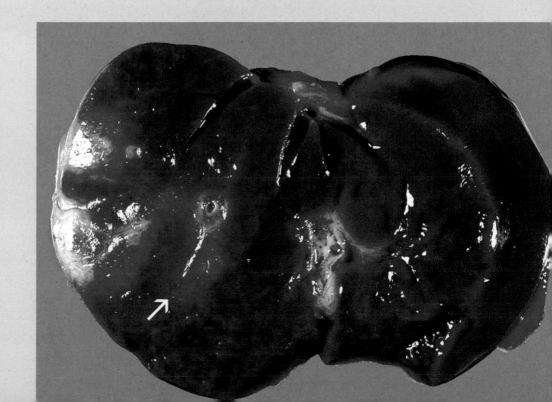

Case 5.6

A female was born to a mother with positive syphilis serology. The baby also had positive serology. She died 2 months after birth. X-ray of the baby's lower legs showed the presence of thickening of the periosteum of both tibiae (see Fig. 5.51).

At post-mortem examination, the thickening of the periosteum of the tibiae could be seen grossly (shown in Fig. 5.52).

Microscopic examination showed irregularity in the pattern of formation of the columns of cartilage cells in the metaphysis of the tibiae (see Fig. 5.53). Similar changes occurred in the cartilage of the vertebrae (shown in Fig. 5.54). The thickening of the periosteum was due to fibrosis and an inflammatory infiltration of lymphocytes and plasma cells as illustrated in Figure 5.55 overleaf).

The vasa vasora in the periosteum showed a florid endarteritis and a perivascular infiltration of lymphocytes and plasma cells (see Fig. 5.56).

Microscopic examination of the brain showed thickening of the meninges by an inflammatory cell infiltration consisting of plasma cells and lymphocytes (shown earlier in Fig. 5.38, see page 122).

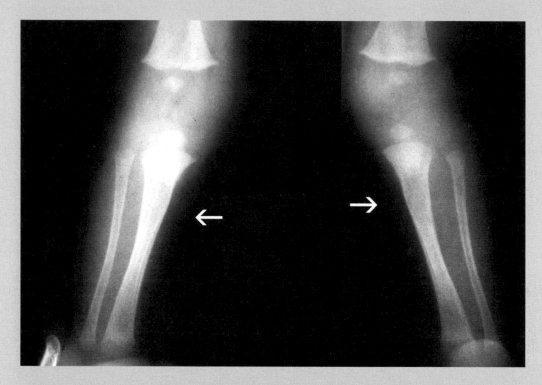

◄ **Fig. 5.51** X-ray of the lower legs showed thickening of the periosteum of both tibiae.

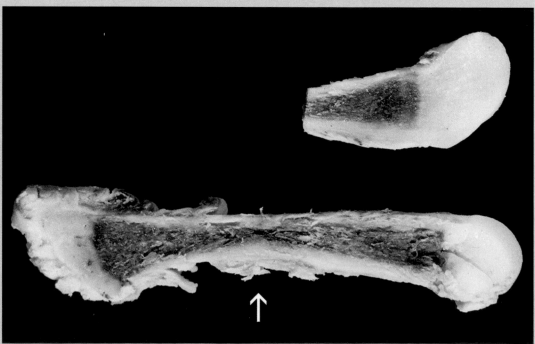

◄ **Fig. 5.52** In the gross specimen, the thickening of the periosteum can be seen.

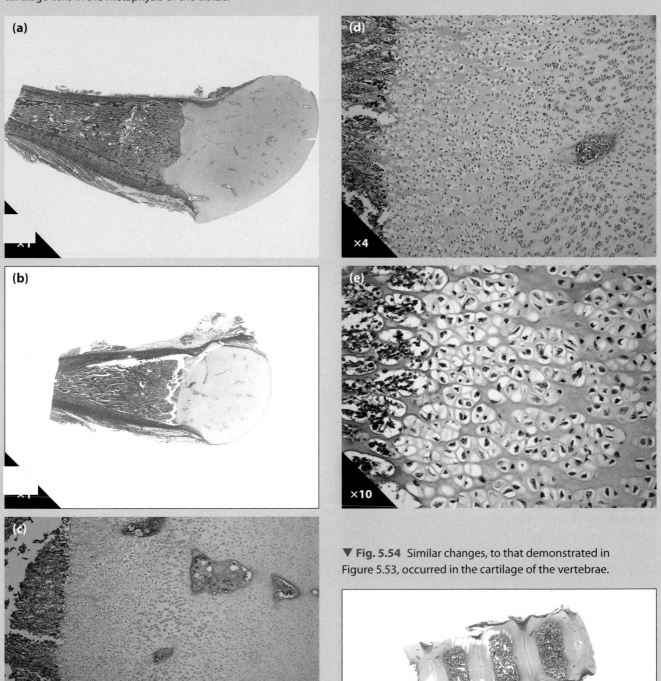

▼ ▶ **Figs 5.53(a), (b), (c), (d) and (e)** Microscopic examination showed irregularity in the pattern of formation of the columns of cartilage cells in the metaphysis of the tibiae.

(a)

×1

(b)

×1

(c)

×2

(d)

×4

(e)

×10

▼ **Fig. 5.54** Similar changes, to that demonstrated in Figure 5.53, occurred in the cartilage of the vertebrae.

×1

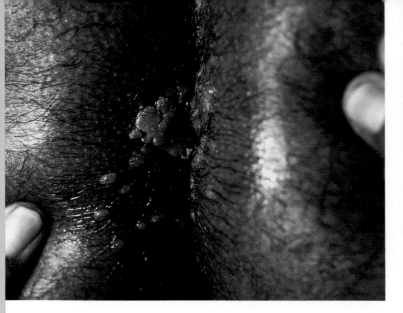

▲ **Fig. 5.58** Donovanosis. 'Condylomatous' lesions around the anus.

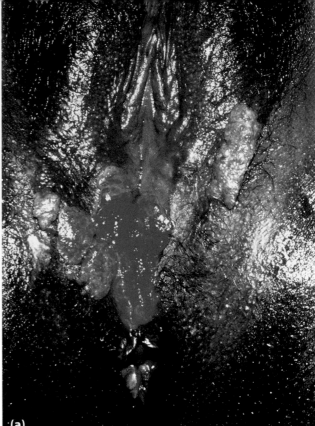

(a)

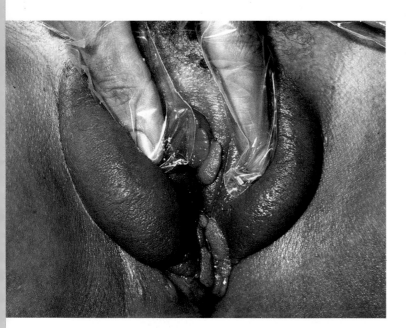

▲ **Fig. 5.59** Donovanosis. A 30-year-old female with hypertrophic lesions on the perineum and labia minora.

▼ **Fig. 5.60** Donovanosis. A 20-year-old female with an ulcerated lesion of the right labia majora.

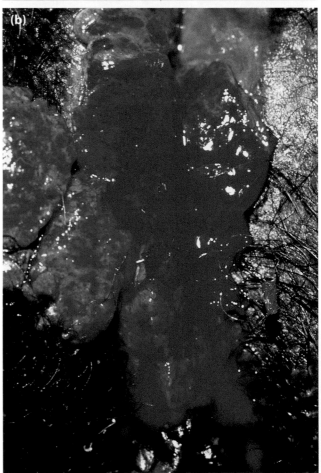

(b)

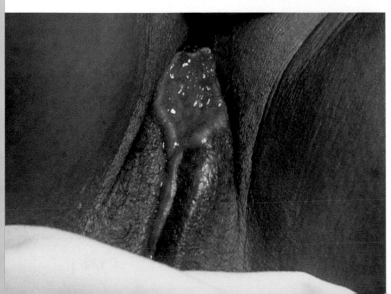

▲ **Fig. 5.61(a) and (b)** Donovanosis. A 22-year-old female with 'condylomatous' hyperkeratotic and ulcerated lesions on the vulva presented in labor. It was decided to perform a Caesarian section in the interests of both the mother and the baby.

Organisms can spread beyond the skin. Sometimes, female patients present with endometrial lesions or with a 'frozen pelvis' from inflammatory masses that mimic a malignant lesion. Biopsies from such cases show a chronic inflammatory reaction with numerous histiocytes with clear cytoplasm, in which the diagnostic organisms can be demonstrated by Warthin Starry stain (see Fig. 5.62) and electron microscopy (EM) (see Fig. 5.63).

In donovanosis, occasional cases with bone lesions are encountered.

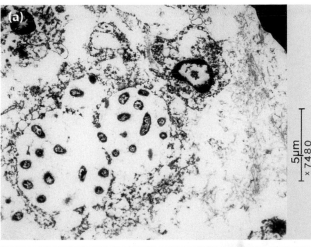

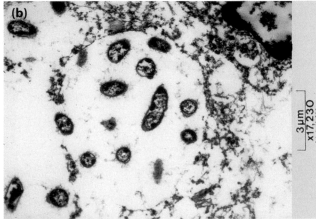

▲ **Fig. 5.63(a) and (b)** Donovanosis. Low and higher magnification electron microscopic examination shows the slightly bent, rod-shaped appearance of the organisms.

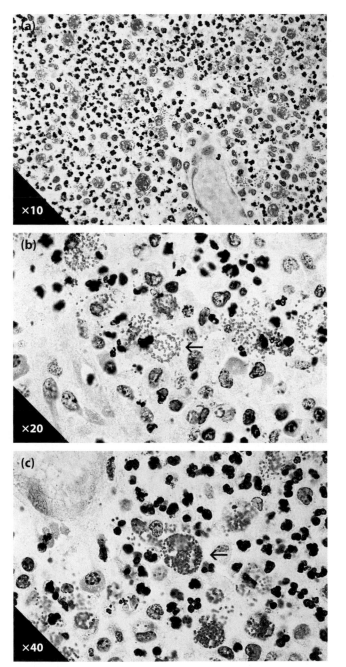

▲ **Fig. 5.62(a), (b) and (c)** Donovanosis. Warthin Starry stain showing the rod-shaped organisms of *C. granulomatis* in the cytoplasm of the histiocytes.

Laboratory diagnosis

Imprints stained with Giemsa stain may be diagnostic (see Fig. 5.64), but a simple smear taken from the surface of the lesion is usually not diagnosable because—unlike syphilis where the organisms are on the surface in the thick stratum corneum—the organisms are in histiocytes in the dermis: a superficial smear consists of pus and debris only.

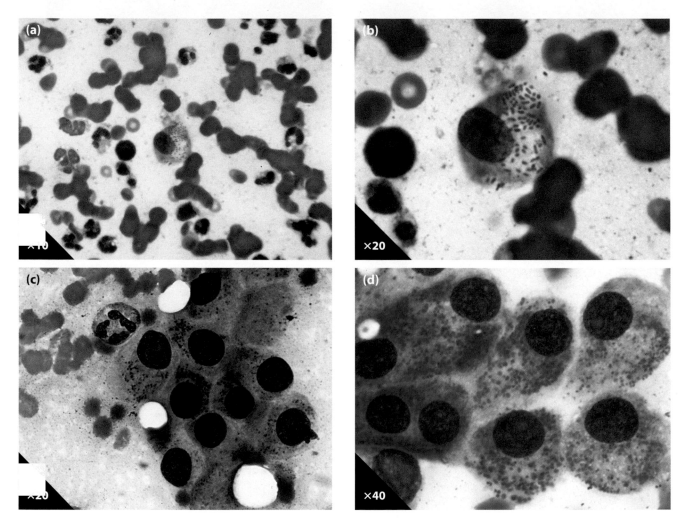

▲ ▶ **Fig. 5.64(a), (b), (c) and (d)** Donovanosis. Imprint smear stained with Giemsa stain. It shows the relative sizes of the histiocytes in comparison with red blood cells and lymphocytes, and the appearance of the intracellular organisms.

Correct procedure for laboratory diagnosis

1. Take a tiny biopsy snip. Dab it gently on a glass microscope slide in a few places. Immediately fix the smear in absolute alcohol.
2. Allow it to dry.
3. Send it to the laboratory for Giemsa staining.
4. Put any remaining tissue into a specimen bottle of formalin for histologic examination.
5. In a positive imprint smear, characteristic intracellular organisms are seen in the cytoplasm of histiocytes.

Formal skin biopsy results

A formal skin biopsy shows the following features.

- Surface ulceration with some epithelial hyperplasia in the epithelium adjacent to the ulcer.
- In the dermis, there is a heavy infiltration of acute and chronic inflammatory cells and numerous histiocytes with foamy cytoplasm (shown in Figs 5.65 and 5.66, continued overleaf).
- The *C. granulomatis* organisms are seen with a Warthin Starry stain in the cytoplasm of the histiocytes (seen earlier in Fig. 5.62 on page 135).
- The *C. granulomatis* organisms may also be seen by electron microscopy (seen earlier in Fig. 5.63 on page 135).
- Some medical professionals—who have written knowledgably about this area—recommend Giemsa stain on tissue sections as the best stain to demonstrate organisms, but this author prefers a Warthin Starry stain (seen earlier in Fig. 5.62 on page 135). A Giemsa stain (see Fig. 5.67, overleaf) is included here to compare with the Warthin Starry stain.
- The concentration of organisms varies from case to case.

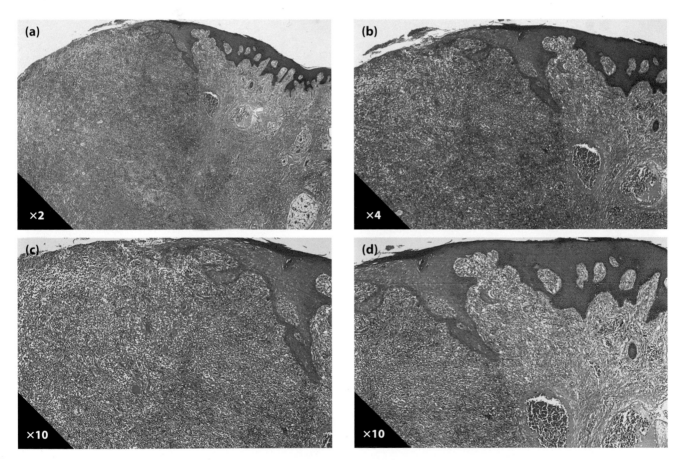

▲ ▶ **Fig. 5.65(a), (b), (c) and (d)** Donovanosis. Microscopic section of a biopsy of a lesion on the penis. It shows the ulceration, the epitheliomatous hyperplasia and the pattern of the inflammatory infiltration which extends throughout the dermis.

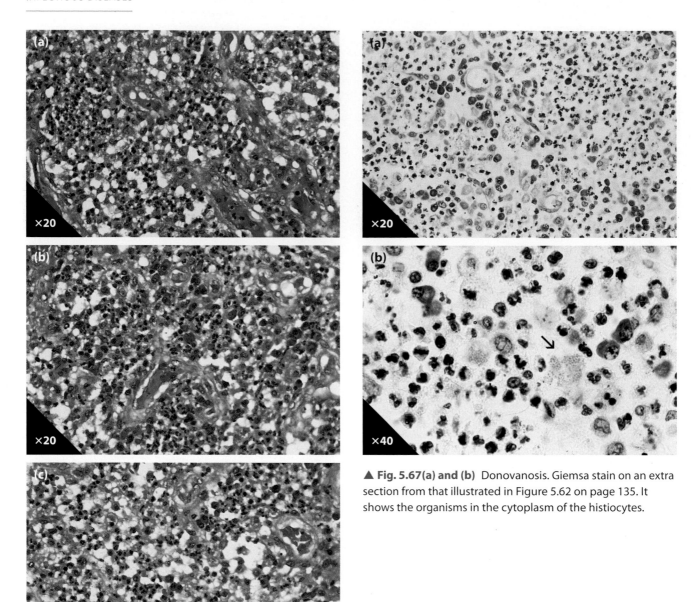

▲ **Fig. 5.67(a) and (b)** Donovanosis. Giemsa stain on an extra section from that illustrated in Figure 5.62 on page 135. It shows the organisms in the cytoplasm of the histiocytes.

▲ **Fig. 5.66(a), (b) and (c)** Donovanosis. Biopsy shows inflammatory infiltration and the histiocytes with foamy cytoplasm.

Case 5.4

A 23-year-old woman presented with pelvic pain and menorrhagia. Examination revealed that she had a 'frozen pelvis'.

Biopsy showed the presence of a chronic inflammatory reaction that included many histiocytes with foamy cytoplasm. Warthin Starry stain showed the presence of organisms consistent with *C. granulomatis* in the cytoplasm of the histiocytes, confirming a diagnosis of donovanosis (shown in Figs 5.68 and 5.69).

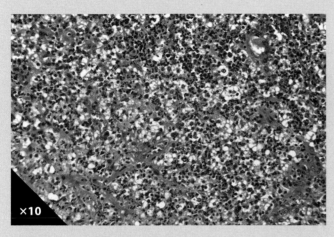

▲ **Fig. 5.68** Donovanosis. Biopsy of a pelvic lesion in a 23-year-old woman. The section showed the presence of a chronic inflammatory reaction that included many histiocytes with foamy cytoplasm.

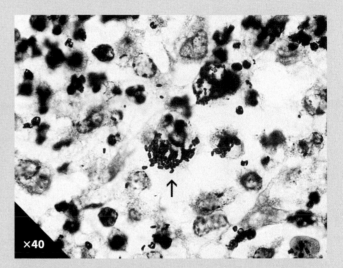

▲ **Fig. 5.69** Donovanosis. Warthin Starry stain showed the presence of organisms consistent with *C. granulomatis* in the cytoplasm of the histiocytes, confirming a diagnosis of donovanosis.

Case 5.5

A 30-year-old Caucasian male from Papua New Guinea, visiting Australia on his honeymoon, complained of ulcerated lesions at the base of his penis shortly after his marriage (see Fig. 5.70). A diagnosis of donovanosis was made.

The patient's new wife had similar lesions on the vulva (see Fig. 5.71). They were both treated with the appropriate antibiotic.

▼ **Fig. 5.70(a) and (b)** Donovanosis. A 30-year-old male complained of ulcerated lesions at the base of his penis.

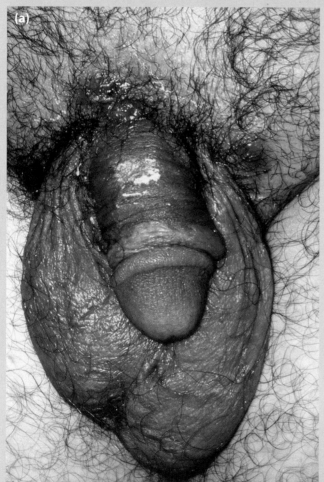

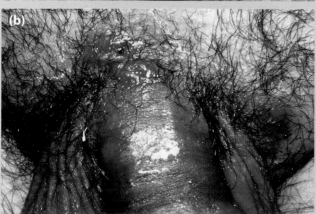

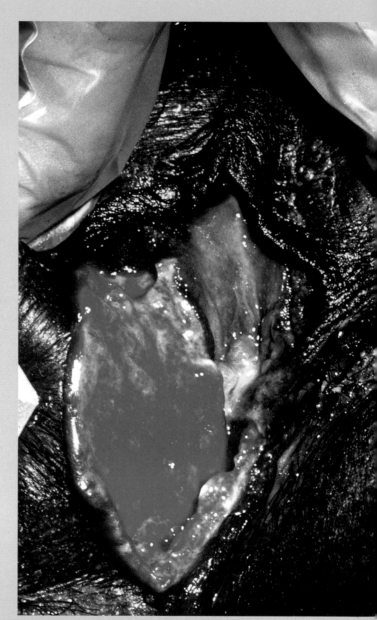

▲ **Fig. 5.71** Donovanosis. The wife of the patient in Figure 5.70 had a large, ulcerated lesion on the vulva.

Pubic lice

The louse *Phthirus pubis* attaches itself to the pubic hairs and causes itching (see Figs 5.72–5.75). The female louse attaches her eggs to the hair shafts. It is transmitted by direct contact or via contaminated clothing.

Scabies

Scabies is caused by the mite *Sarcoptes scabiei*. It is transmitted by direct contact or simply by contaminated clothing. The female mite burrows through the stratum corneum of the skin causing irritation and itching. The linear burrows can be seen on the surface of the skin (shown in Figs 5.76 and 5.77, overleaf).

By dissecting a burrow, a mite can be found at the advancing end (shown in Fig. 5.78 overleaf): this only serves to confirm the clinical diagnosis.

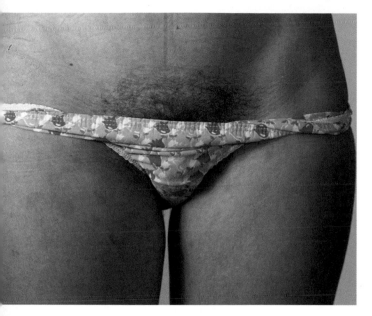

▲ **Fig. 5.72** An 18-year-old female complained of itching in the pubic area. Examination revealed the presence of scratch marks, and lice were recovered from the pubic hair.

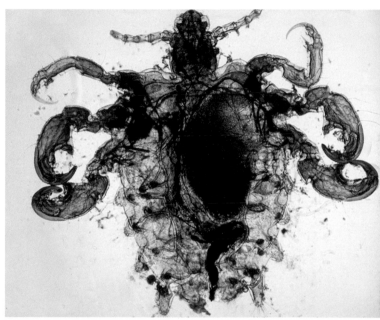

▲ **Fig. 5.74** Pubic louse (*Phthirus pubis*)—recovered from the pubic hair.

▼ **Fig. 5.75** Pubic louse and an egg attached to a pubic hair.

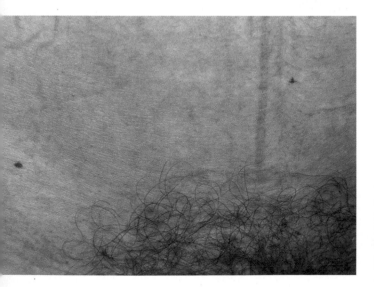

▲ **Fig. 5.73** Close inspection shows lice and eggs attached to the pubic hair.

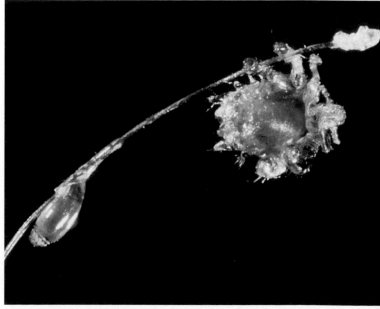

Case 5.6

A female, aged 86 years, had an itchy rash all over her body for some months. On close inspection, the rash consisted of multiple, linear, slightly elevated lesions. These had the appearance of linear burrows characteristic of scabies (shown in Figs 5.76 and 5.77). She was living alone which would have explained why she did not seek attention earlier.

One of the burrows was dissected and a mite was removed which confirmed the diagnosis (see Fig. 5.78). She was given appropriate curative treatment.

▶ **Fig. 5.76** Scabies rash. A female, aged 86 years, had an itchy rash all over her body for some months. She was living alone.

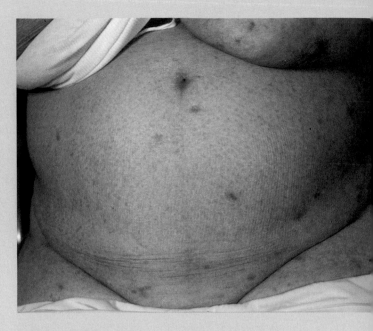

(a)

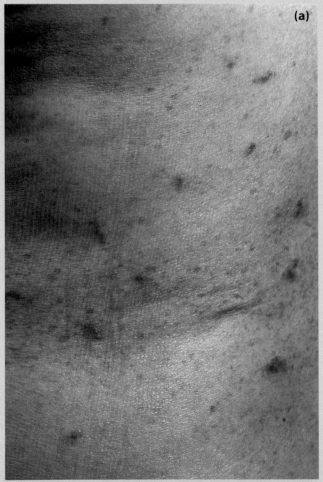

◀ **Fig. 5.77(a) and (b)** Red, linear burrows made by the scabies mites.

▼ **Fig. 5.78** *Sarcoptes scabiei* mite. Removed from one of the burrows on the abdomen of the patient shown in Figure 5.76.

(b)

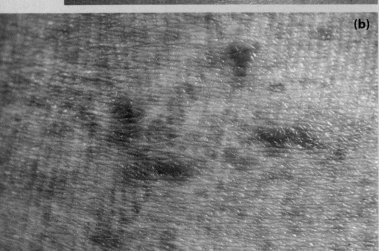

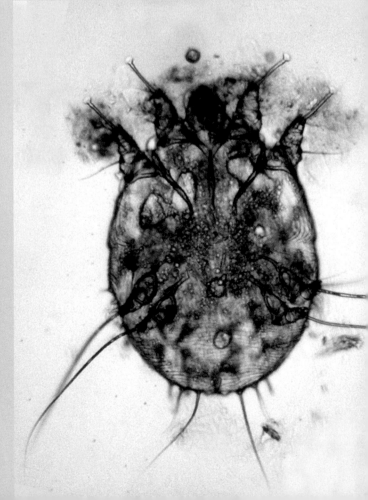

The *Sarcoptes scabiei* mites may occur anywhere on the body, and may sometimes be found on the penis (see Fig. 5.79).

A skin biopsy of a scabies lesion will show the presence of one or more mites in the stratum corneum of the skin (shown in Fig. 5.80). In the dermis, there may be little change, or there may be changes that occur in any arthropod infection, namely a mixed inflammatory cell infiltration that contains many eosinophils.

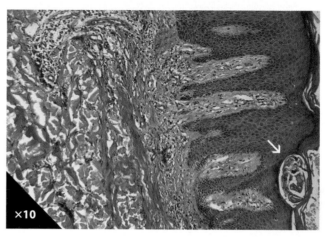

▲ **Fig. 5.80** Skin biopsy of a scabies lesion. The mite can be seen in cross section in the stratum corneum. There is virtually no inflammatory reaction in the dermis in this case.

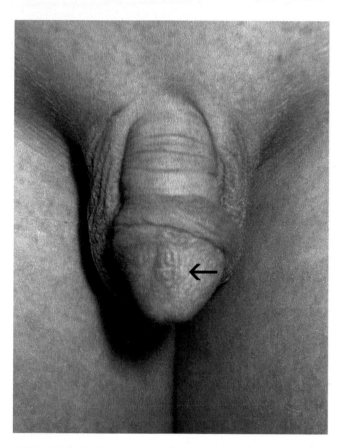

▲ **Fig. 5.79** Scabies lesion on the penis. The typical linear burrow can be seen on the penis of this male, aged 25 years. This infection was acquired by sexual contact.

Case 5.7

A 50-year-old man, living in the Solomon Islands in Melanesia (a nation east of Papua New Guinea), developed a rash on his left buttock. In 6 weeks, it had spread to involve his whole body—except his face. The skin was extremely itchy and the stratum corneum was markedly thickened. This condition is illustrated in Figure 5.81, overleaf.

The superficial layer of the skin was beginning to peel off and the thickened skin was riddled with burrows containing scabies mites. Microscopic examination of a piece of the shed skin showed grossly thickened stratum corneum that contained numerous burrows in which there were scabies mites.

No obvious cause was found as to why this patient developed such a severe infection.

Case 5.7 is a severe form of scabies, called Norwegian scabies. It was first described by the Norwegian leprologist Danielssen in 1848. It results in marked thickening of the skin all over the body. The thick keratin layer is riddled with burrows that contain numerous mites (illustrated in Fig. 5.81, overleaf). This condition may occur in patients who are malnourished or immune suppressed.

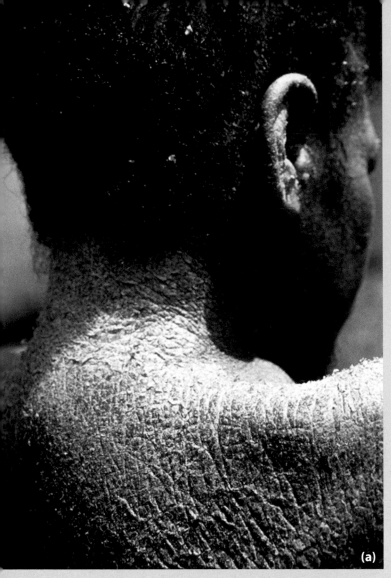

(a)

▲ **Fig. 5.81(a)** Scabies. This 50-year-old man from the Solomon Islands developed a rash on his left buttock. In 6 weeks, it had spread to involve his whole body—except his face. The skin was extremely itchy and the stratum corneum was markedly thickened.

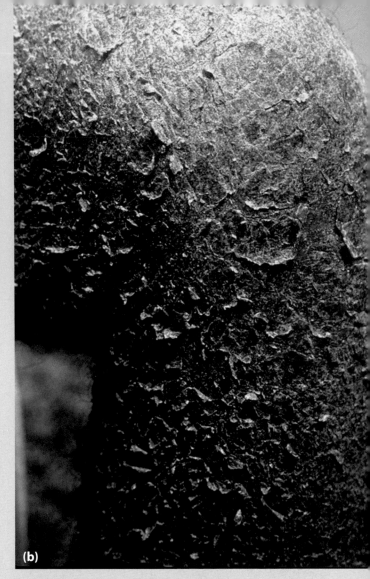

(b)

▲ **Fig. 5.81(b)** Scabies. The superficial layer of the skin was beginning to peel off.

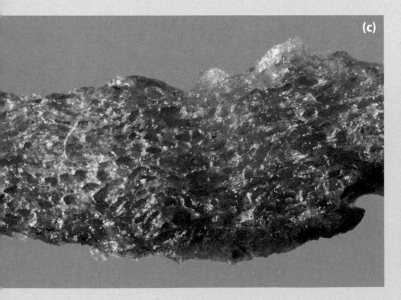

(c)

▲ **Fig. 5. 81(c)** Scabies. Piece of thickened skin that was riddled with burrows containing scabies mites.

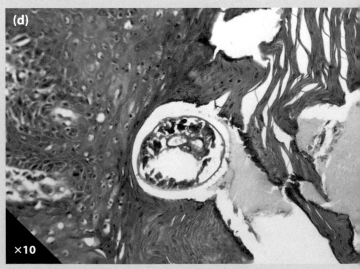

(d)

×10

▲ **Fig. 5.81(d)** Scabies. View of the skin biopsy of this patient showing two scabies mites in burrows at different levels in the thickened stratum corneum.

Mobiluncus

Mobiluncus is a newly recognized species of organism that can be seen in vaginal smears from sexually active women who present with a nonspecific vaginitis, which is recognized by the presence of a milky type of foul-smelling discharge. The diagnostic feature is the presence of epithelial cells, on whose surface are clustered numerous small, V-shaped or crescent-shaped bacilli that are variably Gram positive. These cells are called 'clue cells' (shown in Fig. 5.82).

The organisms on electron microscopic examination are curved with tapered ends and are motile by subpolar flagellae. They contain no lipopolysaccharide.

The organisms cannot be cultured and their etiologic role has not been established with certainty. However, the condition responds to treatment with ampicillin.

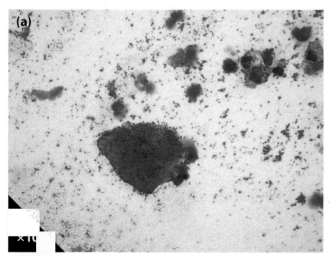

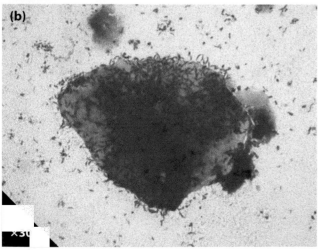

▲ **Fig. 5.82(a) and (b)** Mobiluncus. A 'clue cell' in a Gram stain from a high vaginal swab.

Acknowledgments

- Fig. 5.1 Courtesy of Margaret Mobbs, Brisbane, Australia.
- Fig. 5.2 Courtesy of Ross Forgan-Smith, Brisbane, Australia.
- Fig. 5.6 Courtesy of Margaret Mobbs, Brisbane, Australia.
- Figs 5.7, 5.8 and 5.10 Courtesy of Barry Smithurst, Brisbane, Australia.
- Fig. 5.14 Courtesy of Joan Faoagali, Brisbane, Australia.
- Fig. 5.15 Courtesy of Barry Smithurst, Brisbane, Australia.
- Fig. 5.17 A patient of John Richens, Papua New Guinea, photographed by Robin Cooke.
- Fig. 5.18 Courtesy of Barry Smithurst, Brisbane, Australia.
- Fig. 5.19 Courtesy of Anthony Moore, Townsville, Australia.
- Figs 5.20 and 5.21 Courtesy of John Tyrer, Brisbane, Australia.
- Fig. 5.23 Photographed courtesy of the Curator, Hunterian Museum, London.
- Figs 5.24 and 5.25 Photographed courtesy of the Curator, Dupuytren Museum, Ecole de Medicine, Paris.
- Figs 5.27 and 5.37 From Cooke, R.A. and Stewart, B., *Colour Atlas of Anatomical Pathology*, third edn, Churchill Livingstone, Edinburgh, 2004.
- Fig. 5.40 Courtesy of Ian Davies, Brisbane, Australia.
- Fig. 5.41 Courtesy of John Earwaker, Brisbane, Australia.
- Fig. 5.42 Courtesy of Walter Wood, Brisbane, Australia.
- Fig. 5.61 Courtesy of John Biggs, Brisbane, Australia.
- Fig. 5.63 Courtesy of Geoffrey Strutton, Brisbane, Australia.
- Figs 5.68 and 5.69 Case report. Courtesy of Prasantha Murthy, Papua New Guinea & Griffith, Australia.
- Figs 5.70 and 5.71 Courtesy of John Biggs, Brisbane, Australia.
- Figs 5.72–5.75 Case report. Courtesy of Veronica Hart, Brisbane, Australia.
- Figs 5.76–5.78 Case report. Courtesy of Veronica Hart, Brisbane, Australia.
- Fig. 5.79 Courtesy of Graeme Beardmore, Brisbane, Australia.
- Fig. 5.81 Case report. Courtesy of Ian Wilkey, Papua New Guinea and Brisbane, Australia.
- Fig. 5.82 Courtesy of Joan Faoagali, Brisbane, Australia.

6

Atypical mycobacterial infections, rickettsial infections, yaws and colonic spirochetosis

Atypical mycobacterial infections

Atypical mycobacteria are a group of acid-fast bacilli (AFB) that have different properties and different pathogenicity from *Mycobacterium tuberculosis*. They were recognized at about the same time as the *M. tuberculosis*, in 1882, but it is only in the past 40 years that their clinical and pathologic manifestations have been clarified. The clinical and pathologic features of some of these infections are illustrated here.

The atypical mycobacteria are environmental organisms, which when inoculated through the skin cause infection—with skin and connective tissue suppurative, granulomatous or necrotic inflammation. If they are inhaled, they can cause pulmonary infection.

In Australia:

- The most common causes of skin infections are the rapidly growing atypical mycobacteria, which include *Mycobacterium abscessus*, *Mycobacterium chelonae* and *Mycobacterium fortuitum*.
- The most common cause of respiratory infections is the *Mycobacterium avium* complex.
- *Mycobacterium marinum* is an important cause of skin and connective tissue infection in the setting of marine or fish tank exposure.
- Lymphadenitis in children is commonly caused by *Mycobacterium avium* complex and *Mycobacterium scrofulaceum*.

In many tropical countries:

- *Mycobacterium ulcerans* is an important cause of aggressive debilitating necrotizing ulceration of the skin.

Worldwide:

- In immunosupressed patients, in particular those with human immunodeficiency virus (HIV)/AIDS, disseminated infection with *M. avium* complex was common prior to the advent of effective antiviral therapy.

Mycobacterium ulcerans

In 1897 the English physician Albert Cook working in Uganda, Africa, described skin ulcers that were characterized by the presence of marked undermining of the skin. In 1948 a group headed by Peter MacCallum at the Alfred Hospital in Melbourne, Australia, reported a series of 6 patients with this type of skin ulceration from the small town of Bairnsdale, north of Melbourne. Glen Buckle, the microbiologist at the hospital, was unable to grow an organism using ordinary culture techniques. However, he did grow an organism that was identified as *M. ulcerans* on Lowenstein Jensen media that was left at room temperature on the laboratory bench. It was then realized that this was a disease with a worldwide distribution, particularly in certain tropical countries.

The source of the organism in nature is not known for certain. It has been postulated that some native fauna may provide an animal reservoir for the organism. Recent research has shown the presence of *M. ulcerans* DNA in the salivary glands of some insects, but transmission by this means has not been proven.

Clinical appearance

The *M. ulcerans* lesion begins as a small ulcer, usually on a limb, that rapidly expands by necrosis of the subcutaneous tissue caused by the toxin mycolactone. This expansion is recognized by the redness that extends well beyond the ulcer itself (illustrated in Figs 6.1, 6.2 and 6.3, continued overleaf).

Case 6.1

A young child was referred from remote north Queensland, Australia, to a Brisbane hospital. She presented with a small ulcer, surrounded by a wide area of redness on the right upper arm. This is a typical *M. ulcerans* ulcer (see Fig. 6.1).

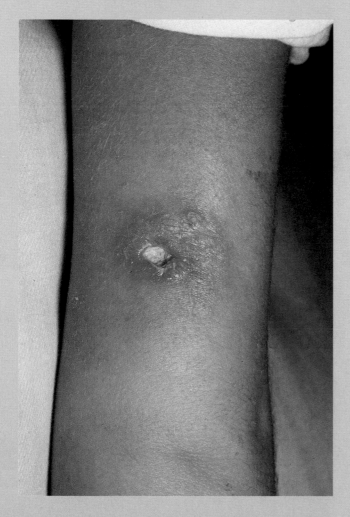

◀ **Fig. 6.1** *M. ulcerans* ulcer. This young child from north Queensland, Australia, presented with a typical *M. ulcerans* ulcer on her right upper arm. The ulcer is small but there is a wide area of redness around it. This indicates the extent of the necrosis of the subcutaneous tissue around the ulcer.

Case 6.2

A child from Papua New Guinea presented with an extensively undermined ulcer over the sacral region of his lower back (see Fig. 6.2).

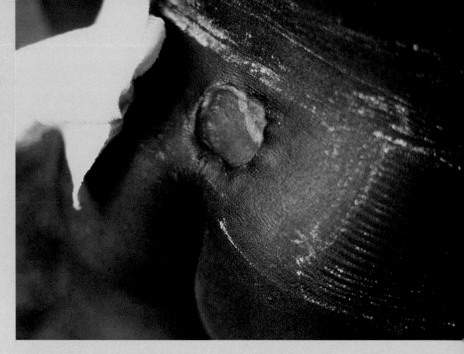

▶ **Fig. 6.2** *M. ulcerans* ulcer. A child from Papua New Guinea presented with an *M. ulcerans* ulcer over the sacral region of his lower back.

Case 6.3

A young child from Papua New Guinea presented with multiple, communicating, undermined ulcers on his right thigh—extending over the knee and into the upper lower leg. This condition and the extent of the undermining is illustrated in Figure 6.3.

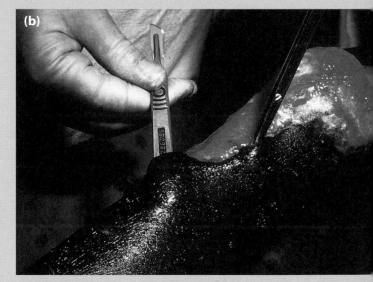

▲ **Fig. 6.3(b)** The extent of the undermining of this *M. ulcerans* ulcer was assessed prior to surgery.

▼ **Fig. 6.3(c)** The affected area was widely excised in readiness for a skin graft to be applied.

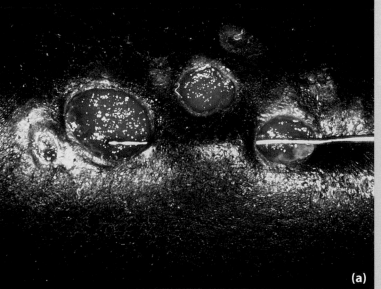

(a)

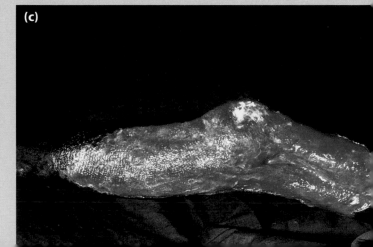

(c)

▲ **Fig. 6.3(a)** *M. ulcerans* ulcers on the thigh. A child from Papua New Guinea has multiple undermined *M. ulcerans* ulcers on his thigh.

Diagnosis

- Acid-fast bacilli (AFB) can be identified in a smear made from the necrotic tissue in the undermined area at the edge of the ulcer.
- Skin biopsy taken from the edge of the ulcer shows extensive necrosis of subcutaneous tissue with little inflammatory cell reaction (see Fig. 6.4). Myriads of AFB are present in the necrotic tissue (see Fig. 6.5). In longstanding ulcers, the inflammatory reaction is granulomatous and organisms are sparse or absent.
- Culture on Lowenstein Jensen media incubated at room temperature yields a growth of the infecting organism (see Fig. 6.6).
- Rapid polymerase chain reaction (PCR) tests are being developed.

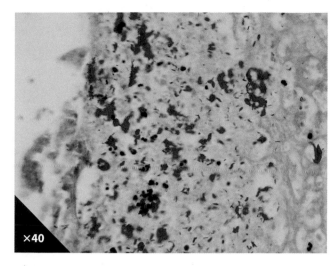

▲ **Fig. 6.5** Ziehl Neelsen (ZN) stain shows myriads of acid-fast bacilli are present in the necrotic tissue.

▼ **Fig. 6.4(a) and (b)** Skin biopsy viewed at low and medium magnification shows extensive necrosis of subcutaneous tissue with little inflammatory cell reaction.

▼ **Fig. 6.6** Lowenstein Jensen slope with a culture of *M. ulcerans* incubated at room temperature 86–95°F (30–35°C) yields a growth of the infecting organism.

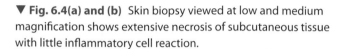
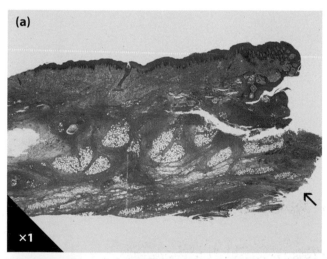

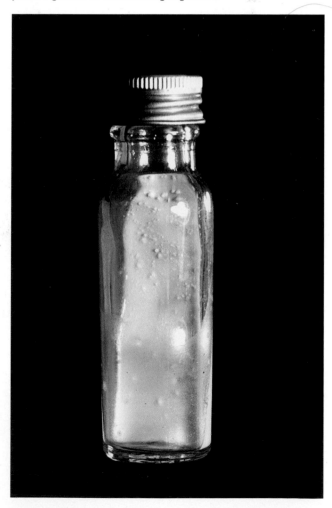

Treatment

The *M. ulcerans* lesion must be excised widely to remove all the affected skin and subcutaneous tissue, as shown in Figure 6.3(c) on page 148.

Mycobacterium scrofulaceum

Lymphadenopathy in children is usually caused by *M. avium* complex or *M. scrofulaceum*. Typically, this presents as an inflammatory mass near the angle of the mandible (see Fig. 6.7). The mass is often adherent to the skin, and it may sometimes form a discharging sinus. It is cured by surgical excision.

The clinical and pathologic appearances of lymphadenopathy are illustrated in Figures 6.7–6.11.

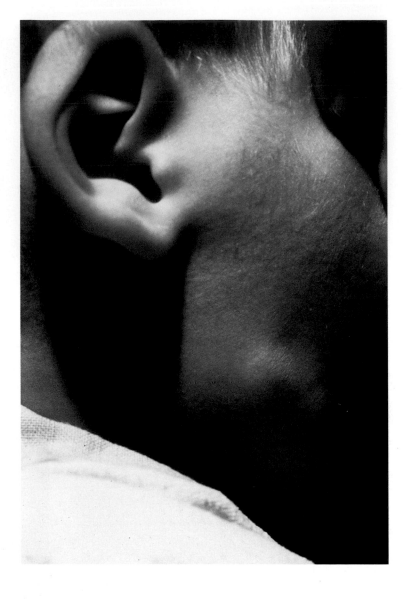

▶ **Fig. 6.7** Lymphadenopathy. This child has a well-circumscribed, subcutaneous, inflammatory mass attached to the skin, just anterior to the angle of the right mandible.

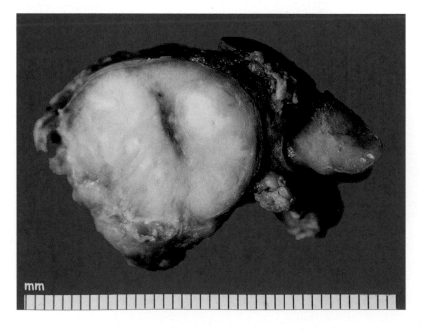

◀ **Fig. 6.8** Lymphadenopathy. The inflammatory mass (seen in Fig. 6.7) was excised and it consisted of a lymph node that had been replaced by a mass of firm, white tissue.

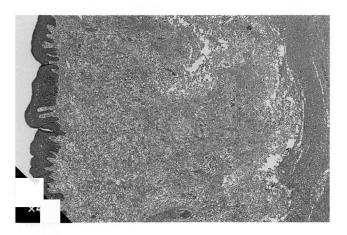

▲ **Fig. 6.9** Lymphadenopathy. The inflammatory tissue can be seen in the dermis of the skin that overlies the lymph node.

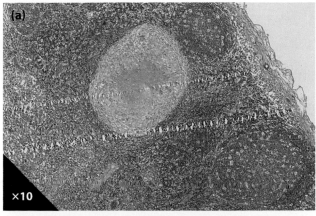

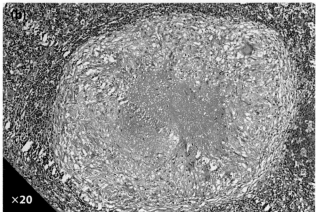

▲ **Fig. 6.11(a) and (b)** Lymphadenopathy. The granulomas can be seen to have nercotic centers in which there are very few cells. Acid-fast bacilli are found only very infrequently in tissue sections, but culture is more likely to be positive for the organism.

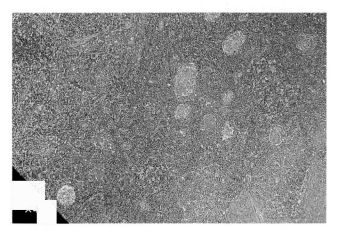

▲ **Fig. 6.10** Lymphadenopathy. The lymph node can be seen to be infiltrated by multiple pale granulomas.

Mycobacterium marinum

Infection with *M. marinum* occurs from injuries inflicted by the fins of fish and crustaceans. It is most likely to be acquired by people who fish or people who keep fish in domestic fish tanks. The lesions appear as red, indolent nodules on hands or elbows. The clinical and pathologic appearances of this condition are illustrated in Figures 6.12 and 6.13 overleaf.

Case 6.4

An elderly lady developed red, nodular lesions on the dorsum of her left hand over the metacarpophalangeal joint of her index finger, as illustrated in Figure 6.12(a) and (b).

She also had a nodular, ulcerated lesion on the outer aspect of her right, upper arm—just above the elbow joint, as illustrated in Figure 6.12(c) and (d). These lesions developed some time after cleaning her fish tank.

The microscopic appearance of a biopsy of the lesion on this patient's upper arm is demonstrated in Figure 6.13.

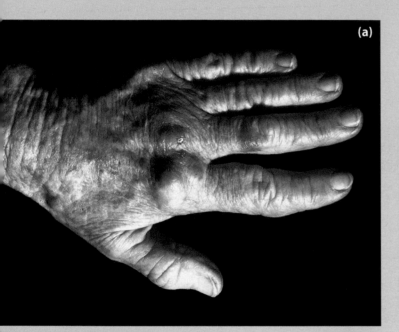

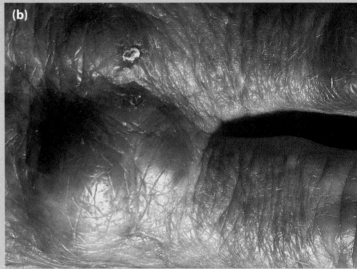

◀▼ Fig. 6.12 *M. marinum*—red nodular lesions. An elderly lady, after cleaning her fish tank, developed red, nodular lesions on her left hand and right elbow. **(a) and (b)** Dorsum of left hand and metacarpophalangeal joint of index finger. **(c) and (d)** Right elbow.

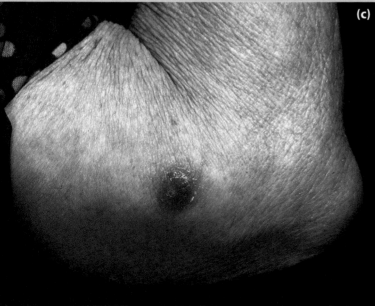

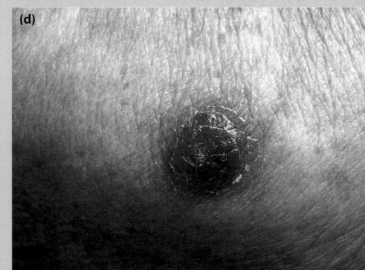

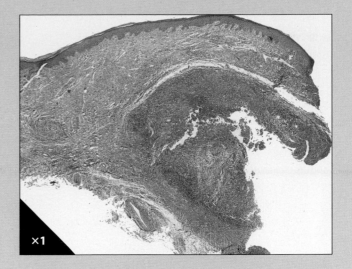

▶ **Fig. 6.13** *M. marinum*—skin biopsy. Extensive necrosis of the mid and lower dermis and upper subcutaneous tissue, with little inflammatory cell infiltration. Acid-fast bacilli were present in the necrotic tissue. (The microscopic appearances in an *M. marinum* skin biopsy are similar to those seen in *M. ulcerans* lesions.)

×1

Mycobacterium avium complex

M. avium has appeared as one of the many opportunistic infections in patients with AIDS. AIDS patients have T-cell immune deficiency similar to that encountered in lepromatous leprosy. The microscopic reaction caused by *M. avium* is similar to that in lepromatous leprosy in that it consists of a proliferation of histiocytes filled with acid-fast bacilli and there are virtually no other inflammatory cells in the reaction.

Two cases of *M. avium* infection are illustrated here. Figures 6.14, 6.15 and 6.16, overleaf, describe an AIDS patient with abdominal infection and Figures 6.17, 6.18 and 6.19, overleaf, describe an AIDS patient with infection of the liver.

Case 6.5

A young man with AIDS had a computed tomography (CT) scan of the abdomen as part of the assessment of his condition. This showed marked enlargement of his para aortic lymph nodes (see Fig. 6.14, overleaf).

Malignant lymphoma is a common complication of AIDS and the question asked was 'Does he have a malignant lymphoma?' A biopsy of one of the enlarged nodes was done and the microscopic appearances of this are illustrated in Figures 6.15 and 6.16, overleaf.

When a pathologist is examining biopsy material from any patient with AIDS, M. avium *infection is one of those that must be considered. In gut biopsies from almost anywhere in the gastrointestinal tract, for example, nodules formed by collections of histiocytes filled with acid-fast bacilli appear in the lamina propria of mucosal biopsies.*

Sometimes, the organisms induce a fibroblastic reaction that produces a 'pseudo soft tissue tumorous mass' that may cause diagnostic difficulties for the pathologist.

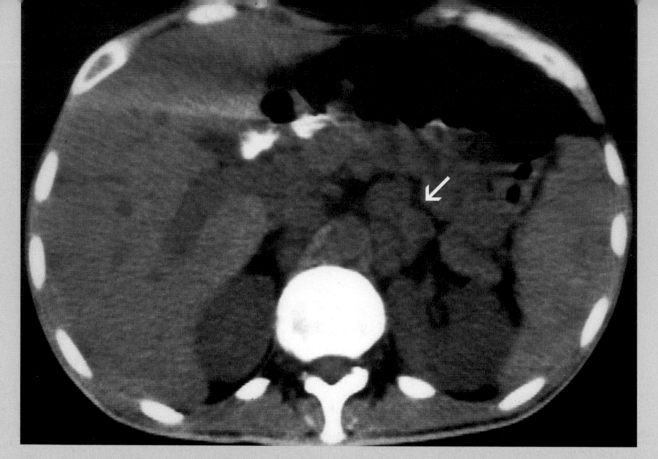

▲ **Fig. 6.14** CT scan of the abdomen of a young man with AIDS. It shows marked enlargement of his para aortic lymph nodes.

▼ **Fig. 6.15(a)** Biopsy of one of the lymph nodes was done. At this low magnification, the shape of the lymph node is retained, but no blue staining lymphoid tissue can be seen. It is staining a pink color.

▼ **Fig. 6.15(b)** At higher magnification, it can be seen that the infiltration consists of histiocytes with clear cytoplasm. Small numbers of lymphocytes were present, too.

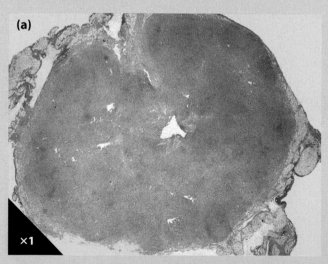

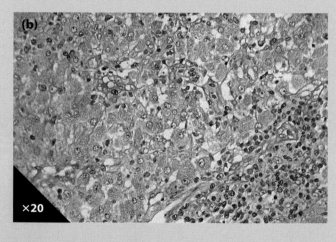

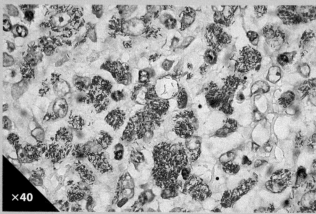

▶ **Fig. 6.16** Ziehl Neelsen (ZN) stain showed that the histiocytes were packed with acid-fast bacilli. The pattern of involvement was consistent with an *M. avium* infection.

| **154** |

Case 6.6

A young man with AIDS was found to have a palpably enlarged liver and mildly abnormal liver function tests. A CT scan showed multiple lucent lesions through his liver (see Fig. 6.17).

The microscopic appearances of the liver biopsy are illustrated in Figures 6.18 and 6.19.

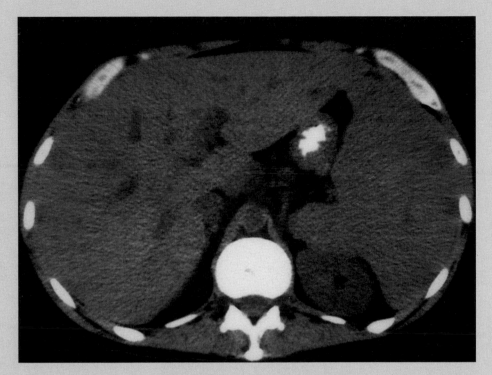

▲ **Fig. 6.17** CT scan of the liver of a young man with AIDS. It shows a palpably enlarged liver. Multiple lesions through the liver are seen.

◄ **Fig. 6.18(a) and (b)** Liver biopsy showed multiple granulomas distributed through the liver.

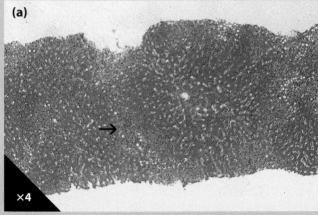

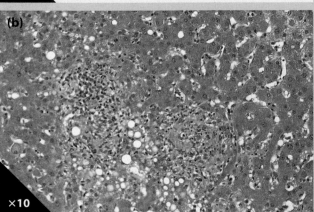

▼ **Fig. 6.19** ZN stain showed the presence of acid-fast bacilli in the granulomas, confirming the presence of *M. avium* infection.

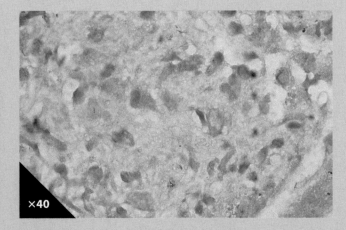

Vibrio vulnificus

V. vulnificus is not an atypical mycobacterium, but its clinical features, microscopic appearances and treatment are similar to those of *M. ulcerans*.

It usually occurs in fishermen who scratch themselves on the spiny shells of crustaceans. The ulcer spreads rapidly, with extensive undermining of the skin caused by necrosis of the subcutaneous tissue. The salient features of this infection are illustrated in Figure 6.20. Diagnosis is confirmed by culture of the organism. These ulcers are cured by wide excision (see Fig. 6.21).

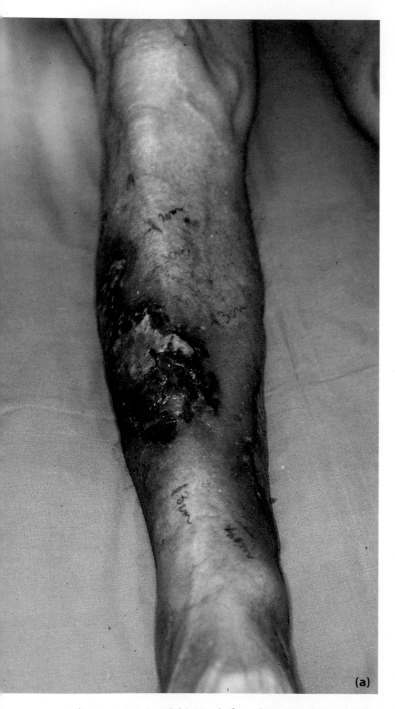 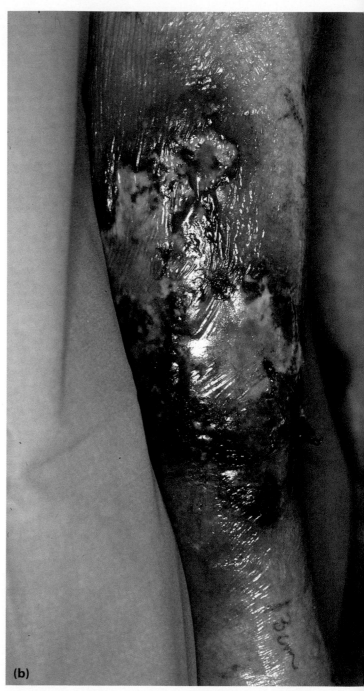

(a) **(b)**

▲ ▶ **Fig. 6.20(a) and (b)** *V. vulnificus* ulcers. This fisherman scratched his arms and legs on the spiny shells of crustaceans. (Similar lesions may follow scratches from coral.) He developed ulcers that spread rapidly.

▼ ▶ **Fig. 6.21(a), (b) and (c)** The *V. vulnificus* ulcers of the patient shown in Fig. 6.20 were cured by wide excision, followed by skin grafting.

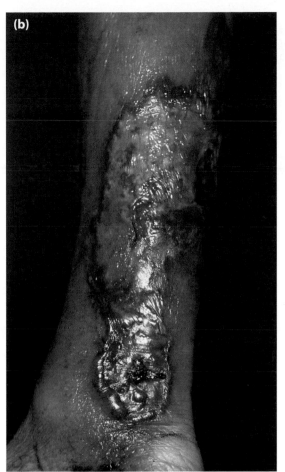

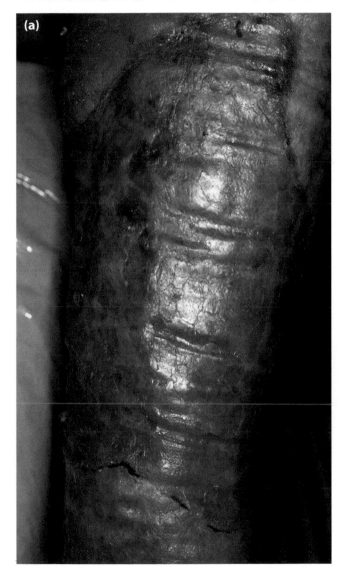

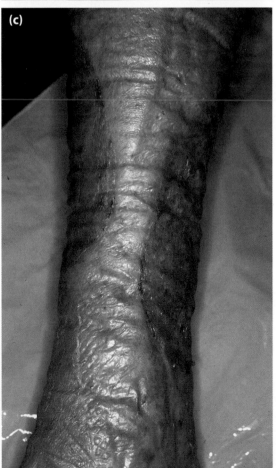

Rickettsial infections

Rickettsiae are small, intracellular organisms that can just be seen by a light microscope. Rickettsial infections can be considered as falling into four groups. These infectons are all transmitted by an arthropod vector, except Q fever (*Coxiella burnetii*)—which is transmitted by aerosols.

The four groups of Rickettsial infections are as follows.

- **Spotted fever group**
  Rocky Mountain spotted fever (*Rickettsia rickettsii*). Transmitted by ticks.
  Other rickettsiae—one of which is Australian spotted fever (*Rickettsia australis*). Transmitted by ticks.
- **Typhus group**
  Epidemic typhus (*Rickettsia prowazekii*). Transmitted by body louse.
  Murine (endemic) typhus (*Rickettsia typhi*, formerly *Rickettsia mooseri*). Transmitted by fleas.
- **Scrub typhus**
  Scrub typhus (*Orientia tsutsugamushi*. Formerly *Rickettsia tsutsugamushi*). Transmitted by mites.
- **Q fever**
  Q fever (*Coxiella burnetii*). Transmitted by aerosols.

Three rickettsial diseases are presented here, each one from a different group of organisms: Australian spotted fever, scrub typhus and Q fever.

Australian spotted fever (*R. australis*)

Tickborne spotted fever has been formally recognized in Australia since 1946, when a case series was reported in army recruits training in north Queensland. A Rickettsia was isolated and named *Rickettsia australis*. The name 'Queensland tick typhus' (QTT) has been used to describe the illness characterized by eschar, rash, fever and headache following tick bite.

Subsequent reports indicate that the geographic range of *R. australis* infection extends along virtually the whole eastern seaboard of Australia, east of the Great Dividing Range, including parts of suburban Sydney, leading to the more general term of Australian spotted fever (ASF).

The *Ixodes holocyclus* tick is the main vector of ASF (see Figs 6.22, 6.23 and 6.24). In 1991, cases of ASF acquired on Flinders Island in Bass Strait, in the south-eastern waters of Australia, were shown to be caused by a new rickettsial species (*Rickettsia honei*). Other clusters of spotted fever have been recognized on mainland Tasmania, as well as in parts of South Australia and Western Australia.

The most common manifestations of ASF are local reaction at the bite site, with local necrosis producing an eschar (ulcer) or 'tache noire' as shown in Figure 6.25(a), with a generalized rash as shown in Figure 6.25(b), and headache, fever, myalgia and arthralgia. The rash may be absent. When present, it varies from macular to maculopapular, vesicular,

▶ **Fig. 6.22** *R. australis* infection. Site of a tick bite on the mid-anterior neck of a middle-aged male. The *Ixodes holocyclus* tick and the surrounding skin was excised *in toto* for sectioning.

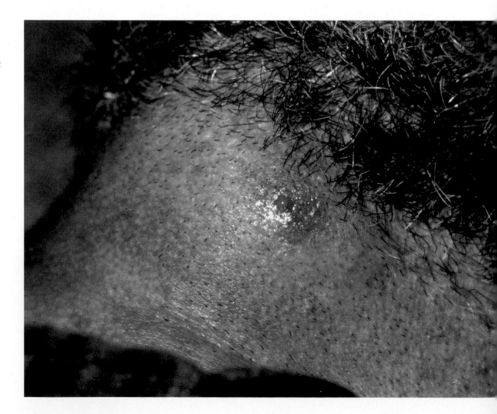

pustular or hemorrhagic in nature. Commonly, the vesicular rash is misdiagnosed as chickenpox or staphylococcal skin infection.

Death from ASF is rare, with most persons recovering over 14 days without treatment. Resolution of illness is generally more rapid when treated with doxycycline, but the rash may take a week or more to completely resolve with or without treatment.

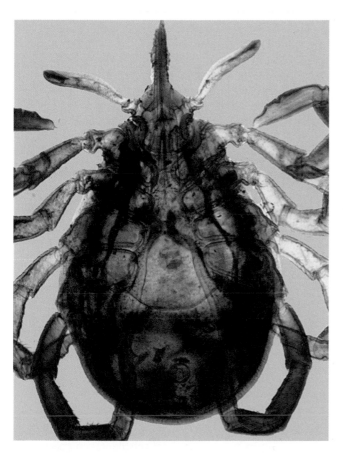

▲ **Fig. 6.23** *Ixodes holocyclus* tick is the vector of *R. australis*.

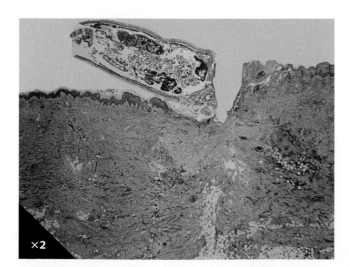

▲ **Fig. 6.24** *R. australis* infection. View of an *Ixodes holocyclus* biting tick on the skin surface of the patient in Figure 6.22. It is causing a tissue reaction in the dermis.

▼ **Fig. 6.25(a)** Eschar on the back, where a young woman from Sydney, Australia, had been bitten by a tick. **(b)** The typical erythematous, maculopapular rash caused by infection with *R. australis*.

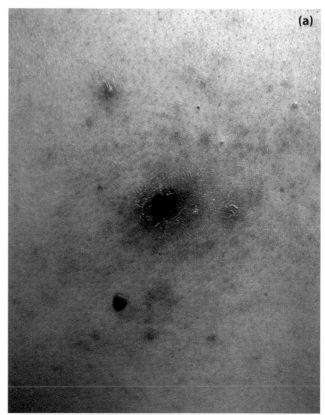

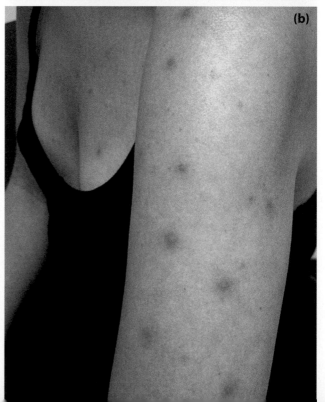

Scrub typhus (*Orientia tsutsugamushi*)

Scrub typhus is a debilitating febrile illness that is transmitted to humans by the bite of a mite. The *O. tsutsugamushi* organism is endemic in a number of different species of wild rodents and is transmitted by the bite of the mites. It is prevalent in the islands of the Western Pacific Ocean, in the northern parts of Australia, and in many parts of South-East Asia. Humans become infected when they enter the habitat of the mites.

Case 6.7

A 30-year-old male presented in Papua New Guinea with a high fever, headache and muscle pain. Examination revealed an eschar (ulcer) on his left leg, at the site where he would have been bitten by a mite (see Fig. 6.26). He had been working in dense forest when bitten.

Following treatment with chloramphenicol (the only broad-spectrum antibiotic available at the time in the hospital), his fever fell rapidly and he recovered (see Fig. 6.27).

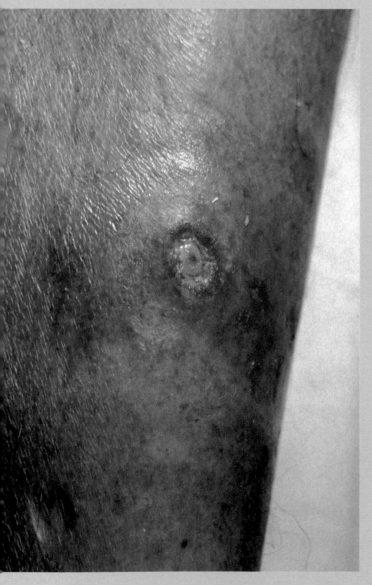

▲ **Fig. 6.26** Eschar (ulcer) caused by the bite of a mite. A 30-year-old male, who was working in Papua New Guinea, presented with fever and an eschar (ulcer) on his left leg.

▼ **Fig. 6.27** Temperature chart from the patient in Figure 6.26, shows the rapid drop in temperature that resulted from treatment with chloramphenicol.

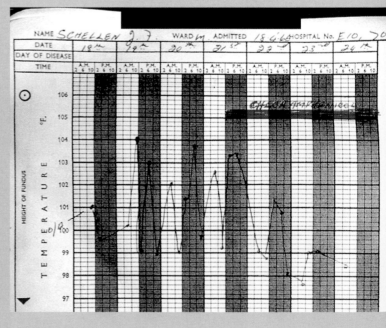

During the war in the Pacific Ocean in the 1940s, the soldiers of the opposing armies were often attacked by mites that gave them scrub typhus. It is a debilitating illness and often there were many soldiers rendered unfit for duty as a result of this illness.

Q fever (*Coxiella burnetii*)

Q fever is a serious disease of abattoir workers and farmers. Residents living near an abattoir, particularly if they are 'downwind' of it, are also at risk of infection. Humans are infected by aerosol droplets from placentas of infected cattle, sheep, goats and pigs and, occasionally, by aerosol droplets from indigenous marsupial animals. The *C. burnetii* organism is very resistant to drying, and can also be spread to humans by dust that was contaminated—often months before the human infection—by aerosol droplets from placentas and the birth fluids of the above-named animals.

The clinical presentation of Q fever is with fever, severe photophobia, headache and muscle pain. Unlike other rickettsial diseases, there is no skin rash.

Pneumonia may sometimes be a presenting symptom. Diagnosis is confirmed by serologic testing. The disease responds to doxycylcine. Most patients recover completely, but there is an occasional death from fulminant hepatitis.

Increasingly, long-term complications are being recognized. These include bacterial endocarditis; some low-grade hematologic lymphoma-like conditions; and some chronic granulomatous conditions, for example granulomatous orchitis.

An effective vaccine is now available to prevent infection and workers at risk of infection are being vaccinated.

Q fever was identified, and its organismal cause found, by Edward Derrick (1898–1976), a pathologist in Brisbane, Australia. He thought that it was a peculiar disease confined to a small area in Australia, but it soon become clear that it had a worldwide distribution.

Just before the definitive paper* on Q fever was published in 1937, Derrick performed a post mortem on his first encounter with a fatal case of Q fever. The patient was a young butcher who worked at the Brisbane abattoir. He had died from liver failure and his liver showed changes (shown in Fig. 6.28), now known to be caused by Q fever. Derrick confirmed the diagnosis by using the serologic test he had devised for Q fever diagnosis, and found it was positive both on serum taken during life and a sample taken at post mortem.

This was the first fatal case of Q fever to be recognized, and this case was the first instance of Workers' Compensation paid under Australian law for an occupational exposure to Q fever.

Derrick did not publish the case. The liver section and the post-mortem report were found in the archives of the Department of Forensic Medicine, Brisbane, by Dr David Williams.

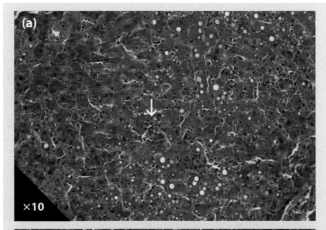

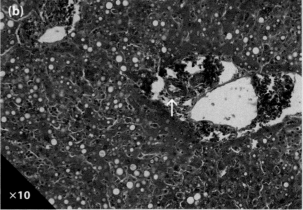

▲ **Fig. 6.28** Section of liver from the post mortem in 1937 of the first recorded death from Q fever. **(a)** There are focal areas of acute hepatitis, as seen by hepatocyte necrosis associated with collections of neutrophils. **(b)** There is hyaline change in the walls of the vessels in portal tracts.

*Derrick, E.H., 'Q' fever, a new fever entity: clinical features, diagnosis and laboratory investigation, Med J Aust 2: 281–299. No. 5. 1937.

Figure 6.29 shows, for comparison with the original Q fever case of 1937, the liver changes in a more recent case, in which the diagnosis was confirmed by modern serologic tests.

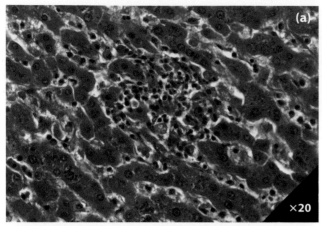

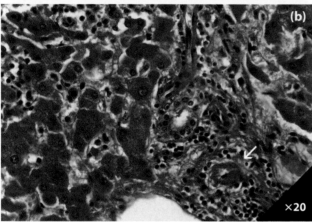

▲ **Fig. 6.29(a) and (b)** Section of liver. A case of Q fever in 2004, proven by modern serologic tests, showing similar changes to those seen in Figure 6.28 on page 161.

Famous early rickettsiologists

The photographs in Figures 6.30–6.35 were found by the author among the papers left in Brisbane by the Australian pathologist Edward Derrick. The papers were sent to him by Derrick's colleagues, who significantly contributed to our understanding of rickettsial diseases. These photographs are of historical interest.

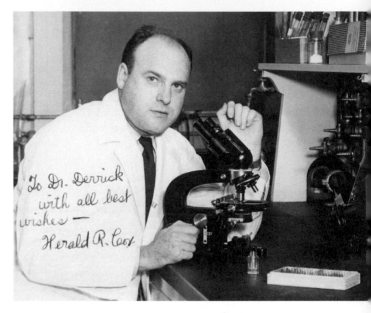

▲ **Fig. 6.30** Herald Cox, associated with Q fever and the name *Coxiella*.

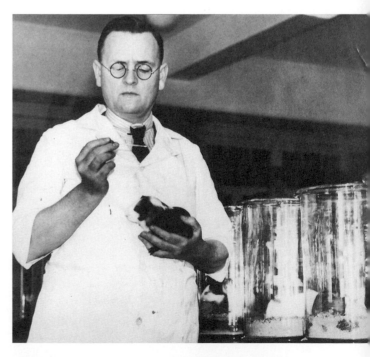

▲ **Fig. 6.31** Edward (Ted) Derrick (1898–1976), who first described the clinical features of Q fever and identified the causative organism. He is measuring the rectal temperature of one of the guinea pigs used to identify the causative organism of Q fever.

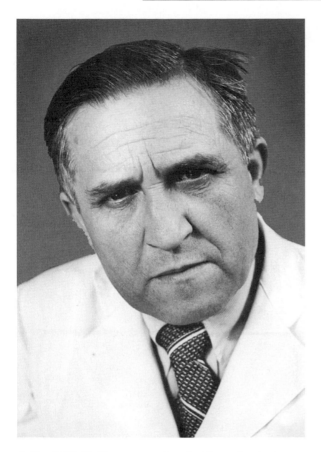

▲ **Fig. 6.32** M. Mooser associated with murine typhus (*R. mooseri* (*R. typhi*)).

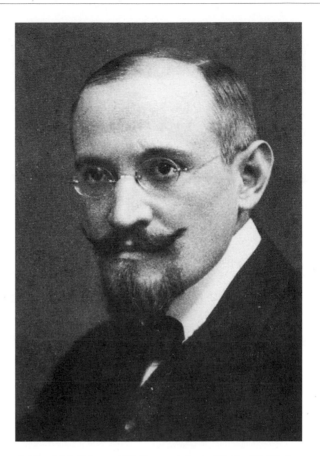

▲ **Fig. 6.34** Edmund Weil, associated with the Weil Felix reaction.

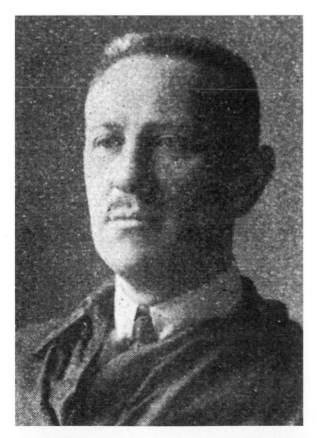

▲ **Fig. 6.33** J.V. Prowazek, associated with epidemic typhus (*R. prowazekii*).

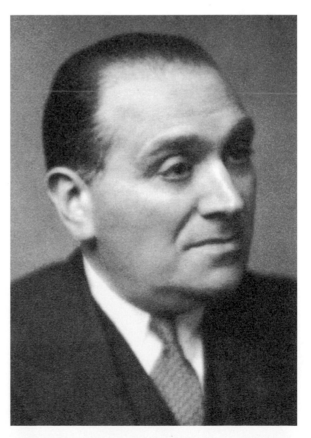

▲ **Fig. 6.35** Arthur Felix, associated with the Weil Felix reaction.

Weil Felix reaction

The Weil Felix reaction was an early test used to diagnose rickettsial infections. It was based on the fact that an antigen of the OXK strain of the Proteus organism cross reacted with antibodies produced by the rickettsiae that caused murine typhus, epidemic typhus, scrub typhus and Rocky Mountain spotted fever. It was negative in Q fever. This test has been superseded by specific antibody tests for the individual causative organisms.

Yaws

Yaws is a disease caused by the spirochete *Treponema pertenue*. The most easily recognized feature of the disease is the presence of one, but more often multiple, ulcerated, hyperkeratotic lesions on the skin. Transmission seems to be by skin-to-skin contact. Thus, in any community many people are affected (as illustrated in Figs 6.36, 6.37 and 6.38).

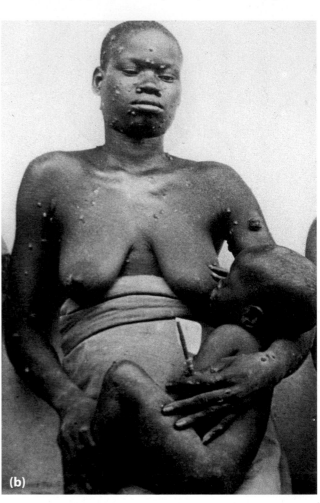

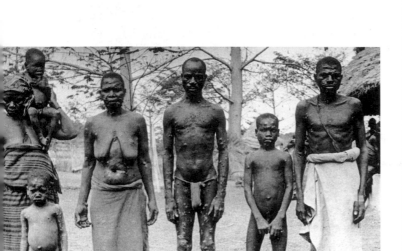

▲ ▶ **Fig. 6.36(a) and (b)** Villagers in tropical Africa in 1934. They are covered with yaws lesions. In those times, yaws was an important and common disease in most tropical countries. It was an uncomfortable and unsightly disease that could be recognized by everyone.

▼ **Fig. 6.37(a) and (b)** Villagers with yaws in the Southern Highlands of Papua New Guinea in 1976.

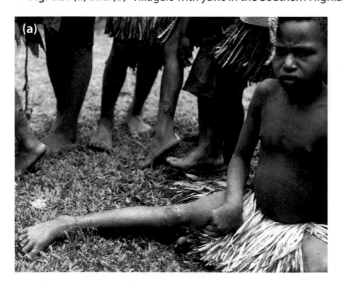

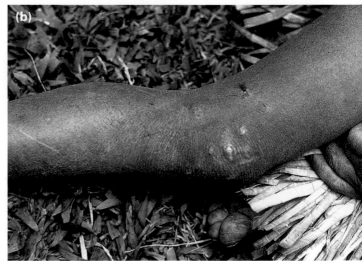

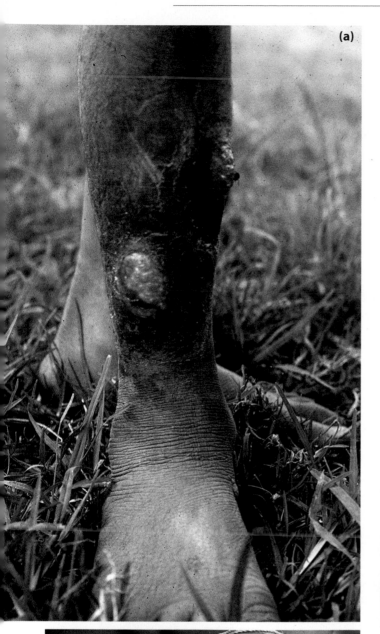

(a)

When the lesions occur on the soles of the feet, it becomes painful to walk, and so the sufferers walk on the sides of their feet with a 'waddling' gait that resembles the movement of a crab—hence the name 'crab yaws' for this type of deformity (see Figs 6.39 and 6.40).

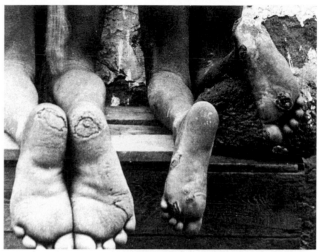

▲ **Fig. 6.39** African patients with 'crab yaws' in 1934.

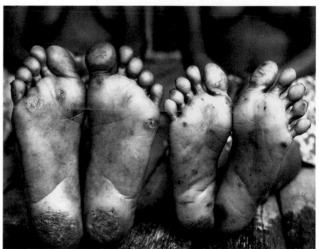

▲ **Fig. 6.40** Papua New Guinean patients with 'crab yaws' in 1967.

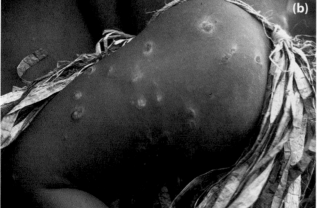

(b)

▲ **Fig. 6.38(a) and (b)** Yaws lesions. Multiple, hyperkeratotic lesions on the body. Many are ulcerated. Flies are attracted to the ulcers. Early medical observers reported that the flies were perhaps the most annoying aspect of this disease.

Involvement of the periosteum of long bones, particularly of the tibia, causes periostitis with a resulting 'anterior bowing of the tibia' and production of a 'sabre tibia' deformity. The microscopic appearance is similar to that of syphilitic periostitis (see Figs 6.41 and 6.42).

▼ ▶ **Fig. 6.41** 'Sabre tibia' in a male, aged about 40 years, from Papua New Guinea. **(a)** Clinical appearance. **(b)** X-ray appearance.

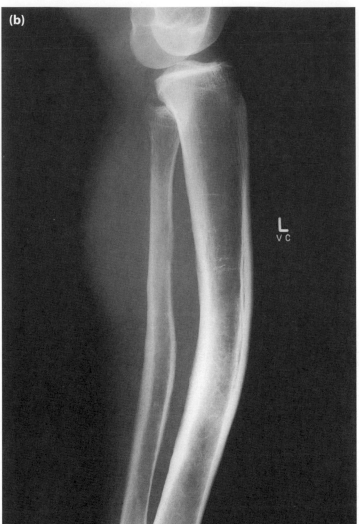

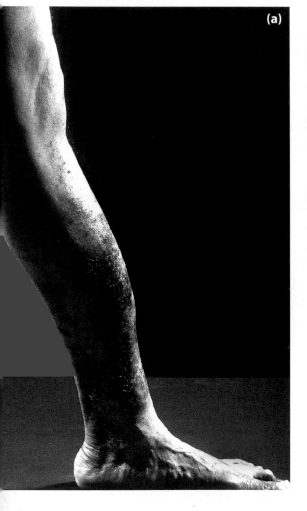

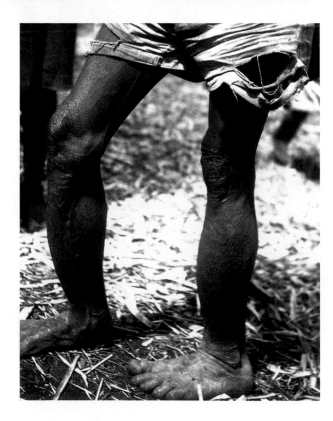

▶ **Fig. 6.42** Both tibiae show the deformity of 'sabre tibia' in a male, aged about 45 years, from Papua New Guinea.

Yaws may result in central face deformities. The cartilage and bone of the central face is destroyed (as illustrated in Figs 6.43 and 6.44).

Very rarely, a peculiar overgrowth of the nasal bones occurs. This results in a 'bossing' type of deformity in which there is bilateral overgrowth of the nasal bones. This has been called 'goundou' (shown in Fig. 6.45, overleaf).

▼ **Fig. 6.43 and Fig. 6.44** Central face deformities due to yaws. They are sometimes called gangosa.

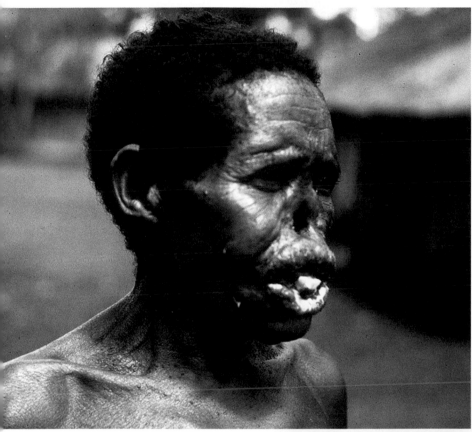

▲ **Fig. 6.43**

▼ **Fig. 6.44**

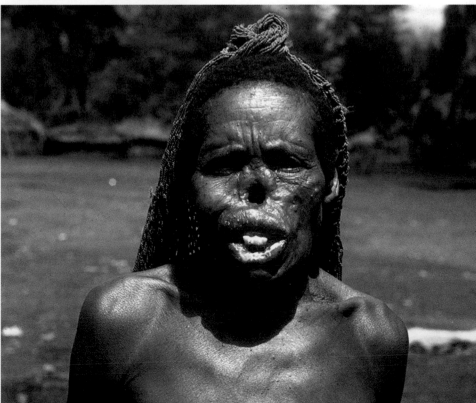

▶ ▼ **Fig. 6.45(a), (b) and (c)**
Goundou. Bilateral overgrowth
of the nasal bones. A skeleton
preserved in the Dupuytren
Museum, Ecole de Medicine,
Paris, France. This was a patient
from the Ivory Coast in West
Africa. The skeleton shows the
typical deformity of the nasal
bones. Both tibiae show the
'sabre tibia' deformity.

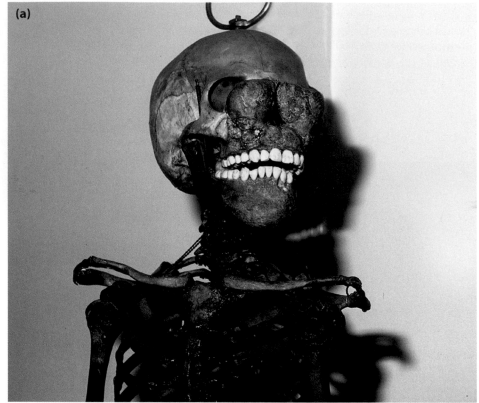

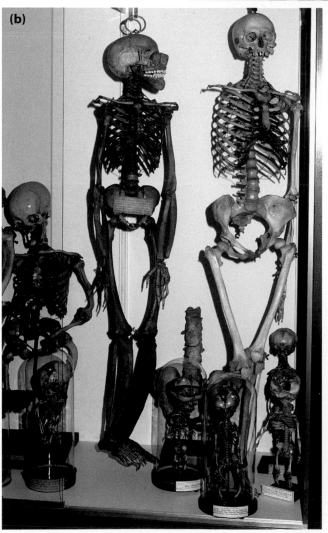

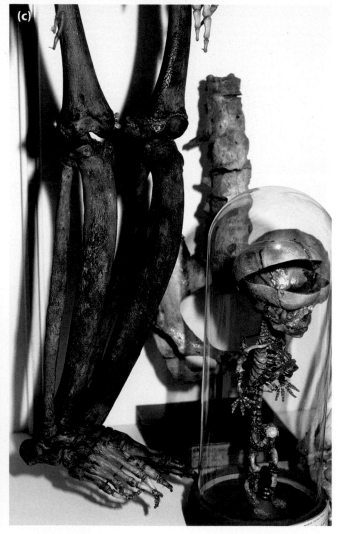

In the 1950s, the newly formed World Health Organization (WHO) distributed penicillin in a campaign aimed at eradicating yaws from the world (see Fig. 6.46). The initial results were dramatic. The yaws lesions disappeared within a day or two of one injection of long acting penicillin. The sufferers were greatly impressed with the effect of this 'wonder' drug and it appeared as though yaws had been eradicated. But from the 1970s, small epidemics of recrudescent yaws have been occurring throughout the tropics.

In Papua New Guinea, for many years after the penicillin campaign, everyone wanted an 'injection' for every conceivable condition. The yaws injection was painful because it was a large volume of an oily, viscous liquid administered through a wide bore needle. Perhaps the pain made it even more impressive as being 'strong' medicine.

In 1976 a team of health workers visited the Southern Highlands of Papua New Guinea. They were responding to a report by the local government administrators that there was an epidemic of what appeared to be yaws in a small village in a remote part of the region. These villagers had not previously had any contact with Western medicine.

The health team found an incidence of yaws that was similar to that encountered before the WHO anti-yaws campaign. This allowed them to document an outbreak of yaws as it used to occur before the introduction of penicillin. The clinical photographs (see Figs 6.37 and 6.38 on pages 164–165) can be compared with those of James McCartney from Africa taken in 1934 (see Fig. 6.36 on page 164). The lesions seen in 1976 responded well to treatment with penicillin.

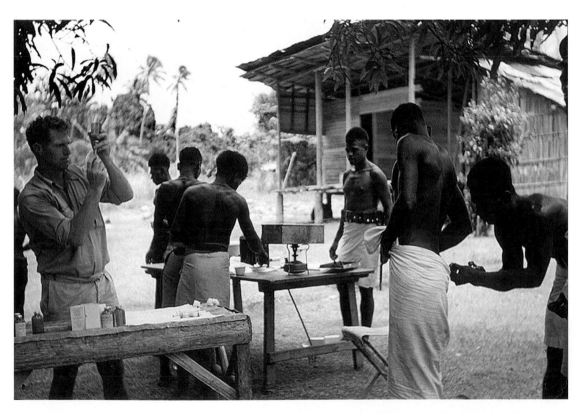

▲ **Fig. 6.46** An Australian medical student on annual vacation in January 1957 and his Papua New Guinean assistants administering injections of long-acting penicillin in New Britain as part of the WHO anti-yaws campaign.

Case 6.8

In 1980, a young boy presented in the Solomon Islands in Melanesia (a nation east of Papua New Guinea), with a round, heaped-up, ulcerated lesion on the dorsum of his right foot (see Fig. 6.47). A biopsy was performed and sent to Brisbane, Australia, for reporting. The biopsy showed the typical appearances of yaws (see Figs 6.48–6.51).

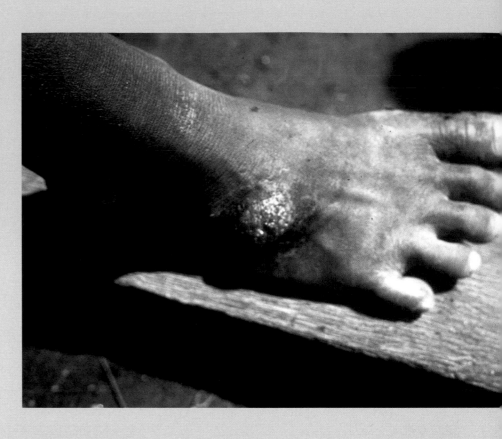

▶ **Fig. 6.47** A young boy presented in the Solomon Islands with a round, heaped-up, ulcerated lesion on the dorsum of his right foot. A biopsy showed this to be yaws.

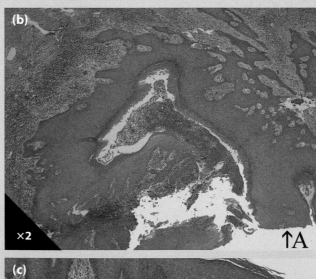

▼ ▶ **Fig. 6.48(a), (b) and (c)** The skin biopsy of the heaped-up ulcerated lesion seen in Figure 6.47 shows thickening of the epidermis (A) with an inflammatory cell infiltration in the dermis (B).

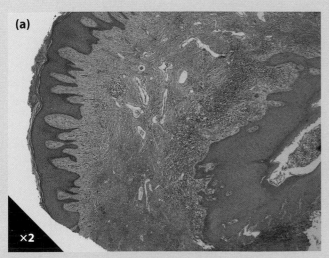

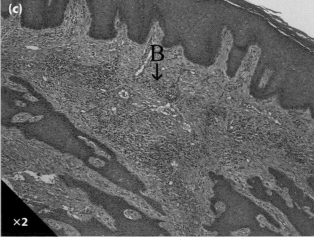

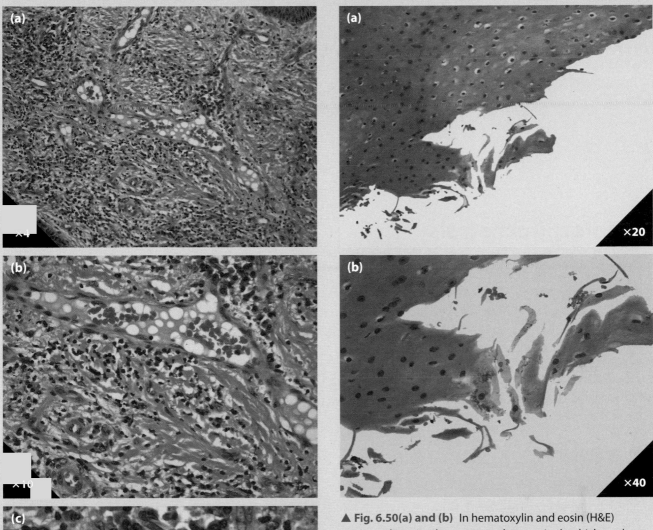

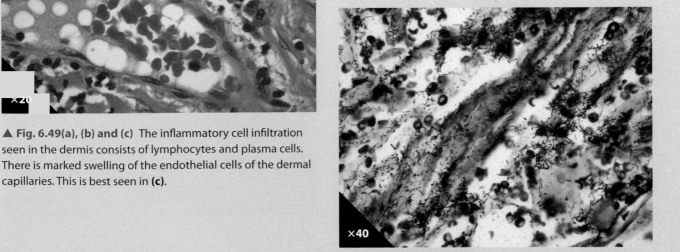

▲ **Fig. 6.50(a) and (b)** In hematoxylin and eosin (H&E) sections, the spirochetes cannot be seen in the thickened keratin layer.

▲ **Fig. 6.49(a), (b) and (c)** The inflammatory cell infiltration seen in the dermis consists of lymphocytes and plasma cells. There is marked swelling of the endothelial cells of the dermal capillaries. This is best seen in **(c)**.

▲ **Fig. 6.51** Warthin Starry stain reveals the spirochetes which stain black with this silver stain. (Note that there are no organisms in the dermis.)

Following receipt of this biopsy report, an epidemiologic survey was conducted by the doctors in the Solomon Islands—10 300 people were contacted. There were 485 cases of yaws—an incidence of 4.5 per cent, and up to 24 per cent in some villages. Penicillin treatment stopped the epidemic.

This is an example of what is happening in many tropical countries where yaws used to be a very common disease. It is an interesting insight into the epidemiology of an old disease that was controlled for a short time, and that has now broken out again.

Colonic spirochetosis

Colonic spirochetosis is a condition in which numerous spirochetal organisms are found attached to the mucosal surface of the epithelial cells of the colon. It is an incidental finding in biopsies from patients who give a history of mild diarrhea, or who are completely asymptomatic and have no evidence of immune deficiency. The observation seems to have no clinical significance. The microscopic appearances are illustrated in Figures 6.52 and 6.53.

▼ ▶ **Fig. 6.52(a), (b) and (c)** A random biopsy of the colon in a patient who had a history of mild diarrhea. In the H&E section, a blue haze can be seen on the mucosal surface. The colon is otherwise normal.

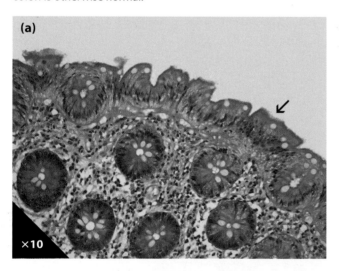

(a) ×10

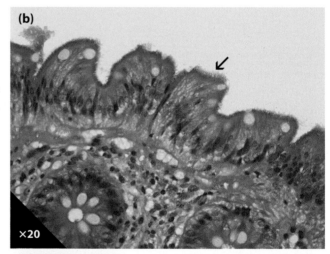

(b) ×20

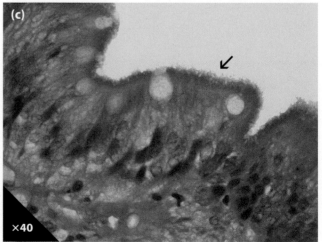

(c) ×40

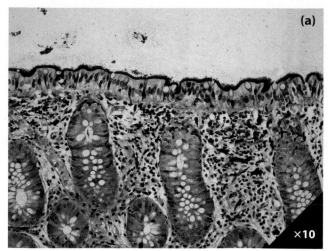

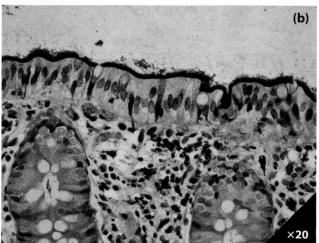

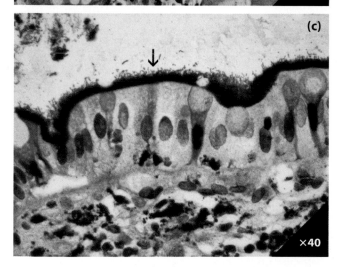

▲ **Fig. 6.53(a), (b) and (c)** Warthin Starry stain shows the morphology of the spirochetes more clearly.

Acknowledgments

- Fig. 6.2 Courtesy of Sandy MacGregor, Papua New Guinea and Gold Coast, Australia.
- Figs 6.3 Courtesy of Ian Reid, Papua New Guinea and Sydney, Australia.
- Fig. 6.7 Courtesy of Fred Leditschke, Brisbane, Australia.
- Fig. 6.12 Courtesy of Graeme Beardmore, Brisbane, Australia.
- Figs 6.20 and 6.21 Courtesy of Trevor Harris, Brisbane, Australia.
- Fig. 6.22 Courtesy of John Sullivan, Brisbane, Australia.
- Fig. 6.25 Case report and photographs. Courtesy of Bernard Hudson, Director of Infectious Diseases Department, Royal North Shore Hospital, Sydney, Australia.
- Figs 6.26 and 6.27 Courtesy of Leonard Champness, Papua New Guinea and Geelong, Australia.
- Fig. 6.28 Case report. Courtesy of David Williams, Brisbane, Australia.
- Fig. 6.29 Case report. Courtesy of Anthony Ansford, Brisbane, Australia.
- Figs 6.30–6.35 Reproduced with permission of Michael Good, Director, Queensland Institute of Medical Research.
- Fig. 6.36 Courtesy of James and Peggy McCartney, Adelaide, Australia.
- Figs 6.37 and 6.38 Courtesy of Sandy Macgregor, Papua New Guinea and Gold Coast, Australia.
- Fig. 6.39 Courtesy of James and Peggy McCartney, Adelaide, Australia.
- Fig. 6.40 Courtesy of Anthony Radford, Papua New Guinea and Adelaide, Australia.
- Fig. 6.42 Courtesy of Sandy Macgregor, Papua New Guinea and Gold Coast, Australia.
- Figs 6.43 and 6.44 Courtesy of Leonard Champness, Papua New Guinea and Geelong, Australia.
- Fig. 6.45 Photographed courtesy of the Curator, Dupuytren Museum, Ecole de Medicine, Paris.
- Fig. 6.46 Courtesy of Maurice Cave, Papua New Guinea and Rockhampton, Australia.
- Fig. 6.47 Courtesy of Bernard Hudson, Director of Infectious Diseases Department, Royal North Shore Hospital, Sydney, Australia.

7

Fungal infections

Fungal organisms are extremely prevalent in the natural world. There are thousands of species, only a few of which are pathologic to humans. Most of the fungi that cause human disease are found in all parts of the world. However, there are some that occur in only localized geographical areas.

The main function of fungi is that they act as 'recycling organisms'. Their invading filaments help to digest dead vegetable and animal material.

Some fungi act synergistically in helping plants to absorb nutrients that their roots unaided cannot absorb. These are called mycorhizal fungi. Some produce medicinally useful material—the best known of these being the *Penicillium notatum*, which produces penicillin.

Fungi cause disease in every living thing, including humans. As pathogens of plants in particular, fungi play a significant role in affecting the lives of human beings. The outbreak of potato mold in Ireland in the 1800s caused severe damage to the potato crops and shortage of a staple food. This resulted in widespread hunger, and the death and emigration of millions of people from Ireland. Similar epidemics of fungal disease in food crops continue to cause disruption to human communities.

While fungi are prevalent in the natural environment, they also occur as commensals on our skins and in our alimentary systems. Most fungal infections are not life threatening, but they do cause serious infection in people whose immune systems are impaired. In recent years, there have been increasing numbers of people whose immune systems have been depressed by chemotherapy or as a result of human immunodeficiency virus (HIV)/AIDS, and they are all susceptible to infection with fungal organisms that are not pathogenic to people with normal immune systems. This type of infection is called 'opportunistic' infection.

The presence of a fungal infection is often first recognized by a histopathologist examining surgical or post-mortem material. Many fungi can be recognized as characteristic by their histologic appearances, but for accurate species diagnosis, in most cases, there needs to be a close collaboration between clinician, microbiologist and histopathologist.

Fungal infections are usually divided into superficial mycoses and deep mycoses:

- superficial mycoses affect the skin.
- deep mycoses affect the internal organs.

There is considerable overlap between the two types of disease.

Superficial mycoses

The most common superficial mycosis is also called a dermatophyte infection. The most common clinical manifestation of a dermatophyte infection is tinea or 'ringworm'.

The fungal species most commonly isolated from dermatophyte infections, namely *Microsporum canis*, *Microsporum gypseum*, *Trichophyton mentagrophytes* and *Trichophyton rubrum*, are discussed in the next section.

Tinea

Tinea (also known as ringworm) presents as single or multiple, round, red, itchy and scaly lesions on the trunk and limbs. It may affect the skin between the toes, the hair and the nails (as shown in Figs 7.1, 7.2 and 7.3, continued overleaf).

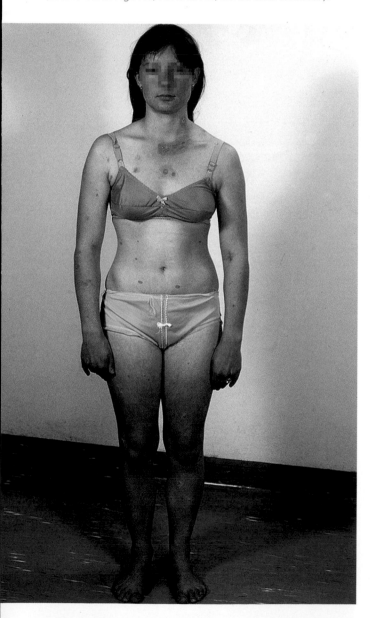

▲ **Fig. 7.1** Tinea corporis. A female, aged 21 years, presented with a number of tinea lesions on her limbs and trunk. These had developed over the previous 6 days. Mycologic culture grew *Microsporum canis*.

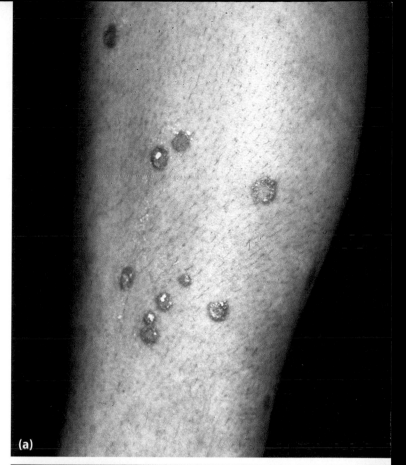

(a)

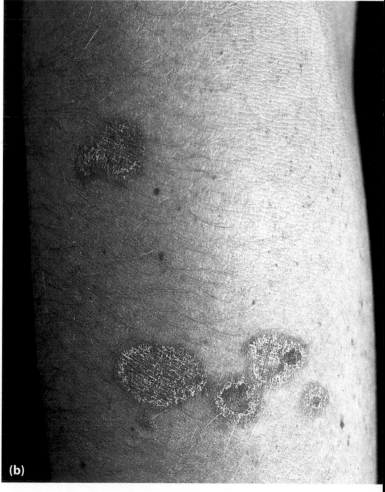

(b)

▲ **Fig. 7.2** Closer view of the lesions demonstrated in Figure 7.1 show the features of the round, red, itchy and scaly lesions. **(a)** Right calf. **(b)** Left forearm.

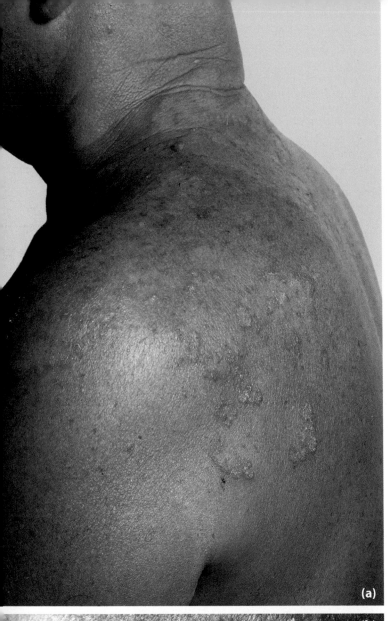

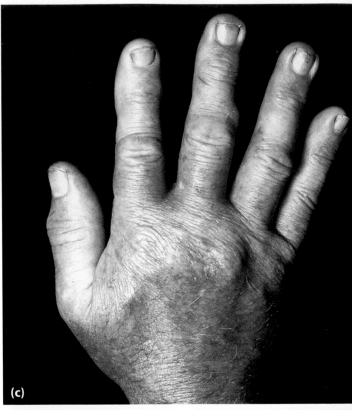

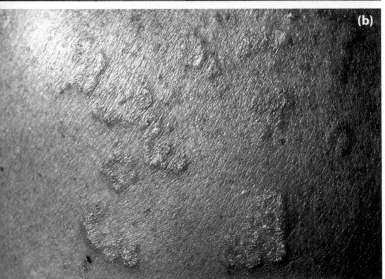

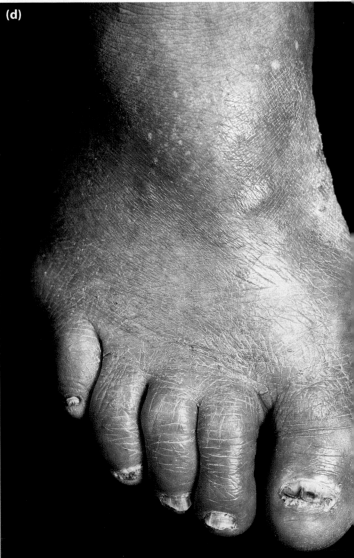

▲ **Fig. 7.3(a), (b), (c) and (d)** Tinea. A male, aged 58 years, presented with tinea of the body (tinea corporis), tinea of the hands and tinea of the feet (tinea pedis). *Trichophyton rubrum* was cultured from the lesions.

People from countries with temperate climates who move to live in hot, moist, tropical countries may suffer from severe tinea that affects the buttocks and groins. This is sometimes called 'tinea cruris'. It can be a very debilitating condition (see Fig. 7.4).

When the infection involves the hair of the scalp, it may cause alopecia, also called tinea capitis (shown in Figs 7.5 and 7.6). Dermatologists use a 'Wood's lamp' to demonstrate fluorescence of a fungal infection of hair under the influence of ultraviolet light (see Figs 7.7 and 7.8 overleaf).

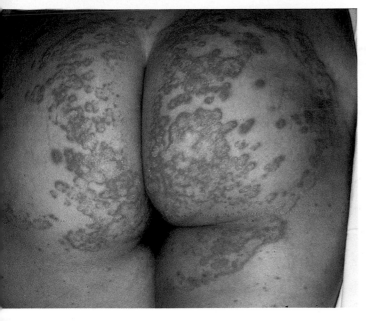

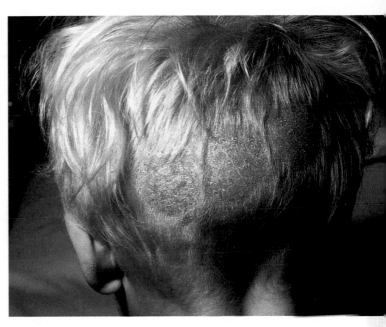

▲ **Fig. 7.4** Tinea cruris. A female, aged 20 years, presented with severe tinea affecting her buttocks. The lesions were also present in her groins. *T. rubrum* was cultured.

▲ **Fig. 7.5** Tinea capitis. A male, aged 5 years, has extensive alopecia from tinea affecting his scalp. *M. canis* was cultured.

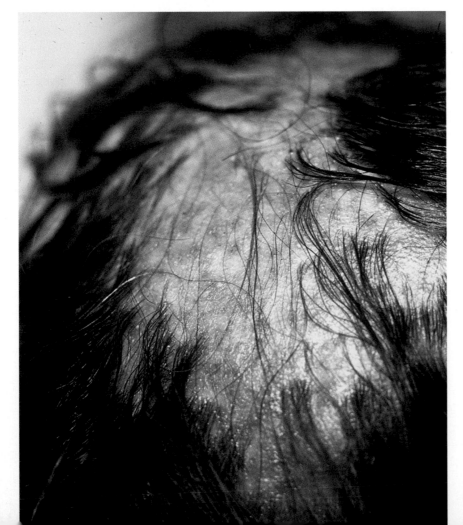

◀ **Fig. 7.6** Tinea capitis. A male, aged 7 years, with extensive alopecia from tinea affecting his scalp. *Trichophyton mentagrophytes* was cultured.

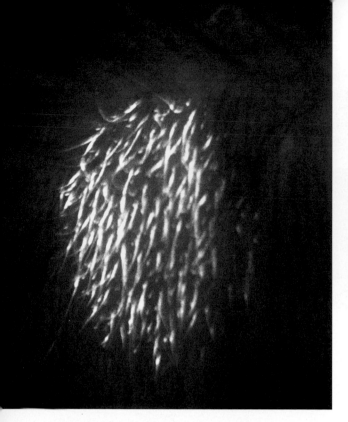

▲ **Fig. 7.7** Tinea capitis. Dermatologists use a 'Wood's lamp' to demonstrate fluorescence of a fungal infection of hair under the influence of ultraviolet light.

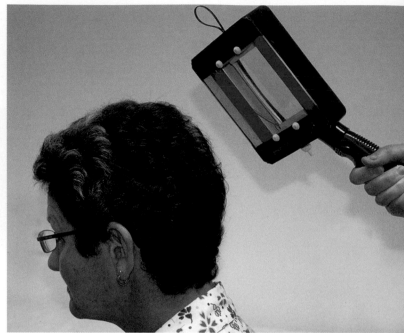

▲ **Fig. 7.8** Wood's lamp being demonstrated.

Diagnosis of superficial mycoses

The process of diagnosis of superficial mycoses involves the following.

- Skin scrapings from the scaly surface of the lesion and including hairs—to demonstrate fungal filaments (hyphae).
- Culture on Sabouraud's dextrose agar, which is 'incubated' at room temperature—growth occurs slowly over many days.
- Skin biopsy of a rash that is not characteristically fungal in appearance.

Skin scrapings

1. A skin scraping is performed by scraping the surface of the scaly lesion with a sterile scalpel blade and directing the scrapings into a sterile Petri dish. The dish is labeled with the patient's details and partially sealed with cellotape to prevent the lid from separating during transport to the pathology laboratory.
2. On arrival at the laboratory, a sample of the scaly material is mixed with a drop of potassium hydroxide (KOH) on a glass microscope slide and stained with blue dye—Parker Quink ink. The KOH digests the keratin of the superficial layer of the skin and makes the fungal hyphae more easily visible (see Fig. 7.9).
3. The hyphae may be septate or nonseptate and branching or nonbranching. The morphology of hyphae is more clearly seen on smears taken from culture plates of the fungus and stained with lactophenol cotton blue (see Fig. 7.10).

Microscopic examination of hairs affected by tinea shows the presence of spores on the surface of the hairs: this is called an ectothrix infection (see Fig. 7.11). Sometimes, the spores occur within the hair: this is called an endothrix infection.

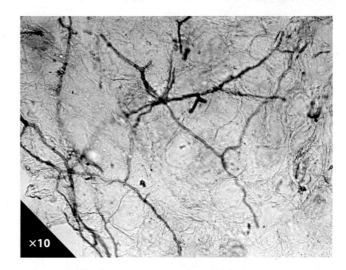

▶ **Fig. 7.9** Skin scraping mounted in KOH and stained with Parker Quink ink—shows the presence of fungal hyphae.

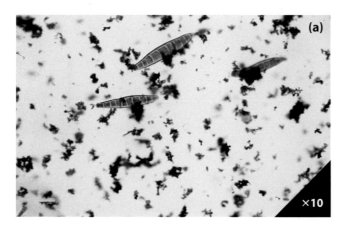

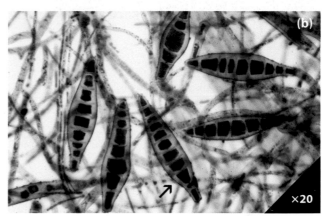

▲ **Fig. 7 10(a) and (b)** Sample smear made from the surface of the *M. canis* culture plate, stained with lactophenol cotton blue. *M. canis* is characterized by the presence of numerous, large septate macroconidia, as shown here.

▶ **Fig. 7.11** Hair mounted in KOH and stained with Parker Quink ink. Spores are present on the surface of the hair. This is known as an ectothrix infection.

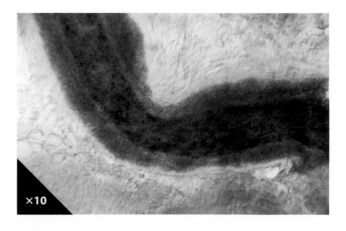

Culture

Diagnosis of the exact species of fungus is made by the cultural appearances of the 'giant colony' as it grows on Sabouraud's dextrose agar.

> *Raymond Sabouraud (1864–1938), the inventor of the specialized culture medium that bears his name, was one of the founders of dermatology in France. He worked at the Hopital St Louis, the dermatology hospital in Paris. He is honored by a bust in the foyer of the Moulage Museum at the hospital (see Fig. 7.12).*

The fungal species most commonly isolated from dermatophyte infections are:

- *Microsporum canis*
- *Microsporum gypseum*
- *Trichophyton mentagrophytes*
- *Trichophyton rubrum*.

When examining the culture plate of a fungal culture, the microbiologist looks at both the front and the back of the culture plate to note its appearance and color. Both of these features vary with the species (illustrated in Figs 7.13–7.16).

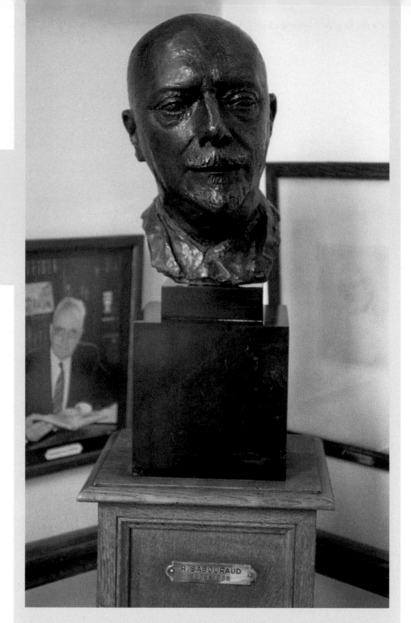

▲ **Fig. 7.12** Bust of Raymond Sabouraud (1864–1938), the inventor of the specialized culture medium that bears his name, sits in the foyer of the Moulage Museum at the Hopital St Louis in Paris.

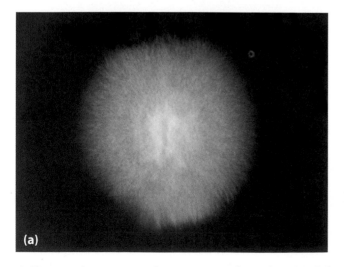
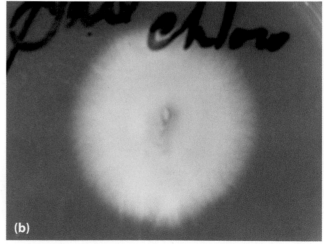

▲ **Fig. 7.13** Appearances of *M. canis* on a culture plate. **(a)** Surface of the culture is filamentous. **(b)** Back of the plate shows a light yellow color.

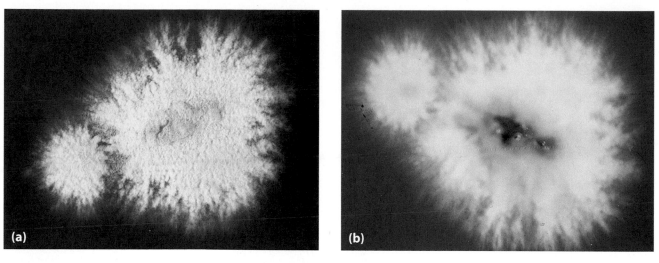

▲ **Fig. 7 14** Appearances of *M. gypseum* on a culture plate. **(a)** Surface of the culture is rough. **(b)** Back of the plate shows a much lighter yellow color than that seen with *M. canis.*

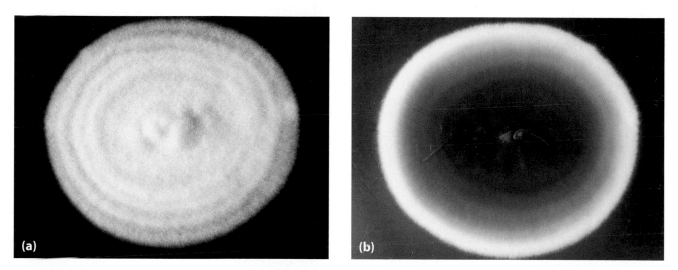

▲ **Fig. 7.15** Appearances of *T. mentagrophytes* on a culture plate. **(a)** Surface of the culture is white and appears 'fluffy'. **(b)** Back of the plate shows a yellow, brown color.

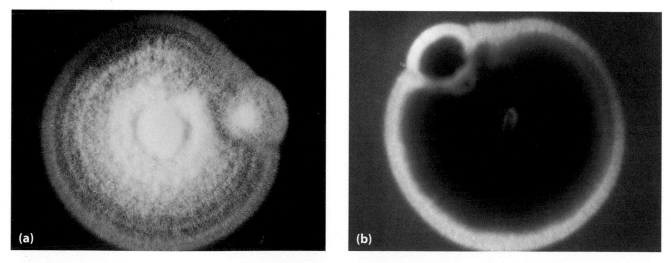

▲ **Fig. 7.16** Appearances of *T. rubrum* on a culture plate. **(a)** Surface of the culture is white and appears 'fluffy', with a red background. **(b)** Back of the plate shows a rich red color.

Further species' diagnostic features are seen on microscopic examination of a scraping made from the surface of the colony.

The features most helpful in diagnosis are:

- the appearances of the hyphae, and
- the presence and morphology of spores and macroconidia (shown in Fig. 7.10 on page 179).

Skin biopsy

A skin biopsy characteristically shows little inflammation in the dermis, but there are microscopic abscesses in the stratum corneum, which is usually slightly thickened (illustrated in Figs 7.17 and 7.18).

Periodic Acid Schiff (PAS) stain shows fungal hyphae in the microabscesses and in the thickened stratum corneum (illustrated in Figs 7.19 and 7.20).

It is not possible to make a species diagnosis on the biopsy appearances. For this, a culture is necessary.

A 'rule of thumb' for histopathologists examining skin biopsies is 'beware a normal-looking skin biopsy of a skin rash'. Always do a PAS stain because, otherwise, the diagnosis of a dermatophyte fungal infection may be missed.

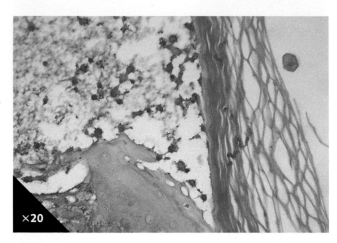

▲ **Fig. 7.19** PAS stain shows fungal hyphae in the microabscess.

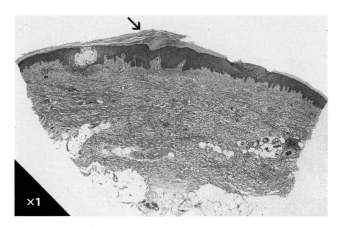

▲ **Fig. 7.17** Skin biopsy, which shows thickening of the stratum corneum at this magnification, with very little inflammation in the dermis.

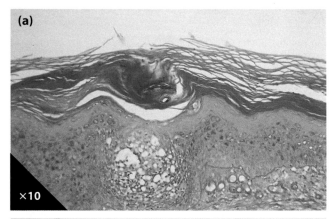

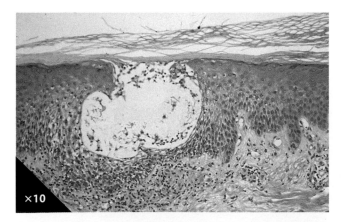

▲ **Fig. 7.18** Microabscess present in the stratum corneum.

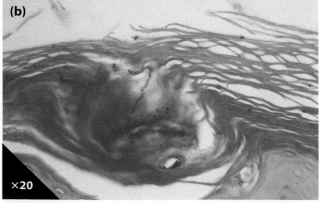

▲ **Fig. 7.20(a) and (b)** PAS stain showing fungal hyphae in the thickened stratum corneum.

Tinea imbricata

Tinea imbricata is caused by the fungus *Trichophyton concentricum*. This clinical condition is characterized by the presence of circular, gyrate, scaly, fungal lesions all over the body (shown in Figs 7.21 and 7.22).

The appearance of the culture is characteristic (see Fig. 7.23, overleaf). The skin biopsy is nearly always 'normal' in appearance until a PAS stain is done (see Fig. 7.24, overleaf).

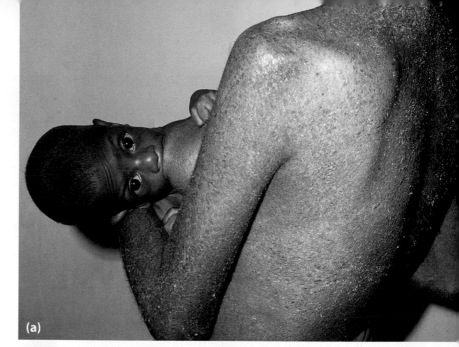

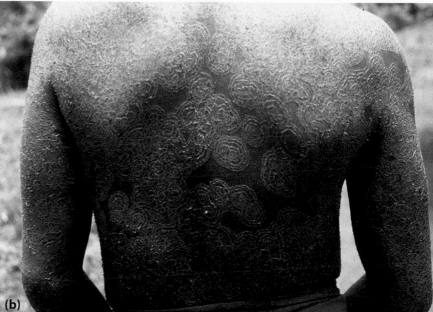

▶ **Fig. 7.21** Tinea imbricata. Two patients from Papua New Guinea (PNG) in the mid-1960s present with very advanced disease. **(a)** Scaling all over the body. **(b)** Particularly in this second patient, the circular appearance of the scaly skin can be seen. (This advanced disease is now uncommon in PNG.)

(a)

(b)

▼ **Fig. 7.22** Tinea imbricata. A patient from Australia.

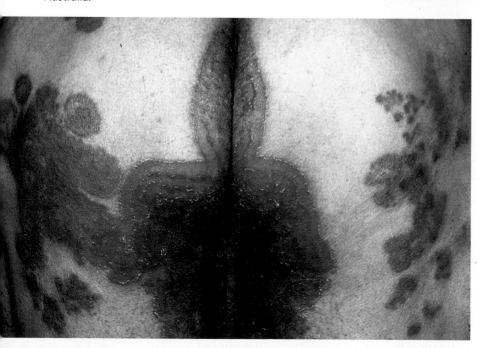

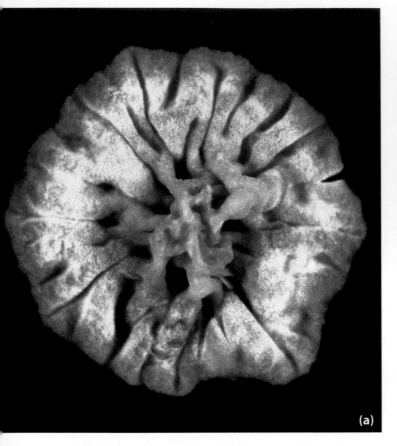

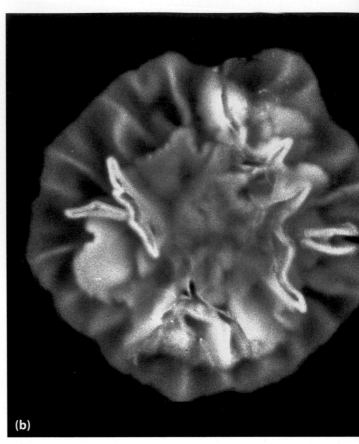

▲ **Fig. 7.23** Cultural characteristics of *T. concentricum*. **(a)** Surface of the culture is deeply furrowed. **(b)** Back of the plate shows a brown color.

▼ ▶ **Fig. 7.24(a) and (b)** Skin biopsy taken from a patient with *Tinea imbricata*. It appears to be normal, but PAS stain, shown in **(c)** reveals the presence of numerous hyphae in the stratum corneum.

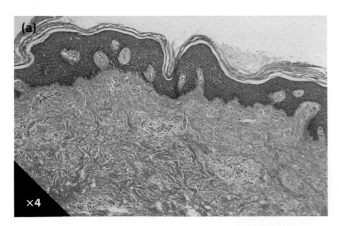

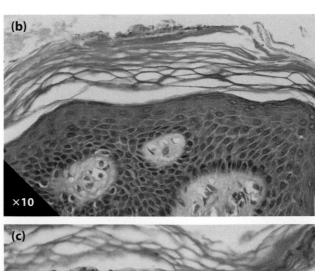

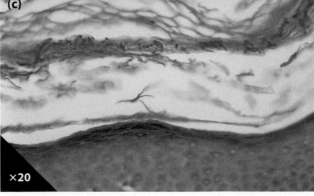

This species of fungus *T. concentricum* is interesting in that it occurs more commonly in some countries than in others. For example, while very rare in Australia, it is the most common species of dermatophyte encountered in Papua New Guinea. It is also common in some South-East Asian countries.

Tinea versicolor

The *Tinea versicolor* lesion consists in white (sometimes pinkish) macules, mainly on the trunk (shown in Fig. 7.25). It is usually asymptomatic, but may sometimes be scaly and itchy. In brown skins, areas of depigmentation can be seen (see Fig. 7.26, overleaf).

Unstained smear of the skin scrapings mounted in KOH from the patient illustrated in Figure 7.25 showed numerous fungal elements—hyphae and spores (demonstrated in Fig. 7.27, overleaf). The causative organism is *Malassezia furfur* (see Figs 7.28 and 7.29, overleaf).

▶ ▼ **Fig. 7.25(a), (b) and (c)** *Tinea versicolor*. A male, aged 49 years, had mildly itchy, reddish, macular lesions on his trunk.

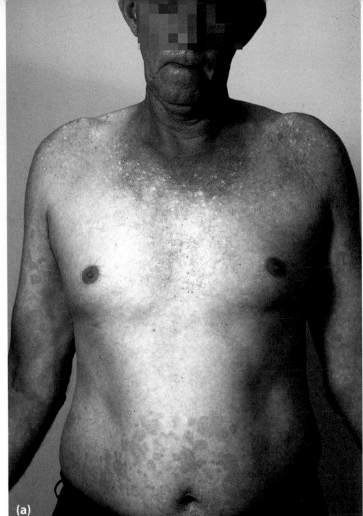

(a)

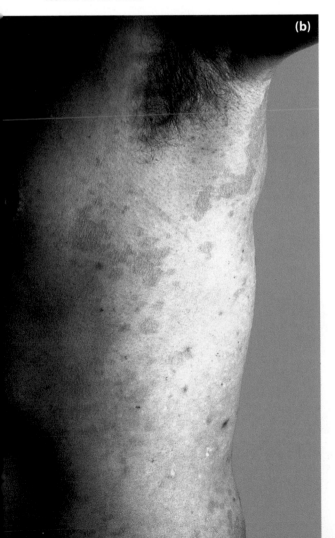

(b)

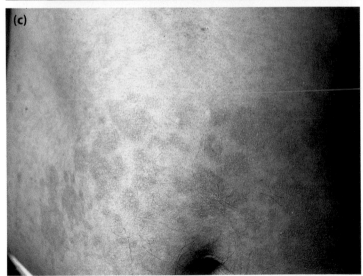

(c)

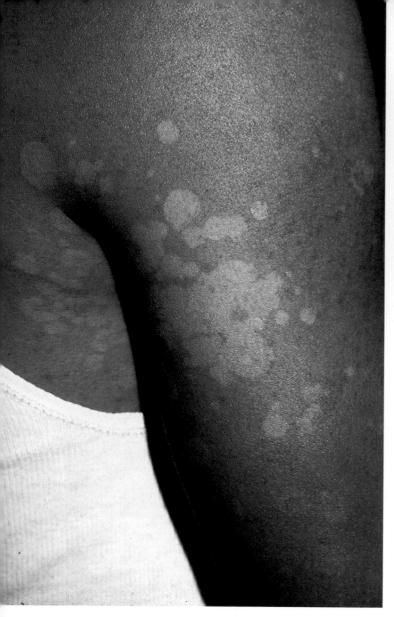

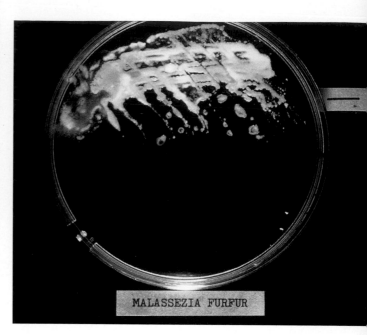

▲ **Fig. 7.28** Culture plate of *M. furfur*, the causative organism of *Tinea versicolor*.

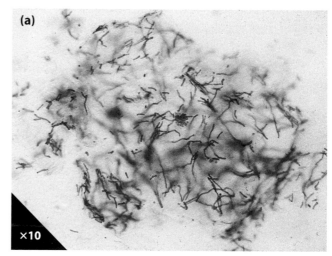

▲ **Fig. 7.26** *Tinea versicolor*. A male, aged 31 years, from Papua New Guinea, has a brown skin and the fungus causes areas of depigmentation.

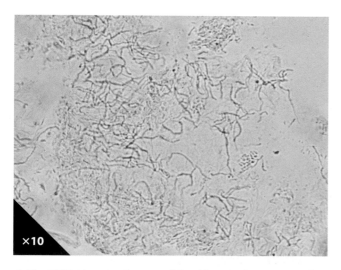

▲ **Fig. 7.27** Unstained smear of the skin scrapings mounted in KOH from the patient illustrated in Figure 7.25 on page 185. Numerous fungal elements—hyphae and spores—can be seen.

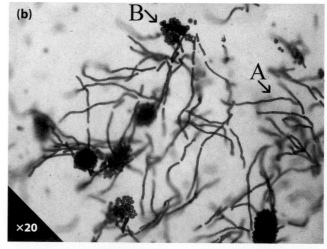

▲ **Fig. 7.29(a) and (b)** Smear made from the culture plate of *M. furfur* stained with lactophenol cotton blue stain. Hyphae (A) and spores (B) can be seen.

Yeasts

Yeasts are usually included with fungi for purposes of discussion. The organisms discussed here are candida, chromoblastomycosis and sporotrichosis.

Candida

Candida albicans is a common form of yeast. It is regarded as being a 'dimorphic fungus' because it grows as a yeast on culture; while in tissues It adopts a filamentous form (pseudohyphae).

Candida is both a superficial mycosis and a deep mycosis. In its superficial form, candida affects healthy people, but infections—both superficial and deep—are more common in diabetics and in people whose immune systems are impaired.

Superficial mycosis

Candida infection may be the first indication of the presence of diabetes or AIDS. As a superficial mycosis, it:

- commonly affects the angles of the mouth, the tongue and the fingers (illustrated in Fig. 7.30)

▼ ▶ **Fig. 7.30** Candida infections seen in a male aged 11 years. **(a)** Left angle of the mouth. **(b)** Tongue. **(c), (d)** and **(e)** Fingers.

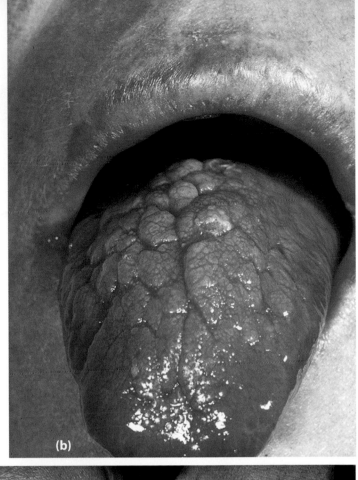
(b)

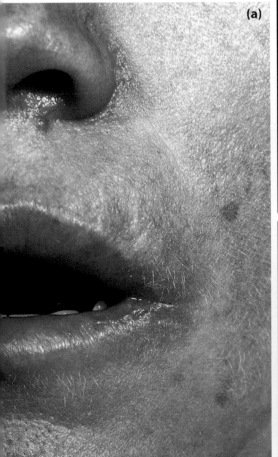
(a)

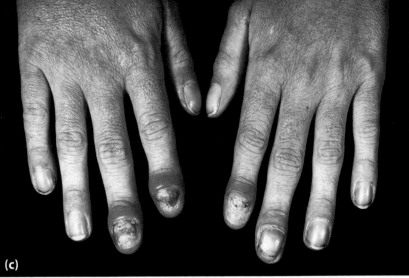
(c)

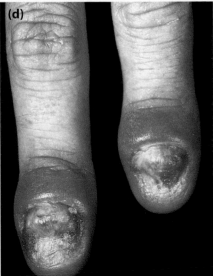
(d)

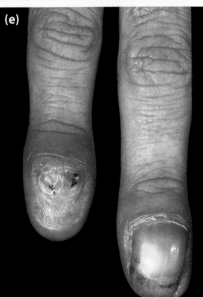
(e)

- causes a red, painful rash in the groin and around the anus
- causes vaginitis in pregnant women.

Deep mycosis

As a deep mycosis, candida may affect any organ.

- Infection of the esophagus and the stomach is shown in Figures 7.31 and 7.32. In both of these organs, there is ulceration and acute inflammation of the mucosa, and a thick plaque forms on the mucosal surface (see Fig. 7.33).
- Infection of the eye is illustrated in Figure 7.34.
- Infection of the liver is illustrated in Figures 7.35 and 7.36, overleaf.
- Intrauterine candidiasis is an uncommon infection, which occurs particularly in diabetic women. White plaques of candida can be seen on the umbilical cord and on the surface of the placenta (shown in Figs 7.37 and 7.38, overleaf).

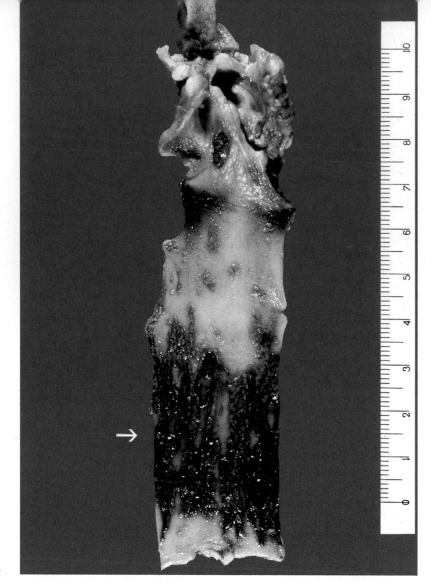

▶ **Fig. 7.31** Candida esophagitis. Post-mortem specimen of a female, aged 6 months, who died from acute leukemia. The hemorrhagic plaques cover a considerable extent of the mucosa of the esophagus. The patient was immune suppressed from both the leukemia and its treatment. Thus, the candida was an opportunistic infection.

▼ **Fig. 7.32** Candida in the stomach. In the stomach, dark greenish plaques occur in a linear fashion along the mucosal folds.

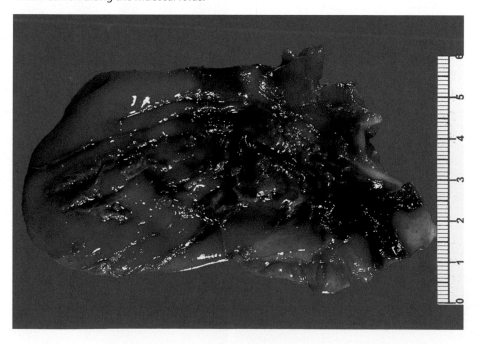

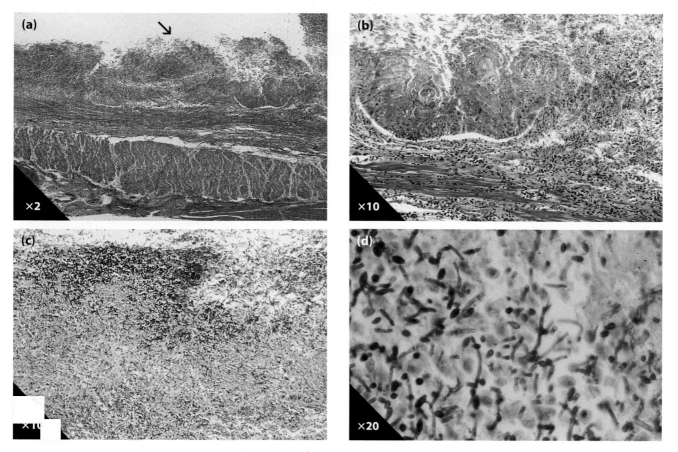

▲ **Fig. 7.33** Candida esophagitis. **(a) and (b)** Microscopic sections show the inflammatory membrane on the mucosal surface of the esophagus. **(c) and (d)** Pseudohyphae can be seen in this hematoxylin and eosin (H&E) stain **(c)** but they are more easily seen in a PAS stain **(d)**.

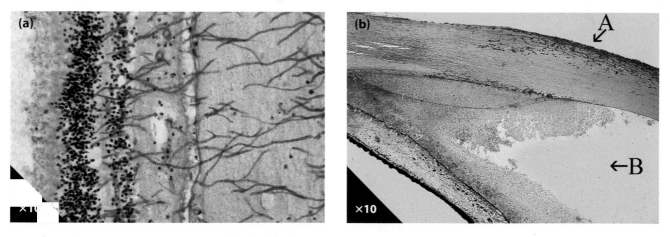

▲ **Fig. 7.34** Candida ophthalmitis. A diabetic patient had an eye removed for treatment of intractable candida infection. The panophthalmitis can be seen involving: **(a)** the retina, and **(b)** the cornea (A) and anterior chamber of the eye (B).

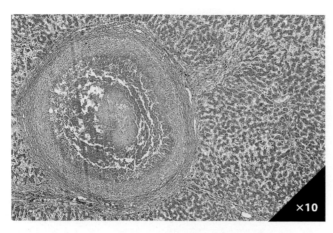

▲ **Fig. 7.35** Candida infection in the liver. A male, aged 20 years, died of acute leukemia. He had disseminated candidiasis. Within a liver abscess, there was an artery whose wall was invaded by candida pseudohyphae.

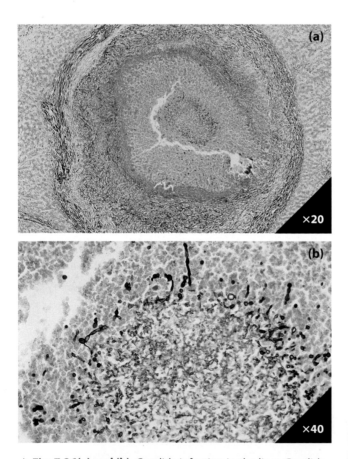

▲ **Fig. 7.36(a) and (b)** Candida infection in the liver. Candida pseudohyphae are better seen in a Grocott silver stain, in which they stain black.

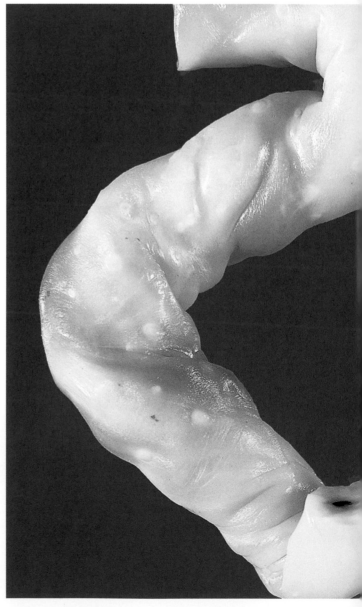

▲ **Fig. 7.37** Intrauterine candidiasis. Umbilical cord showing white plaques of candida.

▶ **Fig. 7.38** Intrauterine candidiasis.
(a) and (b) Microscopically, the white plaques of candida consist of collections of neutrophils on the surface of the umbilical cord, forming microabscesses. Within these abscesses, there are numerous pseudohyphae of candida.
(c) They are better seen in the PAS stain.

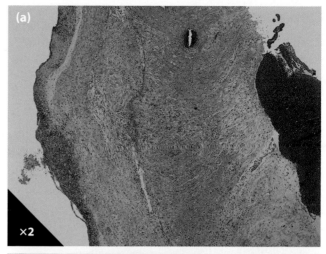

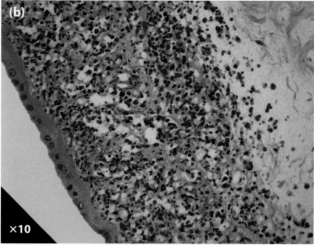

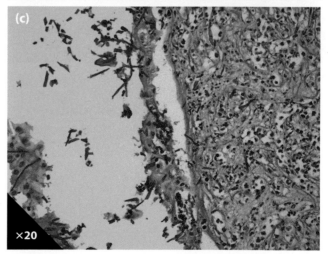

Some things that a pathologist needs to remember about candida.

- *Candida infection of deep organs may be a first presentation of AIDS.*
- *Whenever one sees a few neutrophils on the mucosal surface in a biopsy from the oropharyngeal region or the vagina, one must do a PAS stain. (It is surprising how often one finds pseudohyphae of candida.)*

Chromoblastomycosis

Clinically, the lesions of chromoblastomycosis look like hyper-keratotic, solar-induced lesions of the skin. They usually occur on the hands or limbs. In northern Australia, where this fungal infection is fairly common, and solar-induced lesions are much more common, the fungal lesions (see Fig. 7.39) are often biopsied or excised as skin cancers. When the tissue biopsy is examined, the characteristic brown, planate dividing bodies can be seen (illustrated in Fig. 7.40).

▼ ▶ **Fig. 7.39** Three different patients with skin lesions of chromoblastomycosis. **(a)** Lesion above the knee. **(b) and (c)** Lesions on the hand.

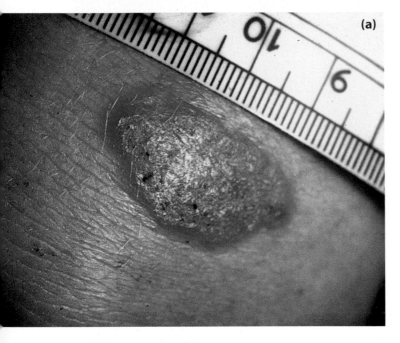

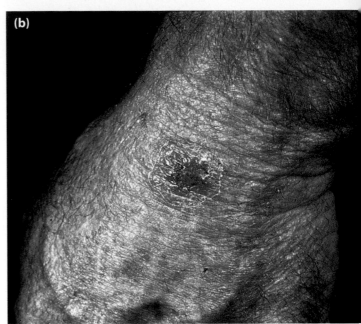

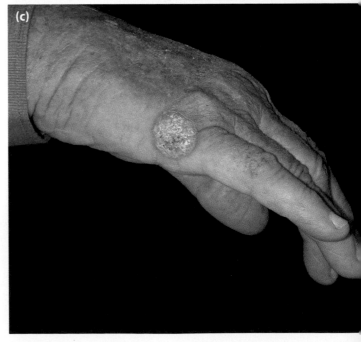

▼ ▶ **Fig. 7.40** Tissue biopsy of chromoblastomycosis.
(a) Microscopically, the skin shows pseudoepitheliomatous
hyperplasia of the epidermis (A) and a chronic inflammation
in the dermis. **(b)** Mixed with this inflammation, there are
microabscesses (B). **(c) and (d)** Within the microabscesses,
there are numerous, brown, planate dividing bodies. **(e)** These
bodies are present in multinucleated giant cells as well. The
appearance of the brown, planate dividing bodies is easy to
see in H&E-stained tissue sections. Special stains for fungi (e.g.
PAS) are not needed.

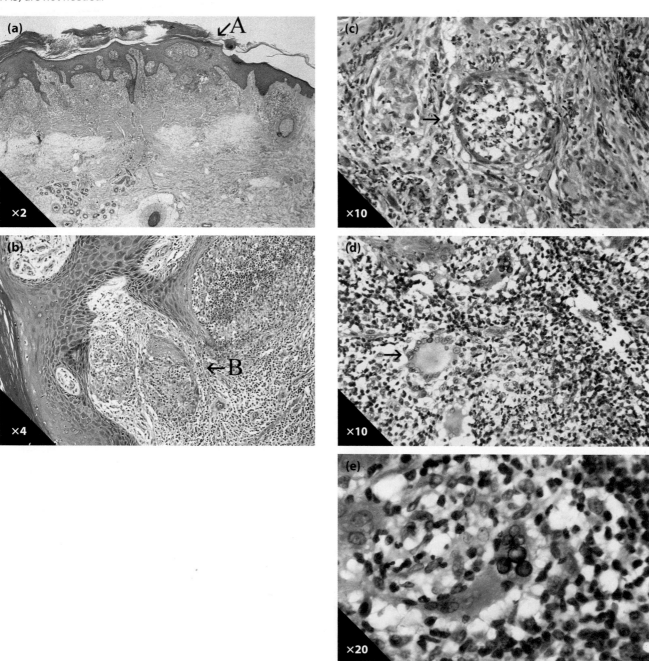

The condition is caused by a dimorphic mold that has both yeast-like forms and filamentous forms in tissue. The dimorphic molds are colored brown because they contain melanin—hence the name 'chromo'.

Infection is usually attributed to a penetrating injury caused by a splinter or a thorn. The lesions are usually single. If left untreated, they continue to spread over the skin of the limbs (illustrated in Fig. 7.41).

A number of different species of yeast, particularly Phialophora and Cladophialophora cause this lesion. The exact species can only be identified by culture (see Figs 7.42 and 7.43).

An example of the filamentous form of this mold is illustrated in Case 7.1.

▼ **Fig. 7.41** Advanced chromoblastomycosis that had been present for many years in a 37-year-old male.

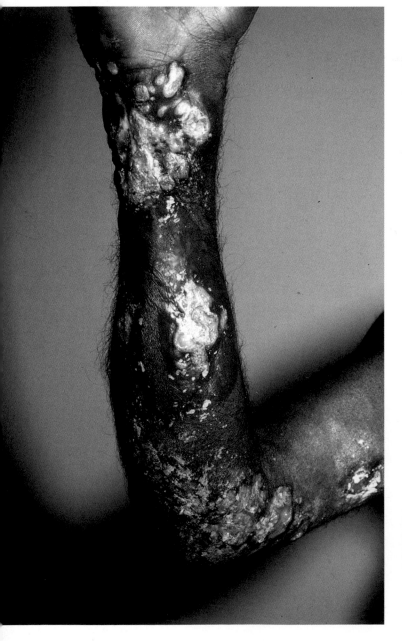

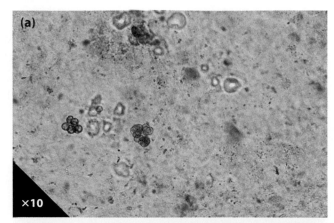

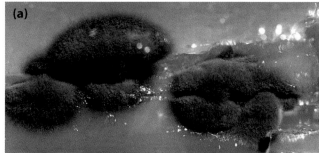

▲ **Fig. 7.42(a) and (b)** An unstained skin scraping mounted in KOH from one of the chromoblastomycosis lesions illustrated in Figure 7.41 showed the presence of brown, planate dividing bodies.

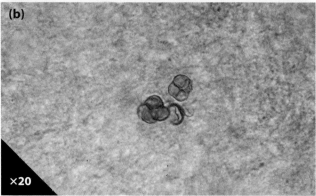

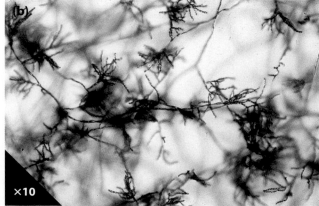

▲ **Fig. 7.43** Chromoblastomycosis. **(a)** Examination of the culture, and **(b)** the slide preparation made from the culture identified the fungus as *Cladophialophora carionii*.

Case 7.1

A 40-year-old female presented with the symptoms and signs of an intracerebral space-occupying lesion that was diagnosed as being a cerebral abscess. This was confirmed on a computed tomography (CT) scan of the brain (shown in Fig. 7.44).

A needle aspiration was performed and fungal hyphae were seen in the KOH-treated smear (see Figs 7.45 and 7.46).

The patient proceeded to a craniotomy for excision of the abscess to obtain tissue for culture and so that a frozen section could be performed to make a confirmatory tissue diagnosis. The frozen section showed the presence of an acute inflammatory reaction, in which there were many brown fungal hyphae (see Fig. 7.47, overleaf).

Tube and plate culture, and the microscopic preparation from the culture plate revealed the species was *Cladophialophora bantiana* (see Fig. 7.48, overleaf).

The abscess was excised with what appeared to be a complete excision (shown in Fig. 7.49, overleaf) and the patient was given a course of Amphotericin B.

The symptoms subsided initially, but the abscess recurred 2 months later and the paient died 1 month after this. The mode of infection was not ascertained.

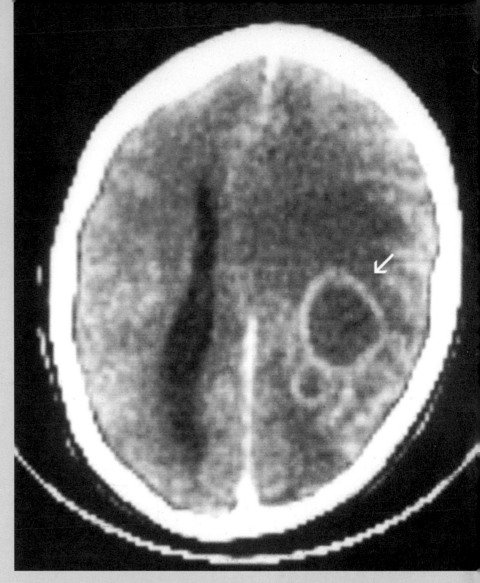

▲ **Fig. 7.44** CT brain scan (enhanced) showed the presence of a left frontal lobe abscess.

▼ **Fig. 7.45** Needle aspiration biopsy was performed and fungal hyphae were seen in the KOH-treated smear.

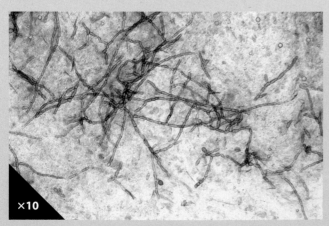

▼ **Fig. 7.46** Gram stain on the smear showed the hyphae more clearly.

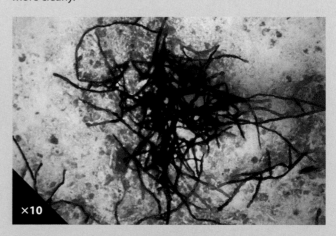

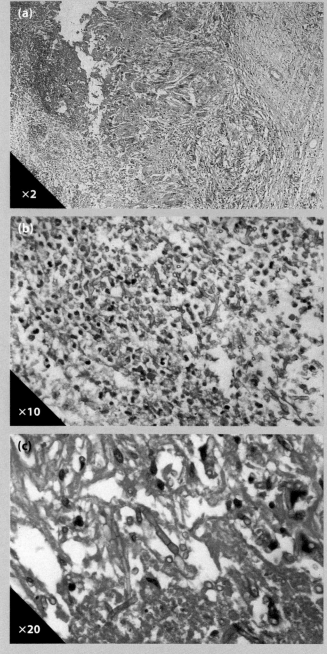

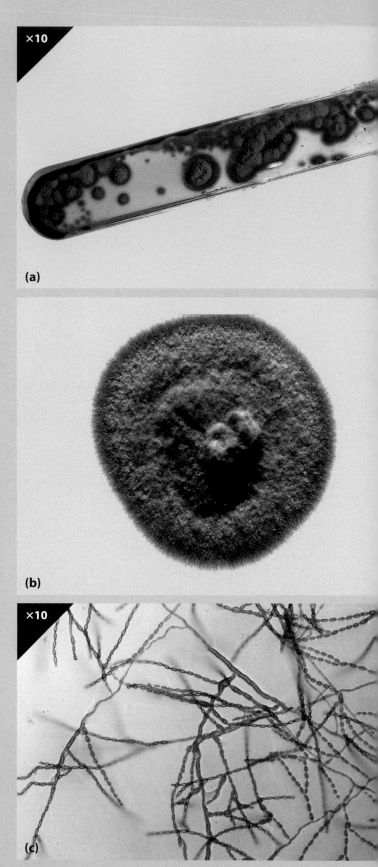

▲ **Fig. 7.47(a), (b) and (c)** Frozen section performed on the brain biopsy showed an acute inflammatory reaction in which there were many brown fungal hyphae.

▲ **Fig. 7.48(a), (b) and (c)** Tube and plate culture, and the microscopic preparation from the culture plate revealed the species was *Cladophialophora bantiana*.

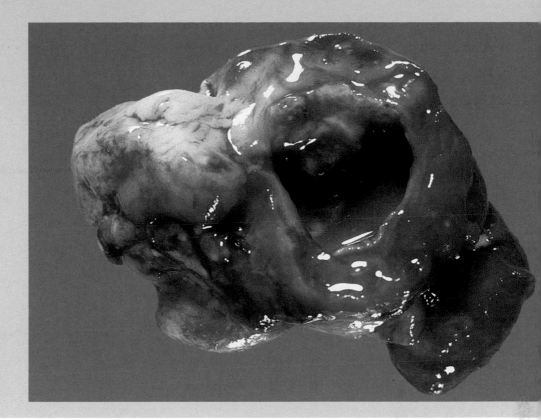

▶ **Fig. 7.49** Excised brain abscess.

Sporotrichosis

Sporotrichosis is caused by the fungus *Sporothrix schenckii*. It causes a hyperkeratotic lesion on the skin that resembles a solar-induced lesion or a squamous cell carcinoma. The first lesion is usually on the hand and follows a penetrating injury from a splinter or a thorn. Further lesions develop and extend up the arm.

Case 7.2

A 54-year-old female had a number of lesions on one arm. They had started on her hand and then extended along the forearm as well. The lesions were red, scarred, scaly and ulcerated in some places (shown in Fig. 7.50).

▼ **Fig. 7.50(a) and (b)** Sporotrichosis. A 54-year-old female had a number of red, scarred and ulcerated lesions on one arm.

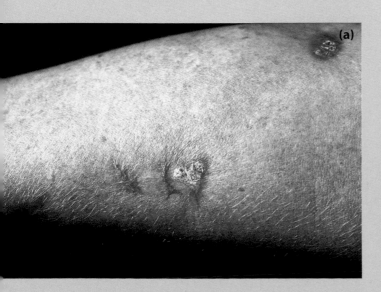

(a)

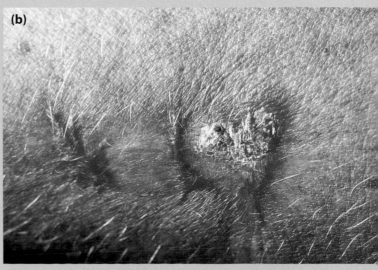

(b)

A skin biopsy showed pseudoepitheliomatous hyperplasia of the epidermis and chronic inflammation in the dermis, with the presence of some microabscesses.

Within the microabscesses, there were a few tiny, single, pink-staining yeasts (see Figs 7.51 and 7.52). These can be seen in H&E stained sections, but they are more clearly seen with PAS stain as small, pink-staining yeasts with tiny projections on their surface. The projections are thought to be a result of an antigen-antibody reaction.

The whole structure has been called an 'asteroid body'. The phenomenon is called the Splendore-Hoeppli phenomenon, after the two scientists who described it.

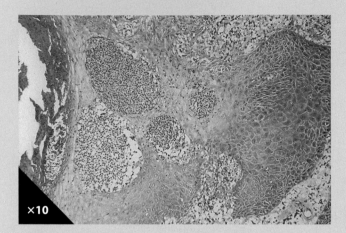

▲ **Fig. 7.51** Skin biopsy showed pseudoepitheliomatous hyperplasia of the epidermis and chronic inflammation in the dermis.

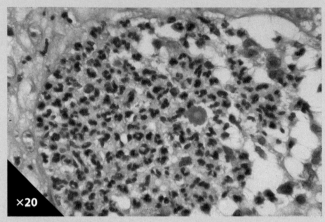

▲ **Fig. 7.52** Microabscess that contains a yeast of sporotrichosis. The yeasts are not present in great numbers and it may be necessary to examine multiple levels through the skin biopsy to find them.

Case 7.3

A 68-year-old man, living in Texas, USA, presented with scaly and ulcerated lesions on the back of his right hand, which was quite swollen (see Fig. 7.53).

The condition had started with a single ulcer after he had visited Mexico, and it slowly spread.

Diagnosis was made after many months of consulting doctors, and when this photograph was taken he had been taking antifungal medication for over 6 months without any significant improvement. Culture of the lesion showed the presence of *Sporothrix schenckii* (shown in Fig. 7.54).

▼ **Fig. 7.53** Sporotrichosis. A 68-year-old man, living in Texas, USA, presented with scaly and ulcerated lesions on the back of his right hand.

▼ **Fig. 7.54** Culture plate showing the appearance of *Sporothrix schenckii*.

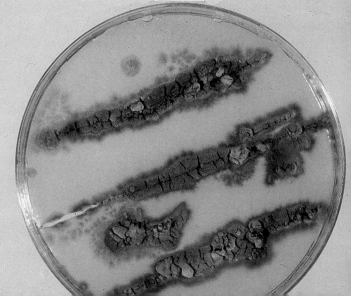

In the 1940s, there was a big epidemic of sporotrichosis among the gold miners in Johannesburg, Republic of South Africa. Sporothrix schenckii fungus was found present in the wooden posts used to support the roofs of the tunnels in the mines. The epidemic was halted by treating the wood with fungicide.

Actinomycosis

Lesions caused by species of the Actinomyces and Nocardia genera have similar clinical and pathologic features to each other. They cause both superficial infections and infections of the deep organs, particularly the liver. Fungi of these genera occur all over the world.

Actinomycotic 'granules' may be seen as commensals in various tissues of the body, notably on the surface of the small intestine (shown in Fig. 7.55) and in the crypts of the tonsils.

Surgically excised material from a lesion consists of firm, rubbery tissue. On the cut surface, one can see multiple, tiny, yellow spots, which on microscopic section are microabscesses that contain 'mycotic granules' (see Fig. 7.56, overleaf). The granules have different appearances in histologic sections, and culture is needed to make a species diagnosis (see Figs 7.57 and 7.58, overleaf).

When taking pus for culture, it is often useful to put the pus into a Petri dish, tilt the dish and allow the pus to trickle down the incline. In this way, the granules (that are heavier than the liquid pus) are left on the bottom of the dish where they can be better seen and then collected for culture.

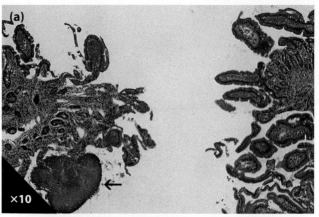

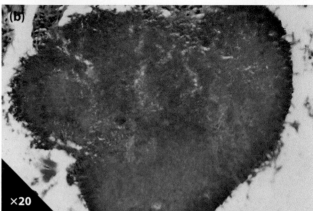

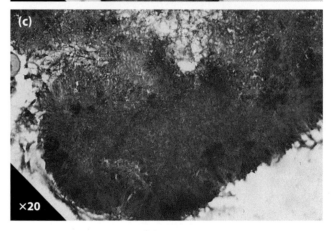

▲ **Fig. 7.55(a) and (b)** Endoscopic biopsy of the small intestine, with an actinomycotic granule on the mucosal surface. The periphery of the granule has a thickened or condensed appearance. This is an example of the Splendore-Hoeppli phenomenon. **(c)** The filamentous nature of the granules is better seen in a PAS stain.

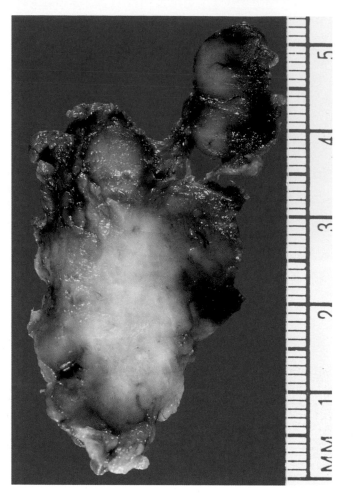

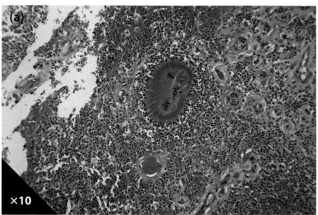

◀ **Fig. 7.56** Actinomycosis. On gross examination, the cut surface of a lesion shows fibrosis in which there are multiple, tiny, yellow spots. On section, these are the characteristic microabscesses, in which the granules of the fungus are found.

▼ **Fig. 7.57(a)** Microscopic examination shows the presence of microabscesses in the dermis and in the fibrotic tissue. A mycotic actinomycotic granule can be seen in the middle of the abscess. **(b)** The detail of the granule is better seen here.

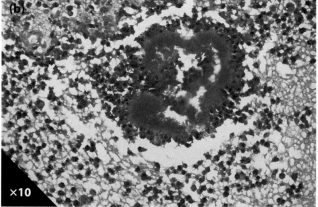

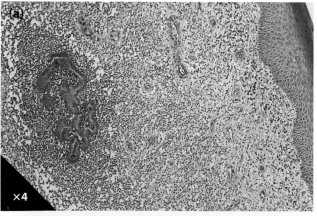

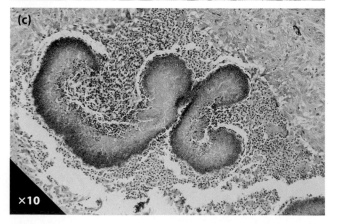

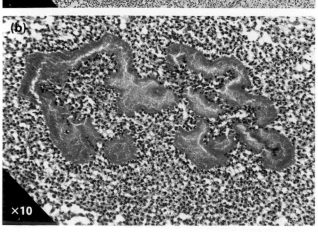

▲ **Fig. 7.58(a), (b) and (c)** Actinomycosis. These histologic sections show the variability in the appearance of the mycotic granule of the fungus in different cases. A number of different species of fungus cause the clinical condition of actinomycosis. It is not possible to diagnose the species on histology alone. One needs to have a culture of the lesion.

Clinical presentation of actinomycosis

Actinomycosis presents as multiple, discharging sinuses on the skin surface (illustrated in Figs 7.59–7.63, continued overleaf). The underlying dermis is thickened by the associated fibrosis.

When the foot is involved, the condition is called Madura foot, named after the town of Madura in India. The two cases illustrated in Figures 7.62 and 7.63, overleaf, were in-patients in Papua New Guinea. They were very advanced and the condition had been present for many years.

The author has photographic records of the patient shown in Figure 7.62, overleaf, over a period of 10 years. During this time, the patient was given intermittent treatment with antifungal medications. At one time, an X-ray of the patient's foot showed that the bones had almost completely disappeared.

The patient shown in Figure 7.63, overleaf, was seen in the 1950s, at the time of first contact between the people of this Stone Age culture and Western medicine. This patient was treated by amputation of his left leg.

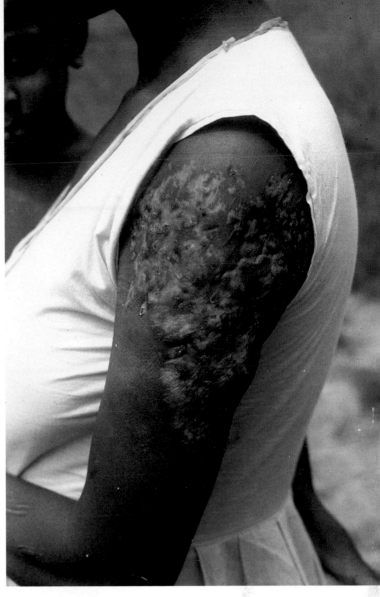

▲ **Fig. 7.60** Actinomycosis involving the left upper arm.

▼ **Fig. 7.59** Actinomycosis involving the lower jaw and neck.

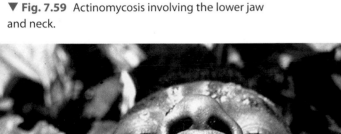

▶ **Fig. 7.61** Actinomycosis involving the back. Note the pallor of the soles of this man's feet. He was paraplegic from involvement of his spinal cord.

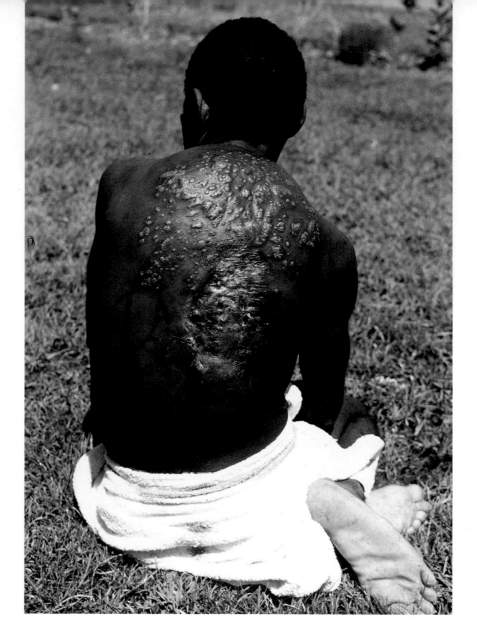

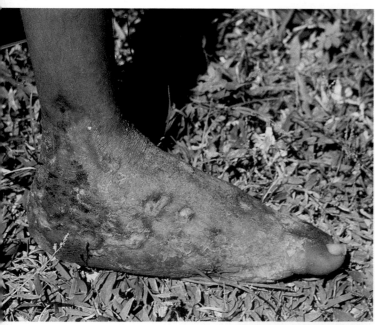

▲ **Fig. 7.62** Actinomycosis involving the left foot. When the foot is involved, the condition is called Madura foot.

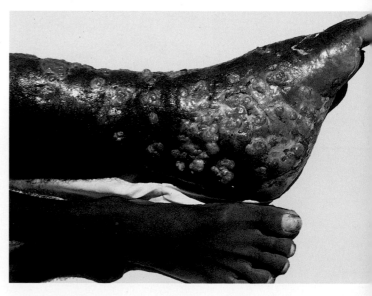

▲ **Fig. 7.63** Actinomycosis involving the left foot and leg, known as Madura foot.

Case 7.4

A 55-year-old female presented with multiple, discharging sinuses in the right groin (see Fig. 7.64), at a hospital in Queensland, Australia. The appearances were consistent with actinomycosis, and the histology and culture confirmed this diagnosis.

During treatment, this case was presented at a surgical clinical meeting at the hospital. A senior surgeon, who had been retired for 15 years, and who regularly attended these meetings, thought he recognized this case as a patient who many years earlier had presented with Madura foot—which he had amputated.

The retired surgeon, excited by the apparent similarity, returned to his home immediately to retrieve the clinical photograph (shown in Fig. 7.65) and reappeared in the office of the pathologist just a few hours later with it.

The original histologic section by this time had been retrieved from the pathology department files, and the retired surgeon was gratified to be shown that the appearances were similar to those in the current lesion.

There had been a 29-year interval between the foot lesion and the one in the groin. This case illustrates the slow progression of this infection

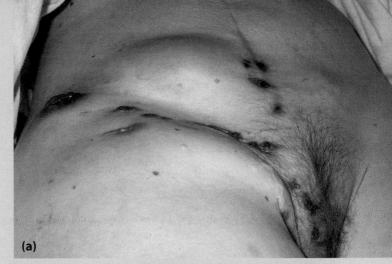

(a)

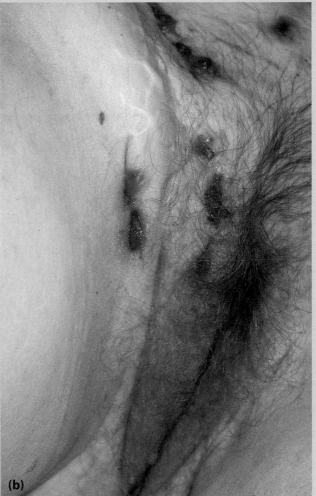

(b)

▶ **Fig. 7.64(a) and (b)** A 55-year-old female presented with multiple actinomycotic discharging sinuses in the right groin.

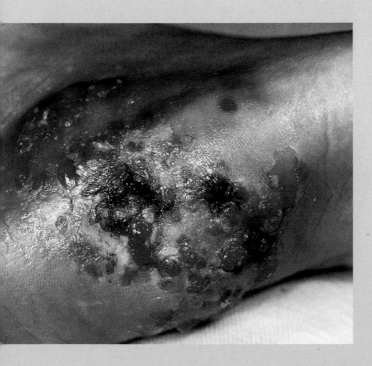

◀ **Fig. 7.65** Madura foot. Amputated 29 years earlier, this is the left foot of the patient in Figure 7.64.

Histoplasmosis

Two species of histoplasma are recognized.

- *Histoplasma capsulatum*—a small yeast surrounded by a thin capsule. It has a universal distribution, with special concentration in the mid west of the United States.
- *Histoplasma duboisii*—a larger yeast, which has a limited distribution in Africa.

Figures 7.66, 7.67 and 7.68 illustrate *H. duboisii*.
Figure 7.69 shows *H. capsulatum* and *H. duboisii* in tissue sections taken at the same magnification. The difference in size between the two can be seen.

▼ **Fig. 7.66** *Histoplasma duboisii.* Lymph node from a patient from central Africa. Its normal structure is replaced by caseous-looking necrotic material.

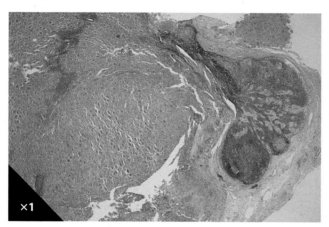

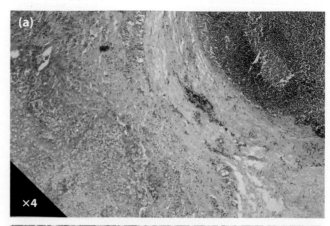

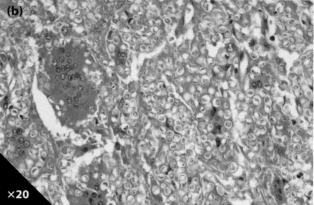

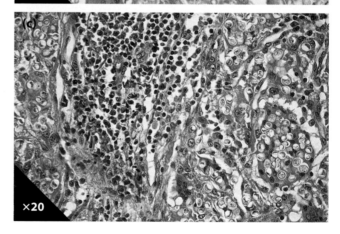

▲ **Fig. 7.67(a), (b) and (c)** *Histoplasma duboisii.* The lymph node from Figure 7.66 examined at higher magnifications. There are many large yeasts within this necrotic material consistent with their being *H. duboisii.*

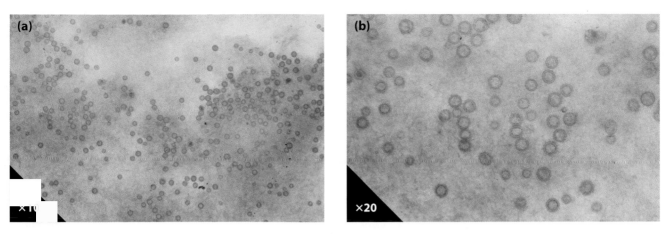

▲ **Fig. 7.68(a) and (b)** *Histoplasma duboisii.* Cotton blue stained smear from a culture of *H. duboisii.*

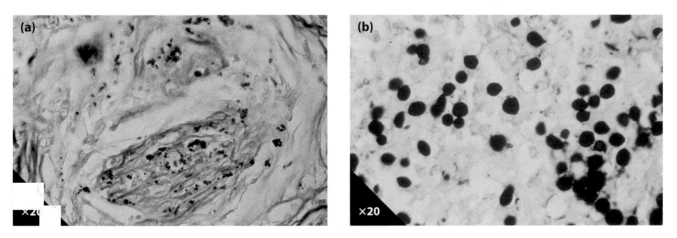

▲ **Fig. 7.69(a)** *H. capsulatum.* **(b)** *H. duboisii.* Tissue sections taken at the same magnification. Note the difference in size.

Clinical presentation of histoplasmosis

Histoplasmosis may involve any organ. In the lung and in the spleen, it produces multiple 'miliary' foci of infection (see Figs 7.70, 7.71 and 7.72). It is particularly seen in patients who are immune suppressed and it is a common infection in patients with AIDS.

▼ ▶ **Fig. 7. 70(a), (b), (c), (d) and (e)** Histoplasmosis. A section of lung showing multiple foci of acute inflammation that contain yeasts of *H. capsulatum*.

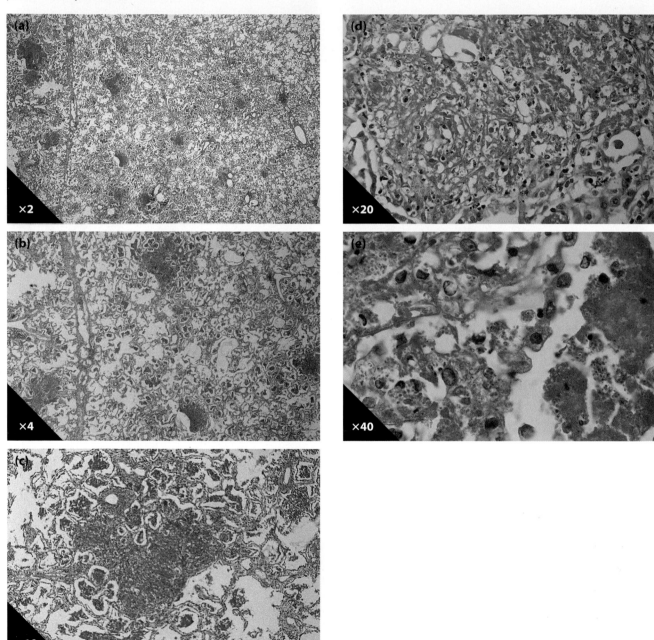

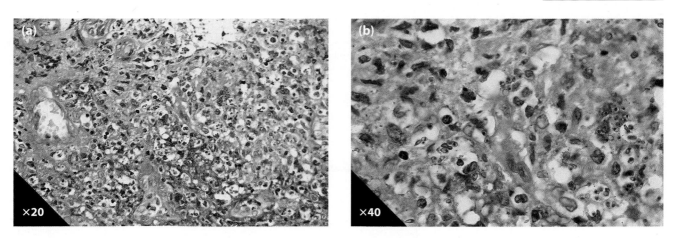

▲ **Fig. 7.71(a) and (b)** *H. capsulatum.* The tiny yeasts are not easily seen in H&E sections. PAS stain makes them more easily visible.

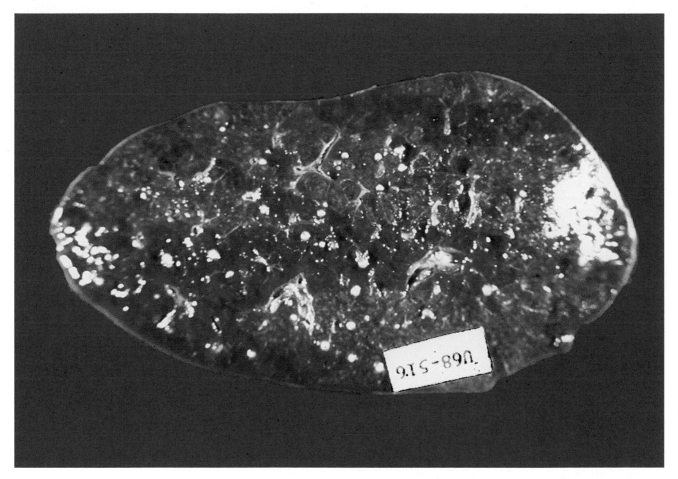

▲ **Fig. 7.72** Spleen removed from an AIDS patient in Winnipeg, Canada. The small granulomas of histoplasmosis can be seen on the cut surface.

Aspergillosis

Aspergillosis is caused by the fungus *Aspergillus fumigatus*. The fungus has a worldwide distribution. It is most commonly seen as an opportunistic infection in immune-suppressed patients. Lungs are the commonest site of involvement, with paranasal sinuses and orbit sometimes being affected (shown in Fig. 7.73).

The fungal hyphae are thin and septate, and they show multiple branching (see Figs 7.74–7.78).

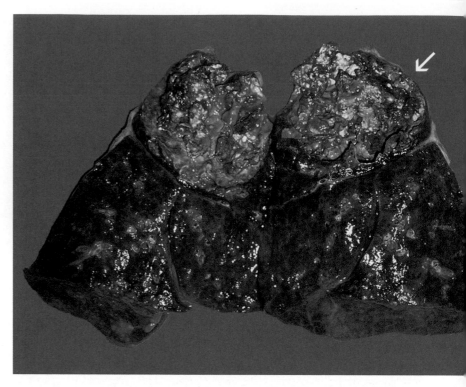

▲ **Fig. 7.73** Lung from a 59-year-old female, who died from acute leukemia complicated by *Aspergillus* infection. The apex of the lung is replaced by a friable mass of grey, necrotic tissue that was forming an abscess.

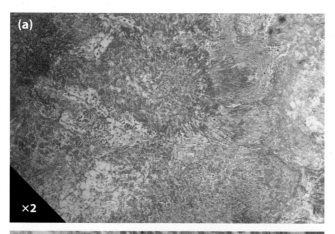

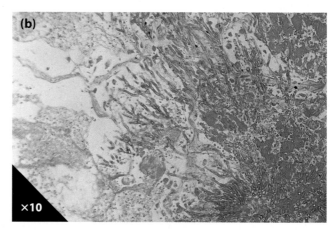

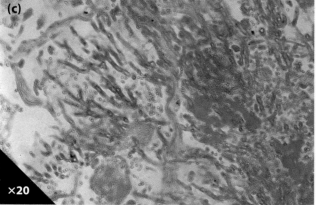

◀ ▲ **Fig. 7.74(a), (b) and (c)** Microscopic section of the lung at low, medium and high magnification shows necrotic tissue in which there is very little cellular reaction and masses of fungal hyphal filaments.

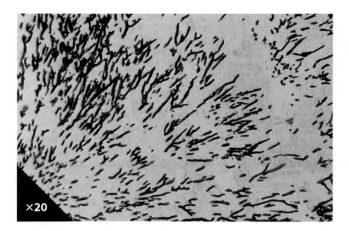

▲ **Fig. 7.75** The fungal hyphae are more clearly seen in a Grocott silver stain.

▼ **Fig. 7.76(a)** Hyphae have invaded the walls of vessels causing thrombosis and infarction of lung tissue. **(b)** The fungal hyphae are better seen in the Grocott silver stain.

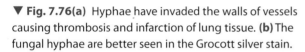

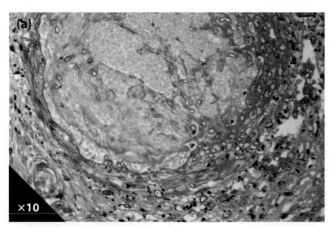

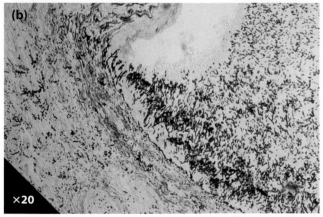

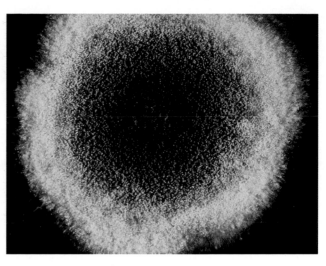

▲ **Fig. 7.77** Sabouraud's dextrose agar culture plate showing the features of the fungus *Aspergillus fumigatus*.

▼ **Fig. 7.78** Lactophenol cotton blue stained smear preparation from the culture shows filaments with specific fruiting bodies—round conidia—with multiple, small, round spores on their surfaces. Fruiting bodies are only occasionally seen in tissue sections of the organism.

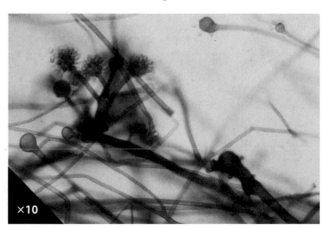

Cryptococcosis

Cryptococcosis is caused by the soil mold *Cryptococcus neoformans*. It has a worldwide distribution and Cryptococcosis can be isolated from soil and from pigeon droppings. The yeast-like organism is surrounded by a thick, mucoid capsule.

Infections occur particularly in the central nervous system and the lung, but any organ, including the subcutaneous tissue may be involved. Normal people may be affected, but it is particularly seen in those who are immune suppressed.

Case 7.5

A 35-year-old female, with no evidence of immune deficiency, presented with the symptoms and signs of meningitis. Cerebrospinal fluid (CSF) examination showed a raised protein; reduced sugar; and an increased cell count, with most of the cells being lymphocytes (shown in Fig. 7.79).

India ink preparation showed the presence of yeasts that had a prominent capsule (see Figs 7.80 and 7.81). Culture confirmed the diagnosis of cryptococcal meningitis. Ophthalmoscopic examination showed 'miliary' lesions in the retina (see Fig. 7.82).

The patient did not respond to treatment and died a few days later. The brain showed a meningitis with opacity of the meninges and pus along its base (illustrated in Figs 7.83 and 7.84, continued overleaf).

Microscopically, the appearances were characteristic of cryptococcosis (that is, a large amount of mucus with little cellular reaction, and numerous yeast-like organisms present).

In H&E sections, the space occupied by the capsule before being dissolved by the solvents used in tissue processing can be seen. PAS stains the organisms pink (see Figs 7.85 and 7.86, overleaf).

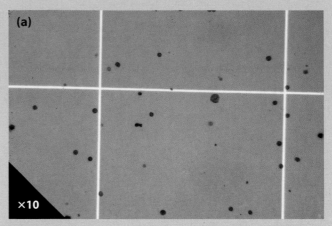

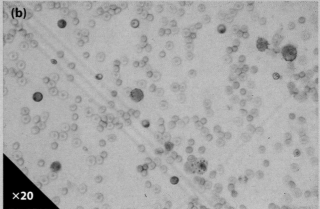

▲ **Fig. 7.79(a) and (b)** Examination of the CSF on a white cell counting chamber showed a slight increase in cells, mainly lymphocytes. There were some round structures slightly larger than lymphocytes seen on the counting chamber.

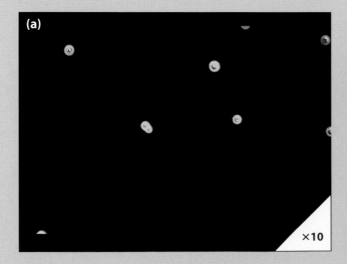

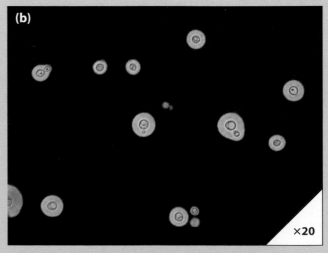

▲ **Fig. 7.80(a) and (b)** CSF India ink preparation positive for cryptococci—yeasts, some of them budding, with a thick capsule.

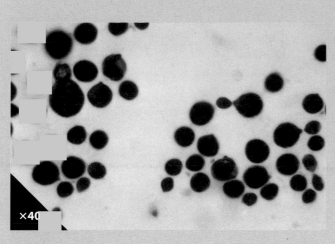

×40

▲ **Fig. 7.81** Gram stain also showed the budding yeast-like organisms.

▼ **Fig. 7.82** Ophthalmoscopic examination showing papilledema and 'miliary' tubercles in the retina in a patient with cryptococcosis.

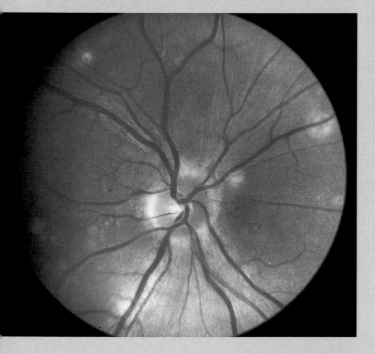

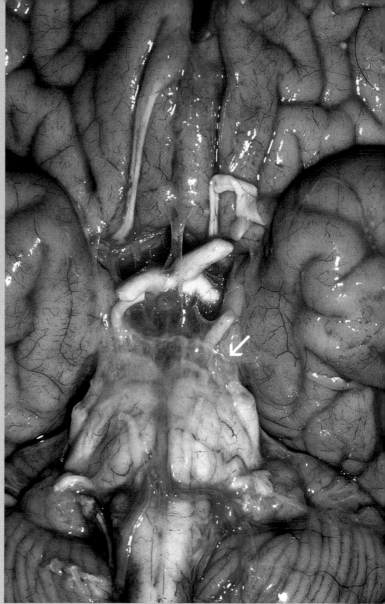

▲ **Fig. 7.83** Cryptococcal meningitis. Pus has settled along the base of the brain causing opacity of the interpeduncular space.

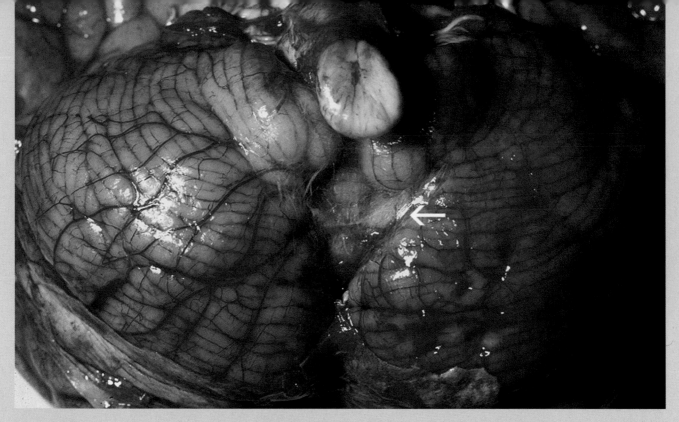

▲ **Fig. 7.84** Pus in the cisterna magna at the base of the cerebellum caused obstruction to the flow of CSF.

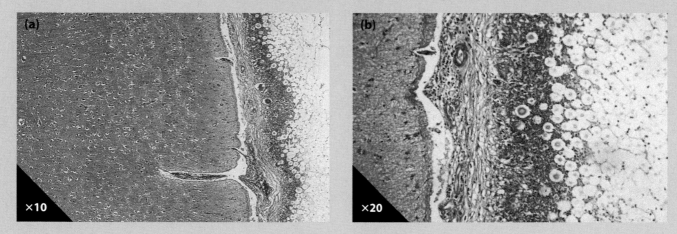

(a) ×10

(b) ×20

▲ **Fig. 7.85(a) and (b)** Microscopically, the appearances are characteristic of cryptococcosis. There is a large amount of mucus with little cellular reaction, and numerous yeast-like organisms are present.

▶ **Fig. 7.86** The yeast-like organisms are well shown with a PAS stain.

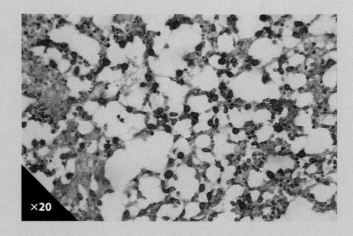

×20

Sometimes the inflammatory reaction in cryptococcosis forms a solid mass that has the features of a tumor. Such a lesion is called a cryptococcoma. Examples of such lesions in a brain are illustrated in Figures 7.87 and 7.88. Cryptococcoma of the lung is shown in Figures 7.89 and 7.90, overleaf. A mediastinal lymph node is illustrated in Figure 7.91, overleaf.

▶ **Fig. 7.87** Enhanced CT brain scan in a male, aged 50, shows the presence of two tumorous lesions. The patient died soon after admission to hospital.

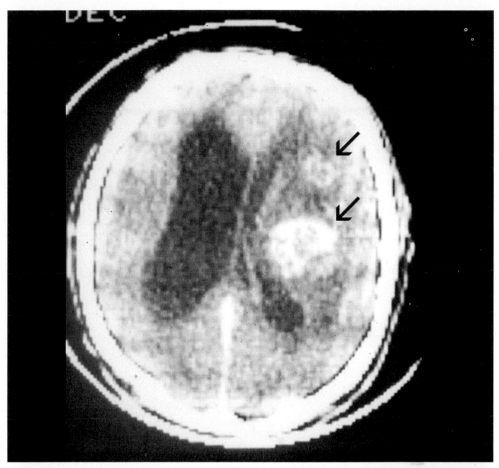

▶ **Fig. 7.88** Post-mortem specimen of the brain confirms the presence of the two areas of cryptococcoma.

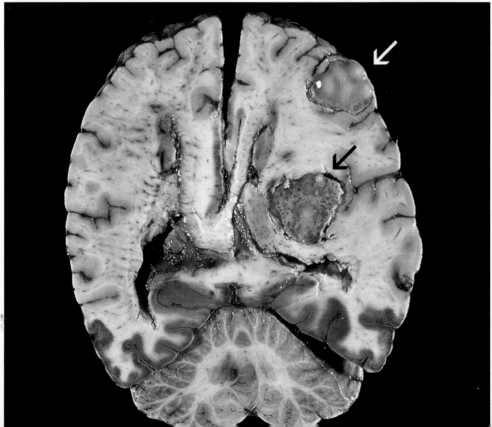

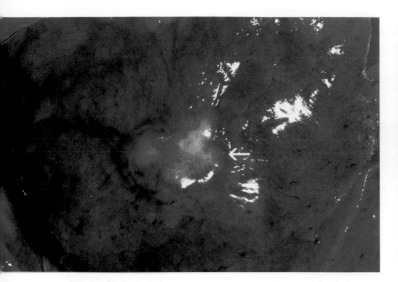

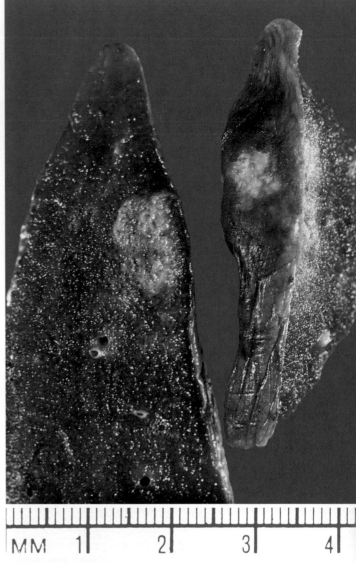

▲ **Fig. 7.89** Lung from a 66-year-old male shows a localized tumor, which had a somewhat mucoid appearance when sliced across. Microscopic section showed it to be a cryptococcoma.

▶ **Fig. 7.90** Lung slice from the postmortem examination on a 67-year-old female. It shows a localized cryptococcoma. This patient had been treated with high-dose steroids for myasthenia gravis caused by a thymoma.

▼ **Fig. 7.91** Mediastinal lymph node, which shows the mucoid appearance of a mass of cryptococcal inflammatory tissue.

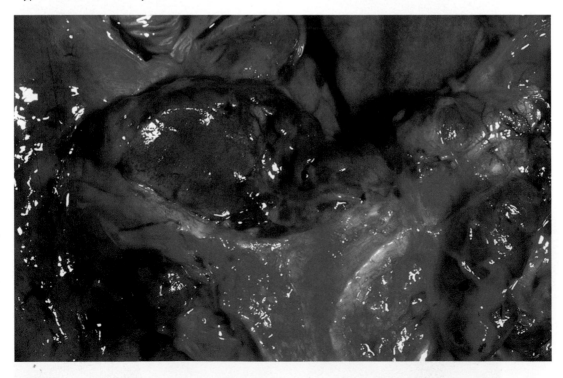

A noninvasive method for distinguishing between a lung tumor and a pulmonary cryptococcoma of the lung is a Fine Needle Aspiration (FNA), as illustrated in Figure 7.92.

Material from the FNA can be used to culture the organism.

A culture of C. neoformans *is shown in Figure 7.93.*

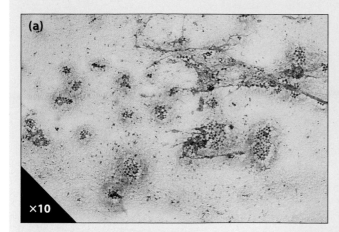

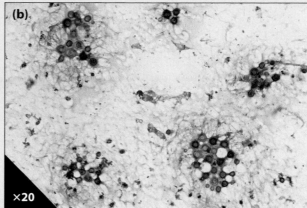

▲ **Fig. 7.92(a) and (b)** FNA of a solid lesion in the lung shows the presence of budding yeast-like organisms consistent with cryptococci.

▶ **Fig. 7.93** Cultural characteristics of *C. neoformans* on a Sabouraud's dextrose agar plate.

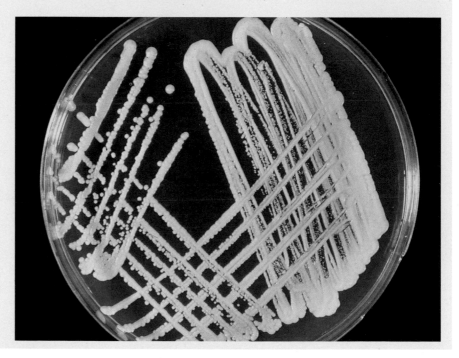

Mucormycosis

Mucormycosis is best regarded as a pathologic entity, with similar features being caused by a number of different species of the common mold fungi that are found on many different fruits and vegetables. The fungi affect immune-suppressed people, alcoholics and people with diabetes. In particular, the fungal hyphae invade the walls of pulmonary and orbital veins causing thrombosis and infarction of tissue in the drainage areas of the veins. These pathologic features are demonstrated in Figures 7.94–7.99, continued overleaf.

Case 7.6

A 54-year-old male alcoholic presented with a sudden onset of jaundice, diarrhea and vomiting. Chest X-ray showed the presence of an abscess in the mid zone of the left lung (see Fig. 7.94). The patient died 3 days after admission to hospital.

Post-mortem examination showed the presence of cirrhosis and esophageal varices. There was thrombosis of the left pulmonary vein with infarction of the lung it drained (see Fig. 7.95).

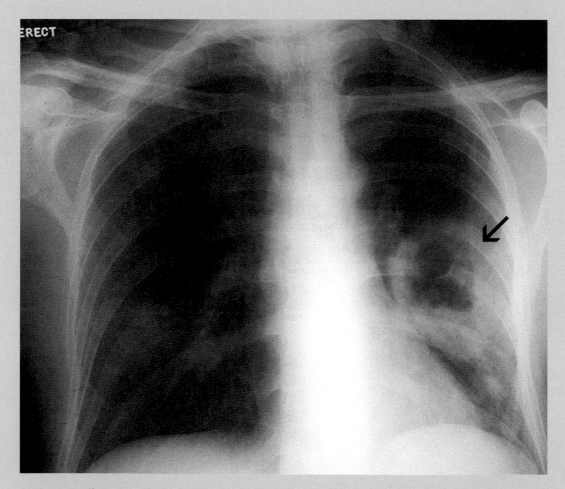

▲ **Fig. 7.94** Chest X-ray showed the presence of an abscess in the mid zone of the left lung.

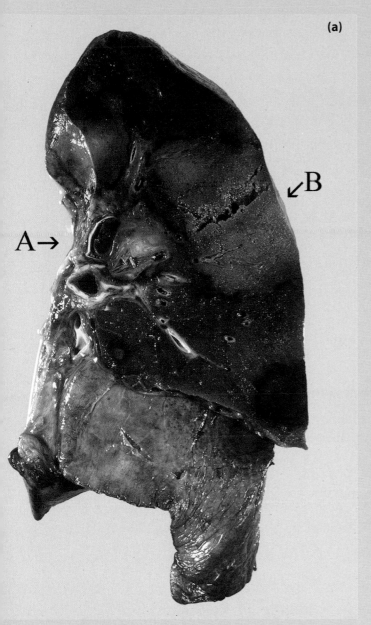

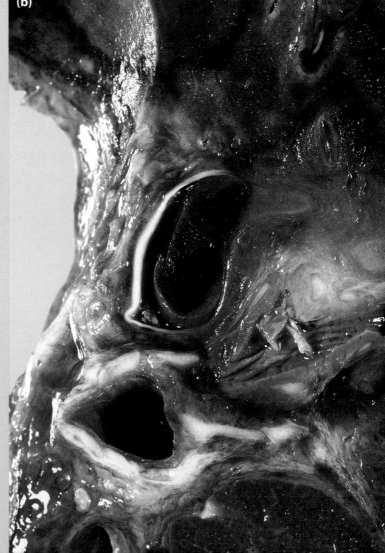

▲ ▶ **Fig. 7.95(a) and (b)** Left lung shows thrombosis of the left pulmonary vein (A), with infarction of the mid zone of the lung (B).

Microscopic sections of the lung showed an area of infarction with little cellular response. Fungal hyphae with very thick walls and no septae were seen in the H&E stained sections, in the infarcted lung, in the thrombus and in the wall of the pulmonary vein (see Fig. 7.96).

The fungal hyphae in the wall of the vein were seen more clearly in the Grocott silver stains (shown in Fig. 7.97).

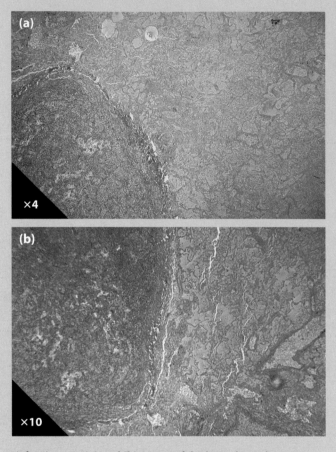

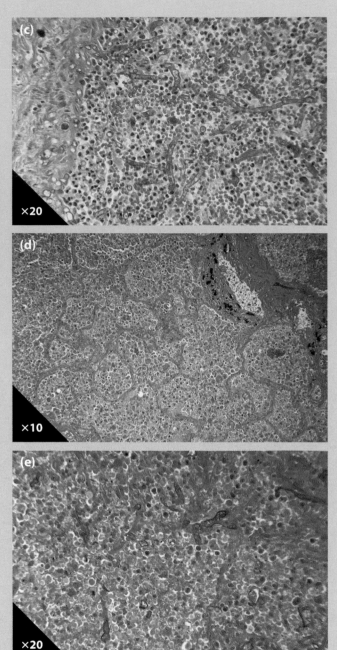

▲ ▶ **Fig. 7.96(a) and (b)** Views of the lung show the area of infarction and the thrombosed vein. There is little cellular response, but fungal hyphae with very thick walls. **(c) and (d)** No septae can be seen in the H&E stained sections, in the infarcted lung, in the thrombus, and **(e)** in the wall of the pulmonary vein.

▼ **Fig. 7.97(a) and (b)** The fungal hyphae in the wall of the vein can be seen more clearly in the Grocott silver stains.

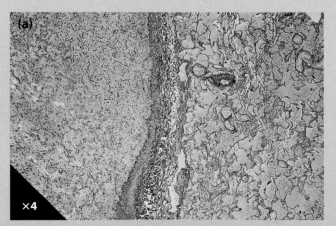

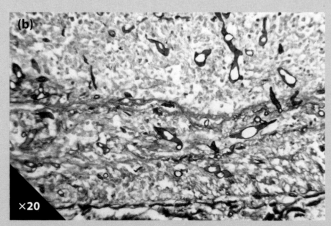

Case 7.7

A 68-year-old female with longstanding diabetes developed a disseminated infection with a Mucor-like fungus (a Zygomycetous fungus). At the time of death, she had thrombosis of the left orbital vein (shown in Fig. 7.98).

A culture plate of the usually saprophytic fungus Mucor is shown in Figure 7.99.

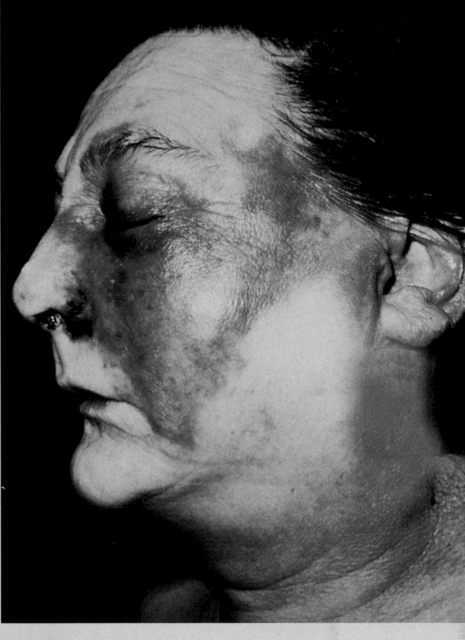

▶ **Fig. 7.98** A 68-year-old female with longstanding diabetes died of disseminated mucormycosis infection. At the time of death, she had thrombosis of the left orbital vein.

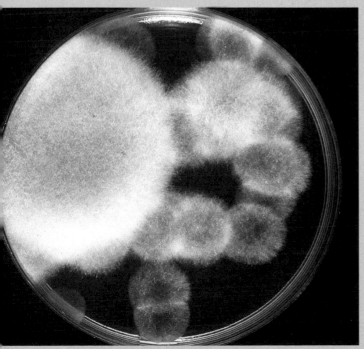

◀ **Fig. 7.99** Culture plate of the usually saprophytic fungus Mucor.

Fungal infections that occur in specific geographic regions

Up to this point, fungal infections that have a worldwide prevalence have been discussed. Now a few examples of fungal infections that occur in specific geographic regions will be presented.

Coccidioidomycosis

Coccidioidomycosis is caused by the fungus *Coccidioides immitis*. The organism is found in soil in certain parts of the world, especially in the San Fernando Valley, north of Los Angeles (and Hollywood). The organism typically causes pneumonia, but inflammation in other organs is also common.

Within the areas of pneumonic consolidation, spherules that contain endospores are seen. They consist of thick-walled structures that contain small, round spores. When the spherules rupture, endospores are spread and inhaled in the dust.

Case 7.8

A male, aged 50 years, with Hodgkin's disease, went on holidays to southern California from Winnipeg, Canada. When he returned, he had a pneumonia from which he died. The spherules of *C. immitis* were easily seen in the pneumonic areas in the lungs.

The histologic features of the lung tissue are illustrated in Figures 7.100, 7.101 and 7.102.

▼ **Fig. 7.100(a), (b) and (c)** Views of the necrosis and chronic inflammation caused by the fungus. Sporangia filled with spores can be seen in the inflammatory reaction.

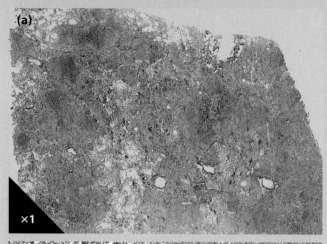

(a) ×1

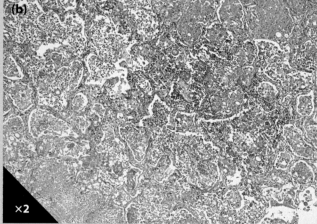

(b) ×2

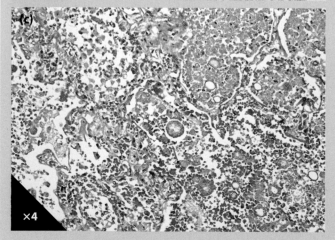

(c) ×4

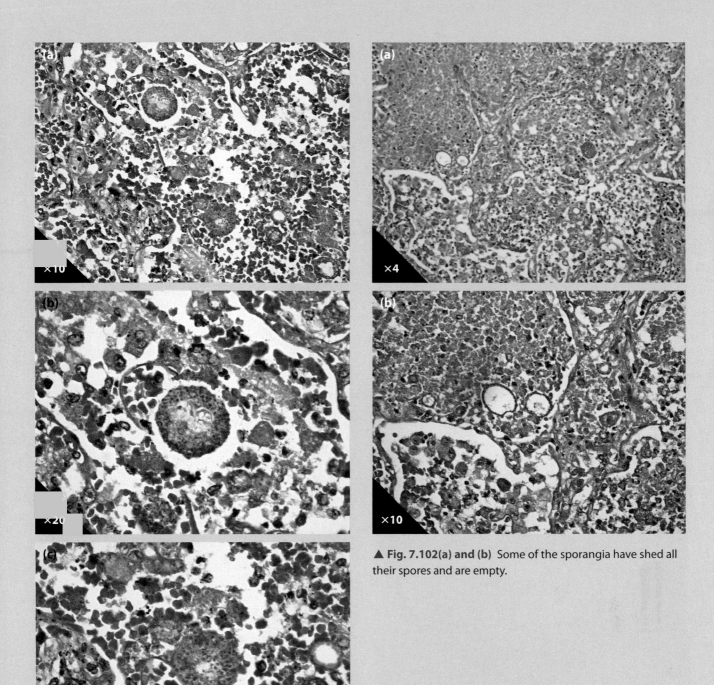

▲ Fig. 7.102(a) and (b) Some of the sporangia have shed all their spores and are empty.

▲ Fig. 7.101(a), (b) and (c) Sporangia filled with spores.

Rhinosporidiosis

Rhinosporidiosis infection is caused by a fungus—*Rhinosporidium seeberi*—that causes an inflammatory mass in the nose and nasopharynx (see Fig. 7.103). It appears to be confined to the southern states of India and the island of Sri Lanka. Its source is not known and it has not been cultured.

Histologic examination of the biopsy tissue shows the presence of multiple spherules that contain endospores that presumably are the infective agent (see Fig. 7.104).

▼ **Fig. 7.103(a) and (b)** This Sri Lankan male, aged 31 years, has a tumor in the left nostril.

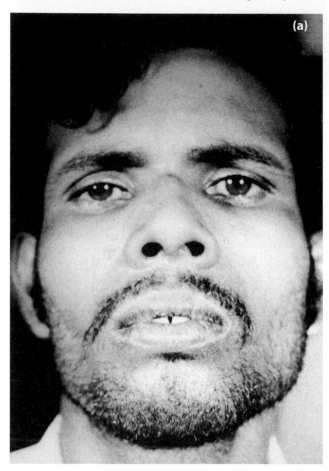 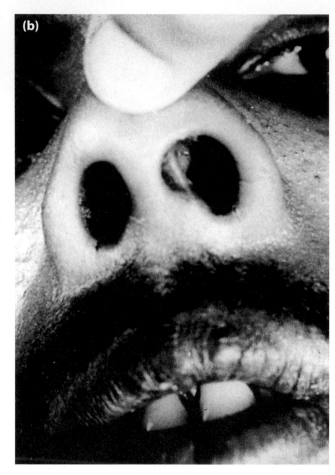

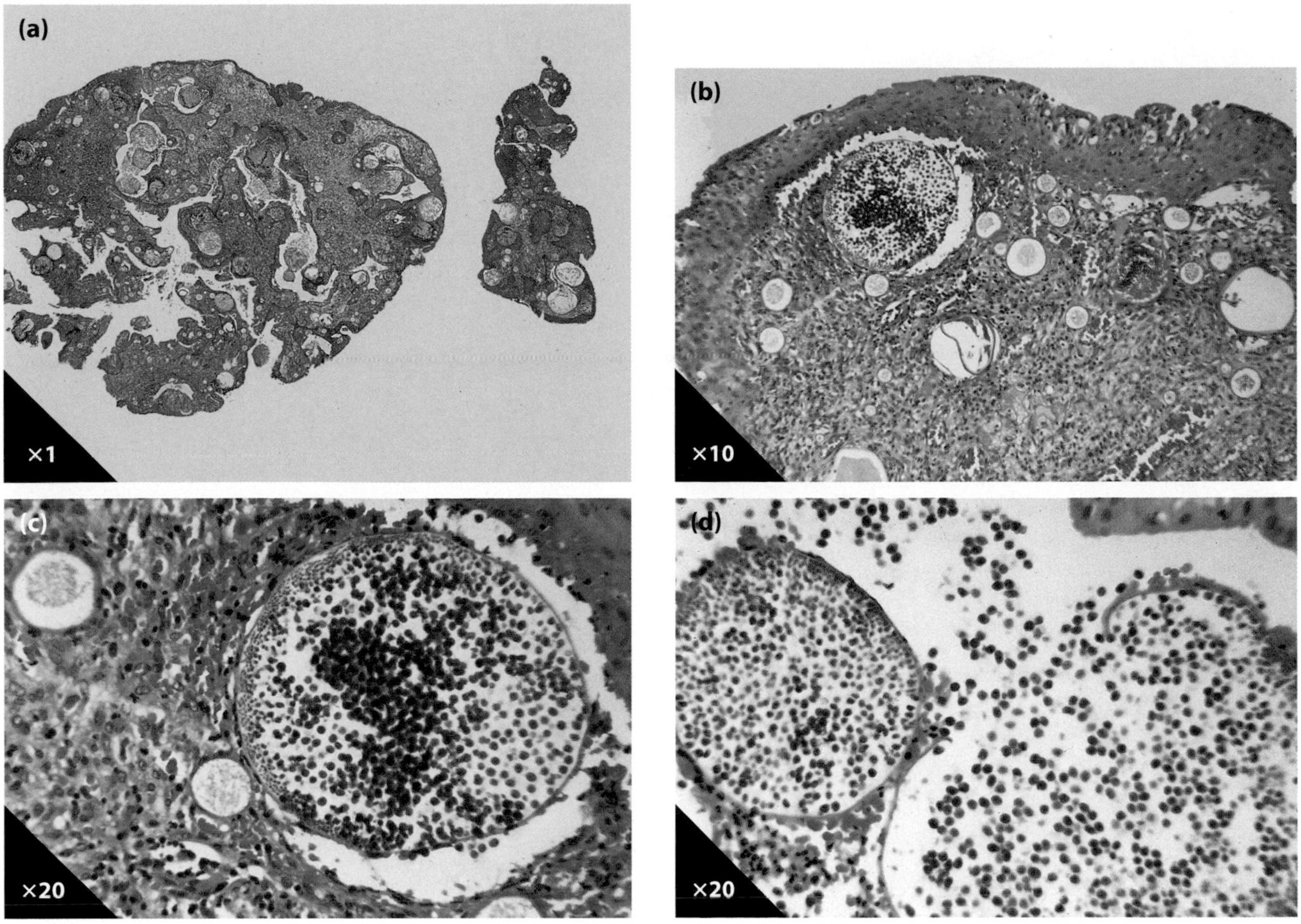

▲ ▶ **Fig. 7.104(a), (b) and (c)** The spherules of *R. seeberi* are easily seen. **(d)** The endospores can be seen escaping from the spherule.

North American blastomycosis

North American blastomycosis—caused by the fungus *Blastomyces dermatitidis*—is a rare infection found particularly in some parts of North America. Cases have also been reported from Central Africa and elsewhere. It causes pneumonia in which thick-walled budding yeasts are seen.

Occasional cases of skin infection have been reported.

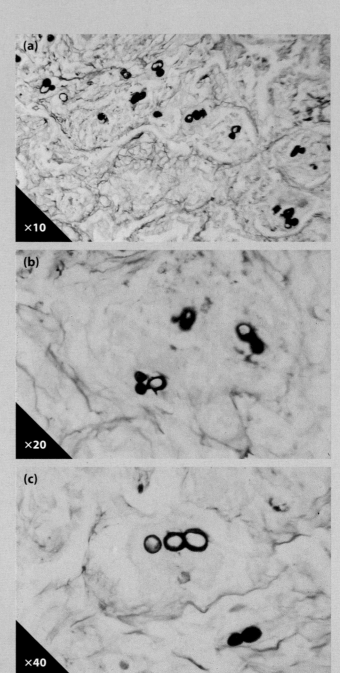

Case 7.9

A male child from central Africa died from pneumonia. The pneumonia had a 'miliary' pattern. Budding yeasts consistent with *Blastomyces dermatitidis* were identified in the pneumonic inflammatory infiltrate (see Figs 7.105 and 7.106).

▲ **Fig. 7.106(a), (b) and (c)** The morphology of the yeasts can be better seen in the Grocott stain.

▲ **Fig. 7.105(a), (b), (c) and (d)** Section of lung shows a 'miliary' type pneumonia. Multinucleated, giant cells can be seen at high magnification. Thick-walled, budding yeasts can be seen in association with the giant cells. These appearances are consistent with a diagnosis of North American blastomycosis.

South American blastomycosis

South American blastomycosis is caused by *Paracoccidioides braziliensis*. This yeast infection causes granulomatous inflammatory skin lesions and, occasionally, pneumonia.

It is found in most countries of South America, especially around the city of Sao Paulo, in the south of Brazil. In tissue sections, the organism appears as a yeast with numerous buds on its surface (see Figs 7.107 and 7.108, continued overleaf).

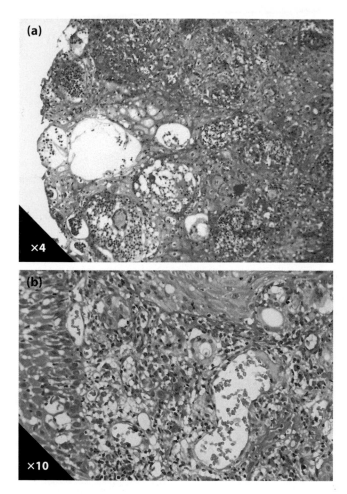

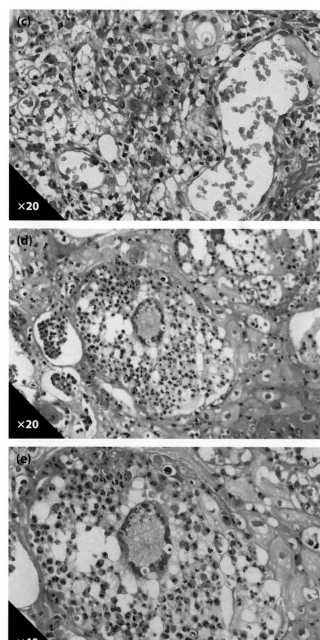

▲ ▶ **Fig. 7.107(a), (b), (c), (d) and (e)** South American blastomycosis. Skin biopsy from the dorsum of the foot of an adult male from Sao Paulo, Brazil. It shows a granulomatous inflammatory reaction in the dermis and some pseudoepitheliomatous hyperplasia. Microabscesses are present and within them, and within some of the multinucleated giant cells, one can see yeast-like organisms.

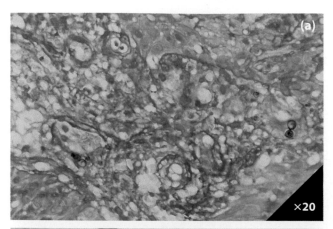

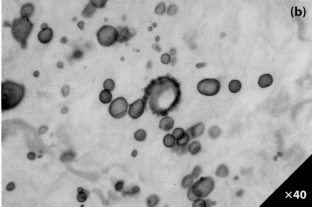

▲ **Fig. 7.108(a) and (b)** South American blastomycosis. Grocott stain shows more clearly the morphology of the yeasts with multiple surface budding.

Basidiobolus

The Basidiobolus fungus belongs to the class Zygomycetes, which also includes the Mucorales. It occurs in a number of countries in central Africa. Only very rarely has it been reported from elsewhere. Infection involves the nose and nasal sinuses. It has an indolent course over many years and may cause severe disfigurement.

Diagnosis is based on the observation of fungal hyphae, surrounded by a typical eosinophilic mantle, within the granulomata. Mycologic culture should be done to confirm the exact species of fungus involved.

Case 7.10

A 21-year-old male from Cameroon presented with swelling across the middle of his face and involving the bridge of his nose. The swelling began about 2 years previously. He was treated with corticosteroids but the swelling continued to advance (see Fig. 7.109).

Microbiology, serology and hematology tests were negative. CT scans revealed marked soft tissue thickening of the nasal bridge and mid face. Biopsy was performed. Part of the tissue was sent for microbiologic testing and the rest was processed for histopathologic examination (see Figs 7.110, 7.111 and 7.112). The fungus *Conidiobolus coronatus* was cultured.

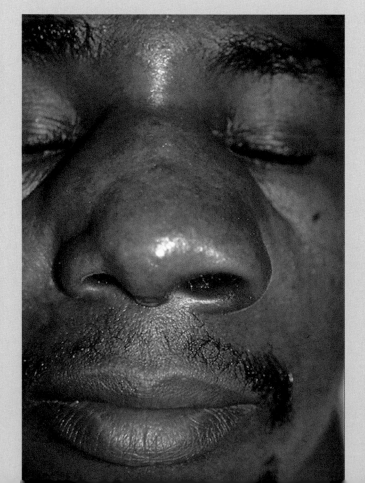

▶ **Fig. 7.109** This 21-year-old male from Cameroon had swelling across the middle of his face and involving the bridge of his nose. It had been present for about 2 years.

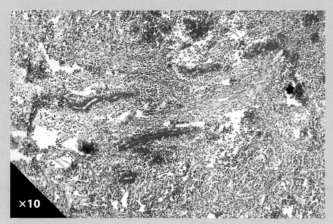

▲ Fig. 7.110 Biopsy shows a suppurative granulomatous inflammation containing a number of bright red-staining structures.

▶ Fig. 7.111(a), (b) and (c) The bright red structures are fungal hyphae which show the Splendore-Hoeppli phenomenon around fungal hyphae in the granulomatous reaction.

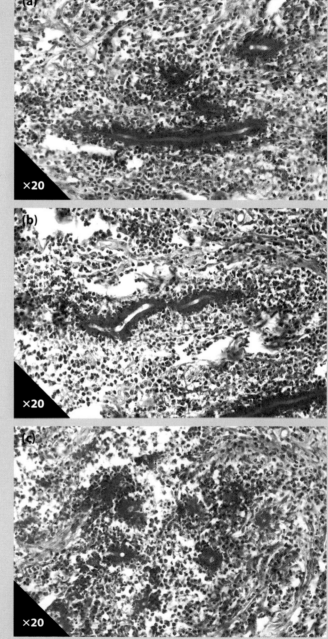

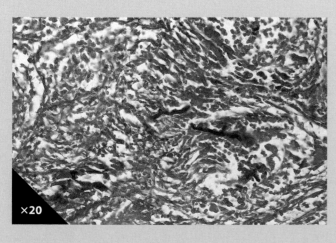

◀ Fig. 7.112 Grocott stain demonstrates fungal hyphae which show occasional branching.

Pneumocystosis

Pneumocystosis is an opportunistic infection caused by *Pneumocystis carinii*. The organism infects lungs of malnourished infants and people suffering from immune suppression from whatever cause. The source of infection and the mode of transmission are not known. Pneumocystis used to be classified as a protozoan parasite but it is now classified as a fungus. Its new name is *Pneumocystis jirovecii*.

Pneumocystis pneumonia changed from being a relative rarity to being an important and relatively common condition with the onset of the worldwide AIDS pandemic. The first symptoms of AIDS may be a candida infection of the esophagus and a pneumocystis infection of the lungs.

With the advent of highly effective, modern chemotherapy for the treatment of cancer, there emerged another group of patients susceptible to pneumocystis infection. Patients being treated for cancer often develop diffuse mottling of their lungs. The three main causes of this are secondary cancer, interstitial fibrosis and pneumocystis.

Bronchial lavage, Fine Needle Aspiration (FNA) and or open-lung biopsy are performed in order to make the correct diagnosis. Smears from bronchial lavage or FNA of the lung are usually satisfactory for diagnosing pneumocystis infection without going through the trauma of an open-lung biopsy.

Other methods used in diagnosis are direct immunofluorescence and polymerase chain reaction (PCR) tests.

The pathologic features of pneumocystis pneumonia are illustrated in Figures 7.113 to 7.117, continued overleaf.

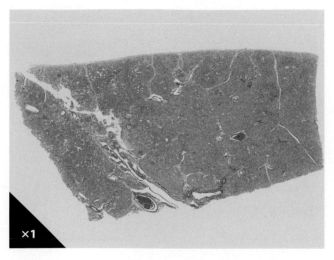

▲ **Fig. 7.113** View of an almost solid lung from a female 4 months of age who died from pneumocystis pneumonia.

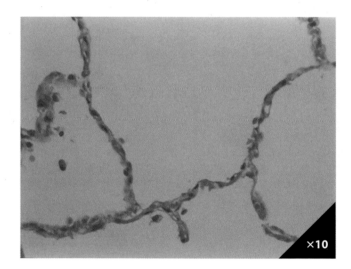

▲ **Fig. 7.114** View of the alveolar part of a normal lung (for comparison with the abnormal lung).

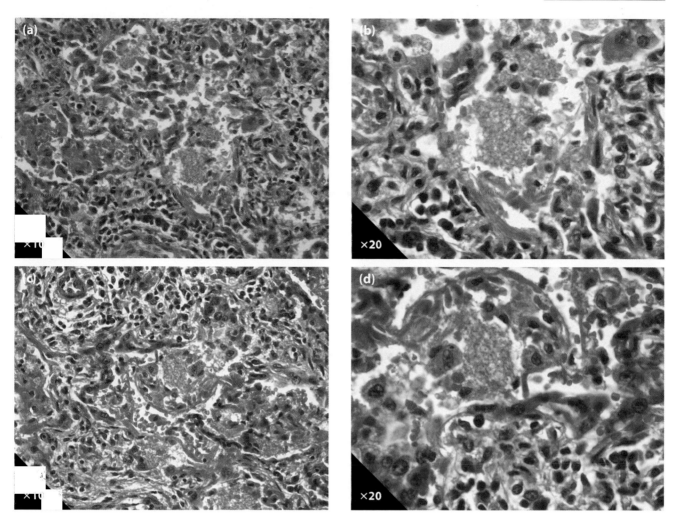

▲ **Fig. 7.115(a), (b), (c) and (d)** Views of the lung showing thickened alveolar septae, an infiltration of chronic inflammatory cells, (especially plasma cells) and pink-staining material filling the alveolar spaces. The exudate in the alveolar spaces is speckled with small 'dots'.

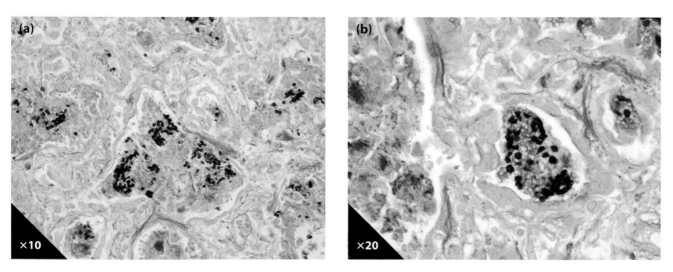

▲ **Fig. 7.116(a) and (b)** Views of a sliver stain that shows the 'dots' (seen in Fig. 7.115) are tiny cysts that contain the infecting organism.

▶ **Fig. 7.117** View of a Grocott stained group of pneumocystis cysts in a bronchial lavage specimen. The cyst walls and the trophozoites within the cysts are clearly seen.

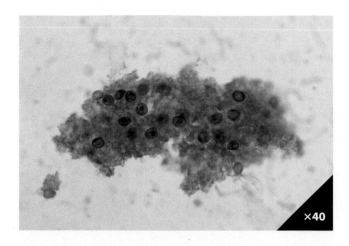

×40

Mimics of fungal infections

There are diseases that look as though they should be fungal in origin, but the nature of the 'organism' that can be seen in tissue sections cannot be determined.

One such disease that demonstrates these characteristics has been called 'sago palm disease'. It is a condition that shows typical and reproducible clinical and pathologic features. New cases have been encountered over a period of at least 30 years. Cases have occurred in a localized area near the Sepik River in the north of the island of Papua New Guinea.

Clinically, the cases have shown nodular lesions on the face, trunk and limbs of teenagers and adults of both sexes (see Figs 7.118, 7.119 and 7.120, continued overleaf). All of the clinical cases demonstrated in this section came from the Sepik River area of Papua New Guinea. Various forms of drug therapy have not been successful.

When excised, the cut surface of the nodules is a yellow color (see Figs 7.121 and 7.122, overleaf). Microscopically, the lesions are easily recognized. There is a chronic inflammatory reaction in the dermis with a cellular infiltration of lymphocytes and plasma cells.

Accompanying this, there is a prominent homogeneous, amorphous mass of material through which there are numerous small, round bodies that look as though they should be organisms. They are PAS positive, but other special investigations to try to identify their nature have been unsuccessful (see Figs 7.123 and 7.124, overleaf).

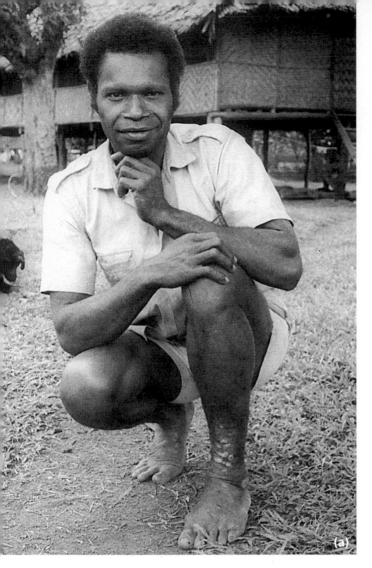
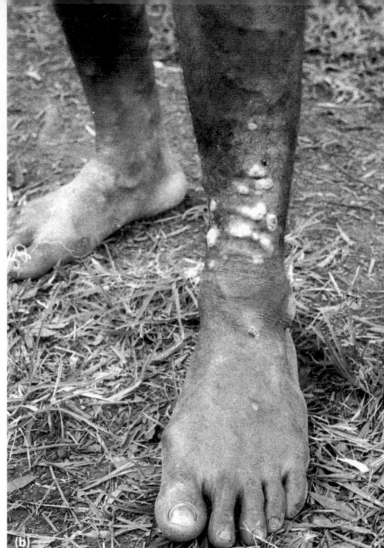

▲ **Fig. 7.118(a) and (b)** This young man has multiple nodular lesions on the anterior aspect of his left lower leg.

▶ **Fig. 7.119** This young man has multiple nodular lesions on his left arm.

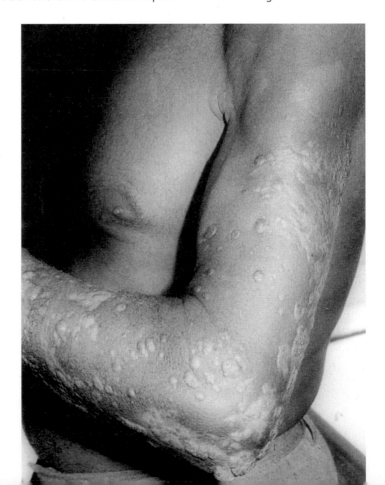

▶ ▼ **Fig. 7.120(a) and (b)** Multiple nodular lesions on the left leg of a young woman.

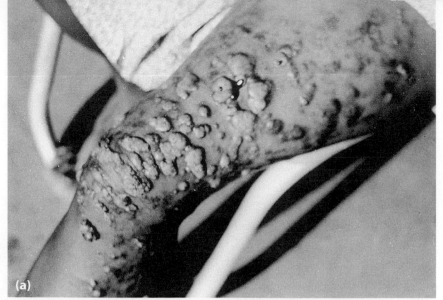

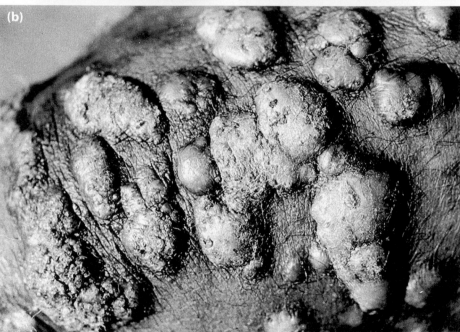

▶ **Fig. 7.121** Two lesions excised from the back of the leg from a male aged 30 years. He had a number of other similar lesions on his legs.

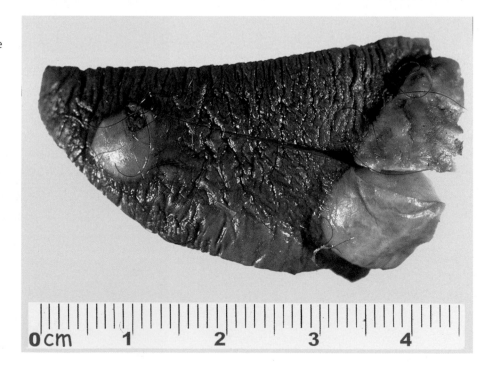

▶ **Fig. 7.122** The cut surface of the larger nodule shows a homogeneous yellow tumor.

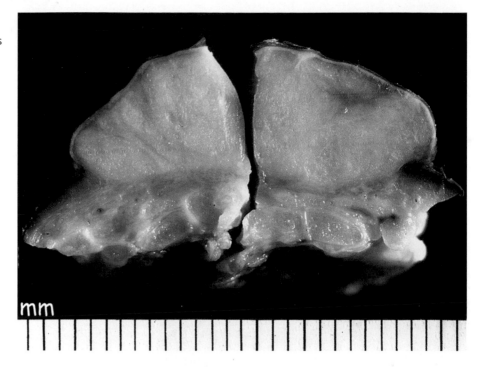

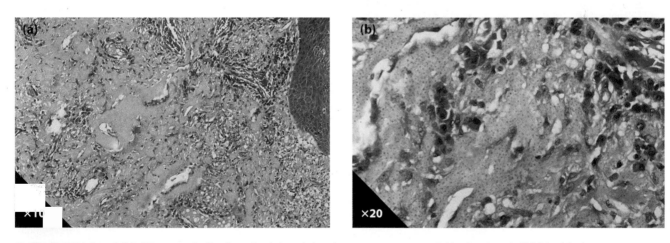

▲ **Fig. 7.123(a) and (b)** Microscopically, there is pink-staining, homogeneous material in the dermis. Within this there are numerous small, blue-staining 'dots.' Surrounding this pink material there is an infiltration of lymphocytes and plasma cells.

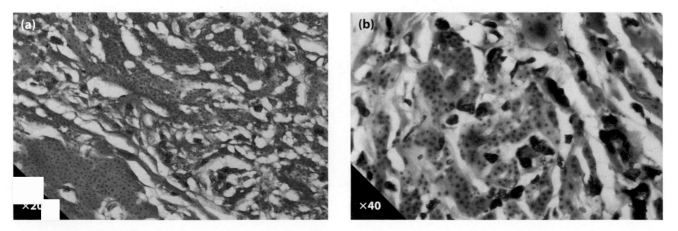

▲ **Fig. 7.124(a) and (b)** PAS stain stains the 'dots' a bright pink color.

Lesions that look superficially like fungal diseases but are not

Fungal balls

Fungal balls consist of masses of laminated 'fleshy' material that are found in association with chronic urinary tract infection. Microscopic examination shows that they consist of amorphous acellular material (see Figs 7.125 and 7.126).

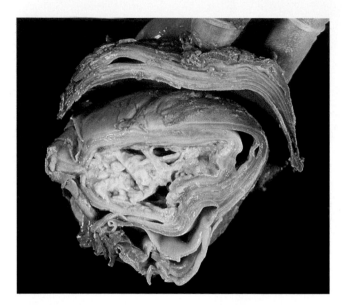

▲ **Fig. 7.125** A mass of laminated 'fleshy' amorphous material removed from the bladder of an 82-year-old female. No organism was grown from this material. She had been suffering from chronic cystitis.

Acknowledgments

- Fig. 7.12 Photograph taken with permission of the Curator of the Moulage Museum, Paris, France.
- Fig. 7.23 Courtesy of David Ellis, Adelaide, Australia.
- Fig. 7.37 From Cooke, R.A. and Stewart, B., *Colour Atlas of Anatomical Pathology*, third edn, Churchill Livingstone, Edinburgh, 2004.
- Fig. 7.39(c) Courtesy of Wayne Pederick, Rockhampton, Australia.
- Figs 7.59–7.61 Courtesy of Maurice Cave, Papua New Guinea and Rockhampton, Australia.
- Fig. 7.63 Courtesy of Leonard Champness, Papua New Guinea and Geelong, Australia.
- Fig. 7.65 Courtesy of Konrad Hirschfeld, Brisbane, Australia.
- Fig. 7.66 Courtesy of Victor Harrison, London, England.
- Fig. 7.72 Courtesy of David Buntine, Brisbane, Australia.
- Fig. 7.73 From Cooke, R.A. and Stewart, B., *Colour Atlas of Anatomical Pathology*, third edn, Churchill Livingstone, Edinburgh, 2004.
- Fig. 7.82 Courtesy of Barry Appleton, Brisbane, Australia.
- Fig. 7.103(a) and (b) and case report. Courtesy of Prof. Mrs Bhaskaran, Colombo, Sri Lanka.
- Fig. 7.105 Courtesy of Victor Harrison, London, England.
- Fig. 7.107 Case courtesy of Marcello Franco, Sao Paulo, Brazil.
- Figs 109 and 110 Case courtesy of Michel Huerre, Chief, Histopathology Unit, Pasteur Institute, Paris, France.
- Fig 7.117 Courtesy of Peter Dash, Brisbane, Australia.
- Figs 7.118–7.124 Courtesy of Ian Wilkey, Prasantha Murthy and Kamal SenGupta, all formerly of Papua New Guinea and now in Australia.

▶ **Fig. 7.126** A mass of laminated 'fleshy' amorphous material in a hydronephrotic kidney from a 73-year-old female.

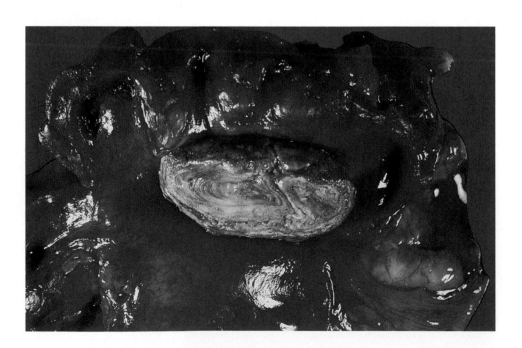

Viral infections

Viruses are infectious agents that multiply within living cells. Most of them are too small to be seen with a light microscope and are visible only under an electron microscope. The Russian biologist Dimitry I. Ivanovsky (1864–1920) from Rostov-on-Don, the center of the Cossack area in southern Russia, is given the credit for identifying this group of organisms.

The incidence of many of the viral diseases has been greatly reduced in the second half of the twentieth century by the progressive introduction of increasing numbers of effective vaccines, many of which are administered to children in the first few years of life as part of immunization programs. Vaccines to prevent specific diseases (such as yellow fever and rabies) in known areas of occurrence are also available. Vaccines are available for the following viruses: influenza, hepatitis A and hepatitis B, polio, human papilloma virus, chickenpox, measles, mumps, rubella, rotavirus, smallpox and yellow fever.

Viruses are divided into two broad groups.

- Those that contain only deoxyribonucleic acid (DNA).
- Those that contain only ribonucleic acid (RNA).

Prion diseases (a group included here for convenience) used to be called 'slow viruses'—so named because the disease becomes apparent only some months after infection. These contain no nucleic acid—only protein.

DNA viruses

Varicella zoster (VZV) (see page 236)
Herpes simplex virus (HSV-1 and HSV-2) (see page 252)
Human papilloma virus (HPV) (see page 259)
Molluscum contagiosum (see page 262)
Cytomegalovirus (CMV) (see page 263)
Hepatitis B virus (HBV) (see page 266)
Epstein–Barr virus (EBV) (see page 279)
Smallpox virus (see page 458)
Monkeypox virus (see page 478)
Adenovirus
Parvovirus

RNA viruses

Mumps (see page 252)
Measles (see page 244)
Rubella (see page 264)
Hepatitis A virus (HAV) (see page 266)
Hepatitis C virus (see page 269)
Yellow fever (see page 269)
Rabies (see page 271)
Australian bat lyssavirus (ABLV) (see page 274)
Poliovirus (see page 283)
Enteroviruses (polio (see page 283), coxsackie, echo)
Influenza (see page 460)
Human immunodeficiency virus (HIV) (see page 466)
Severe acute respiratory syndrome (SARS) (a coronavirus) (see page 473)
Dengue fever
Parainfluenza
Rhinovirus
Rotavirus
Henipavirus (see page 480)

Prion diseases

Creutzfeldt-Jacob Disease (CJD) (see page 276)
Iatrogenic CJD (see page 278)
Bovine spongiform encephalopathy (BSE) (mad cow disease) (see page 278)
CJD variant type (see page 278)
Kuru (see page 278)
Mink encephalopathy
Scrapie (in sheep)

Structure of viruses

Each virus has a DNA or an RNA genome. This is surrounded by a protein envelope called a capsid. The capsid is sometimes intimately wrapped into the nucleic acid. In many viruses, this complex is surrounded by a lipid envelope. This entire structure is the infective virus particle. The virus particle is called a virion. The virion of each genus of virus has a distinctive size, shape and antigenic properties.

How does a virus enter a cell?

When the envelope of the virion of the infecting virus fuses with the host cell membrane, the envelope is dissolved and the capsid is injected into the cytoplasm of the cell. The capsid is removed from the nucleic acid particle and the virus takes over the host cell and uses its synthetic mechanisms to replicate the nucleic acid of the virus.

- DNA viruses replicate within the nucleus of the host cell (for example, cytomegalovirus (CMV) and pox viruses).
- RNA viruses replicate in the cytoplasm (for example, measles and influenza).

The viral inclusions can be seen in these sites in microscopic sections of human tissues, as will be demonstrated in the examples of these diseases.

Ultimately, the newly formed viral nucleic acid is covered by a protein capsid and a lipid envelope, and released from the host cell to reinfect further cells.

Chickenpox

Caused by the chickenpox virus—varicella-zoster virus (VZV)—this disease is spread by respiratory droplet infection or by contact with fluid from the vesicles. It is highly contagious and occurs in epidemics which particularly involve children of primary school age.

The incubation period is 17 days (range 9–21 days) and symptoms are mild. It lasts for about 7–10 days. The incidence of chickenpox has been greatly reduced by the introduction of an effective vaccine.

Clinical features

The clinical features of chickenpox are demonstrated in Figure 8.1. The patient seen here is a male, aged 10 years. He shows numerous groups of vesicles, of varying size, which are mainly on his trunk. These vesicles occur in recurring crops that appear every 24–48 hours.

The vesicles are small, and in the early stage they are filled with clear fluid. The skin around the vesicles is red. The vesicles are itchy. When they rupture, a scab forms and healing occurs. Secondary bacterial infection may occur.

Chickenpox pneumonia

A few patients develop chickenpox pneumonia as a complication of the chickenpox disease. Very rarely death occurs from this complication, in both children and adults. When death does occur, it is usually in immunocompromised patients.

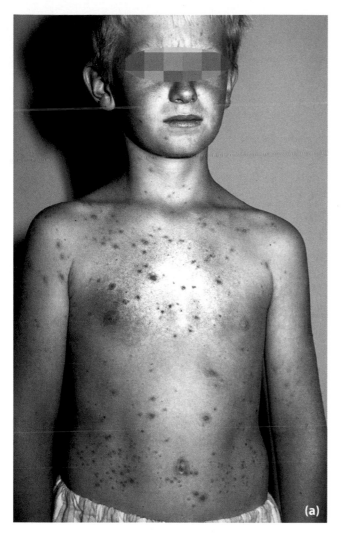

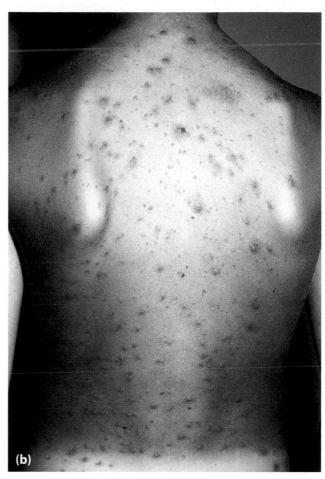

▲ **Fig. 8.1(a) and (b)** Chickenpox. Groups of vesicles that appear as recurring crops every 24–48 hours are present, mainly on the trunk.

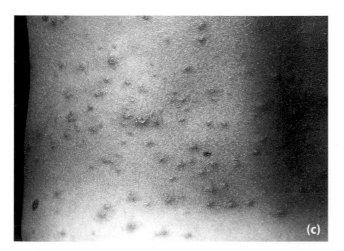

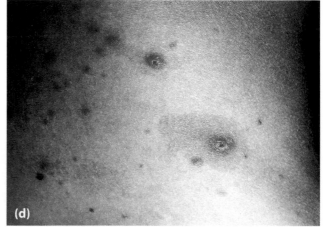

▲ **Fig. 8.1(c) and (d)** Chickenpox. The vesicles are in various stages of development. Some have been secondarily infected as a result of scratching.

Case 8.1

A female, aged 13 years, developed a sore throat, nasal obstruction and malaise. Three days later, a chickenpox rash appeared mainly on her trunk. She deteriorated with severe headaches and became delirious. She was admitted to hospital on the sixth day of symptoms.

Steroids and antibiotics were given but she continued to deteriorate. The rash became hemorrhagic (shown in Fig. 8.2). She died 14 days after the onset of symptoms.

A post-mortem examination was performed. A section of the skin rash showed suprabasal vesicles with features of poxvirus invasion of the epidermal cells; that is, enlargement of nuclei and formation of multinucleated cells with the presence of intracytoplasmic viral particles (shown in Fig. 8.3).

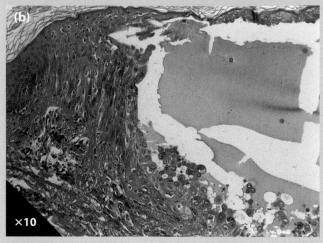

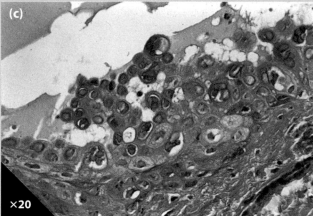

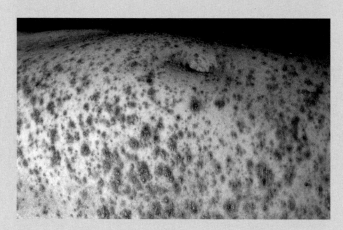

▲ **Fig. 8.2** Hemorrhagic vesicular rash in a fatal case of chickenpox in a female 13 years.

▲ **Fig. 8.3(b) and (c)** Base of the vesicle shows the enlarged epithelial cells, some of which are multinucleated and contain intracytoplasmic viral inclusions.

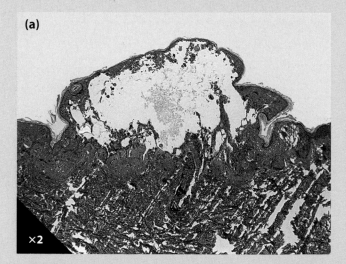

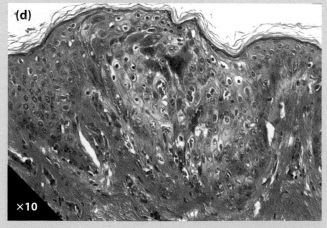

▲ **Fig. 8.3(a)** Skin biopsy of a vesicular lesion from this fatal case of chickenpox.

▲ **Fig. 8.3(d)** The epithelium adjacent to the vesicle shows changes of enlargement of the epithelial cells and the beginning of multinucleated, giant cells.

Grossly, the lungs were heavy, firm and rubbery, with hemorrhagic focal lesions noted through the pleura. Microscopically, they showed multiple areas of necrosis with edema fluid in the alveolar spaces and very little inflammatory cell reaction (see Figs 8.4 and 8.5).

Multiple hemorrhagic areas were present throughout the liver (as shown in Fig. 8.6, overleaf). Microscopically, these were focal areas of necrosis without any significant cellular reaction (see Fig. 8.7, overleaf).

Similar focal areas of necrosis were present in other organs as well (for example the adrenal gland, shown in Fig. 8.8, overleaf).

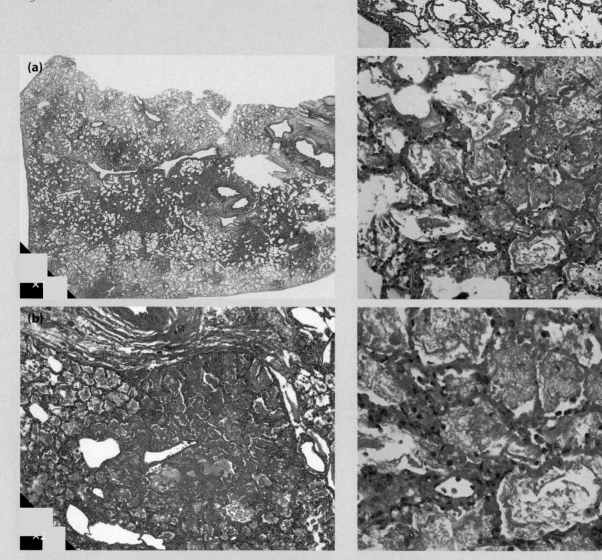

▲ **Fig. 8.4(a) and (b)** Views of lung showing a large area of necrosis, from this fatal case of chickenpox.

▲ **Fig. 8.5(a), (b) and (c)** Views of one of the smaller focal areas of necrosis in the lung.

Fig. 8.6 Cut surface of liver showing multiple hemorrhagic foci of necrosis, from this fatal case of chickenpox.

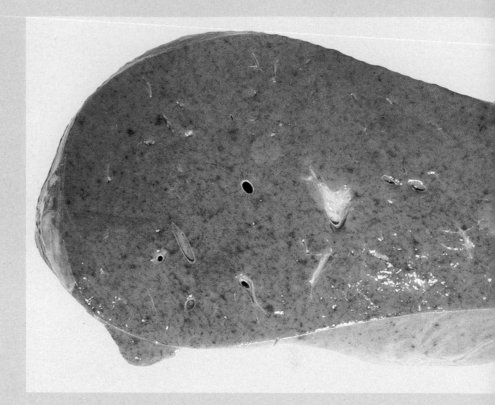

Fig. 8.7(a) and (b) Views of a focal area of necrosis in the liver.

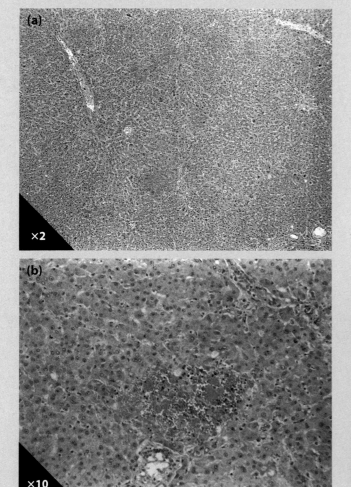

(a)

×2

(b)

×10

Fig. 8.8 Focus of necrosis in the adrenal gland.

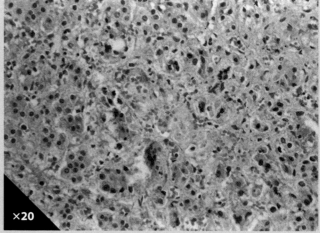

×20

In the early 1960s, some patients who attended a hospital in Brisbane, Australia, were found to have developed multiple, calcified nodules through their lungs (see Fig. 8.9), some years after they had had an attack of chickenpox. It was considered that these nodules may have resulted from calcification of the areas of acute necrosis.*

One such case came to autopsy, the patient having died from another cause. The chest X-ray and the pleural surface of the lungs showing the calcified nodules are demonstrated in Figure 8.10.

Microscopic section of one calcified nodule appears to support the hypothesis that it resulted from calcification of a focal area of necrosis in the acute phase of chickenpox pneumonia (see Fig. 8.11).

*Abrahams, E.W., Evans, C., Knyvett, A.F. and Stringer, R.E. Varicella pneumonia: a possible cause of subsequent pulmonary calcification. Med J Aust 2: 781–782, 1964.

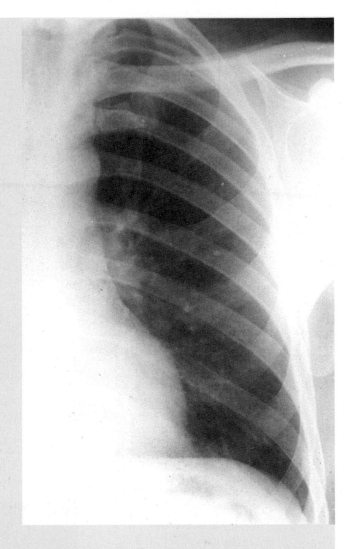

▶ **Fig. 8.9** Chest X-ray showing multiple, small foci of calcification in the lung. These appeared some years after the patient had had an acute attack of chickenpox.

▼ **Fig. 8.10** At post-mortem examination, the calcified nodules can be seen through the pleural surface of the lung.

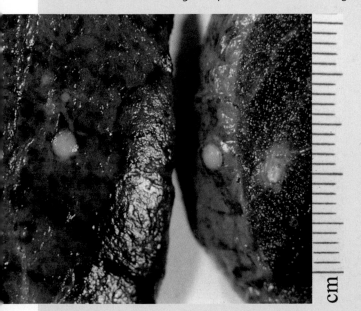

▼ **Fig. 8.11** View of a nodule seen in Fig. 8.10. The surrounding lung is normal.

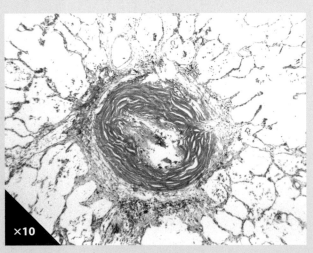

Herpes zoster virus

Herpes zoster (also known as shingles) is a condition that results from recurrence of a latent infection of chickenpox virus—varicella zoster (VZV). The disease may affect children, but it is more commonly seen in older adults, especially those over 65 years of age. In older adults, it may occur after contact with a child who has chickenpox or at times of stress.

Clinical features

The first indication of herpes zoster disease is usually severe pain in the distribution of a nerve root. Redness follows; then the vesicles appear. The nerve roots most frequently involved are the thoracic and lumbar ones. The involvement is usually unilateral. The rash first appears on the back and extends a variable distance around the trunk to the midline anteriorly (as shown in Fig. 8.12).

The individual branches of the fifth cranial nerve may be involved (see Fig. 8.13). When the first branch of the fifth nerve is involved, the eye usually is affected as well. This may result in serious damage to the cornea.

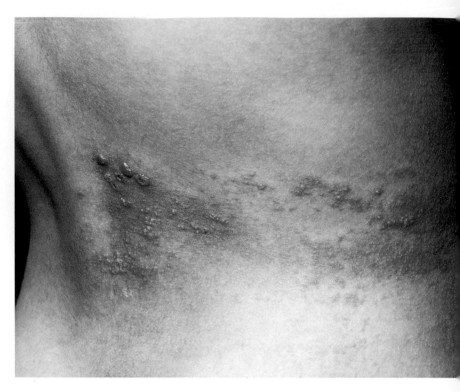

▲ **Fig. 8.12** This patient has the typical vesicular rash of herpes zoster, affecting the right first lumbar nerve.

▼ **Fig. 8.13** This young boy has herpes zoster affecting the second branch of his right fifth cranial nerve.

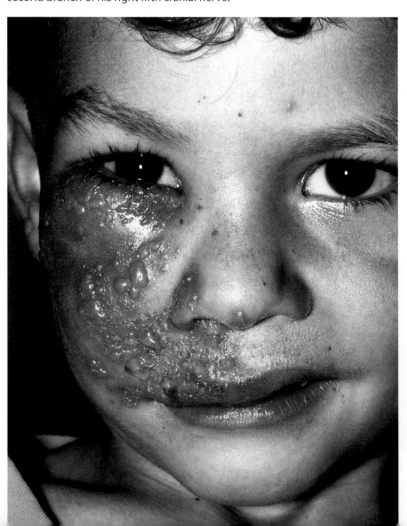

Severe pain (post herpetic neuralgia) may be felt for a long time (months) after the rash has subsided. Early treatment (within 72 hours of onset of symptoms) with an antiviral drug (for example acyclovir) may abort the symptoms.

The virus invades the posterior root ganglion of one or more cranial or spinal nerves. Here, it causes necrosis of the ganglion cells with a chronic inflammatory cell infiltration (see Fig. 8.14).

The disease usually occurs in people whose immune system is normal, but it is a recognized complication in patients with any type of immune deficiency.

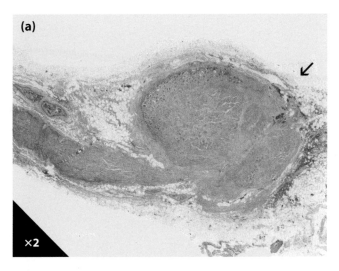

(a) ×2

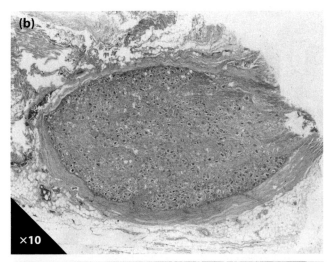

(b) ×10

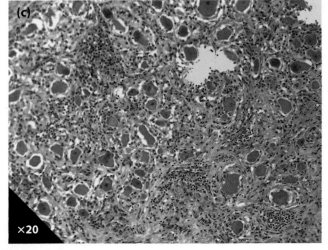

(c) ×20

▲ ▶ **Fig. 8.14(a), (b) and (c)** Views of the posterior nerve root ganglion of an adult patient who had a herpes zoster rash and died from a malignant lymphoma. There is necrosis of ganglion cells and an infiltration of mononuclear inflammatory cells.

Measles

Measles occurs in epidemics mainly in young children. Spread by droplet infection, it begins as what appears to be an ordinary upper respiratory tract infection. The child is miserable. After a day or two, a blotchy red rash appears all over the body (see Fig. 8.15). This is often accompanied by conjunctivitis (see Fig. 8.16).

The incubation period is 8–12 days. An attack usually lasts about 7 days, with full recovery. The incidence of measles has been greatly reduced by the introduction of an effective vaccine.

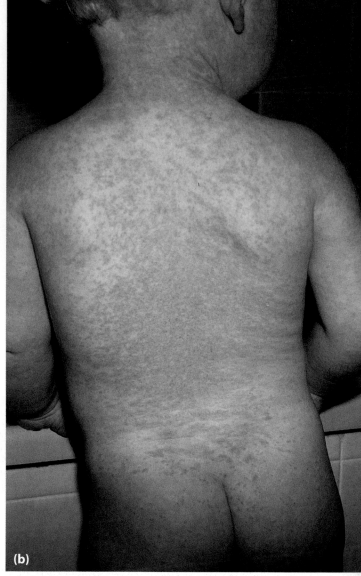

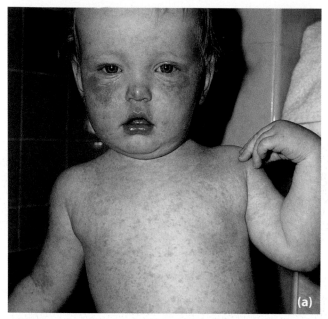

(a)

(b)

▲ **Fig. 8.15** Measles. **(a)** This female, aged 2 years, looks sick and miserable. **(b)** A blotchy red rash is present all over the body.

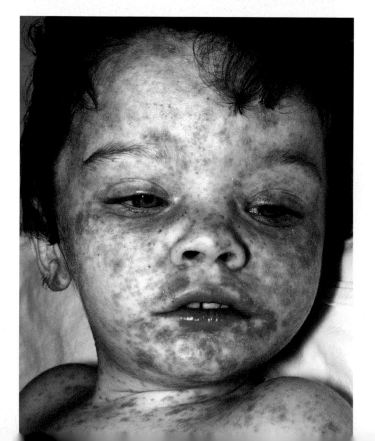

◀ **Fig. 8.16** Measles. This female, aged 2 years, has a severe rash. Note the conjunctivitis.

Complications of measles

Complications of measles are rare.

- The most common are bacterial bronchopneumonia and otitis media (about 1/100 of cases).
- More rarely, there is a measles virus pneumonia.
- Very rarely, an acute encephalitis occurs a week or so after the rash (about 1/1000 of cases).
- More rarely still, post measles subacute sclerosing panencephalitis occurs (about 1/300 000 of cases).

Case 8.2

A 3-year-old female was being treated with chemotherapy for a malignant lymphoma.

While in hospital, she was visited by a sibling, who developed measles the next day. A few days later, the patient developed a measles pneumonia and she died. The measles pneumonia is seen in an X ray taken when she became sick—shown in Figure 8.17.

The child's lung showed the pathologic features of measles pneumonia. These features are illustrated in Figures 8.18, 8.19, 8.21 and 8.22, continued overleaf.

For comparison, Figure 8.20, overleaf, shows a view of the alveolar portion of a normal lung.

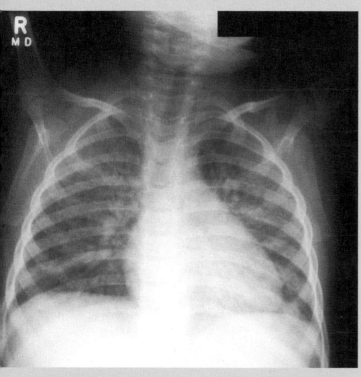

▲ **Fig. 8.17** Measles pneumonia. Chest X-ray taken when the child became sick. It shows the presence of increased lung markings consistent with pneumonia.

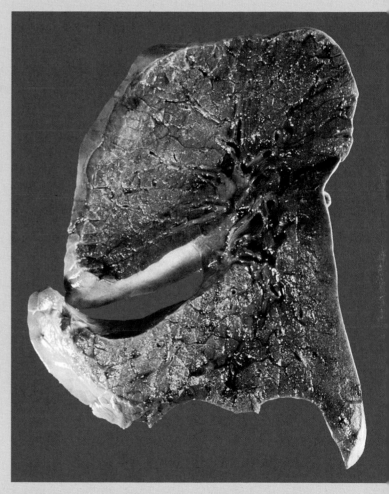

▲ **Fig. 8.18** Measles pneumonia. The lung at post-mortem examination was firm and rubbery.

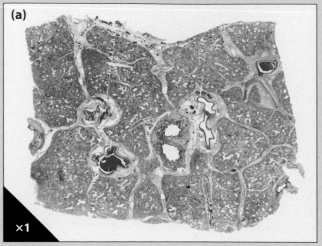

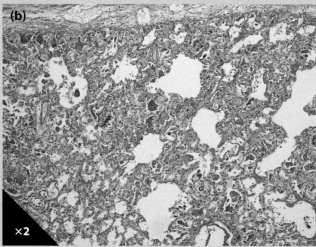

▲ **Fig. 8.19(a) and (b)** Measles pneumonia. Microscopic views show an almost solid lung.

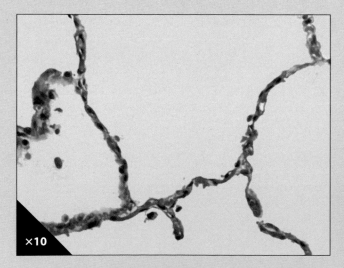

▲ **Fig. 8.20** View of the alveolar portion of a normal lung.

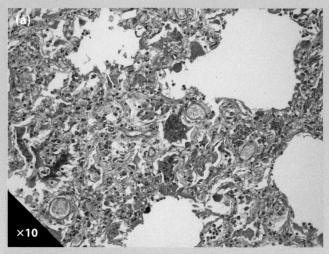

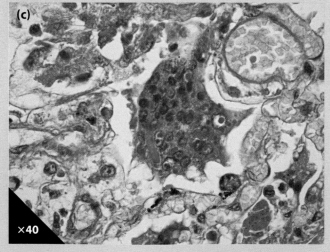

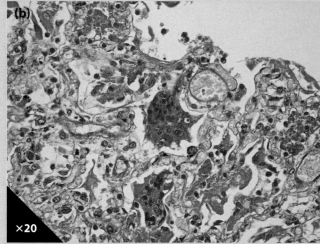

▲ **Fig. 8.21(a), (b) and (c)** Measles pneumonia. Solid-looking lung with thickened alveolar septae, a chronic inflammatory cell infiltration and multinucleated giant cells containing virus inclusions.

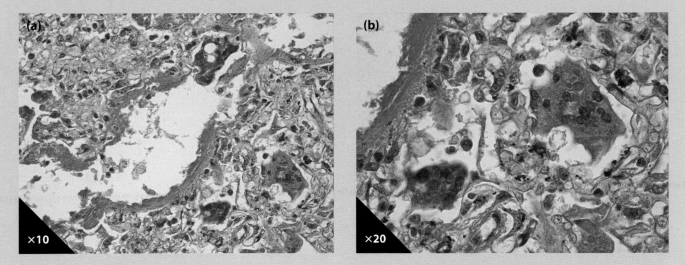

▲ **Fig. 8.22(a) and (b)** Measles pneumonia. Views that show hyaline membranes lining alveolar walls and multinucleated, giant cells containing virus inclusions.

Case 8.3

A male, aged 14 years, developed an acute encephalitis a few weeks after he had an attack of measles. He deteriorated rapidly and died. Post-mortem examination revealed the features of measles encephalitis (see Fig. 8.23).

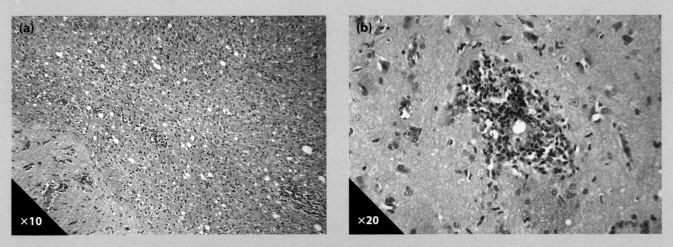

▲ **Fig. 8.23(a) and (b)** Brain sections show the features of a nonspecific encephalitis. In accordance with the history, this was interpreted as being a measles encephalitis.

Case 8.4

A female, aged 4 years, with leukemia, had contact with a child who had measles during an epidemic in her school. The child's pediatrician was examining the 4 year old daily for early signs of measles.

Koplik spots appeared on the mucosal surface of her mouth. These multiple, small, white patches are characteristic early signs in the prodromal stage of measles (see Fig. 8.24).

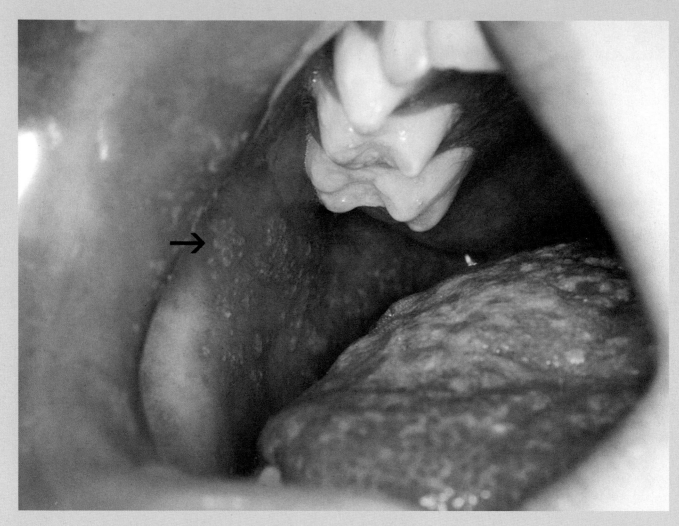

▲ **Fig. 8.24** Koplik spots on the buccal mucosa in the prodromal stage of measles.

Case 8.5

A male, aged 4 years, had surgery to remove a dysplastic lobe of a lung.

Microscopic examination of the surgical specimen showed that some bronchial epithelial cells were proliferating and contained intracytoplasmic viral inclusions (see Fig. 8.25).

Sections of lymphoid tissue in the lung showed numerous multinucleated giant cells with the characteristics of Warthin-Finkeldey giant cells (see Fig. 8.26). These cells are seen in sections of lymphoid tissue throughout the body in the prodromal stage of measles. This child developed clinical evidence of measles a few days after the surgery.

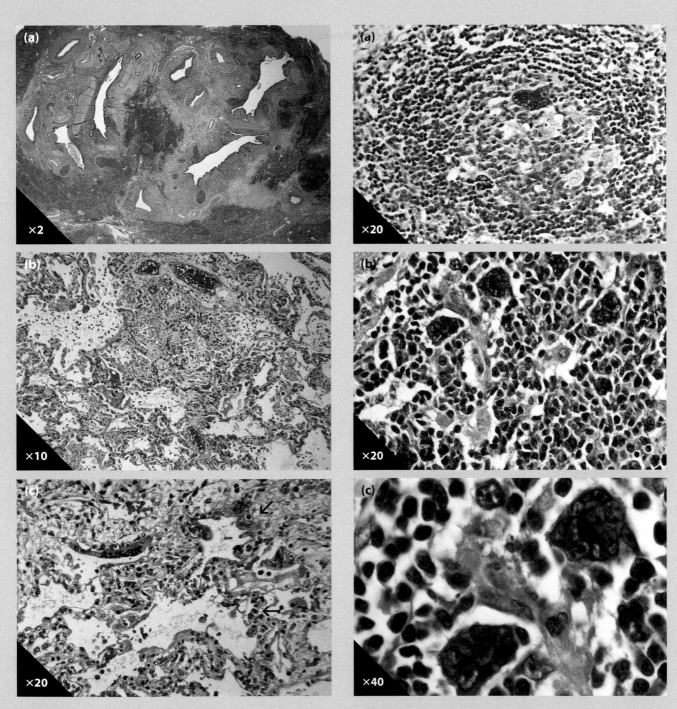

▲ **Fig. 8.25(a), (b) and (c)** Dysplastic lobe of a lung showing proliferation of bronchial epithelial lining cells.

▲ **Fig. 8.26(a), (b) and (c)** Numerous multinucleated giant cells with the characteristics of Warthin-Finkeldey giant cells are present in lymphoid tissue.

Case 8.6

Measles is a serious disease in communities that have not been exposed to the virus before. There are many reports of measles epidemics in communities living on islands in the South Pacific Ocean region after the visit of a ship carrying Europeans. Such epidemics resulted in many deaths. In the middle of the twentieth century, similar epidemics among children in Papua New Guinea caused serious illness, with a significant mortality.

The measles rash in a dark skin (see Fig. 8.27) has a different appearance from that in a fair-skinned person. Doctors who are not aware of this difference are often confused about the diagnosis.

▼ **Fig. 8.27(a) and (b)** This male, aged 5 years, in Papua New Guinea, has measles. Note that he is very sick. He has an oxygen tube in his nose because he has bronchopneumonia. Note also the appearance of the rash: the spots are black. The appearance is very different from that in children with fair skins. Doctors who are not aware of this difference are often confused about the diagnosis.

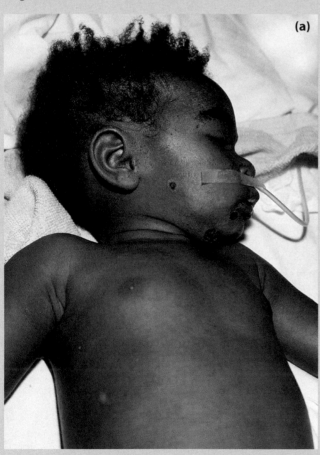
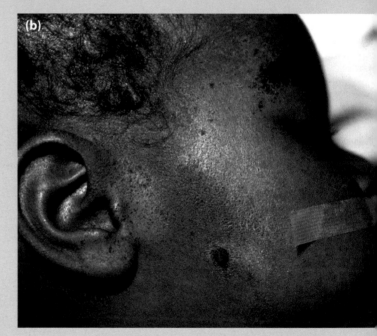

(a) (b)

Case 8.7

A male, aged 19 years, began to have mental deterioration about 2 years before coming to medical attention. His school work began to deteriorate. Then he developed myoclonic seizures. Mental deterioration continued.

He had had measles during his early childhood. Measles antibodies were present in high titre in his serum. He deteriorated further and died.

The clinical diagnosis was subacute sclerosing pan-encephalitis. Post-mortem examination was performed and the changes seen in the brain are illustrated in Figures 8.28, 8.29 and 8.30.

▼ **Fig. 8.28(a) and (b)** Section of the brain, stained to accentuate the glial proliferation, shows some widening of sulci (A) and atrophy of the white matter (B).

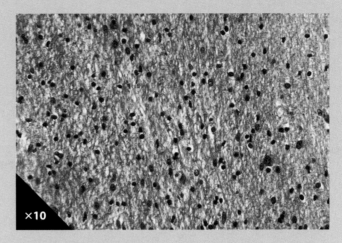

▲ **Fig. 8.29** Section through the white matter shows gliosis.

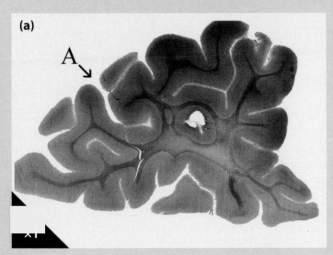

▼ **Fig. 8.30(a) and (b)** Phosphotungstic acid hematoxylin (PTAH) stain accentuates the glial fibers.

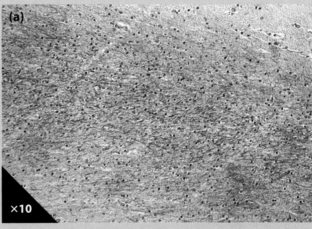

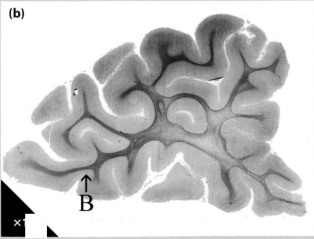

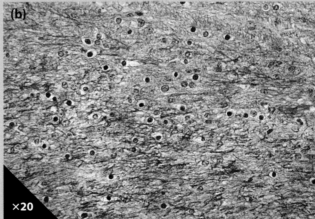

Mumps

Mumps is caused by infection with the mumps virus, which causes painful enlargement of one or more salivary glands—most frequently the parotid gland (see Fig. 8.31). It is spread by respiratory droplet infection.

The incubation period is about 18 days. The incidence of mumps has been greatly reduced by the introduction of an effective vaccine.

Children are usually not very sick and the only abnormality is the swollen face. The symptoms last for a few days and then regress.

Mothers may complain that their infants have stopped eating. The reason for this is that when they open their mouths, the angle of the mandible hits the tender parotid gland and they respond to this by not wanting to open their mouths.

Adults who become infected may be quite sick, and they are more prone to the complications of acute orchitis and acute pancreatitis than are children.

▼ **Fig. 8.31** This female, aged 8 years, shows the clinical features of mumps with bilateral swelling of the parotid and submandibular glands.

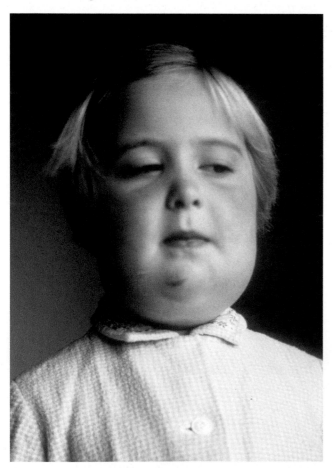

Herpes simplex virus (HSV)

Herpes simplex virus (HSV) invades the skin and mucous membranes of the mouth and the nose (herpes labialis), and the skin of the genitalia (herpes genitalis). This invasion produces multiple, small, fluid-filled, painful vesicles that last for about a week and then they heal.

The virus is spread by direct contact. The incubation period is 1–2 weeks after contact.

Healing occurs spontaneously, but repeated attacks continue for many years afterwards. It is not known what precipitates the repeat attacks.

Symptoms are more severe in some people than in others but they are particularly severe in people who are immune suppressed.

There are two subtypes of herpes simplex virus—HSV-1 and HSV-2 .

- Type 1 infects predominantly the mouth and skin (15% of oral herpes is type 2).
- Type 2 predominantly causes genital herpes (15% of genital herpes is type 1).

Clinical features of HSV

Herpes simplex infection consists in a vesicular eruption around the mouth and nose (see Fig. 8.32). Other parts of the skin may be affected. The onset of the rash is somewhat painful. Vesicles form and rupture, and may become secondarily infected. The rash appears from time to time without any specific precipitating cause. It subsides within a week or two. In some cases, the lesions are more severe and last longer, particularly in immune-suppressed patients.

Before the introduction of the routine use of gloves when examining and treating patients, infections of the fingers of health professionals occasionally occurred (see Fig. 8.33).

Genital herpes appears as a sexually transmitted infection (shown in Fig. 8.34).

▶ **Fig. 8.32** This female, aged 18 years, has recurrent herpes simplex lesions around her mouth. These particular lesions are in the healing phase.

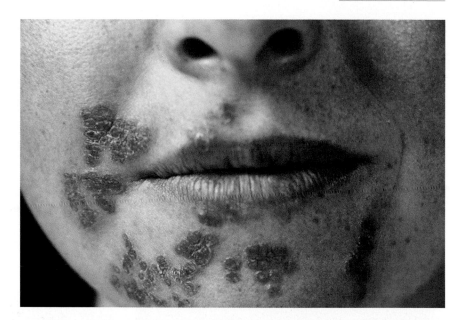

▶ **Fig. 8.33** This female, aged 23 years, has a herpes simplex lesion on her right thumb. She was, as a nurse, attending to the laryngeal airway of a patient with a tracheostomy. This infection occurred before the wearing of gloves became mandatory while doing such procedures, which are now recognized as being an occupational hazard.

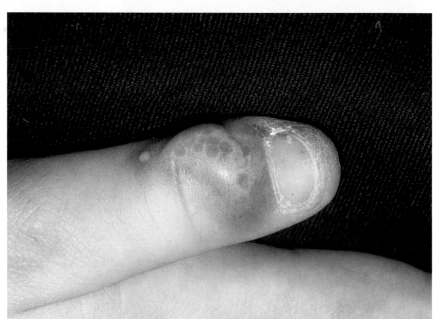

▶ **Fig. 8.34** This female, aged 19 years, has genital herpes with vesicular skin lesions on the labia.

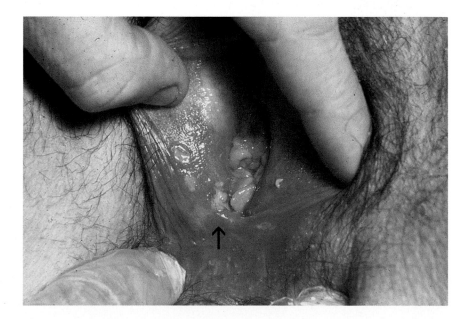

Microscopic appearances of HSV skin infections

The histologic appearances of the herpes simplex vesicular skin lesion are demonstrated in Figure 8.35.

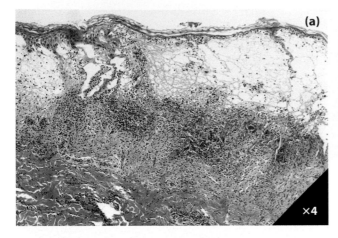

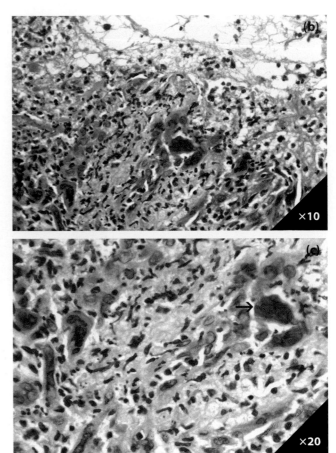

▲ ▶ **Fig. 8.35(a), (b) and (c)** Skin biopsy of a herpes simplex lesion in a male, 35 years. It shows a suprabasal, vesicular lesion. Some epithelial cells in the basal layer of the lesion are multinucleated and contain viral particles. This appearance is similar to that seen in herpes zoster, chickenpox and smallpox lesions.

▼ **Fig. 8.36** This male, aged 18 months, had a dendritic ulcer on the cornea of one eye caused by herpes simplex virus. This is an uncommon complication. The outline of the ulcer is accentuated by staining with fluorescein dye.

Complications of HSV
Dendritic ulcer on the cornea

An occasional complication of HSV is a dendritic ulcer on the cornea (illustrated in Fig. 8.36).

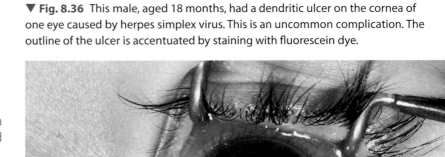

Herpes encephalitis

In many countries, the commonest cause of encephalitis is herpes simplex. The virus causes hemorrhage and necrosis in the brain, particularly in the temporal lobes.

The damaged temporal lobes can be visualized using magnetic resonance imaging (MRI) scanning. The mortality rate is significant, but patients with cases diagnosed early and treated with antiviral agents may recover completely.

People of all ages are susceptible, and the clinical and pathologic features are similar across all ages.

The gross and microscopic appearances in the brain of a female, 8 months of age, who died of herpes encephalitis, are illustrated in Figures 8.37–8.41, continued overleaf. This infant had a viral meningitis in association with the encephalitis. This case history illustrates most of the features of herpes encephalitis.

Case 8.8

A female, aged 8 months, presented at a country hospital in Australia with a 4-day history of pyrexia and twitching of the right arm. Soon all four limbs were twitching and her level of consciousness deteriorated. Both eyes were deviated to the left and nystagmus was present. She was transferred to a hospital in the city of Brisbane, where she was noted to have raised intracranial pressure with papilledema and separation of the sutures on a skull X-ray.

Chest X-ray was normal and a lumbar puncture showed clear cerebrospinal fluid (CSF) with normal protein and sugar, and 40 leukocytes per cubic mm, most of them being lymphocytes. The child deteriorated rapidly and died 24 hours after admission.

A post-mortem examination was performed. There was no skin rash and all the organs except the brain were normal. The brain was edematous and abnormally soft to feel. Changes were maximal in the left temporal lobe, in which there was marked necrosis with some hemorrhage.

There was a lesser degree of edema and hemorrhage in the right temporal lobe, as shown in Figure 8.37.

A small piece of brain from the right temporal lobe was submitted for viral culture but this was negative. Immunoperoxidase stains for herpes simplex virus type 1 (HSV-1) were positive.

Microscopic examination showed the presence of hemorrhage and necrosis in the brain substance, together with an inflammatory cell infiltration that was mainly mononuclear in cell type (see Figs 8.38 and 8.39, overleaf). Occasional intranuclear viral inclusions could be seen in astrocytes within the areas of inflammation (see Fig. 8.40, overleaf).

Meningitis was present as well, as indicated by the expansion of the subarachnoid space by inflammatory cells, mainly mononuclears (illustrated in Figs 8.38, 8.39, 8.40 and 8.41, overleaf).

▼ **Fig. 8.37** This cut slice of the formalin fixed brain of a female, 8 months of age, viewed from the anterior aspect, shows marked necrosis of the left temporal lobe and lesser but similar changes in the right temporal lobe.

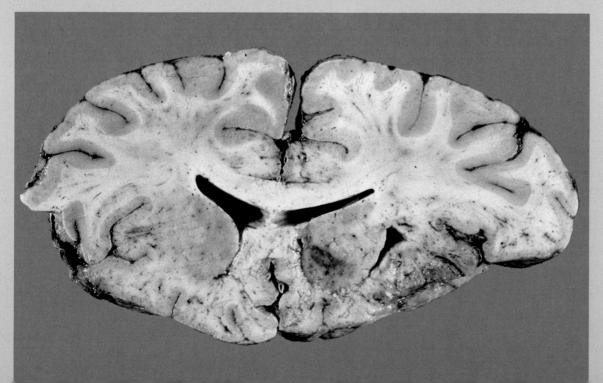

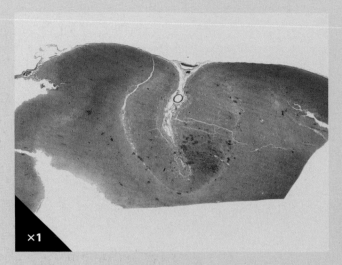

▲ **Fig. 8.38** This low magnification view shows an area of hemorrhage and necrosis at the base of the sulcus on the right side of the image.

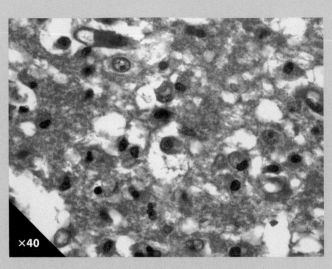

▲ **Fig. 8.40** There is an intranuclear inclusion in an astrocyte in the middle of the picture.

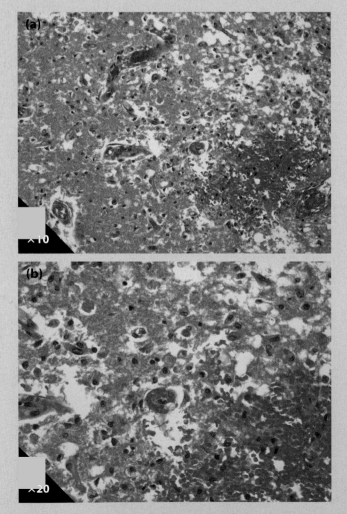

(a)

(b)

▲ **Fig. 8.39(a) and (b)** At higher magnifications, the hemorrhagic necrosis together with a mild infiltration of mononuclear inflammatory cells can be better seen.

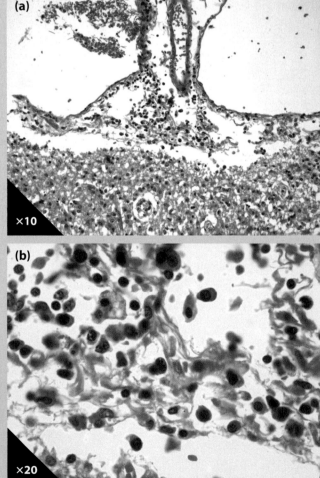

(a)

(b)

▲ **Fig. 8.41(a) and (b)** There is a mononuclear inflammatory cell infiltration in the subarachnoid space consistent with a viral meningitis in association with the encephalitis.

Disseminated neonatal herpes

Occasionally, when the mother has an active herpes genitalis infection, babies may be infected during delivery. Quite often, infection in the mother is unrecognized. About 75 per cent of infections are caused by HSV-2 and the other 25 per cent by HSV-1.

The baby may have lesions involving the skin and the oral cavity; or encephalitis may be the predominant manifestation; or most rarely of all, there are disseminated herpes lesions in many organs, for example the adrenal and the liver. Pathologic changes in the adrenal and the liver are illustrated in Figures 8.42 and 8.43, overleaf.

Skin lesions are frequently not found in association with encephalitis and disseminated lesions.

Case 8.9

A 7-day-old male infant, who had had an uneventful term delivery, began to have cyanotic attacks. In one of these, he was cold and blue and was resuscitated by his father by mouth-to-mouth resuscitation. There was no fever and no localizing signs could be found.

The next day, the infant was admitted to a child-minding facility, because his mother had to be readmitted to the obstetric hospital where he was born for treatment of acute vulvitis that was ulcerative rather than vesicular.

The staff of the child-minding center quickly realized that the infant needed expert medical attention and he was admitted to a Brisbane hospital, where he was found to be partially conscious and still having cyanotic attacks.

There were no localizing neurological signs and the only clinical abnormality of significance was an enlarged liver (of three fingers breadth below the right costal margin).

Chest X-ray was normal. The electrocardiogram was 'low voltage' and the lumbar puncture produced blood-stained CSF, which was sterile on bacterial and viral culture. He was started on intravenous antibiotics but he began to fit, and he deteriorated and died 24 hours after admission to the hospital.

Post-mortem examination showed that he had no skin rash or any other physical abnormality. The liver was enlarged and attached to the slightly enlarged spleen by fibrinous adhesions. The cut surface of the liver revealed the presence of multiple, focal, yellowish areas. The cut surfaces of both adrenal glands showed the presence of multiple yellowish, areas edged by hemorrhage. Pathologic changes in the adrenal and the liver are illustrated in Figure 8.42, overleaf.

The spleen showed some perisplenitis at the point of attachment to the liver and there were a few yellowish spots in the adjacent splenic tissue. The other organs showed no abnormality.

Microscopic examination of the liver showed focal areas of necrosis that were becoming confluent. There was no inflammatory reaction. Many of the damaged hepatocytes contained intranuclear inclusions (see Fig. 8.43, overleaf). Similar changes were seen in the adrenal glands.

Electron microscopic examination of the liver and adrenal showed that the intranuclear inclusions were viral particles with the appearance of herpes virus. Viral culture of liver was negative. Immuno-peroxidase stains for herpes virus were not available at that time, but when they were performed later the tissue was positive for herpes virus type 2.

> *In retrospect, it is likely that the mother's vulvitis was a herpes simplex infection and this was the source of infection of the baby. This infant demonstrates the usual features of disseminated neonatal herpes in which the symptoms and signs are very vague with respiratory distress, fitting and jaundice, and bleeding from liver failure.*

▶ **Fig. 8.42(a)** Adrenal. **(b)** Liver. These organs show the presence of multiple, focal necrotic lesions that look a little like miliary tuberculosis to the naked eye.

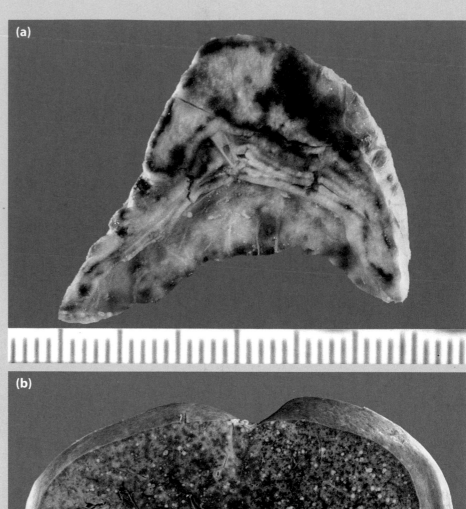

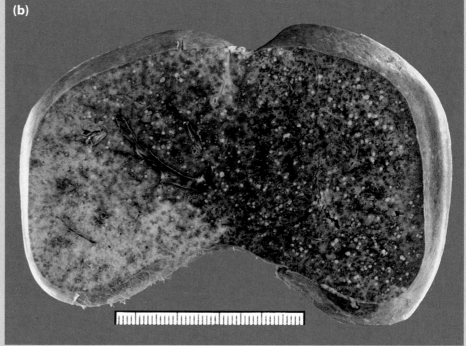

▶ **Fig. 8.43** View of the liver lesion showing necrosis of the liver cells. Some of the necrotic cells contain intranuclear viral inclusions. For example, in the 2 hepatocytes in the middle of the picture.

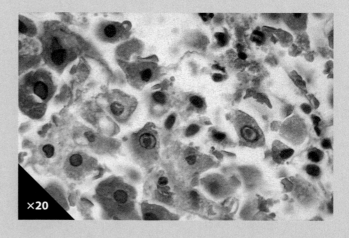

Other sites of herpes infections

Ulcerated lesions may occur at sites such as the oropharynx, the esophagus and the stomach, particularly in immuno-compromised patients. Biopsies of such ulcers show the presence of multinucleated cells containing viral particles.

Multinucleated cells seen in Pap smears also indicate the presence of herpes simplex infection of the cervix and vagina (see Fig. 8.44).

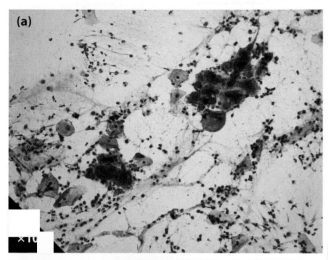

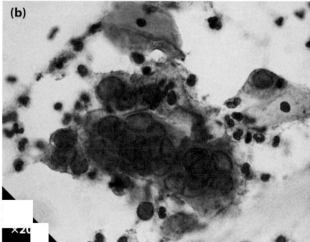

▲ **Fig. 8.44(a) and (b)** Herpes virus infection of the cervix and vagina can be diagnosed in cervical smears (Pap smears) by the presence of multinucleated epithelial cells that have a fairly characteristic appearance. Biopsies of ulcerated lesions in the oropharynx, esophagus or stomach can also be diagnosed as being caused by herpes infection by the presence of these multinucleated epithelial cells. Such ulcers occur particularly in immunocompromised patients.

Human papilloma virus (HPV)

Skin lesions (warts—*verruca vulgaris*)

The wart virus *verruca vulgaris* is a subtype of the human papilloma virus (HPV). There are more than 90 genotypes of HPV that cause warts.

The presence of the various types of HPV can be demonstrated by immuno-peroxidase stains, using the appropriate monoclonal antibodies. Different serotypes show a predilection for different areas of the body.

HPV type 1 causes hyperkeratotic lesions that occur on the fingers (see Fig. 8.45) and, less frequently, on the feet (see Fig. 8.46, overleaf). The lesions are a nuisance and cause discomfort. They may persist for many years but, eventually, they disappear spontaneously.

In immunocompromised patients, large numbers of warts may occur on the hands and feet and elsewhere on the body (see Fig. 8.47, overleaf). The microscopic appearances of a wart are illustrated in Figure 8.48, overleaf.

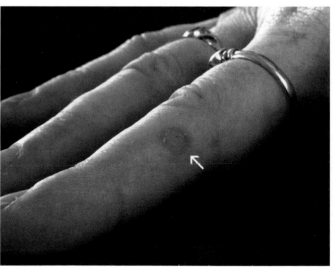

▲ **Fig. 8.45** Wart on the finger of a female, aged 37 years.

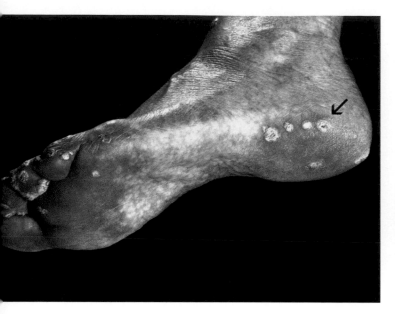

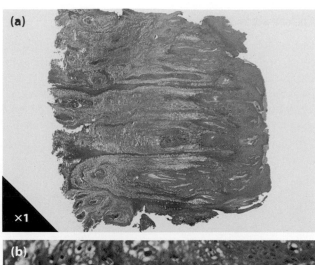

▲ Fig. 8.46 Warts on the sole of the left foot.

▼ Fig. 8.47 Multiple warts on the fingers of an immunocompromised patient.

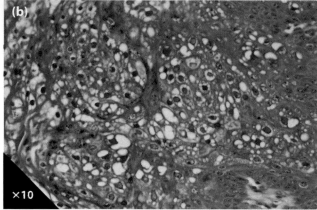

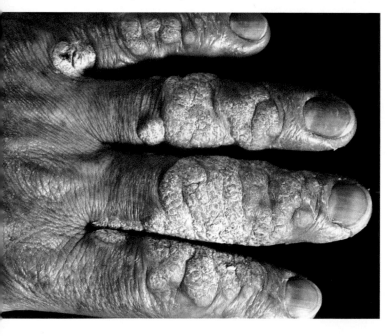

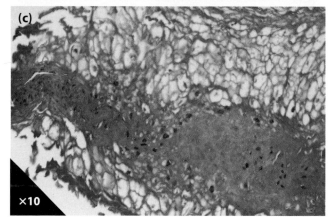

▲ Fig. 8.48 Microscopic appearance of an excised wart. **(a)** The base is cup shaped and there is a plug of markedly thickened stratum corneum on the left of the section. **(b)** The granular layer of the epidermis is prominent. **(c)** In the surface keratin layer, blue virus particles can be seen.

Genital lesions

HPV infection has been shown to be the cause of cervical cancer. The presence of HPV in the cervix can be recognized in Pap smears by the presence of perinuclear vacuolation in the epithelial cells. This vacuolation is often associated with a mild degree of epithelial atypia. These lesions are caused by HPV types 11, 16, 18, 31 and 45.

Ian Frazer and his research group in Brisbane, Australia, engineered a virus-like particle that included HPV types 16 and 18 antigens, and they produced a vaccine against HPV. This was trialled in 2005 and was shown to give almost 100 per cent protection against HPV infection. This exciting result raises the possibility of eliminating cervical cancer.

Males develop similar genital warts and the HPV vaccine may prevent penile cancer as well. The cytologic and histologic appearances of HPV infection are illustrated in Figures 8.49 and 8.50.

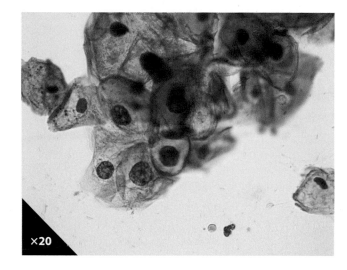

▶ **Fig. 8.49** Papanicolaou smear from the cervix. It shows the effects of HPV infection. The epithelial cells show perinuclear vacuolation and mild nuclear atypia.

▼ **Fig. 8.50(a) and (b)** In cervical biopsies, HPV infection shows itself by the presence of perinuclear vacuolation (koilocytosis) and nuclear atypia. A similar appearance is seen in sections from 'genital warts' in males.

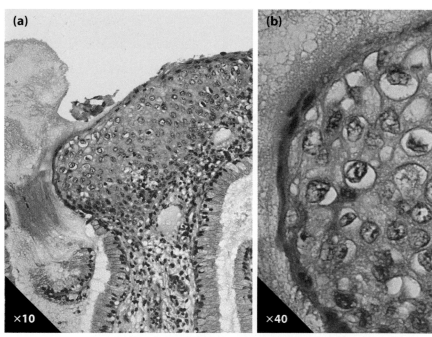

Condylomata accuminata

Condylomata accuminata are hyperkeratotic papillomas that occur in the anogenital region of males and females, particularly in children. They are caused by HPV types 6 and 11. They are not necessarily caused by sexual contact, and they do not become malignant.

Laryngeal papillomatosis

In laryngeal papillomatosis, multiple, thick, keratinized papillomas grow on the vocal cords and adjacent larynx, resulting in varying degrees of laryngeal obstruction. The condition is caused by HPV types 6 and 41.

These lesions occur in children. They are benign and need to be excised surgically. Very occasionally, a cancer follows many years after the first appearance of the lesion.

Molluscum contagiosum

Molluscum contagiosum is a skin lesion caused by a DNA poxvirus. It occurs either singly or as multiple, well-circumscribed, rounded, pinkish papillomatous lesions. They are quite common in children. The clinical and histologic features are illustrated in Figures 8.51, 8.52 and 8.53.

Molluscum contagiosum may be transmitted by sexual contact and it is then regarded as being a sexually transmitted infection.

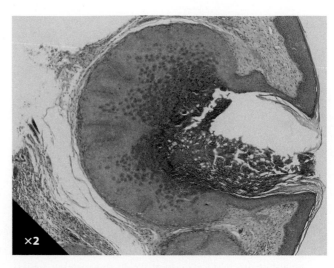

▲ **Fig. 8.52** Molluscum contagiosum. Microscopic section showing the characteristic cup-shaped, well-circumscribed lesion with a keratin plug in the middle.

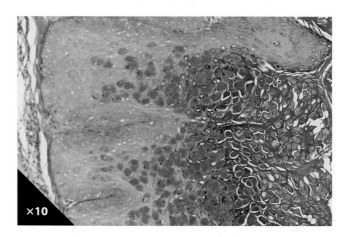

▲ **Fig. 8.53** Molluscum contagiosum. Within the keratin one sees large, eosinophilic virus particles.

▼ **Fig. 8.51** Molluscum contagiosum on the skin. It occurs as a well-circumscribed, elevated, rounded lesion.

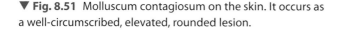
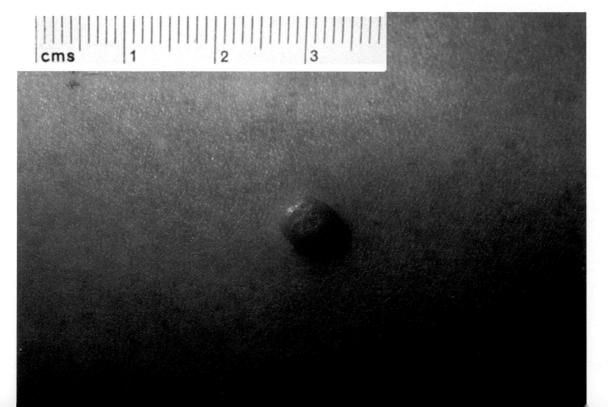

Cytomegalovirus (CMV)

The cytomegalovirus is a member of the Herpes family of viruses. The virus has a universal distribution, and over 50 per cent of adults in the United States have positive serologic tests for the virus. Acute infection usually causes only mild symptoms of disease. Serious disease occurs:

- in neonates when it is a cause of neonatal death
- in organ transplant patients

- as an opportunistic infection in immunocompromised patients and it may infect any or all tissues in the body.

Microscopic examination of infected tissue shows the presence of characteristic large, intranuclear inclusions. The microscopic appearances in various organs are illustrated in Figures 8.54–8.59.

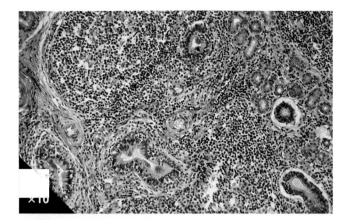

▲ **Fig. 8.54** View of salivary gland. At this magnification, the presence of a CMV infection can be recognized because the infected acinar epithelial cells are much larger than normal.

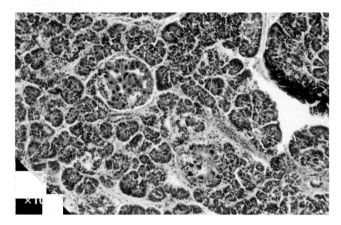

▲ **Fig. 8.55** Intranuclear inclusions are present in the islet cells of the pancreas.

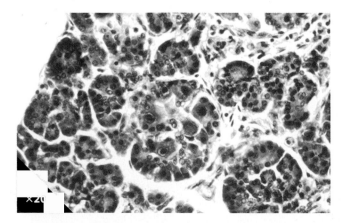

▲ **Fig. 8.56** Intranuclear inclusions are also present in the acinar cells of the pancreas.

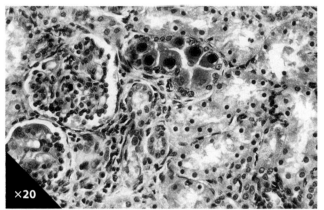

▲ **Fig. 8.57** In the kidney, the epithelial cells of the tubules are infected and enlarged. Cells of the glomeruli may also be infected and become similarly enlarged.

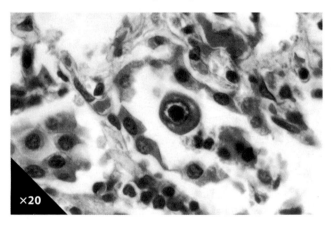

▲ **Fig. 8.58** In the lungs, the pulmonary alveolar macrophages show intranuclear virus particles of CMV.

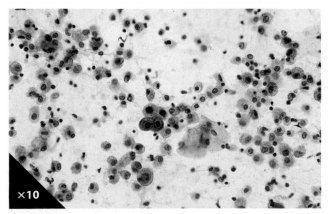

▲ **Fig. 8.59** Infected macrophages are sometimes seen in smears made from bronchial lavage specimens.

Rubella

Rubella is caused by the rubella virus, which is a member of the Togavirus family. Rubella infections may occur either sporadically or in small epidemics. The virus is spread by respiratory droplet infection. The incubation period is 16–18 days (range 14–23 days).

All age groups are affected. The incidence of rubella has been greatly reduced since the introduction of an effective vaccine. In countries that can afford the cost of vaccination, children are now vaccinated against rubella at 12 months of age and again at 4 years of age

Rubella infection is frequently asymptomatic but symptomatically it presents with a blotchy, red rash on the trunk and arms, a mild fever and lymphadenopathy (see Fig. 8.60). The rash makes the skin feel hot.

Some patients develop a painful arthritis (pain, swelling and stiffness) of the small joints of the hands and feet. The rash lasts for a few days and the arthritis lasts for about 2 weeks.

The most serious complication occurs when pregnant women get the disease in the first trimester of a pregnancy. Exposure of the fetus in utero to the rubella virus at this stage of pregnancy results in a high incidence of congenital abnormalities, especially deafness, congenital cataract and congenital heart disease (see Fig. 8.61).

▶ **Fig. 8.60** Rubella. This middle-aged male has a macular (flat), blotchy, dull red rubella rash.

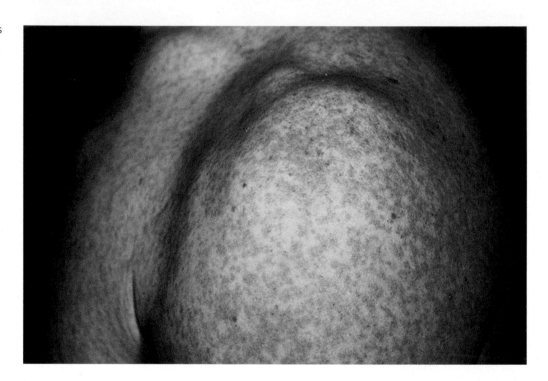

▼ **Fig. 8.61(a) and (b)** These two babies have congenital cataract due to exposure to rubella virus during the first trimester of pregnancy. The lens of the eye is white and opaque.

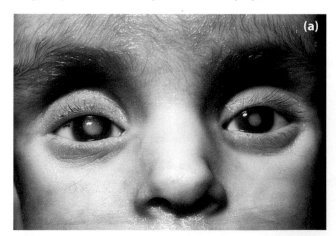

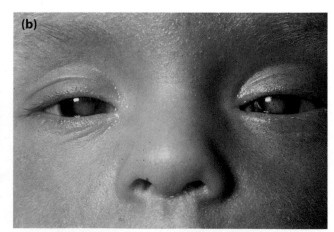

Chlamydia infections

Chlamydia are not viruses, but they are conveniently mentioned in this section. They are nonmotile, obligate intracellular organisms, that are smaller than bacteria. They grow in the cytoplasm of their host cells, forming microcolonies or inclusion bodies. These stain best with Giemsa stain.

Chlamydia trachomatis, Chlamydia psittaci and Chlamydia pneumoniae

There are four species of Chlamydia: three of which cause disease in humans. These three are *C. trachomatis*, *C. psittaci* and *C. pneumoniae*.

- *C. trachomatis* causes:
  - trachoma, an acute conjunctivitis
  - sexually transmitted infections, namely nonspecific urethritis (NSU) and lymphogranuloma venereum (LGV)
  - neonatal pneumonia.
- *C. psittaci* causes Psittacosis, a pneumonia acquired from birds.
- *C. pneumoniae*, a cause of atypical pneumonia.

Trachoma

Trachoma is the name for a severe form of conjunctivitis that progresses to blindness (see Fig. 8.62). The infecting Chlamydia is transmitted by flies. It responds to treatment with broad-spectrum antibiotics.

Diagnosis is confirmed by taking a smear from the surface of the conjunctiva and staining it with Giemsa stain. The large intracellular inclusions are easily seen in the cytoplasm of histiocytes (see Fig. 8.63, overleaf).

Serologic and polymerase chain reaction (PCR) tests are available for diagnosing Chlamydia infections.

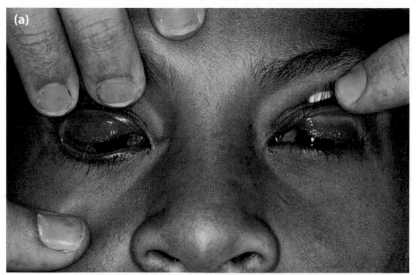

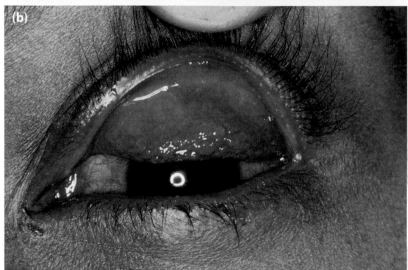

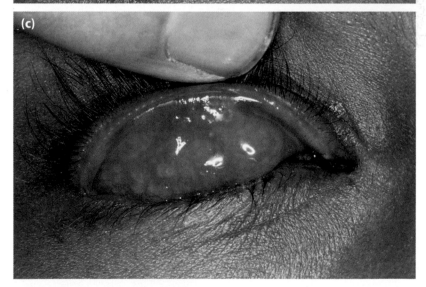

▲ **Fig. 8.62(a), (b) and (c)** Chlamydia conjunctivitis. A female, 4 years of age, with trachoma. The conjunctiva of both eyes is red, edematous and finely nodular.

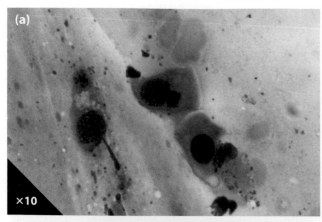

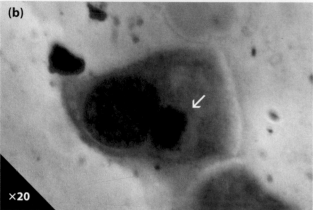

▲ **Fig. 8.63(a) and (b)** Giemsa-stained smear from the conjunctiva of this patient shows the intracellular inclusions of *C. trachomatis*.

Hepatitis viruses

There are a number of subtypes of the hepatitis virus—A, B, C, D and E. The most important of these are A, B and C. They each have slightly different clinical and pathologic features. Serologic tests, PCR tests and liver biopsies help in making an exact diagnosis.

Hepatitis A

The hepatitis A virus (HAV) causes acute hepatitis. It is spread by the fecal-oral route. Infection is particularly common in countries where hygienic standards in handling food are not high.

Recovery after an acute infection is usually complete. Chronic hepatitis, cirrhosis and hepatocellular carcinoma are not as common as after an attack of acute hepatitis caused by hepatitis B virus (HBV).

Hepatitis B

The hepatitis B virus (HBV) is transmitted by parenteral, sexual and maternal-fetal routes. It is more common in some countries than in others. Most infections are asymptomatic, but it does cause acute hepatitis, which has a significant mortality, and it frequently goes on to active chronic hepatitis and cirrhosis.

The cirrhosis caused by HBV results in the liver being smaller than normal and hard, and the normal substance being replaced by large, irregularly sized nodules of liver cells separated by bands of fibrous tissue. The pathologic features of this type of cirrhosis are illustrated in Figures 8.64–8.67.

▶ **Fig. 8.64** Close-up view of the cut surface of a cirrhotic liver. The cirrhotic nodules are large and irregular in size. This pattern of cirrhosis is most often seen in association with hepatis B virus (HBV) infection.

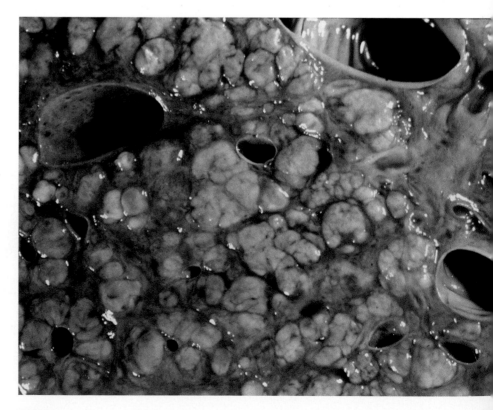

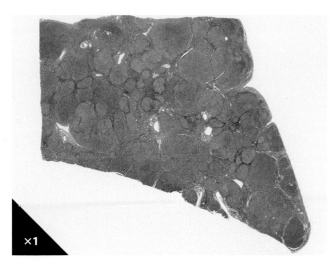

▲ **Fig. 8.65** View of a microscopic section of a macronodular cirrhotic liver.

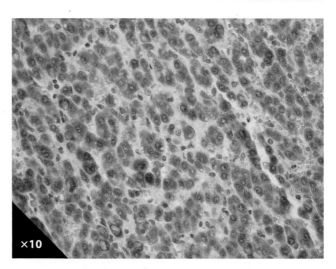

▲ **Fig. 8.67** The presence of HBV can be demonstrated by an immuno-peroxidase stain for hepatitis B surface antigen (HBsAg). The intracytoplasmic antigen stains brown.

▼ **Fig. 8.66(a) and (b)** Views of the liver. The normal architecture has been replaced by nodules of hepatocytes, some of which have homogeneous staining cytoplasm. This so-called 'ground glass' staining appearance is found in HBV infected hepatocytes. In the portal tracts shown in **(a)**, there is some proliferation of small bile ducts and a heavy infiltration of mononuclear inflammatory cells.

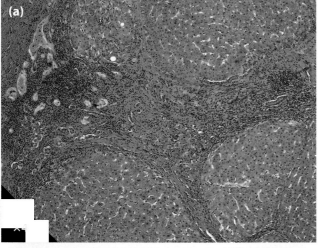

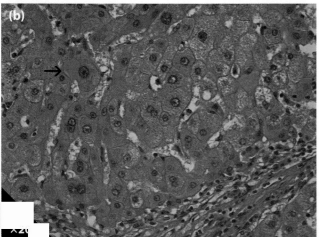

For over 100 years, it was known that there was an inordinately high incidence of cirrhosis and hepatocellular carcinoma in tropical countries but it was not until the scientist Baruch Blumberg (see Fig. 8.68, overleaf) identified the virus in 1964 as being the cause of the cirrhosis and hepatocellular carcinoma that the explanation for this became clear. There is now an effective vaccine for the prevention of hepatitis B infection.

There is a high incidence of hepatocellular carcinoma in cirrhosis caused by HBV. The histologic features of hepatocellular carcinoma are illustrated in Figures 8.69 and 8.70, overleaf.

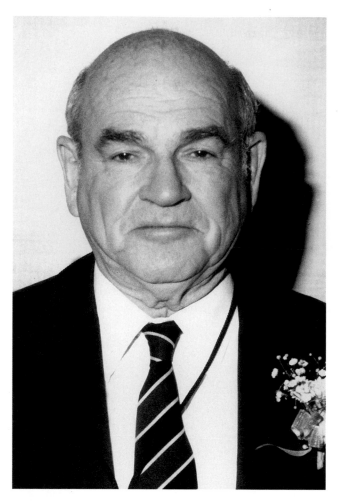

▼ Fig. 8.68 Baruch Blumberg (b. 1925), photographed in 1992. Blumberg identified the hepatitis B virus, which he first called 'Australia antigen' because he found it in the serum of Australian Aborigines. He received a Nobel Prize for this work in 1976.

▼ ▶ Fig. 8.69(a), (b), (c) and (d) This needle liver biopsy shows a hepatocellular carcinoma in a cirrhotic liver. The darker-staining cells are cancer cells of hepatocellular carcinoma.

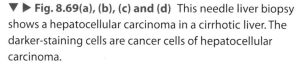

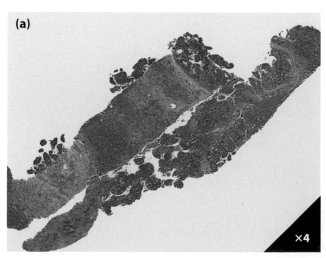

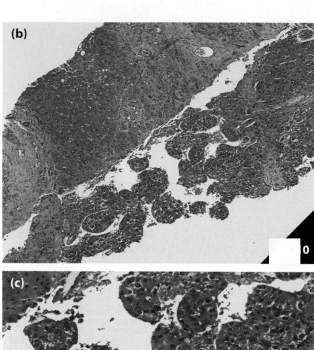

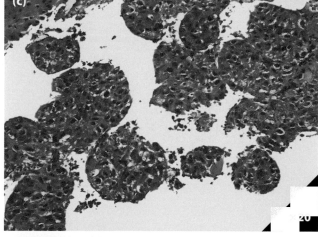

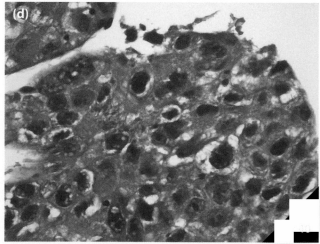

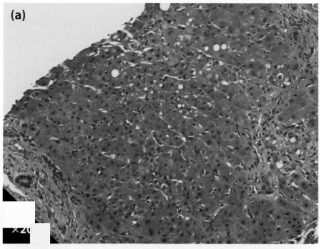

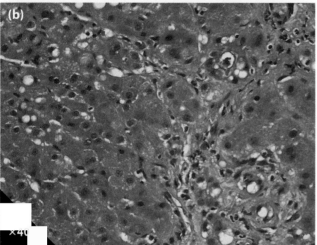

▲ **Fig. 8.70(a)** The pink-staining cells in the HBV liver biopsy are nonmalignant hepatocytes of the cirrhotic liver. **(b)** Note the intracanalicular bile thrombus, which indicates the presence of jaundice.

Hepatitis C

The hepatitis C virus (HCV) is transmitted mainly by blood, that is by intravenous (IV) drug use or by blood transfusion. It may cause acute hepatitis, but more commonly it causes chronic active hepatitis, which progresses to cirrhosis. Of the cirrhoses, 20 per cent progress to hepatocellular carcinoma.

Yellow fever

The yellow fever virus is endemic in the northern countries of South America, the Caribbean, and in the northern countries of Africa. In South America, it is endemic in monkeys. In the other countries, different mammals provide the epizootic focus. Mosquitoes transmit the infection to humans.

Clinical features include fever, jaundice, headache and myalgia. In severe cases, this leads to liver and renal failure. The histologic appearances in the liver are illustrated in Figure 8.71. The mortality is about 50 per cent.

Yellow fever is a quarantinable disease, and many countries will not allow visitors to enter if they have visited an endemic area unless they have had a certified vaccination against the disease.

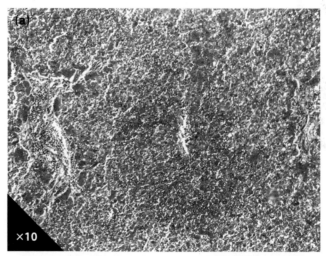

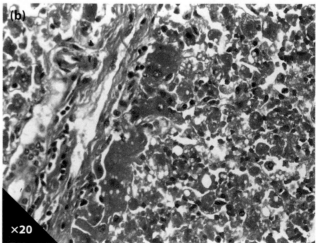

▶ **Fig. 8.71** Views of a liver from a female, aged 35, who died of yellow fever. **(a)** Note the large area of necrosis in the hepatic lobule with preservation of a thin line of hepatocytes around the portal tract on the left side of the image.
(b) An extremely large number of apoptotic hepatocytes (Councilman bodies) can be seen. This appears to be a feature of the changes caused by the yellow fever virus.

The mode of transmission of yellow fever was determined by Walter Reed (1851–1902), a doctor from the Army Medical Corps, Washington, USA. In 1900, Reed investigated an outbreak in an army camp in Havana, Cuba, and demonstrated that yellow fever was spread by the bite of a mosquito.

An assistant in the investigations, James Carroll, who was the first Director of the Armed Forces Institute of Pathology in Washington, allowed himself to be bitten by an infected mosquito and developed yellow fever. He had ill health for some years after this (and probably died of its effects). Another member of the investigating team was infected, too, and he died from yellow fever.

In 1901, in a period of 3 months, William Gorgas (1854–1920), from the Army Medical Corps, Washington, directed army engineers in drainage of Cuban swamps and implemented other measures to control the breeding of mosquitoes. This eradicated yellow fever in Cuba.

In 1904, the first attempt to build a canal through the Isthmus of Panama linking the Atlantic and Pacific Oceans failed for a number of reasons, not the least of which was the high mortality among the workers from malaria and yellow fever.

In 1904, the then President of the United States, Theodore Roosevelt, initiated a second attempt to build the canal (shown in Fig. 8.72). William Gorgas was engaged to control the mosquitoes in the Panama zone. He did this and it contributed significantly to the successful completion of the Panama Canal.

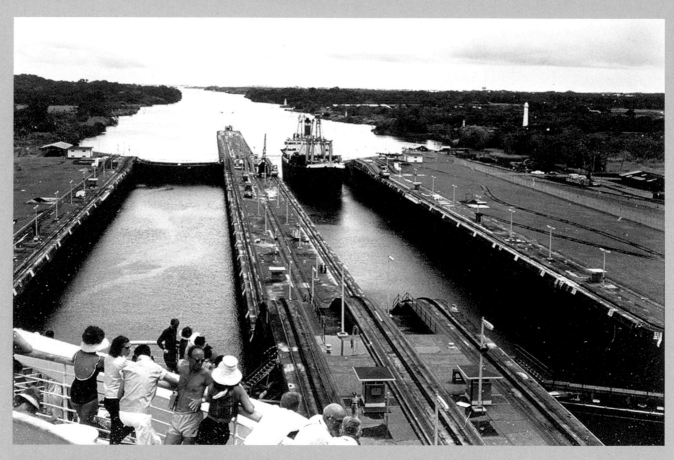

▲ **Fig. 8.72** Panama Canal. Ship leaving one of the locks at the highest point of the canal, 1967.

Lyssaviruses

The best known lyssavirus is the rabies virus, but there are other related viruses in this group, for example the Australian bat lyssavirus

Rabies

In most countries of the world, rabies is endemic in animals, particularly dogs, monkeys and bats. Infection is acquired through the saliva injected by the bite of one of these infected animals. Although symptoms of disease usually occur within a week or so of the bite, they may be delayed for many months and even for years.

Case 8.10

A male, aged 9 years, was admitted to a hospital in Brisbane, Australia, having been sick for about 23 days. This started with fever, malaise and headache and proceeded to muscle weakness, nerve palsies, fitting and gradual deterioration in consciousness to death. In spite of intensive investigations, no diagnosis was made during life.

Post mortem was confined to an examination of the brain. This showed changes of encephalitis—focal areas of necrosis with lymphocytes and perivascular cuffing with lymphocytes infiltrating the Virchow Robin spaces around the capillaries. There was a light infiltration of lymphocytes in the subarachnoid space. In many of the neurons, there were large eosinophilic intracytoplasmic inclusions consistent with rabies inclusions (see Fig. 8.73).

Immunofluorescent tests for rabies virus were positive and electron microscopy showed viral particles consistent with rabies virus (see Figs 8.74 and 8.75, overleaf).

The eosinophilic inclusions in the cytoplasm of affected neurons are called Negri bodies, named after the Italian physician who first described them. Figure 8.76, overleaf, shows his hand drawing of Negri bodies in rabies.

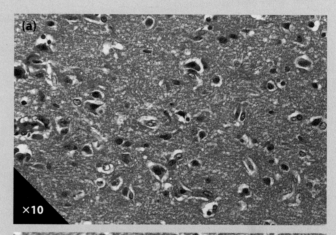

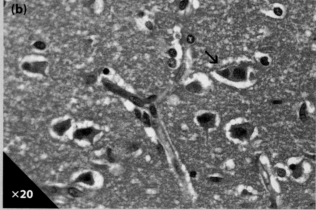

▲ **Fig. 8.73(a) and (b)** Views of the brain, showing the presence of rabies virus particles (Negri bodies) in the cytoplasm of the neurons.

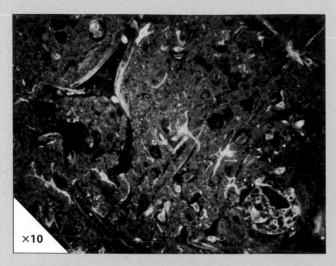

▲ **Fig. 8.74** Positive immunofluorescence test for rabies virus on a section of brain.

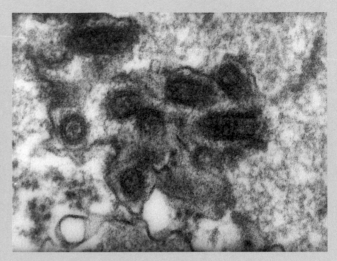

▲ **Fig. 8.75** Electron micrograph showing viral particles consistent with rabies virus.

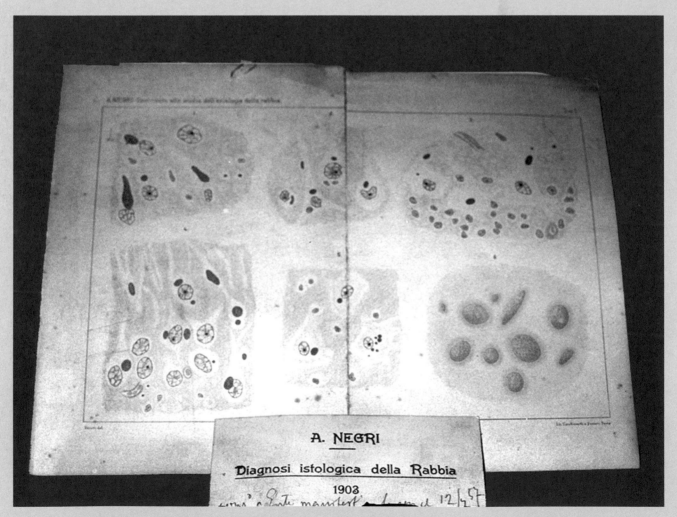

▲ **Fig. 8.76** This hand drawing of Negri bodies in rabies was done by A. Negri, who first described them in 1903. It is displayed in the History of Medicine Museum in Pavia, Italy.

Further history: After the results of the post mortem became known, a more detailed account of the boy's travel history was obtained. He had spent 8 months travelling in India with his mother. During this time, she now remembered, he had indeed been bitten on the finger by a monkey during a visit to a shrine. This occurred about 9 months before the onset of symptoms.

The incubation period for rabies is usually a few months, but it is sometimes much longer as in this case.

The author took the photo shown in Fig. 8.77 on the approach to the tomb of the Mogul Emperor Akbar (1542–1605) in Agra, India, some years before this case appeared in his department at the hospital in Brisbane. The photo was taken specifically to illustrate the setting and method of transmission of rabies—'for when he would encounter the first case in his department': it took a while to happen.

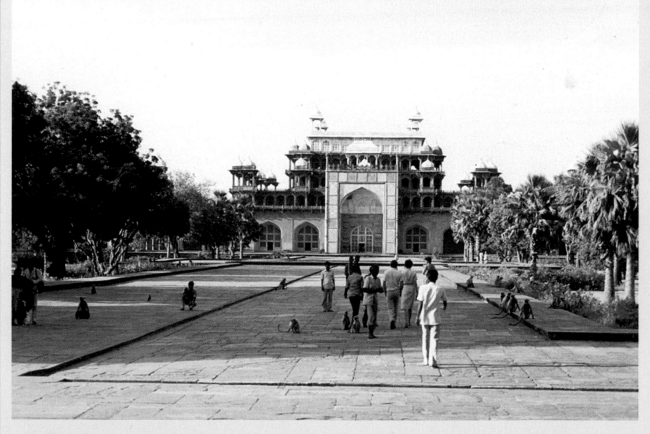

▲ **Fig. 8.77** Monkeys, Agra, India. The monkeys would jump onto visitors in search of food. Some were controlled by 'handlers', who for a small fee would prevent them from doing this.

Australian bat lyssavirus (ABLV)

Case 8.11

A 37-year-old Australian female developed an encephalitic illness that led to her death 14 days later. Subsequent history revealed that she had been bitten by a fruit bat on the left hand 27 months before the onset of her illness.

Permission for post-mortem examination of her brain only was obtained. Sections of the brain showed an encephalitis.

The histologic features of this are illustrated in Figures 8.78, 8.79 and 8.80.

Many of the neurons contained well-defined intra-cytoplasmic inclusion bodies, which resembled the Negri bodies seen in brains infected with rabies.

▼ **Fig. 8.78(a), (b) and (c)** Views showing the presence of encephalitis—perivascular cuffing with mononuclear inflammatory cells and brain necrosis.

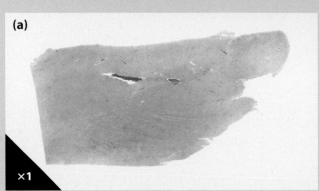

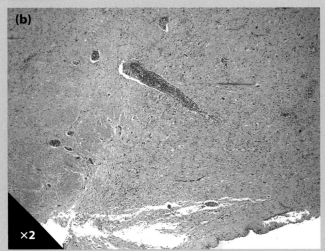

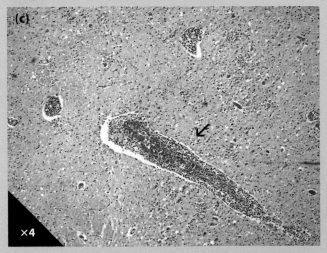

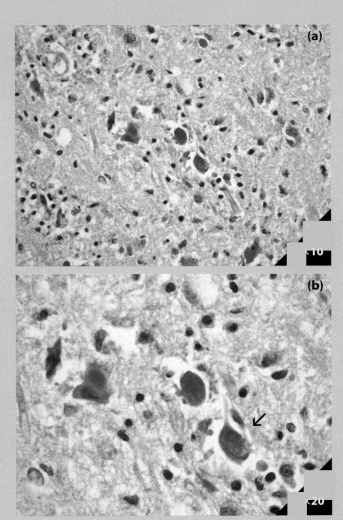

▲ **Fig. 8.79(a) and (b)** Views of the encephalitic reaction and neurons containing Negri bodies.

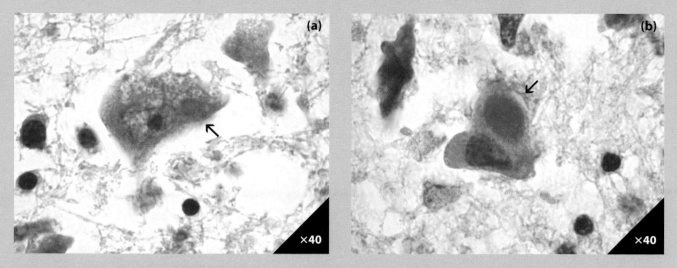

▲ Fig. 8.80(a) and (b) Neurons containing intracytoplasmic eosinophilic inclusions consistent with Negri bodies, viewed at higher magnification.

Diagnosis: The diagnosis of Australian bat lyssavirus encephalitis was confirmed by detecting ABLV-specific nucleic acids by RT-PCR in saliva taken during life.

Throughout the world, many species of fruit bats carry lyssaviruses that have different genotypes from that of rabies, which is the best known lyssavirus. These viruses very occasionally cause a rabies-like illness in humans.

Infections with Australian bat lyssavirus (ABLV) have only recently been reported for the first time. Figure 8.81 shows Australian fruit bats.

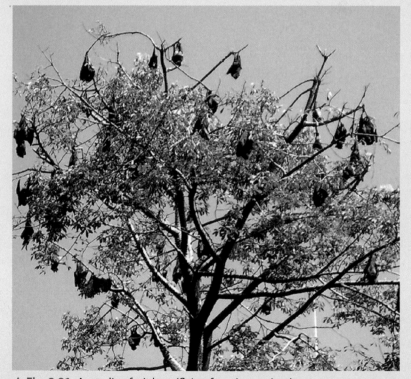

▲ Fig. 8.81 Australian fruit bats (flying foxes), roosting in a tree.

Prion diseases

Prion diseases (a group included here for convenience) used to be called 'slow viruses'—so named because the disease becomes apparent only some months after infection. These contain no nucleic acid—only protein.

Creutzfeldt-Jacob Disease (CJD)

Case 8.12

A 64-year-old female died in a nursing home in Brisbane, Australia. Post-mortem examination of the brain alone was requested by her relatives. The only history available was that she had been demented for the 12 months prior to death.

The brain weighed 1340 grams. The hemispheres were symmetrical but there appeared to be a mild degree of global atrophy of gyri, with some compensatory dilatation of ventricles. No other gross abnormality was noted.

Microscopic examination: At low magnification, the gyral atrophy can be seen by the slightly excessive space between gyral folds (see Fig. 8.82). The striking abnormality is the 'spongiform change', which is present in the cortex and was seen in almost all areas of the brain (see Figs 8.83, 8.84 and 8.85).

Diagnosis: The diagnosis was Creutzfeldt-Jacob Disease (CJD), sporadic type.

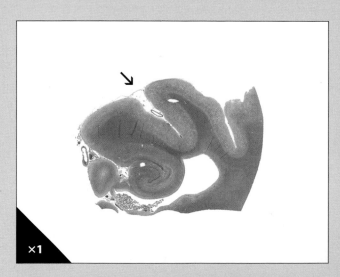

▲ **Fig. 8.82** View showing gyral atrophy, which can be seen by the slightly excessive space between gyral folds.

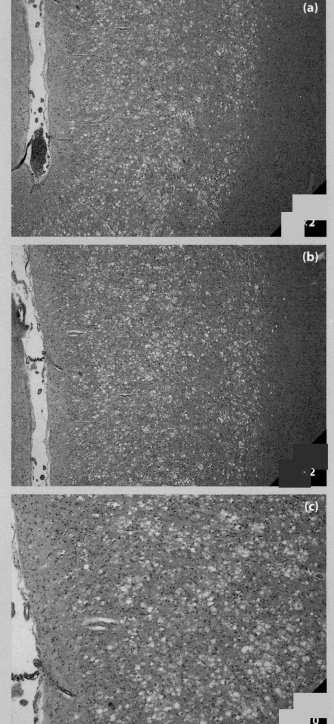

▲ **Fig. 8.83(a), (b) and (c)** Views that show the appearances of the widespread spongiform change.

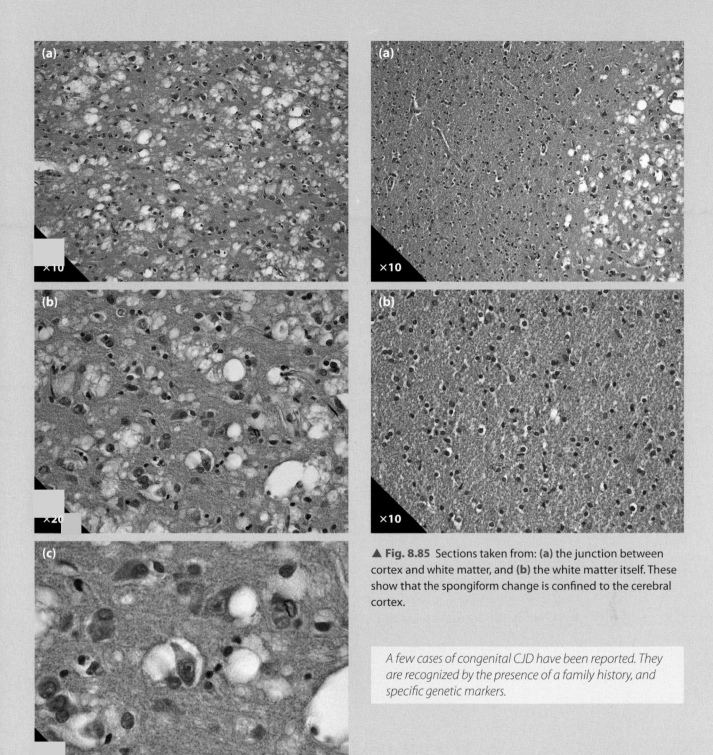

▲ **Fig. 8.85** Sections taken from: **(a)** the junction between cortex and white matter, and **(b)** the white matter itself. These show that the spongiform change is confined to the cerebral cortex.

A few cases of congenital CJD have been reported. They are recognized by the presence of a family history, and specific genetic markers.

▲ **Fig. 8.84(a), (b) and (c)** The spongiform change at higher magnification.

Iatrogenic CJD

Cases of CJD occurred in some recipients of tissue harvested from post mortems on patients who must, in retrospect, have been asymptomatic carriers of the prion. This happened in some patients who received corneal transplants harvested from post mortems, and others who had injections of human growth hormone prepared from pituitary glands harvested from post mortems. This condition is called iatrogenic CJD.

Bovine spongiform encephalopathy (BSE)

Bovine spongiform encephalopathy (BSE), also known as mad cow disease, is a disease that occurs in cattle and is sometimes transmitted to humans. It was first recognized in the United Kingdom (UK) in 1986.

CJD variant type

CJD variant type is the name given to the human disease that is acquired from eating BSE-infected beef.

The first cases of human disease occurred in the United Kingdom in 1995. The vast majority of reported cases have also come from the United Kingdom.

It differs from sporadic CJD, which affects older people (of over 60), by affecting younger patients (of average age 28 years). Sporadic CJD presents with neurologic symptoms while CJD variant presents with psychiatric symptoms.

Kuru

Kuru was a disease that manifested itself as ataxia that progressed to death in about 1 year from its onset. It affected young women, and children of both sexes, and was confined to a small linguistic group (the Fore) in the Eastern Highlands of Papua New Guinea. The most striking pathology was the presence of amyloid plaques in the brain (Figs 8.86).

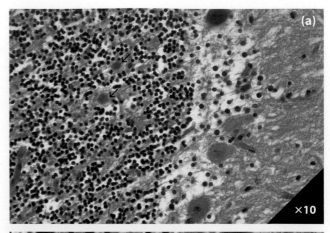

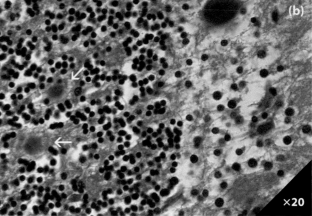

▲ **Fig. 8.86(a) and (b)** Amyloid plaques in the cerebellum of a patient who died of Kuru.

Kuru was defined by Carlton Gajdusek (shown in Fig. 8.87) and his co-workers in the late 1950s. It was transmitted by the custom (mainly of women) of eating the brains of the dead. This custom has now been abandoned and the disease has died out.

From his clinical and epidemiologic studies, and the reproduction of the symptoms and signs of Kuru by injecting fresh frozen human brain from deceased sufferers of Kuru into chimpanzees, Gajdusek developed the concept of a slow virus infection. For this he was awarded the Nobel Prize in 1976.

Epstein–Barr virus (EBV)

The Epstein–Barr virus was identified by Anthony Epstein (shown in Fig. 8.88) and Yvonne Barr. It causes infectious mononucleosis. It is associated with endemic Burkitt lymphoma, nasopharyngeal carcinoma and, recently, it has been identified in association with a group of lymphoproliferative disorders in immunosupressed patients.

In the latter three conditions, virus particles can be seen in tissue culture of the tumor cells but the virus has not been shown to actually cause the diseases.

▼ **Fig. 8.87** Carlton Gajdusek (b. 1923), photographed by the author during a visit to Gajdusek's laboratory at the National Institutes of Health (NIH), Washington, 2 weeks after the award of his Nobel Prize was announced.

▼ **Fig. 8.88** Anthony Epstein (b. 1921), photographed during a visit to Brisbane, Australia.

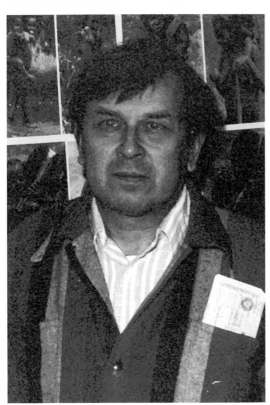

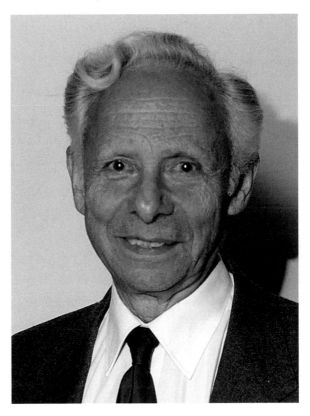

Infectious mononucleosis

Infectious mononucleosis (also known as glandular fever) presents with fever, malaise (which is often severe) and cervical lymphadenopathy (which is often accompanied by tonsillitis). Patients may have a maculopapular rash. It is spread by respiratory droplet infection.

It occurs either sporadically or in small epidemics, particularly in teenagers and young adults.

Diagnosis is confirmed by performing a full blood count, which shows a moderately elevated white cell count consisting mainly of lymphocytes. A significant number of the lymphocytes are abnormal in that they are large, with an abundant, blue-staining cytoplasm and they have mildly atypical nuclear morphology. These 'atypical' lymphocytes are reactive T-cell lymphocytes (see Figs 8.89 and 8.90).

A 'monospot' serologic test for heterophile antibodies is positive in about 85 per cent of cases.

Recovery from infectious mononucleosis usually occurs within a week or two. Sometimes, however, the disease continues for a considerably longer time. It is sometimes followed by a period of depression.

Asymptomatic biochemical hepatitis is noted in most cases, and occasionally this becomes clinically apparent. Rarely, 'spontaneous' rupture of the spleen occurs.

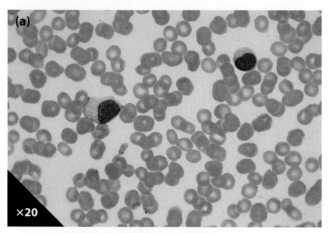

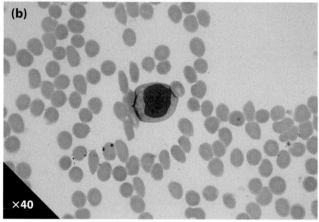

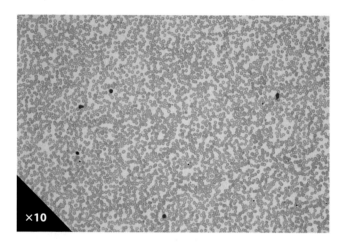

▲ **Fig. 8.89** Peripheral smear from a patient with infectious mononucleosis. It shows a mild lymphocytosis.

▲ **Fig. 8.90(a) and (b)** Views showing the morphology of the 'atypical lymphocytes' (reactive T-cells) of infectious mononucleosis. In **(a)** a normal lymphocyte is included at the top right for comparison with an 'atypical lymphocyte'.

Burkitt lymphoma

The condition known as Burkitt lymphoma was identified by Denis Burkitt (see Fig. 8.91), a surgeon who worked in Uganda, in central Africa, from the late 1950s to the mid 1970s. Burkitt found that this was the most common form of tumor in children in that part of the world.

The most common presentation of Burkitt lymphoma in Africa was with a jaw tumor that involved one or more quadrants of the jaw. Other sites for the tumor were the alimentary system, the kidneys, the orbit of the eye, the spinal cord, both breasts in girls, the ovary and the testis.

Burkitt's pathologists said the tumor did not resemble anything they were used to seeing, but it looked most like a malignant lymphoma. This was so in spite of the fact that its anatomical distribution was not like any lymphoma then known, and the histologic appearance was not like any then known malignant lymphoma.

Burkitt noticed that the tumor occurred below 5000 feet altitude. Because of its geographical distribution he thought that it might be transmitted by a vector, and might be caused by a virus. He sent tissue for culture to Anthony Epstein, a virologist in London, who was able to show that the tumor cells contained what looked like a virus. This became known as the Epstein–Barr virus.

Millions of dollars of research money have been spent on trying to show that the EBV virus causes Burkitt lymphoma, but without success. But it has been shown to cause infectious mononucleosis and to be associated with nasopharyngeal carcinoma, and more recently with a group of lymphoproliferative disorders in immunosupressed patients. No vector has yet been identified.

However, Burkitt lymphoma cells in tissue culture have been a successful experimental tool in the study of the biology of cancer.

Soon after Burkitt's discovery in Africa, a tumor that closely resembled the features of African Burkitt lymphoma was found in Papua New Guinea (see Fig. 8.92, overleaf). The similarities included a similar histologic appearance (see Fig. 8.93, overleaf) and the presence of EBV in tissue culture (see Fig. 8.94, overleaf). This was the first report of Burkitt lymphoma occurring outside Africa. Since then, it has been found that Burkitt lymphoma is found in most other countries, but it is only in 'endemic' cases (from Africa and Papua New Guinea) that the EBV can be found in tissue culture of the tumor.

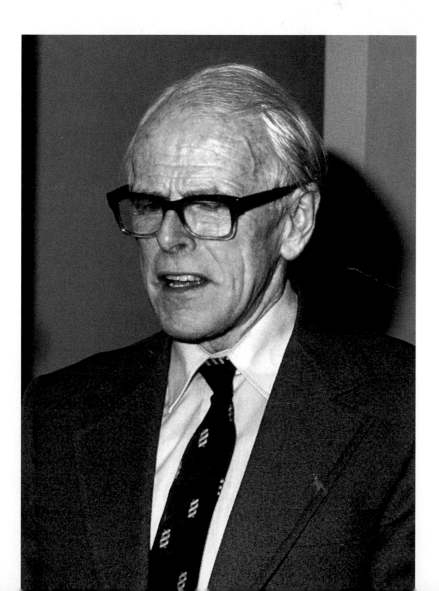

▶ **Fig. 8.91** Denis Burkitt (1911–1993), photographed in Brisbane, Australia in 1982.

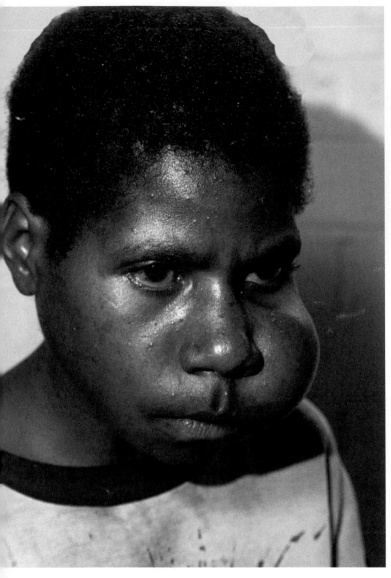

▲ **Fig. 8.92** Child from Papua New Guinea has a jaw tumor that on biopsy was a Burkitt lymphoma.

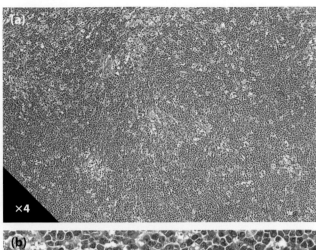

▲ **Fig. 8.93(a) and (b)** Burkitt lymphoma. Views of a Papua New Guinean case, showing the so-called 'starry sky appearance' described by the pathologists from Africa. This is due to the blue-staining tumor cells which form a blue background to the pale histiocytes proliferating among the tumor cells.

▼ **Fig. 8.94** Electron micrograph of the EBV in tissue culture from a Papua New Guinean case of Burkitt lymphoma.

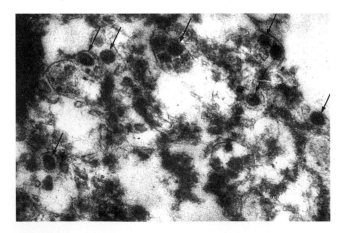

Poliomyelitis

The poliovirus is normally a nontroublesome inhabitant of the alimentary canal. It has three distinct serologic subtypes—type 1, type 2 and type 3. Before the introduction of the Salk vaccine in 1955, epidemics of polio occurred every few years. Transmission of the virus is from anus to mouth (fecal-oral transmission).

The clinical features were fever, headache, photophobia and neck stiffness, suggesting a diagnosis of meningitis. CSF examination showed a moderately high lymphocyte count as in any other viral infection of the central nervous system (CNS). During an epidemic, most infections were mild and were followed by immunity. However, immunity to one serologic subtype did not confer immunity to any of the others.

Of those who developed serious disease, the majority survived without sequelae. A small proportion of sufferers developed flaccid paralysis of muscles innervated by nerves arising from segments in the spinal cord in which the anterior horn cells were destroyed by the virus. The muscles affected were usually in one leg or one arm. The failure of muscle movement resulted in 'disuse' atrophy of the limb bones. This gave rise to the presence of a 'withered arm' or a 'withered leg'. This condition is illustrated in Figures 8.95, 8.96 and 8.97.

People with polio deformities were easily identified throughout the world before the introduction of polio vaccines. Now, they are only seen in medically underserved countries. Such cases will become less common there, too, in years to come, as a result of the recent worldwide campaign of polio vaccination by governments and private funding agencies.

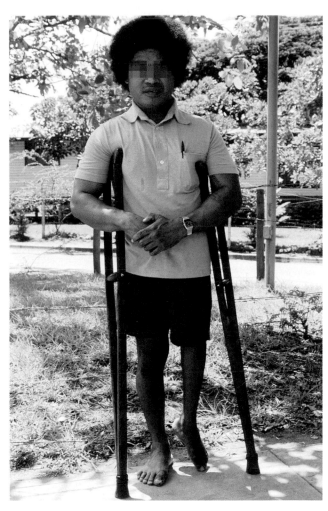

▶ **Fig. 8.95** Young man in Port Moresby with a withered leg. He is a survivor of the polio outbreak in the area in 1962.

▼ **Fig. 8.96** Transverse section of a grossly atrophic calf muscle.

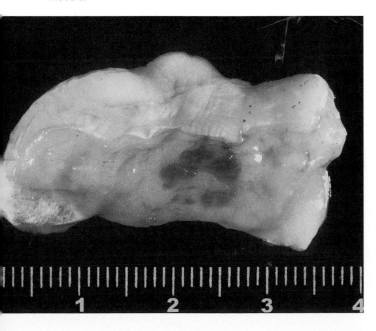

▼ **Fig. 8.97** View of a transverse section from muscle that shows the effects of motor-nerve damage. There is atrophy of groups of muscle fibers (the small, dark, red-staining fibers), while the rest of the muscle appears to be normal.

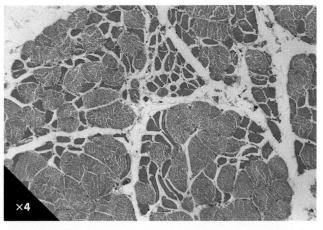

×4

During an epidemic, some patients developed 'bulbar palsy'—resulting in an inability to breathe, speak or swallow. This was caused by destruction by the virus of the motor neurons of the cranial nerves 9–12 that arise from the brain stem. This was usually associated with complete muscle paralysis of arms and legs as well. Such patients were kept alive by artificial, external life-support systems.

In the 1940s and 1950s, the main machine that made this possible was a large and cumbersome 'iron lung' (shown in Fig. 8.98). Some patients survived on continuous life support until the 1990s. In the last decade of the twentieth century, a syndrome called 'post polio syndrome' has become recognized. It affects patients who had polio in the 1940s and 1950s. As they are getting older, they find that their 'withered limb' is becoming a little weaker and some of them are developing incontinence of urine. The cause of this is not clear but it may be due to a further loss of motor neurons occurring as part of the aging process.

The pathology of poliomyelitis is demonstrated in Figures 8.99, 8.100 and 8.101.

▶ **Fig. 8.98** An iron lung from the 1950s, in the historical museum in the Medical School of Mahidol University, Bangkok, Thailand.

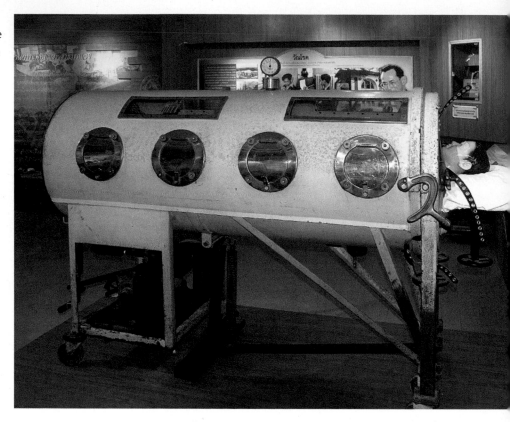

▶ **Fig. 8.99** View of a transverse section of spinal cord of a patient who died during the polio epidemic in Brisbane, Australia, in the years 1952 and 1953. At this magnification, the posterior nerve roots (A), which are sensory conductors, are of normal size. The anterior nerve roots (B), that carry motor impulses to the muscles, are smaller and quite atrophic. This has been caused by the destruction by the polio virus of the motor neurons in the anterior horns of the spinal cord.

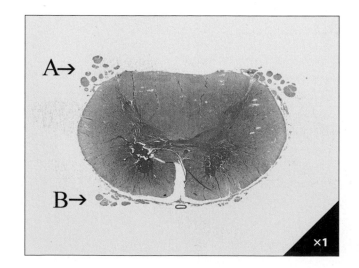

▼ ▶ **Fig. 8.100(a), (b), (c), (d) and (e)** Views of the right anterior horn of the spinal cord. In **(a)** the circled area shows almost complete loss of motor neurons. In **(d)** and **(e)** a few remaining degenerate neurons are arrowed, and some gliosis can be seen.

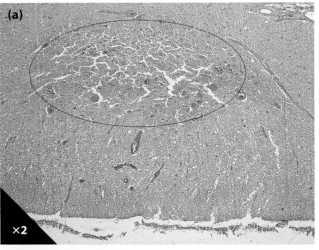

(a) ×2

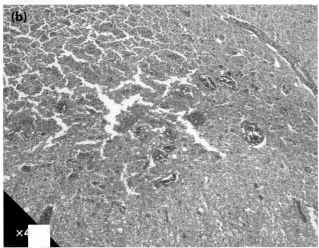

(b) ×4

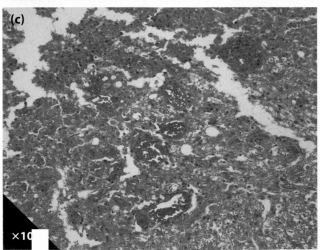

(c) ×10

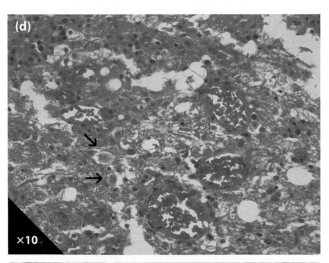

(d) ×10

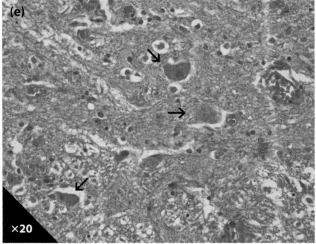

(e) ×20

▼ **Fig. 8.101** This blood vessel shows lymphocytes In the perivascular space (perivascular cuffing). There are also a few lymphocytes in the tissue above the vessel. In acute polio, there is an infiltration of lymphocytes in association with the necrosis of the motor neurons, and a CSF examination reflects this with an increased number of lymphocytes being present. The changes seen in this section probably represent the remains of this lymphocytic reaction.

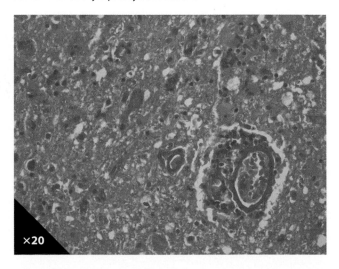

×20

A short history of the polio vaccine

John Enders, Frederick Robbins and Thomas Weller were awarded a Nobel Prize in 1954 for their successful cultivation of poliovirus in tissue culture of human embryonic tissue. This made possible the studies on the virus that led to the production of successful polio vaccines.

Jonas Salk (1914–1995) developed the first effective vaccine, which was released to the market in 1955. It was a killed virus administered by subcutaneous injection.

Albert Sabin (1916–1993) developed an oral vaccine made from an attenuated virus. It was released to the market in 1960.

Sabin vaccine is dispensed as a liquid. Because it has a bitter taste, it is administered mixed with a sugar solution. This is very convenient for use in countries where highly trained medical staff are in short supply.

Both the Salk and Sabin vaccines contain antigens to polio virus type 1, type 2 and type 3.

The author was at school when the last polio epidemic occurred in Australia in the years 1951 and 1952. The majority of polio patients survived, some with no sequelae but most with a wasted leg or arm. There were a few deaths. A few fellow students needed total life support for the rest of their lives, most of them living for about 40 years after their acute illness.

In 1962, the author was the pathologist in Port Moresby, Papua New Guinea, when an epidemic of polio occurred among the local population. Within a week or two, the children's wards of the 300-bed hospital were overcrowded with polio patients. The newly invented Sabin vaccine had just reached Australia. A large quantity of this was urgently flown to Port Moresby. All available staff of the Health Department were mobilized to undertake a mass vaccination of the children in the area. Within a week, the epidemic was halted. This was an unforgettable experience of the power of an effective vaccine to control an epidemic disease.

It is disturbing to note that in 2005 a few small epidemics have arisen in various countries in which polio vaccinations have been ceased for political or religious reasons. As with any epidemic disease, it is important that the level of vaccination be maintained so that the 'herd immunity' does not fall far enough for a new epidemic to occur.

Acknowledgments

- Fig. 8.24 Courtesy of Ray Tiernan, Brisbane, Australia.
- Fig. 8.34 Courtesy of Ian Wilkey, Brisbane, Australia.
- Fig. 8.71 Courtesy of Jaime Rios-Dalenz, La Paz, Bolivia.
- Fig. 8.73 Case courtesy of Hema Samaratunga, Brisbane, Australia. Photographed by Robin Cooke.
- Fig. 8.74 Courtesy of the Australian Animal Health Laboratory, Geelong, Australia.
- Fig. 8.76 Photo taken with permission of the Curator of the History of Medicine Museum, Pavia, Italy.
- Figs 8.78–8.80 Case courtesy of Tom Robertson, Brisbane, Australia. Photographed by Robin Cooke.
- Figs 8.82–8.85 Case courtesy of Tony Tannenberg, Brisbane, Australia. Photographed by Robin Cooke.
- Fig. 8.86 glass slide. Courtesy of Ross Anderson, Melbourne, Australia.
- Fig. 8.94 Courtesy of John Pope, Brisbane, Australia.
- Figs 8.95 and 8.96 From Cooke, R.A. and Stewart, B., *Colour Atlas of Anatomical Pathology*, third edn, Churchill Livingstone, Edinburgh, 2004.
- Fig. 8.98 Photograph taken with permission of the Curator, Mahidol University Medical School Museum, Bangkok, Thailand.

9

Parasitic infections
Protozoa

As the concept of the microbial cause of diseases became established in the late 1800s, another major class of organisms began to be discovered—parasites. These infectious agents mainly occurred in tropical countries, so the study of parasitic infections became synonymous with tropical medicine.

Unlike most of the infectious agents identified up to this time, they were transmitted by vectors, mainly insect vectors, and many of them had very complicated life cycles. Thus, scientists with a wide range of interests and expertise were needed, as well as medical personnel interested in the clinical features and pathology of the diseases. Laboratory scientists, entomologists, sanitation engineers, public health personnel and others all became involved in the investigation of parasitic diseases.

The earliest investigations of parasitic diseases were done mainly in Africa, India, China, South-East Asia, Central America and South America. Institutes of tropical medicine were established in these countries, and also in European countries that had major governmental and economic ties with the tropical world.

Tropical medicine included a study of parasitic diseases, but it expanded to embrace a wide range of other specialty interests, which included the management and epidemiology of all types of infectious diseases, and the geographic distribution of neoplastic and non-neoplastic disease. It was one of the 'glamour' specialties of medicine right into the middle of the twentieth century.

The diseases to be discussed in this chapter are as follows:

- African trypanosomiasis (see page 288)
- American trypanosomiasis (Chagas' disease) (see page 289)
- Leishmaniasis (see page 291)
- Malaria (see page 299)
- Toxoplasmosis (see page 326)
- Amebiasis (see page 334)
- Free-living amebas (see page 347)
- Balantidiasis (see page 350)
- Giardiasis (see page 351)
- Trichomoniasis (see page 352)
- Cryptosporidium (see page 353)
- Microsporidium (see page 354).

These references support the content of chapters 9 and 10:

Binford, C.H. and Connor, D.H., *Pathology of Tropical and Extraordinary Diseases*, vols I and II, Armed Forces Institute of Pathology (AFIP), Washington, DC, 1976.

Kean, B.H., Mott, K.E. and Russell, A.J., *Tropical Medicine and Parasitology Classic Investigations*, vols I and II, Cornell University Press, New York, 1978.

Protozoa

Trypanosomiasis

The Trypanosome organism is elongated, with a distinct nucleus and a smaller body called a kinetoplast. The kinetoplast is situated at the distal end of the organism and is the point of origin of a flagellum, which passes along the length of the organism and projects anteriorly. This is a mechanism for motility.

Two types of trypanosomiasis can be recognized on geographic and clinical grounds, and on grounds of the appearance of the infecting organisms. They are called:

- African trypanosomiasis, and
- American trypanosomiasis.

African trypanosomiasis

African trypanosomiasis is an infection caused by two species of Trypanosome:

- *Trypanosoma gambiense*—the cause of West African 'sleeping sickness', and
- *Trypanosoma rhodesiense*—the cause of East African 'sleeping sickness'.

The organisms are indistinguishable morphologically, but the species can be differentiated by serologic tests. The disease is transmitted by the bite of the tsetse fly of the genus Glossina (see Life cycle 9.1). The flies live in the vegetation near rivers and lakes. Humans become infected by the bite of tsetse flies when they come to the water (see Fig. 9.1). The trypanosome form occurs both in humans and in the fly.

African trypanosomiasis

humans
(game animals
the natural reservoir)

tsetse fly
(Glossina)
(lives in vegetation near
fast-flowing streams)

▲ **Life cycle 9.1** African trypanosomiasis.

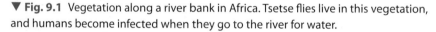

▼ **Fig. 9.1** Vegetation along a river bank in Africa. Tsetse flies live in this vegetation, and humans become infected when they go to the river for water.

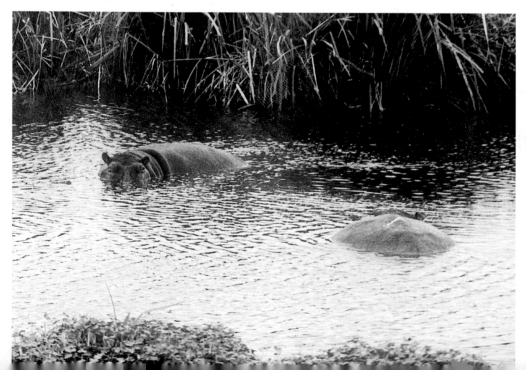

Humans are the main reservoir host for *T. gambiense*, with some animals also acting as hosts. Wild game animals are the main reservoir for *T. rhodesiense*.

The site of the bite of the tsetse fly usually results in a local area of ulceration. This is followed by fever, lymphadenopathy and splenomegaly. At this time, trypanosomes may be found in the peripheral blood (shown in Fig. 9.2).

In the later stages of the infection, meningo-encephalitic symptoms occur, namely headache and somnolence, going on to coma and, if untreated, death. These symptoms gave the disease the name 'sleeping sickness'. Post mortem examination of the brain shows the nonspecific features of encephalitis (see Fig. 9.3).

In the early 1900s in central Africa, there were severe epidemics of trypanosomiasis with a high mortality rate. In other parts of the world, it is a disease of travelers. For example, in Brisbane, Australia, there have been a few reported cases of *T. rhodesiense* in travelers returning from East Africa.

American trypanosomiasis (Chagas' disease)

Chagas' disease is caused by the organism *Trypanosoma cruzi*. It occurs in Central America and South America. It occurs in a number of animal hosts, as well as in humans. The organism is spread from person to person by the bite of blood-sucking triatomine bugs. A flagellate form occurs in the bugs. When they bite humans, they inject the flagellate forms into the bloodstream (see Fig. 9.4). The organisms invade tissues, particularly the cells of the myocardium, where they transform into a nonflagellate (amastigote or leishmania) form (see Figs 9.5 and 9.6, overleaf).

The leishmania organisms multiply in the tissue cells and then rupture and form flagellate forms again. These may be seen in the peripheral blood (see Fig. 9.4). The flagellate forms are taken up by the next triatomine bug to bite the patient and the cycle is repeated.

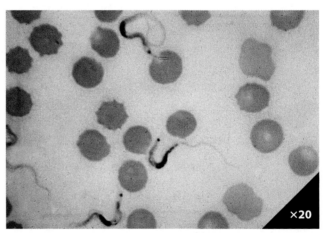

▲ **Fig. 9.4** *T. cruzi* organisms in a peripheral blood smear from a child, who had acute Chagas' disease. Note the acute U-shaped bend in the organism, the prominent kinetoplast and the long flagellum. Compare this with the shape in Figure 9.2.

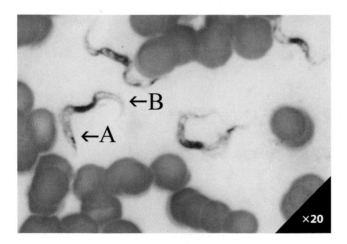

▲ **Fig. 9.2** African trypanosomiasis. A peripheral blood smear, showing the presence of Trypanosomes. (Note the 'open' curved shape, the oval nucleus in the middle of the organism, the kinetoplast at one end (A), and the flagellum at the other (B).

▶ **Fig. 9.3** African trypanosomiasis. This section is from the brain of an African patient, who died from sleeping sickness. There is perivascular cuffing with lymphocytes—the hallmark of encephalitis. Trypanosomes are not seen in tissues.

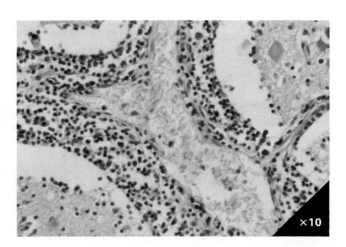

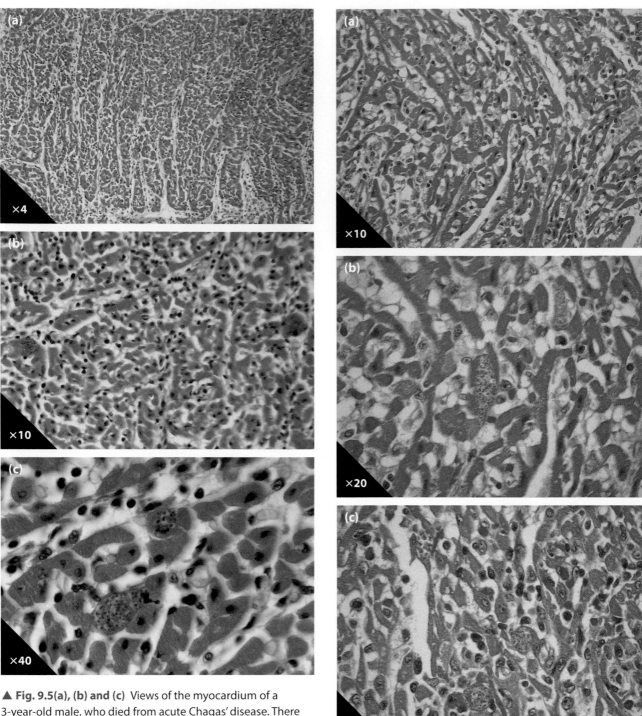

▲ **Fig. 9.5(a), (b) and (c)** Views of the myocardium of a 3-year-old male, who died from acute Chagas' disease. There is a diffuse myocarditis, with mononuclear inflammatory cells infiltrating the myocardium. Organisms can be seen within some of the myocardial cells. At high magnification, the organisms can be seen to have a nucleus and a much smaller kinetoplast adjacent to it.

▲ **Fig. 9.6(a), (b) and (c)** Views of the heart from a case of acute Chagas' disease. There is much less inflammatory infiltration in this case than in the one evident in Figure 9.5. Again, at high magnification, the nucleus and kinetoplast in each of the leishmania forms can be seen easily. These organisms must be distinguished from histoplasmosis in which only multiple single yeast forms are present within the parasitized muscle fibers. The yeasts stain positively with Periodic Acid Schiff (PAS) stain. The leishmania organisms do not stain with PAS.

The organism was first identified in 1909 by the Brazilian scientist Carlos Chagas (1879–1934), after whom the disease is named. Chagas reported the clinical and pathologic features of twenty-nine cases in 1916.

Triatomine bugs live in the fabric walls of village houses (see Life cycle 9.2). They come out at night to feed on the sleeping inhabitants. Bites occur particularly on the face. Marked periorbital edema (a localized, allergic response to the bite of a bug) is a fairly frequent finding in acute cases of Chagas' disease. This clinical feature is called Romana's sign, after the physician who first described it.

There are two clinical forms of American trypanosomiasis.

- The acute form presents with fever, lymphadenopathy and acute myocarditis in young children. Edema of one eye may be seen (known as Romana's sign).
- A chronic form is recognized in adults. It manifests itself as cardiomyopathy and chronic heart failure in patients who had an acute infection during childhood. The gross and microscopic pathology are nonspecific, but serologic tests are usually positive. Megaesophagus and megacolon are also thought to be manifestations of chronic Chagas' disease.

Chagas' disease has been almost completely controlled by eradication of the Triatomine bugs from houses.

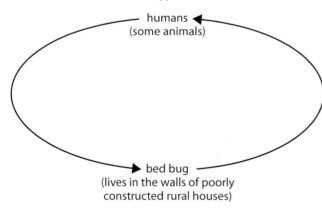

American trypanosomiasis

▲ **Life cycle 9.2** American trypanosomiasis.

Leishmaniasis

Leishmaniasis is transmitted by the bite of sandflies (see Life cycle 9.3). Quite a number of species of leishmania infect a variety of mammals. Morphologically, the organisms from the different species are indistinguishable from one another. However, the different species can be identified by a variety of molecular tests.

There are two readily distinguishable clinical forms of leishmaniasis:

- the cutaneous form (caused by a number of species of leishmania), and
- the visceral form (caused by *Leishmania donovani*).

Both forms occur in many parts of the world, including South America, Asia, India, the Mediterranean region, the Middle East and Africa.

In the sandfly, the organism is in the flagellated, leptomonad form (shown in Fig. 9.7, overleaf). In both forms of the disease in humans, the organism is seen in tissues in the leishmania form.

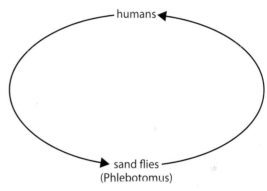

Leishmaniasis

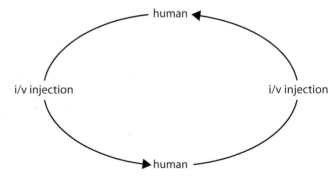

Life cycle in drug users who share unsterilized needles

▲ **Life cycle 9.3** Leishmaniasis.

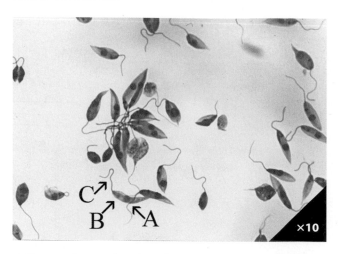

▲ Fig. 9.7 Smear of a culture from a hamster. It shows the flagellated, leptomonad form of leishmania, as it appears in the sandfly vector. The nucleus (A), kinetoplast (B) and flagellum (C) can be seen.

Cutaneous leishmaniasis

In cutaneous leishmaniasis, the patient develops a cutaneous nodule on an exposed area of skin. The original bite may go unnoticed.

Case 9.1

A red nodule developed on the nose of a 27-year-old woman about six weeks after she returned to Australia from a visit to relatives in Sicily, Italy (see Fig. 9.8).

The lesion on the nose was excised and the microscopic appearances of cutaneous leishmaniasis were seen (illustrated in Fig. 9.9). After the initial excision the lesion slowly resolved leaving a scarred area on the nose (Fig. 9.10, overleaf).

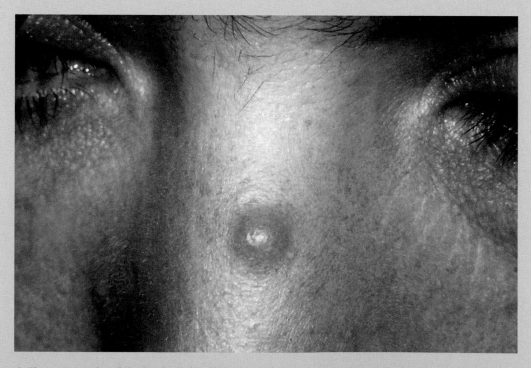

▲ Fig. 9.8 A red nodule developed on the nose of a 27-year-old woman about 6 weeks after she returned to Australia from a visit to Sicily in Italy.

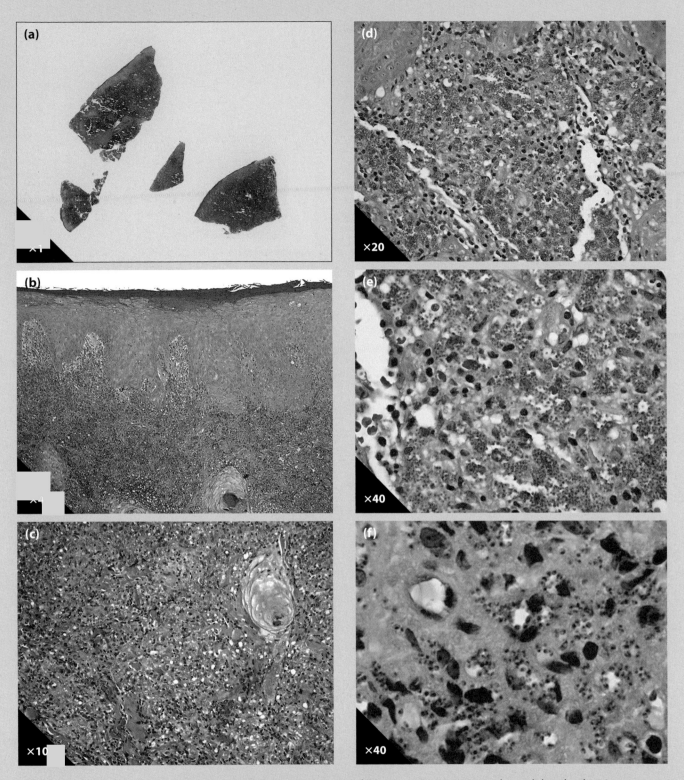

▲ **Fig. 9.9(a), (b), (c), (d) and (e)** The lesion on the nose was excised. Microscopic examination showed that the dermis was extensively infiltrated with an inflammatory cell infiltrate consisting of lymphocytes, plasma cells, eosinophils and histiocytes with pale-staining cytoplasm in which leishmania organisms can be seen. The organisms are round with an eccentric nucleus, and in some of them a small kinetoplast can be seen. The kinetoplast is not visible in every parasite because of the plane of section. **(f)** Giemsa stain. The lesion has not been completely excised.

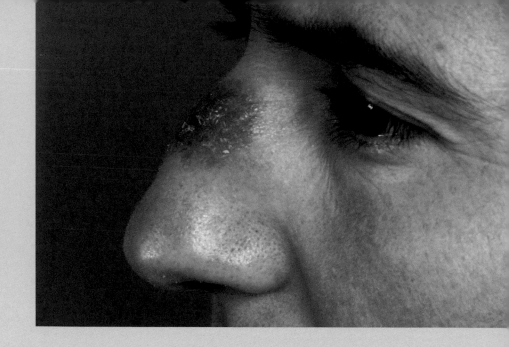

► **Fig. 9.10** After the initial excision, the lesion slowly resolved leaving a scarred area on the nose.

Case 9.2

A 27-year-old female Australian university student developed a lesion with a central area of ulceration and heaped-up edges on her right upper arm (Fig. 9.11). It developed 6 weeks after a visit to north Africa. Biopsy showed the appearances of cutaneous leishmaniasis. The lesion resolved with treatment.

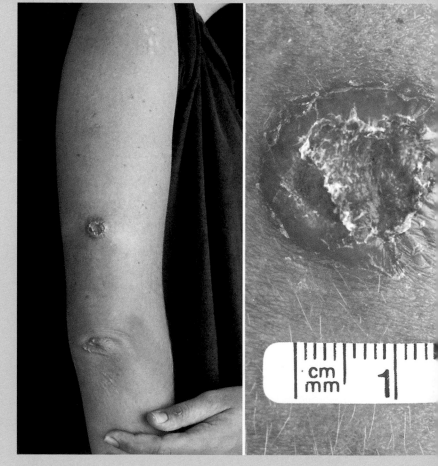

► **Fig. 9.11** Female, aged 27 years, has a lesion of cutaneous leishmaniasis at the lower end of her right upper arm.

Visceral leishmaniasis

In visceral leishmaniasis (also known as kala azar), the brunt of the infection is borne by the hematopoietic system. Patients present with fever, cachexia, hepatosplenomegaly and lymphadenopathy. The leishmania organisms are found in the histiocytes of the sinusoids in the lymph nodes, spleen, liver and bone marrow. As well as being transmitted by the bite of a sandfly, it can be transmitted by intravenous drug users who share needles, and by blood transfusion.

The diagnosis of visceral leishmaniasis can be confirmed by tissue biopsy or by needle aspirate of the spleen or bone marrow (see Figs 9.12 and 9.13). In some parts of the world (for example, in India), a fine needle aspiration (FNA) of spleen is the method of choice.

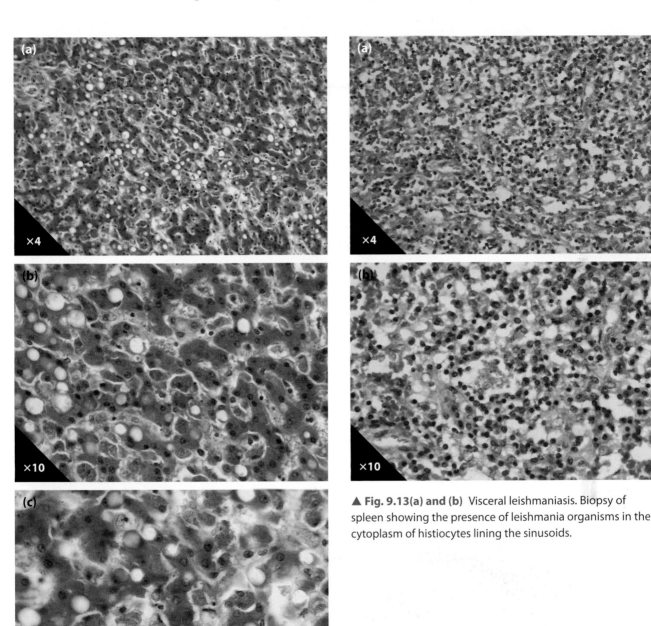

▲ **Fig. 9.13(a) and (b)** Visceral leishmaniasis. Biopsy of spleen showing the presence of leishmania organisms in the cytoplasm of histiocytes lining the sinusoids.

▲ **Fig. 9.12(a), (b) and (c)** Visceral leishmaniasis. Liver biopsy from an AIDS patient in which the hepatocytes are morphologically normal, but the sinusoids are markedly distended by proliferating Kupffer cells filled with leishmania organisms. In this patient, the infection may have been acquired from needles shared with other drug users.

Case 9.3

A male child from Bihar state, in northern India, presented with fever, wasting and splenomegaly (see Fig. 9.14).

The clinical diagnosis was kala azar (visceral leishmaniasis). This diagnosis was confirmed by examining a Giemsa-stained smear made from a fine needle aspirate from the spleen (see Fig. 9.15).

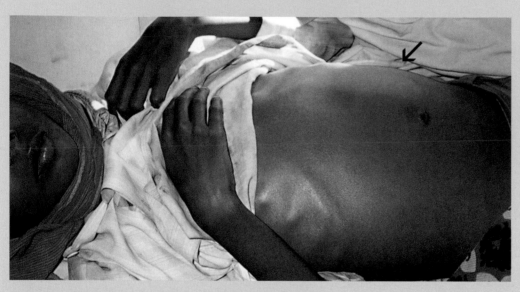

▲ **Fig. 9.14** Male child from Bihar state, in northern India, presented with fever, wasting and splenomegaly. The clinical diagnosis was kala azar (visceral leishmaniasis). This diagnosis was confirmed by examining a Giemsa stained smear made from a fine needle aspirate from the spleen.

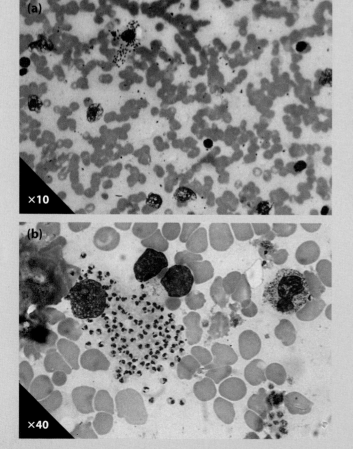

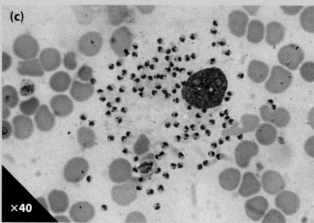

◀ ▲ **Fig. 9.15(a), (b) and (c)** Visceral leishmaniasis. Views of a fine needle aspirate from the spleen of a patient like the one shown in Figure 9.14. The cytoplasm of the monocytes is filled with leishmania organisms. The nuclei and their accompanying kinetoplasts are well seen in this preparation.

Case 9.4

A female, aged 43 years, returned to her hometown of Brisbane, Australia, after traveling in India. She presented with a 'pyrexia of unknown origin'. As part of her investigations, she had a needle aspiration of bone marrow. Leishmania organisms were seen in the cytoplasm of the monocytes (see Fig. 9.16).

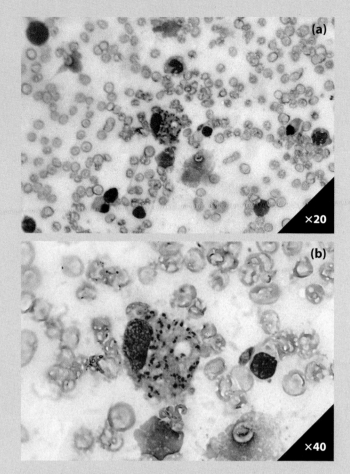

▲ **Fig. 9.16(a) and (b)** Visceral leishmaniasis. Leishmania organisms in the cytoplasm of the monocytes in a smear from a needle aspiration of bone marrow from a traveler who presented in Brisbane, Australia, with a 'pyrexia of unknown origin'.

Case 9.5

A male, aged 25 years, suffering from AIDS presented with diarrhea. One of the investigations was rectal biopsy, which showed the presence of leishmania organisms in histiocytes in the submucosa (see Figs 9.17 and 9.18).

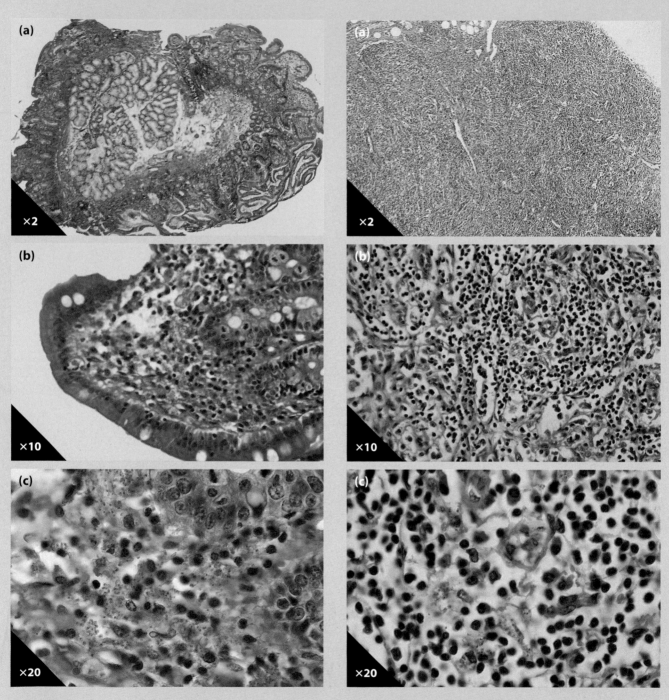

▲ **Fig. 9.17(a), (b) and (c)** Visceral leishmaniasis. Rectal biopsy from an AIDS patient suffering from diarrhea. Leishmania organisms can be seen in the cytoplasm of histiocytes in the submucosa.

▲ **Fig. 9.18(a), (b) and (c)** Visceral leishmaniasis. Views from another area of the rectal biopsy.

Malaria

Malaria is an infection caused by a protozoan parasite of the genus Plasmodium. It is the most important of the tropical diseases because it causes so much mortality and morbidity throughout the tropical countries of the world. Malaria is transmitted by the bite of the female Anopheline mosquito (see Life cycle 9.4).

Four species infect humans: *Plasmodium falciparum*, *Plasmodium vivax*, *Plasmodium malariae* and *Plasmodium ovale*.

- *P. falciparum* and *P. vivax* cause the vast majority of infections.
- *P. malariae* causes a small percentage of infections.
- *P. ovale* is extremely rare.

Malaria

Mosquito cycle

A female Anopheline bites an infected human.

↓

In the stomach of the mosquito, male gametocytes exflagellate and the filaments fuse with female gametocytes to become oocytes.

↓

Oocytes become sporozoites that enter the salivary glands.

↓

The infected mosquito bites an uninfected human.

↓

Human cycle

Sporozoites enter the liver and produce schizonts that rupture. The released merozoites become ring forms that invade red blood cells, and the first attack of fever occurs.

↓

The ring forms (trophozoites) become schizonts.

↓

Schizonts rupture, releasing merozoites that invade red blood cells to become trophozoites.

↓

About 10 days after the first fever, some trophozoites become gametocytes.

↓

Gametocytes are sucked into the stomach of a mosquito that bites an infected human.

↓

The mosquito cycle occurs.

▲ **Life cycle 9.4** Malaria.

Historical aspects of malaria

It appears that the Greek physician Hippocrates (460–377 BC) described the clinical features of malaria. From earliest times, it was known that it occurred particularly in areas of marshland. The French term for malaria is *le paludisme* ('associated with marshes'); and the English term is derived from the Italian *mal* ('bad') and *aria* ('air')—words with a similar connotation.

France—Alphonse Laveran

In 1880, the French physician Alphonse Laveran (1845–1922) (shown in Fig. 9.19), while working as an army doctor in north Africa, demonstrated living organisms in the blood of some of his patients who presented with severe and intermittent fever.

Laveran correctly assumed that these organisms—the malaria parasite—were the cause of the fever. He examined preparations of unfixed, unstained blood from febrile patients using a monocular microscope (see Figs 9.20 and 9.21, overleaf). He also described the phenomenon of exflagellation (see Fig. 9.22, overleaf). He returned to France from north Africa and worked at the Institut Pasteur in Paris. Laveran was awarded a Nobel Prize in 1907.

▼ **Fig. 9.19** Alphonse Laveran (1845–1922), who at the age of 35 years identified the malaria parasite.

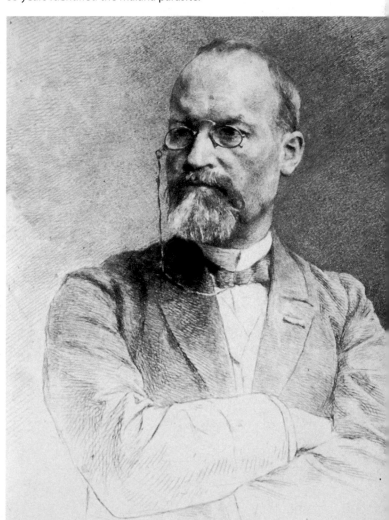

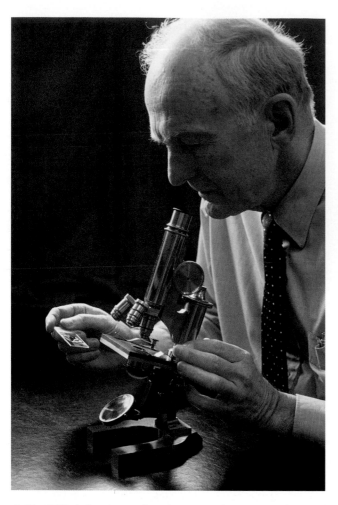

▲ **Fig. 9.20** Leitz monocular microscope. Laveran used a monocular microscope like this vintage Leitz one with a sub-stage mirror for illumination. He examined preparations of unfixed, unstained blood from febrile patients.

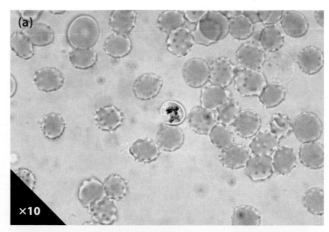

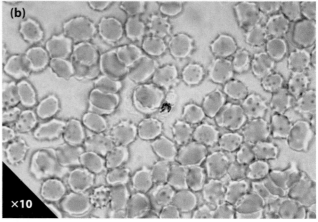

▲ **Fig. 9.21(a) and (b)** Reenactment of Laveran's observations. A drop of anticoagulated blood from a patient with *P. falciparum* malaria was placed on a glass microscope slide and covered by a coverslip. The slide was then examined in the fresh state. **(a)** Shows a round body with a thick capsule. In the preparation, it could be seen that the structures within this capsule were actively and independently motile—just as they were described by Laveran. **(b)** Shows an unstained crescent-shaped gametocyte.

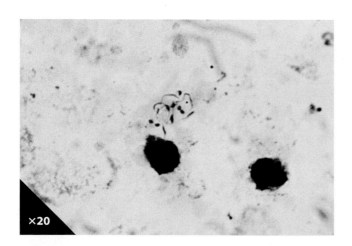

◄ **Fig. 9.22** Exflagellation of a microgametocyte of *P. vivax*. The blood was left on a laboratory bench for a few hours. This is a process that occurs in vivo in the gut of the mosquito. These male gametocytes then fertilize female ones and oocytes develop. This observation was one made by Laveran on one of the crescent bodies—a *P. falciparum* gametocyte. He prepared the blood in a similar way to how this specimen was prepared.

Laveran returned to France from north Africa and worked at the Institut Pasteur, in Paris, where he continued working in bacteriologic and parasitologic research. He was awarded a Nobel Prize in 1907. The Institut Pasteur has honored him and some of its other famous staff members by naming buildings after them (see Fig. 9.23).

Paludism (Le Paludisme), one of Laveran's many publications, which he wrote in 1893, mentions that quinine is better treatment for malaria than is phlebotomy (see Fig. 9.24).

It is very interesting that Laveran thought it was necessary to mention this fact in his book. Perhaps it indicates the extreme strength of the resistance to change that was prevalent in Laveran's time. Then, phlebotomy in its various forms was in widespread use as treatment for all sorts of diseases—a practice persisting for a very long time. Later, the discoveries of Pasteur, Koch, Laveran and others effectively 'killed' phlebotomy.

Laveran also tells the story of a French army officer who led an expedition into the Ivory Coast, where there was a very high incidence of malaria. The standing orders required all military personnel to take prophylactic doses of quinine. The officer died from malaria, but all the others remained well. The officer had insisted that all personnel take quinine, but did not take it himself.

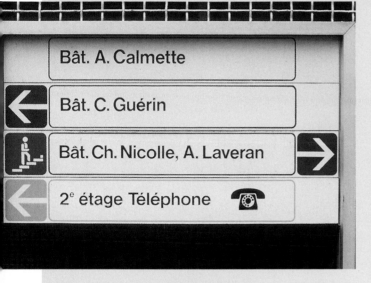

▲ **Fig. 9.23** Laveran returned to France and worked at the Institut Pasteur in Paris.

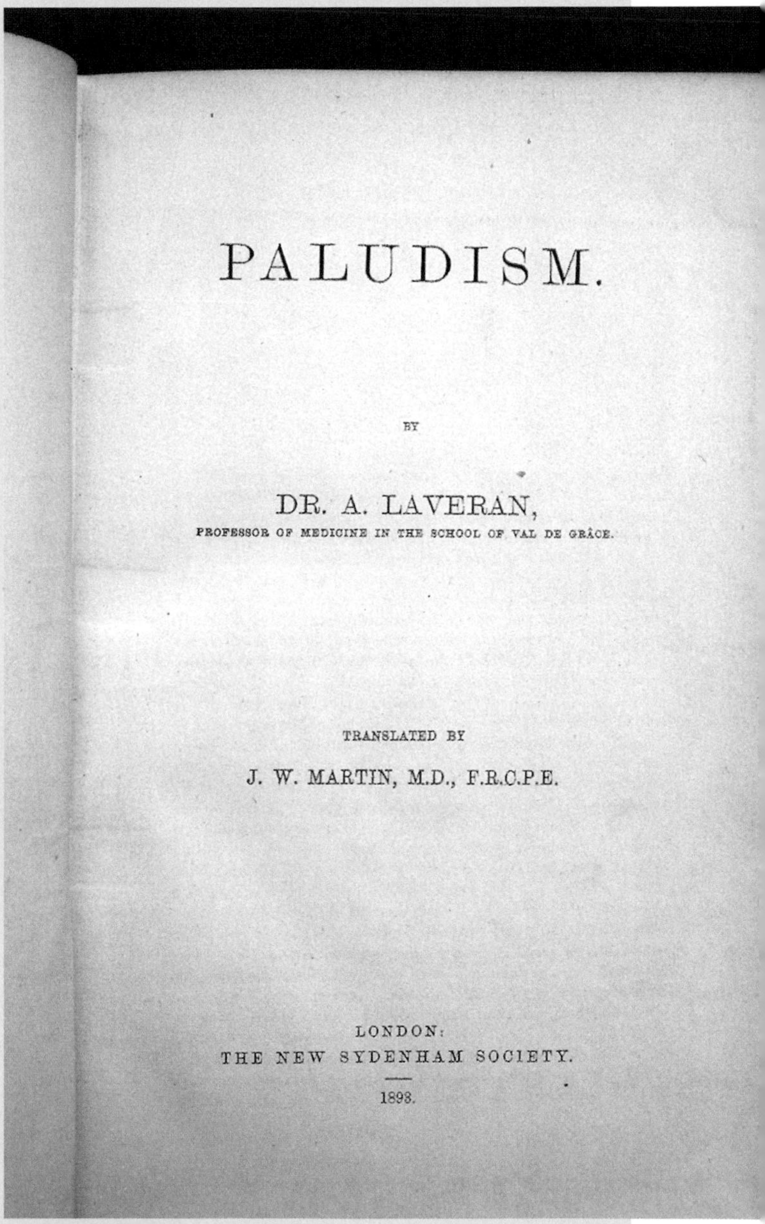

PALUDISM.

BY

DR. A. LAVERAN,
PROFESSOR OF MEDICINE IN THE SCHOOL OF VAL DE GRÂCE.

TRANSLATED BY

J. W. MARTIN, M.D., F.R.C.P.E.

LONDON:
THE NEW SYDENHAM SOCIETY.
1893.

▲ **Fig. 9.24** *Paludism* (*Le Paludisme*) one of Laveran's many publications, which he wrote in 1893, mentions that quinine is better treatment for malaria than is phlebotomy.

Italy—Camillo Golgi, Ettore Marchiafava, Giovanni Grassi and Amico Bignami

Malaria was a common clinical problem in Italy. A group of Italian workers, notably Camillo Golgi (1843–1926), Ettore Marchiafava (1847–1935), Giovanni Grassi (1854–1925) and Amico Bignami (1862–1929), contributed significantly to an understanding of this disease.

Golgi performed microscopic examinations on blood taken from patients in Pavia, in northern Italy, and correlated the appearances of the parasites with the clinical features of the fever. Golgi, commemorated at a museum in Italy (see Fig. 9.25), was dealing with *P. vivax* and *P. malariae* infections, which presented with what he called, respectively, tertian malaria and quartan malaria—because the intermittent fever occurred every third and fourth day respectively. He published the first microphotograph of *P. malariae* in 1890 (see Fig. 9.26).

Marchiafava, Grassi and Bignami worked in Rome, where serious summer epidemics of malaria had occurred for

▶ **Fig. 9.25** Commemoration of Camillo Golgi (1843–1926). Golgi was primarily a neuroanatomist and received a Nobel Prize for this in 1906, but his contributions to the understanding of malaria were also significant. A display of his work is in the Museum of Medical History, University of Pavia, Italy. *(Left)* Citation from the Liverpool School of Tropical Medicine, and to the right is a copy of his Nobel Prize certificate. *(Bottom left)* Slide tray containing some of Golgi's malaria blood films. Behind the tray is a microtome and microscopes of the era. *(Right)* Copy of Golgi's drawings of the nerve cells for which he was awarded the Nobel Prize.

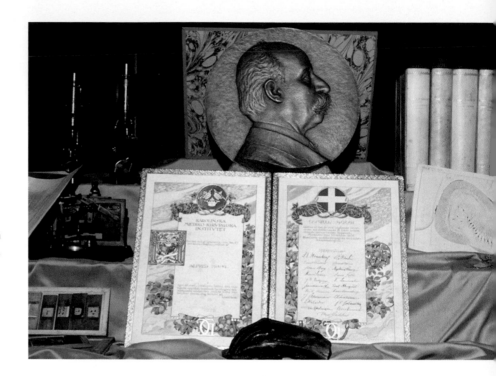

▶ **Fig. 9.26** Temperature charts of patients with malaria, together with copies of the microphotographs Gogli made of *P. malariae* in 1890.

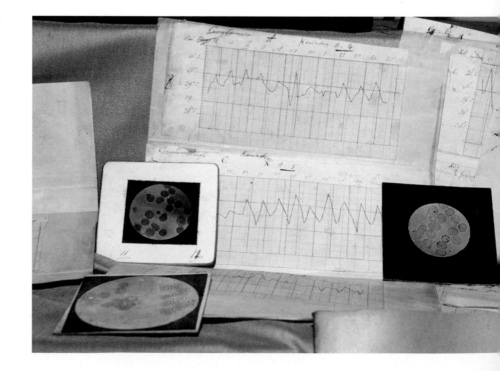

centuries. Their form of malaria was a more severe disease than that which occurred in the north of Italy. It produced intermittent fever that appeared every third day, and the mortality was significant. It came to be called malignant tertian malaria to distinguish it from Golgi's benign tertian malaria. It was caused by *P. falciparum*. These Italian physicians contributed to an understanding of the clinical features of malaria and demonstrated that it was transmitted to humans by the bite of Anopheline mosquitoes. Malaria was eradicated from Rome in the 1930s, when the mosquitoes were controlled by the draining of the Pontine marshes.

> *'Pontine marshes' refers to marsh land associated with the prevalence of recurrent fevers from which many people died every summer. It was a problem in the summer time in Rome for centuries.*
>
> *It is an area of about 175 000 acres (70 875 hectares), which stretches as a broad coastal strip for about 50 miles (80 km) south of Rome. Various rulers tried to drain them but Benito Mussolini was finally successful.*
>
> *Since the marshes were drained, this reclaimed area has become rich farming land that is used for a variety of agricultural purposes.*

Russia—Dimitri Romanowsky

Dimitri Romanowsky (1861–1921) was a graduate of the University of St Petersburg, Russia. In 1891, the year of his graduation in medicine, he introduced a new method for staining blood smears. The stain contained eosin and methylene blue. It was so good that it has been the basis of hematologic stains ever since. Apart from staining the cells of the blood, it also showed the morphology of malaria parasites much more clearly than the stains being used by Golgi and others at the time. Malaria was, then, a significant cause of death in Russia.

Britain—Patrick Manson and Ronald Ross

Patrick Manson (1844–1922) is regarded as being the founder of tropical medicine in Britain. Soon after graduating in medicine, he went to work in Hong Kong, Formosa (Taiwan) and Amoy (Xiamen)—a coastal city in southern Fujian province, from where Taiwan was settled.

In 1877, he showed that filariasis was transmitted by the bite of a mosquito. He returned to London in 1890 and established the London School of Tropical Medicine, which opened in 1899. Manson's *Tropical Diseases* textbook became a standard textbook in tropical medicine (shown in Figs 9.27 and 9.28).

Probably, Manson's most famous pupil was Ronald Ross (1857–1932), a medical officer in the British Indian Army. While on leave, Ross attended some of the classes conducted by Patrick Manson. Manson encouraged him to investigate whether a mosquito was the vector for malaria.

What Manson asked Ross to do was likely to be a difficult problem to solve because nobody knew exactly what form

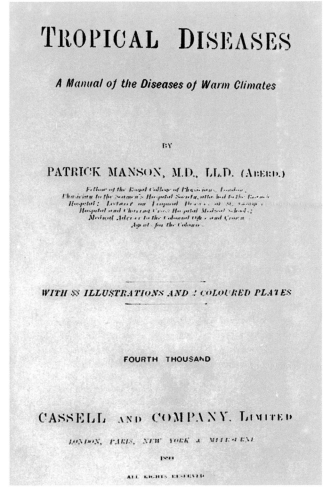

▲ **Fig. 9.27** Manson's *Tropical Diseases*, an edition published in 1899. This was a standard textbook on tropical medicine for over 60 years.

▼ **Fig. 9.28** A section from Manson's *Tropical Diseases* textbook, which refers to the transmission of malaria by a mosquito vector.

The mosquito considered as the extra-corporeal host of the plasmodium.—Further, as the plasmodium whilst in the circulation is always enclosed in a blood corpuscle and is therefore incapable of leaving the body by its own efforts, and as it is never, so far as known, extruded in the excreta, I have suggested that it is removed from the circulation by some blood-eating animal, most probably by some suctorial insect common in the haunts of malaria. This insect, as Laveran has also suggested, I believe to be the mosquito*; an insect whose habits seem well adapted the malaria parasites might take in the body of a vector. Studies of blood films on patients with malaria showed that the parasite could appear in many different forms. A 'marker', which appeared to be relatively constant in all of these forms, was the presence of brown pigment. This could be seen within the parasitized red blood cells, or within the cytoplasm of monocytes in the peripheral blood (see Fig. 9.29). Ross went looking for this marker—that is to 'find the pigment'.

During his first posting in India, Ross dissected many hundreds of mosquitoes without finding any pigment bodies. After holiday leave in England, he returned to India and was posted to Secunderabad (now Hyderabad), on the Deccan, the huge plateau that forms much of central south India. At that time, little was known about the different species of mosquito. In Hyderabad, Ross found a mosquito he had not seen before. It had dappled wings and banded legs. This mosquito was subsequently classified as an Anopheline (Fig. 9.30).

To his joy, he found rounded pigment bodies in the body wall of one these mosquitoes (shown in Fig. 9.31). One can imagine his excitement as he found more mosquitoes with the same appearance. He made sketches of these pigment bodies (now called oocytes) and sent them in letters to Manson in England, in 1897 (see Fig. 9.32(a) and (b)). He then looked for the next stage of the parasite by meticulously examining the heads of infected mosquitoes. He saw numerous, thin, filamentous bodies that were congregated in what he concluded must have been salivary glands. He deduced that these bodies (now called sporozoites) must be the infective form that was transmitted to humans by the bite of the mosquitoes (see Fig. 9.32(c) and (d)). His definitive paper on the topic was published in 1899.

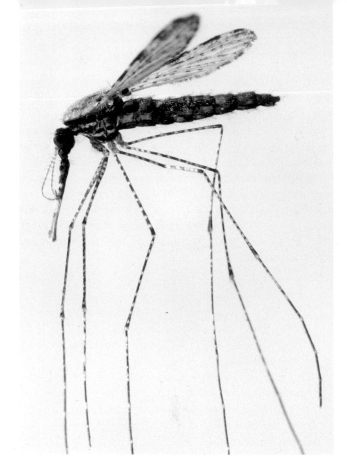

▲ **Fig. 9.30** Anopheline mosquito.

▼ **Fig. 9.31(a) and (b)** Views of a dissected mosquito, showing the rounded bodies (now called oocytes) that Ross saw in his dissections in Secunderabad (now Hyderabad).

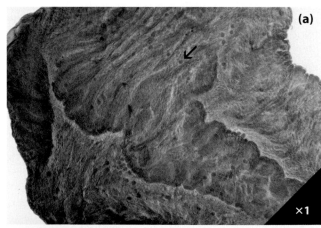

(a)

×1

▼ **Fig. 9.29** Malaria pigment in the cytoplasm of a monocyte in a peripheral blood smear of a patient with malaria. This was the marker that Ronald Ross was looking for in his dissections of mosquitoes.

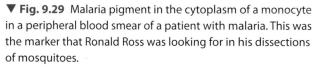

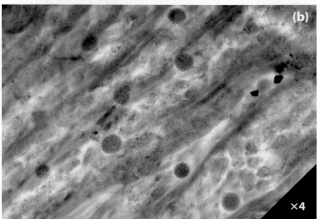

(b)

×4

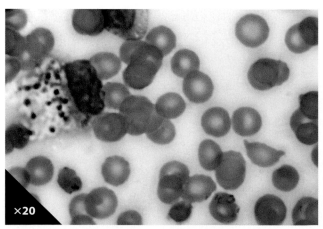

×20

A few months after his discovery of the pigment bodies in the mosquito, Ross took a period of leave and worked in the School of Tropical Medicine in Calcutta (see Fig. 9.33), where he is commemorated (see Figs 9.34 and 9.35, overleaf).

The actual laboratory in which Ross did his experiments is shown in Figures 9.36 and 9.37, overleaf. Here, he demonstrated with elegant, controlled experiments that bird malaria was transmitted by a mosquito, which was probably a Culicine. The laboratory is in the grounds of the Postgraduate Hospital in Calcutta. It has been used for many purposes over the years, including as a common room for medical residents (interns) of the hospital. It is now used as a storage area.

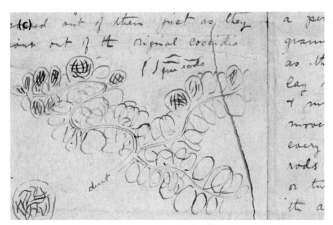

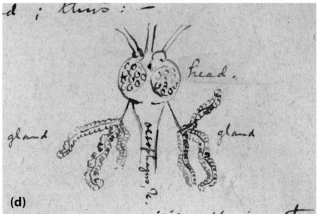

▲ **Fig. 9.32(c) and (d)** This letter from Ronald Ross contained diagrams that show the sporozoites in the salivary gland, ready to be injected into the next person that the mosquito would bite, thus transmitting the malaria to a second host.

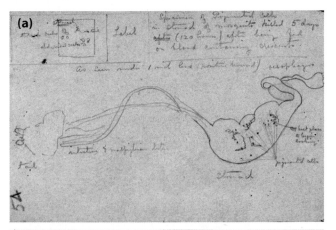

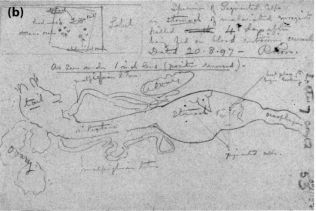

▲ **Fig. 9.32(a) and (b)** An original letter from Ronald Ross to Patrick Manson preserved in the historical collection of the library of the London School of Tropical Medicine, England. The diagrams show the presence of oocytes in the body wall of mosquitoes.

▼ **Fig. 9.33** The School of Tropical Medicine, Calcutta, India.

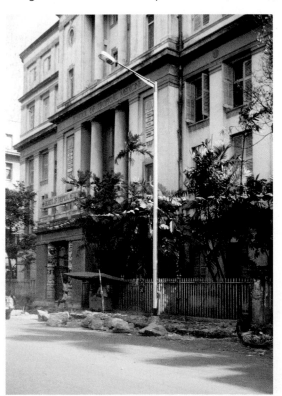

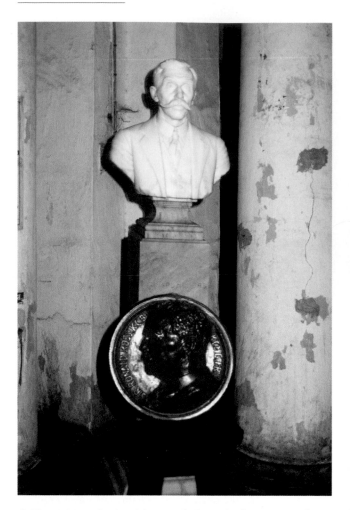

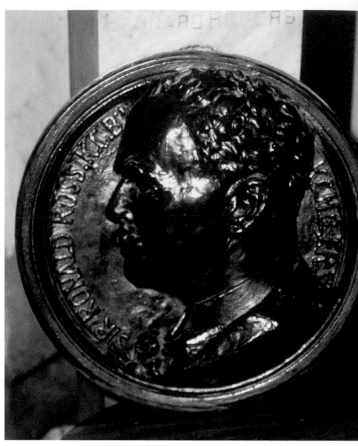

▲ **Figs 9.34 and 9.35** A bust and plaque in the entrance foyer in the School of Tropical Medicine, Calcutta, to honor Ronald Ross.

▼ **Figs 9.36 and 9.37** The laboratory in the grounds of the Postgraduate Hospital in Calcutta where Ronald Ross conducted his experiments that showed definitively that the Anopheline mosquito is the vector of malaria.

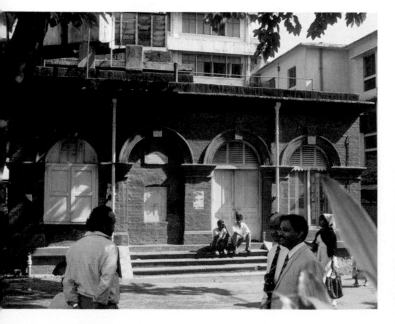

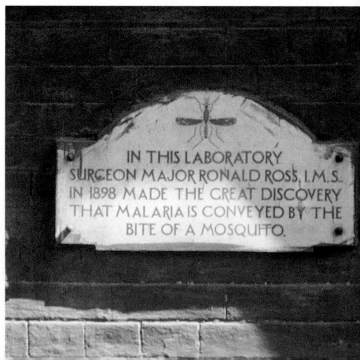

IN THIS LABORATORY
SURGEON MAJOR RONALD ROSS, I.M.S.
IN 1898 MADE THE GREAT DISCOVERY
THAT MALARIA IS CONVEYED BY THE
BITE OF A MOSQUITO.

After his work in India, Ross returned to England and joined the staff of the Liverpool School of Tropical Medicine. He was awarded a Nobel Prize in 1902.

United States—William Gorgas

William Gorgas (1854–1920) (depicted in Fig. 9.38) joined the US Army Medical Corps after graduation from medical school. From 1898 to 1902 he worked as chief sanitation officer in Havana, Cuba, with Walter Reed and others from the Army Hospital, Washington, USA. The group demonstrated that yellow fever was transmitted by mosquitoes. Gorgas drained the swampy land in the vicinity and, thus, destroyed the breeding grounds of the mosquitoes. This in turn eliminated yellow fever.

In 1904, he was transferred to the Panama Zone where American engineers were attempting to complete the Panama Canal that would join the Atlantic and Pacific Oceans, thus making the sea voyage between the east and west coasts of the Americas much shorter and much less dangerous than having to survive the very stormy passage round Cape Horn. French engineers had failed to complete the canal some years prior to this. A major cause for this failure was the extremely high mortality among the workers from malaria and yellow fever.

▼ **Fig. 9.38** Bust of William Gorgas (1854–1920) at the entrance to the Medical Museum at the Armed Forces Institute of Pathology, Washington, USA.

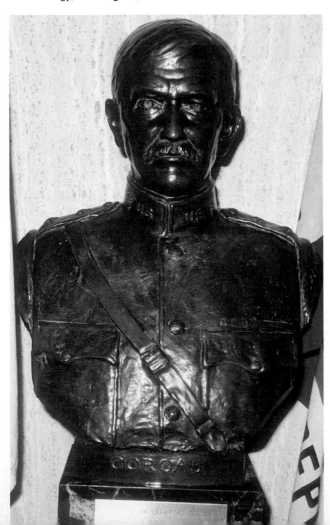

Gorgas managed to control malaria and yellow fever by doing two things. He stopped the spread of infection by isolating patients from the biting mosquitoes by keeping them behind mosquito screens, and he controlled the breeding of the mosquitoes by draining the swampy areas near human habitation.

William Gorgas received many honors for his work: one of these was to have his image appear on stamps from the Panama Zone.

William Gorgas was a member of the Cosmos Club, a prestigious private club in Washington, USA (see Fig. 9.39).

On its walls, the Cosmos Club has displays to commemorate the awards some club members have received, for example the Nobel Prize and the Pulitzer Prize. One of its displays commemorates members who have been honored on stamps, such as Gorgas who was the first club member to be honored in this way (see Fig. 9.40).

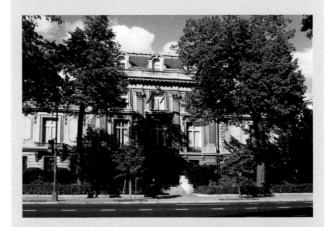

▲ **Fig. 9.39** The Cosmos Club in Washington, USA.

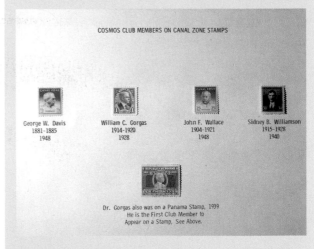

COSMOS CLUB MEMBERS ON CANAL ZONE STAMPS

George W. Davis
1881–1885
1948

William C. Gorgas
1914–1920
1928

John F. Wallace
1904–1921
1948

Sidney B. Williamson
1915–1928
1940

Dr. Gorgas also was on a Panama Stamp, 1939
He is the First Club Member to
Appear on a Stamp, See Above.

▲ **Fig. 9.40** Display of stamps featuring members of the Cosmos Club who have been honored on stamps. Gorgas is commemorated here for his work in the Panama Zone.

Clinical features of malaria

Malaria may present in many different ways. This can cause diagnostic confusion in a country in which it is not an endemic disease, as doctors and other health workers are not experienced in its clinical manifestations. To confirm the presence of malaria a full blood examination is done.

The commonest presentation of malaria is with an acute attack of fever, often associated with severe headache and drenching sweats that occur as the fever subsides.

The patient recovers from one attack of fever after about 8 hours, and then has a period in which he or she feels fairly well, until the fever returns. The fever of malaria is typically cyclical, with 1 or 2 days between bouts of fever, but this is not always the case and it can occur every day.

In acute attacks of malaria, there is often tender enlargement of spleen and liver. Repeated attacks of malaria result in permanent splenomegaly (as illustrated in Fig. 9.41).

In former times, when epidemiologists were assessing the prevalence of malaria in a community, it was common practice to take a blood smear to look for parasites giving a parasitemia rate, and to palpate the spleen in order to estimate the splenomegaly rate.

Any attack of malaria will cause a pancytopenia. There is a drop in hemoglobin, a decreased red cell count, a decreased white cell count and a decrease in the platelets. (Very rarely skin purpura occurs as a result of severe thrombocytopenia.)

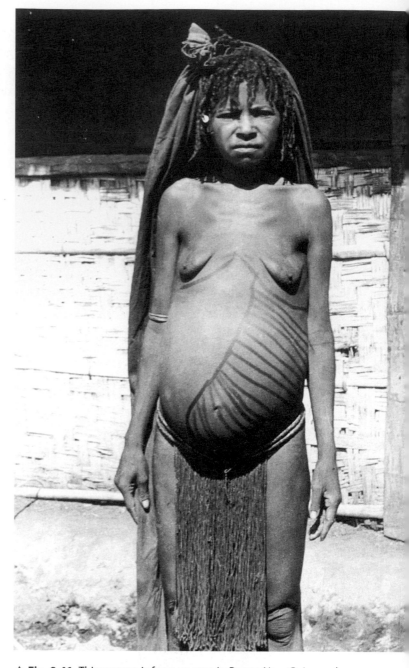

▲ **Fig. 9.41** This woman is from an area in Papua New Guinea where malaria is highly endemic. She has a very large spleen.

The red cell morphology usually shows the features of a hemolytic anemia—anisocytosis, some poikilocytosis and some polychromasia. The presence of malaria parasites can be confirmed, and their species can be determined.

In recent years, various immunologic methods have been introduced to diagnose malaria (shown in Figs 9.42–9.45), but a full blood examination remains the method of choice.

A history of recent travel out of one's own country is an important part of any clinical history. A febrile illness in someone who has recently visited a country where malaria is endemic should awaken the doctor to the possibility of malaria and other tropical diseases. Travel medicine doctors often find that diagnosis has been delayed because the patient was not asked this question at an early stage of their illness.

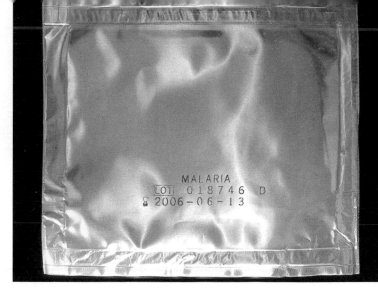

▲ **Fig. 9.42** Immunologic test kit for the diagnosis of malaria. It comes in a sealed packet that is kept refrigerated until used.

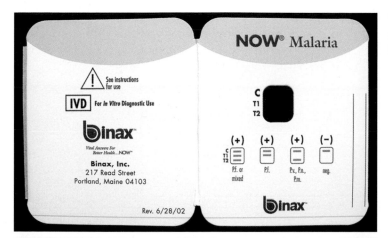

◀ **Fig. 9.43** Immunologic test kit for the diagnosis of malaria. The method for performing the test is illustrated on one side of the test card.

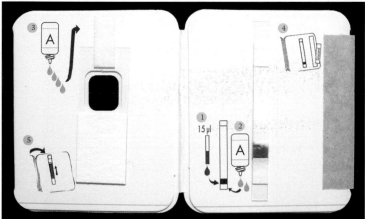

◀ **Fig. 9.44** On the other side of the immunologic test kit (shown in Fig. 9.43), there is a diagram that shows how to interpret the test.

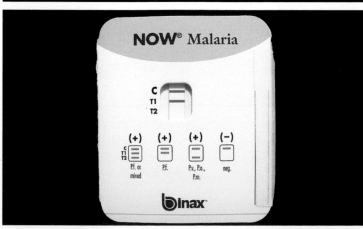

◀ **Fig. 9.45** Immunologic test kit for the diagnosis of malaria shows a positive test for *P. falciparum*.

Case 9.6

A 3-year-old boy from Papua New Guinea presented to a hospital in Brisbane, Australia, with febrile convulsions. His liver and spleen were enlarged (see Fig. 9.46). A blood examination demonstrated parasites of *P. vivax*.

This was a typical presentation and it caused no diagnostic difficulties.

In Brisbane, in the first few weeks after school holidays, there are always a few children who develop malaria after returning from visiting parents who live in malarial countries. Schools that cater for such children are well aware of this problem and quickly seek medical treatment for the students.

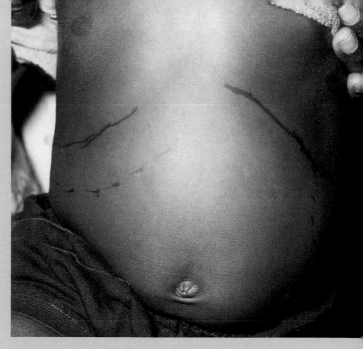

▲ **Fig. 9.46** This 3-year-old boy from Papua New Guinea presented to a children's hospital, in Brisbane, Australia, with febrile convulsions. His liver and spleen were enlarged. A blood examination demonstrated parasites of *P. vivax*.

Case 9.7

A 35-year-old Australian man spent 3 months in rural parts of India. When he returned to Brisbane, he was sick and jaundiced. At first, it was thought he had hepatitis, and the liver function tests supported this diagnosis.

One of the investigations ordered was a blood examination for the presence of malaria parasites. These tests were ordered late each day and were examined by the night staff, who at that time were relatively inexperienced. It was not until his ninth day in hospital that *P. vivax* parasites were seen in his peripheral blood, by a more experienced laboratory scientist.

The patient's temperature chart shows the typical cyclical nature of the fever of malaria (see Fig. 9.47). As soon as he was treated, the temperature rapidly returned to normal, his jaundice disappeared and he recovered.

Liver function tests are often mildly abnormal in any acute attack of malaria but frank jaundice is one of the less common presentations in visitors returning from malarial areas.

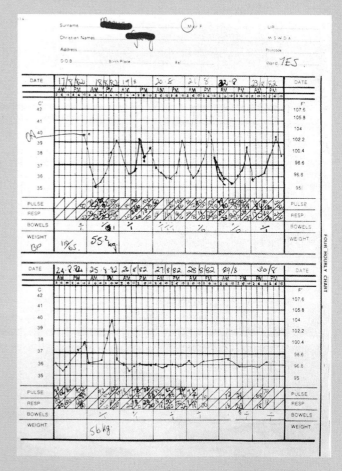

▲ **Fig. 9.47** Malaria. Temperature chart of a 35-year-old Australian man, who spent 3 months in rural parts of India. When he returned to Brisbane, he was sick and jaundiced. (At first it was thought he had hepatitis, and the liver function tests supported this diagnosis.)

The son of one of the medical staff at a hospital in Brisbane, Australia, became jaundiced with all the clinical and biochemical features of acute hepatitis. After he had been ill for about a week, a blood test was performed to look for malaria parasites. P. vivax parasites were found. He was treated and made a quick recovery.

This young man had not been out of Australia since he had returned from a trip to the United Kingdom with his parents 18 years previously. They had returned to Australia by the overland route that included passing through a number of countries in which malaria was endemic. This is an indication of how long the incubation period for malaria can be.

Complications of malaria

The major complications of malaria occur in *P. falciparum* infections. The two most serious of these are renal failure (the so-called blackwater fever) and cerebral malaria. Both of these can cause death if untreated.

Blackwater fever

Case 9.8

A male, aged 25, was transferred from the Solomon Islands (a nation in Melanesia, east of Papua New Guinea) to a hospital in Brisbane, Australia, suffering from blackwater fever (so called because the malaria attack is accompanied by the passing of black colored urine) and severe oliguria. The effects of this are seen in Figure 9.48.

Figure 9.49, overleaf, shows plasma from this patient compared with normal plasma.

His renal shutdown was treated medically without dialysis and he was given treatment for his *P. falciparum* malaria. He recovered and was repatriated.

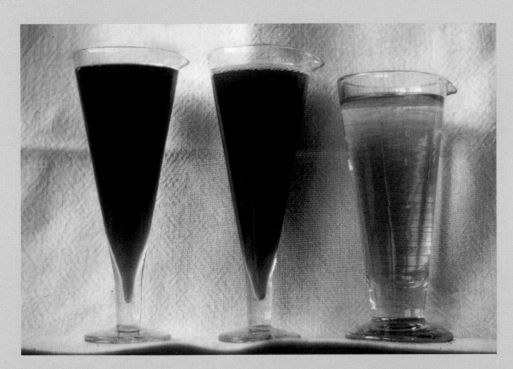

▲ **Fig. 9.48** Renal failure. Urine of the patient with blackwater fever. From left to right, note that the color lightens as his condition improved. The black color resulted from hemoglobinuria.

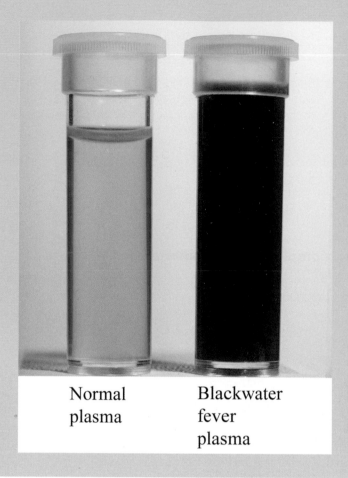

| Normal plasma | Blackwater fever plasma |

▶ **Fig. 9.49** Plasma from the patient in Figure 9.48 *(right)* compared with normal plasma *(left)*. The plasma is also black from the breakdown of hemoglobin. Any patient with acute malaria produces laboratory detectable red cell breakdown products in the blood. These are usually insignificant and cause no change in the color of the plasma.

Cerebral malaria

Cerebral malaria can present in a number of different ways—fever going on to drowsiness and coma—or it may mimic a range of neurological conditions, such as acute psychosis, fitting or abnormal behavior.

These symptoms can progress quite quickly to coma and death. Very often, the post-mortem examination of the brain shows no macroscopic abnormality. The classical abnormality, however, is the presence of multiple petechial hemorrhages throughout the white matter (shown in Fig. 9.50).

Microscopic examination of the areas of petechial hemorrhages shows the presence of capillary thrombosis with rupture of the vessel walls and escape of blood into the surrounding brain substance (see Fig. 9.51, overleaf). The capillaries throughout the brain show brown malarial pigment in the red blood cells, and very occasionally one sees ring forms of the parasite (trophozoites) in the red blood cells in the capillaries (shown in Fig. 9.52, overleaf).

The exact mechanism of cerebral malaria is still not known.

Case 9.9

A 60-year-old Australian male had spent some years working in Papua New Guinea and was about to return to Australia permanently. As was the usual custom, he attended many farewell parties for a few weeks before the day of his departure. As a result, he arrived in Australia in an intoxicated state. He remained in this state for a few days after his arrival in Australia when his neighbors called the police because he was making too much noise. The police officer thought he looked sick and took him to a Brisbane hospital for examination.

The emergency staff were uncertain of his diagnosis and it was not until some hours after admission that a diagnosis of cerebral malaria was made. By this time he was comatose and he died before treatment became effective.

A post-mortem examination was carried out. The pathologic features of his brain are demonstrated in Figures 9.50, 9.51 and 9.52, continued overleaf.

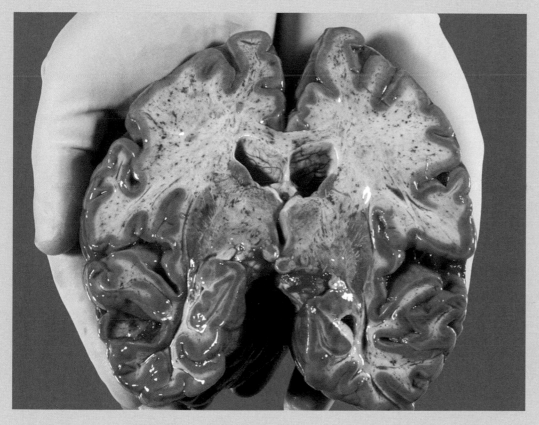

▲ **Fig. 9.50** Cerebral malaria. Slice of the brain from a 60-year-old Australian man, showing multiple petechial hemorrhages throughout the white matter.

This patient had been taking antimalarial prophylaxis but he was lulled into not being as careful as usual by the imminent approach of his retirement and, later, by the effect of the alcohol he had consumed. This resulted in his getting malaria without his noticing it.

The signs of cerebral malaria can be extremely diverse. So, every doctor should be sure to think of malaria and to exclude this in any patient who has recently been residing in or visiting a malarial country, especially when they have any type of neurological symptoms.

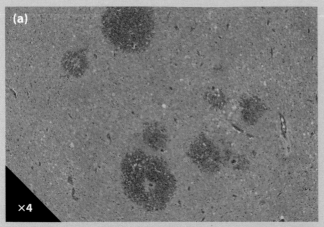

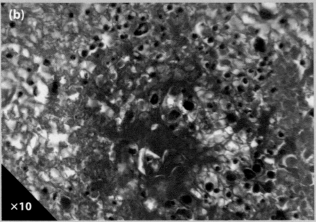

One of the most bizarre psychotic presentations of cerebral malaria seen by the author was a young man admitted to the psychiatric ward of a hospital in Brisbane, Australia.

This man had been acting strangely and he telephoned the police to report that he was being attacked by large cockroaches, and being threatened by some local thugs. The police officers, thinking he might be sick and possibly 'high' on drugs, delivered him to the hospital.

One of the tests on admission to the ward was a blood count, in which ring forms and schizonts of P. falciparum were identified. The author went to see him and found the ward staff trying to do a lumbar puncture test on a wildly resisting patient.

The presence of schizonts of P. falciparum in the peripheral blood is usually a sign of a medical emergency, with death being fairly imminent. The author suggested that they give the patient some intravenous quinine instead. They did this and 2 days later the patient's temperature was down (and the cockroaches and the thugs were leaving him alone). He made a full recovery. Tests for abnormal levels of drugs were negative.

▲ **Fig. 9.51(a) and (b)** Microscopic section from an area of petechial hemorrhages showing thrombosis of blood vessels, damage to the capillary walls and escape of blood into the surrounding brain substance.

▼ **Fig. 9.52** The red blood cells in this brain capillary contain ring forms (trophozoites) of *P. falciparum*. It is unusual to be able to see malarial parasites as clearly as this in capillaries in the brain.

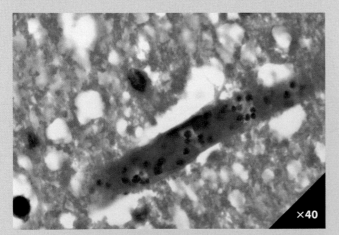

Other complications of malaria

Splenomegaly

Splenic enlargement occurs during all acute attacks of malaria. When the attack subsides, the spleen returns to normal size. In some people living in areas of high malarial endemicity, the spleen remains enlarged and the enlarged spleen is exposed to being ruptured from trauma to the abdomen.

The doctors working in remote areas of Papua New Guinea in the 1950s and 1960s, frequently had to deal with ruptured spleens, particularly during football matches in the newly established schools. A solo doctor would be confronted with the prospect of doing one or more splenectomies independently, with the assistance of variably qualified nursing staff, because it would not be possible to transfer a patient to a hospital that had a surgeon. The doctor would have to arrange for blood donors to be bled, start the anesthetic, perform the operation and then complete the anesthetic.

Tropical splenomegaly (big spleen disease)

In a small percentage of people in an area of endemic malaria, the spleen becomes very large indeed. Such a big spleen is demonstrated in the young woman shown in Figure 9.41 on page 308.

People with spleens of this size develop the syndrome of tropical splenomegaly, in which they suffer from a chronic anemia with very low hemoglobin values and pancytopenia. The anemia is not improved by antimalarial treatment nor by giving hematinics nor by splenectomy.

Malaria during pregnancy

An acute attack of malaria may cause spontaneous abortion. Very occasionally, the parasite may cross the placenta, resulting in malaria in the newborn baby. *P. vivax* is more likely to cause this problem than the other species.

In Brisbane, Australia, a few cases of neonatal jaundice from *P. vivax* infection in the mother have presented between the years 1968 and 2007. Usually, the mother has been living in a malarial area and then returns home for the delivery of the baby. The baby is jaundiced at birth. The cause of the neonatal jaundice is diagnosed when malarial parasites are seen in the baby's blood.

Case 9.10

A 20-year-old woman delivered a baby in Calcutta, India. She became febrile on the day of delivery. A touch preparation was made from the placenta and a histologic section was made of the placenta (see Figs 9.53 and 9.54). She was treated for the malaria and made an uneventful recovery. The baby was quite unaffected.

▼ **Fig. 9.53** Touch preparation from the placenta showing ring forms (trophozoltes) (A) and schizonts (B) of *P. falciparum*.

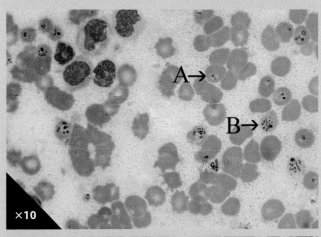

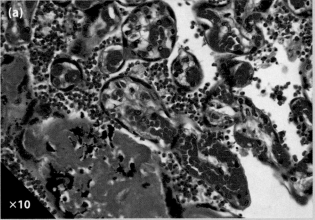

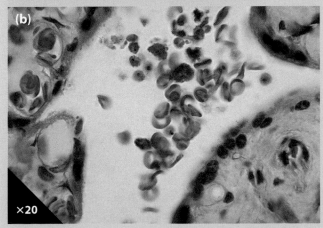

▲ **Fig. 9.54(a) and (b)** Views of the placenta showing 'dots' in the red blood cells in the maternal blood in the intervillous spaces. These are malarial pigment and ring forms of *P. falciparum*.

Case 9.11

A 56-year-old man was referred to a hospital in Brisbane, Australia, from Papua New Guinea because he had developed disseminated purpura, hematuria and oral, nasal and rectal bleeding. Figures 9.55 and 9.56 demonstrate his condition.

He had been febrile for a few days. He was not taking any antimalarial prophylactic drugs. Ring forms of *P. falciparum* were present in his blood. He had a mild pancytopenia with markedly reduced platelets.

He was treated for his malaria. His bleeding stopped after about 24 hours, and all his symptoms subsided within a few days.

◀ **Fig. 9.55(a) and (b)** A 56-year-old man with disseminated purpura from thrombocytopenia due to an acute attack of *P. falciparum* malaria.

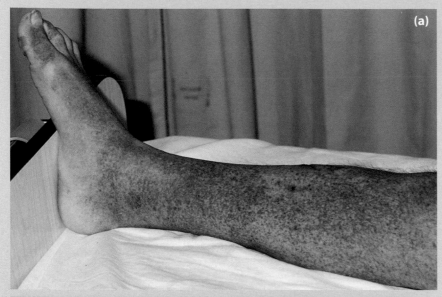

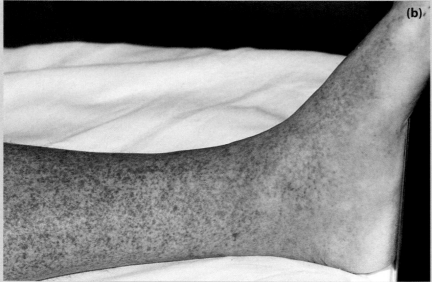

▼ **Fig. 9.56** Purpura developed at the venipuncture site in this man's antecubital fossa.

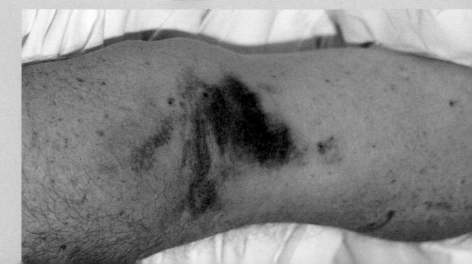

Species diagnosis of malaria

The diagnosis of malaria is confirmed by finding the parasites in the peripheral blood. It is important to be able to identify the species correctly because *P. falciparum* is now resistant to virtually all of the drugs currently available for treatment.

There are numerous charts available that list a myriad of features, which allow one to identify accurately the species of malaria. However, for practical laboratory diagnosis, an exact species can be identified in most cases by taking into account the features illustrated in Figures 9.57–9.74, see pages 317–321.

Features to be considered in making a species diagnosis of malaria

Red blood cell size and shape

- *P. falciparum*—the parasitized red blood cells are the same size and shape as the nonparasitized cells.
- *P. vivax*—the parasitized red blood cells are larger than the nonparasitized ones.
- *P. malariae*—the parasitized red blood cells are not enlarged and are the same size as the nonparasitized ones.
- *P. ovale*—the parasitized red blood cells are enlarged and most of them are oval in shape.

Parasite size and shape

- *P. falciparum*—the trophozoites are all small rings, with a red-staining nuclear dot and a small amount of blue-staining cytoplasm.
- *P. vivax*—the trophozoite may be in a ring form, with a nuclear dot and a crescent of cytoplasm or it may be much larger and have an irregular contour (an ameboid form).
- *P. malariae*—the trophozoite has a large, round nucleus and a solid, blue cytoplasm. Very frequently, this cytoplasm adopts a shape which looks like a thick band across the red blood cell. *P. malariae* has a well-defined blob of brown malarial pigment in the red blood cell.
- *P. ovale*—the trophozoite is large with a large nucleus and abundant irregularly distributed cytoplasm.

Schizonts

- *P. falciparum*—schizonts are present in the peripheral blood only in the preterminal phase of the infection. The schizonts contain 12–24 merozoites (nuclear dots). The red blood cell containing the schizont is not enlarged.
- *P. vivax*—contains 12–24 merozoites and the infected red blood cell is enlarged.
- *P. malariae*—the schizont contains 8–12 merozoites. The infected red blood cell is not enlarged.
- *P. ovale*—the schizont contains 12–24 merozoites. The infected red blood cell is enlarged and is an oval shape.

Gametocytes

- The gametocytes of *P. falciparum* are crescent shaped.
- Gametocytes of *P. vivax*, *P. malariae* and *P. ovale* are round with a large, eccentric nucleus at the edge.

- Gametocytes are about the same size as the schizont for the particular species.
- The size and shape of the infected red blood cells is the same as for the other stages of the parasite.

Most laboratories stain both a thick film and a thin film for identification of malarial parasites. The advantage of the thick film is that it concentrates the parasites about fiftyfold. This is particularly important if there is a light infection, when one would have to spend a large amount of time searching through a thin blood film to find only one or two parasites.

It usually takes about 8 days from the beginning of the first fever until gametocytes appear in the peripheral blood.

These features are illustrated in the following figures

Figures 9.57–9.63: *P. falciparum*, continued overleaf.
Figures 9.64–9.68: *P. vivax*, overleaf.
Figures 9.69–9.72: *P. malariae*, see page 320.
Figures 9.73 and 9.74: *P. ovale*, see page 321.

P. falciparum

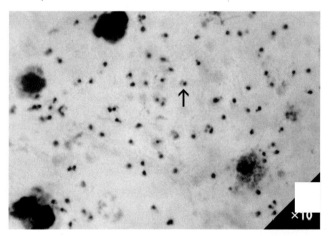

▲ **Fig. 9.57** Thick blood film from a fairly heavy infection of *P. falciparum*. Numerous ring forms (trophozoites) can be seen.

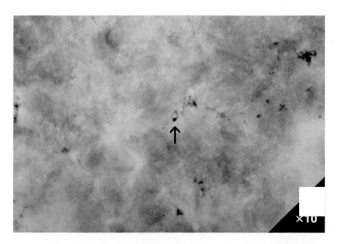

▲ **Fig. 9.58** A very occasional ring form of *P. falciparum* in a thick film. It was very difficult to find any parasites at all in the thin film from this patient.

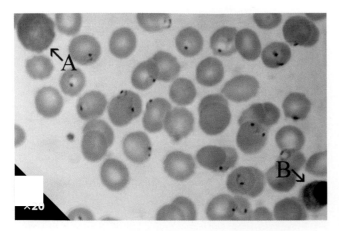

▲ **Fig. 9.59** Thin blood film from a patient with a heavy infection of *P. falciparum*. Malaria causes a hemolytic anemia. The blood film shows the presence of hemolysis, with a polychromatic red cell (A) in the top left corner and a nucleated red cell (B) in the bottom right corner. This is *P. falciparum* because the red cells are all about the same size and shape, and the parasites are all small rings.

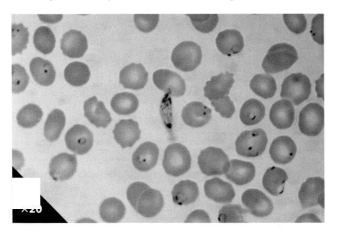

▲ **Fig. 9.60** Another field from the smear shown in Figure 9.59. This shows the presence of a characteristic crescent-shaped gametocyte of *P. falciparum*. It usually takes about 8 days from the beginning of the first fever until gametocytes appear in the peripheral blood, so this patient would have had his fever for at least 1 week.

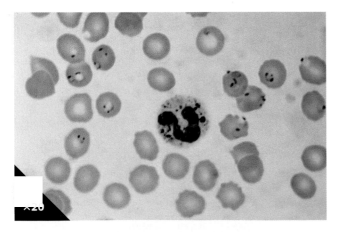

▲ **Fig. 9.61** *P. falciparum*. This is another field from the smear shown in Figure 9.59. It shows a neutrophil with malarial pigment in the cytoplasm.

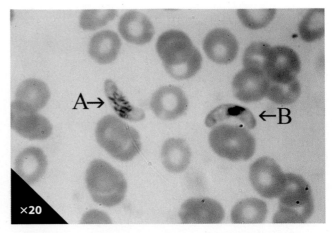

▲ **Fig. 9.62** Blood film from a patient with an infection of *P. falciparum*. In this field, there is a female gametocyte of *P. falciparum* on the left (A) and a male on the right (B). The nuclear material in the female is more diffuse than in the male. The gametocyte stage of the parasite is what develops into the next stage of the cycle (the oocytes) in the body of the mosquito. The male gametocyte undergoes exflagellation and each of the 'sperms' can then fertilize a female gametocyte.

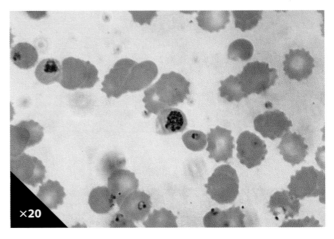

▲ **Fig. 9.63** Thin film of *P. falciparum* infection. It shows a schizont, which contains about sixteen or eighteen merozoites together with some pigment. This patient would have died within a few hours if treatment had not been started at once.

P. vivax

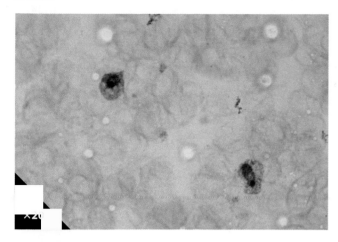

▲ **Fig. 9.64** Thick film of *P. vivax* showing two large ring forms.

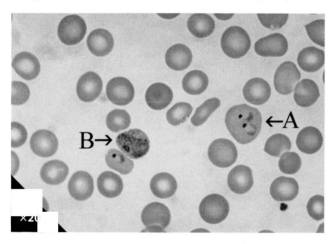

▲ **Fig. 9.65** Thin blood film which shows trophozoites (A) and a gametocyte of *P. vivax* (B). The parasitized red blood cells are larger than their neighbors. The trophozoites are large ring forms. The gametocyte is round and has a single, red nuclear dot.

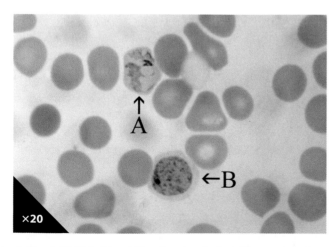

▲ **Fig. 9.66** Thin blood film showing *P. vivax*. The trophozoite (A) is an ameboid form. The lower parasite is a gametocyte (B). Both parasites are in red blood cells which are enlarged.

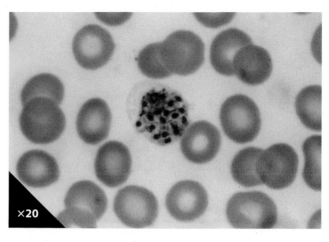

▲ **Fig. 9.67** Schizont of *P. vivax*. The red blood cell is enlarged and there are eighteen merozoites in the schizont.

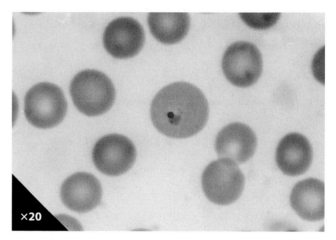

▲ **Fig. 9.68** Small ring form of *P. vivax*. This appearance presents one of the diagnostic problems in the species identification of malaria. The trophozoite is only marginally larger than the trophozoite of *P. falciparum* but it is *P. vivax* because the infected red blood cell is enlarged. In such cases, one usually finds more characteristic trophozoites of *P. vivax* in other areas of the smear.

P. malariae

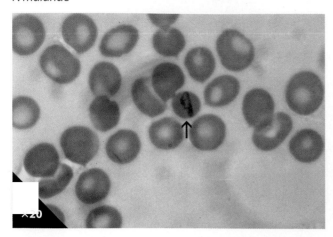

▲ **Fig. 9.69** Blood film from a patient with *P. malariae* infection. The infected red blood cell is not enlarged. The trophozoite is large and is forming a band across the middle of the red blood cell.

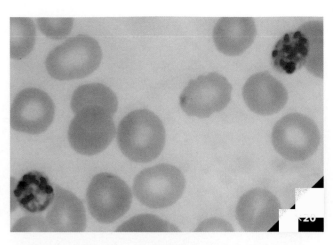

▲ **Fig. 9.71** Blood film showing two schizonts of *P. malariae*. The red blood cells are not enlarged. The schizont has eight merozoites and each schizont has a large blob of pigment within it.

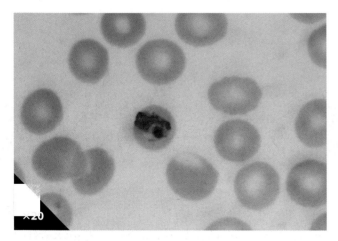

▲ **Fig. 9.70** Blood film from a patient with *P. malariae* infection. The red blood cell is not enlarged. The trophozoite is in a band form and there is a large blob of pigment associated with the parasite. This prominent malarial pigment is a feature of *P. malariae*.

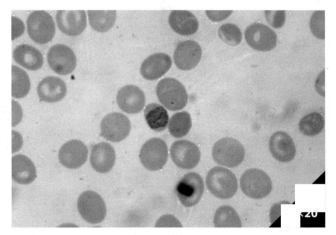

▲ **Fig. 9.72** Gametocyte of *P. malariae*. The red blood cell is not enlarged, the gametocyte is round and there is a single nucleus at one margin.

P. ovale

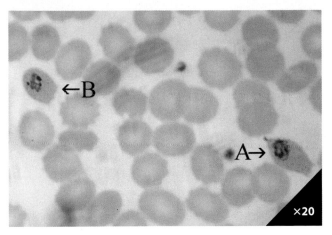

▲ **Fig. 9.73** Blood film which shows *P. ovale* parasites. The red blood cells are enlarged and their shape is changed. One is a definite oval shape and the other is flattened on one edge. The trophozoites are large and ameboid in form.

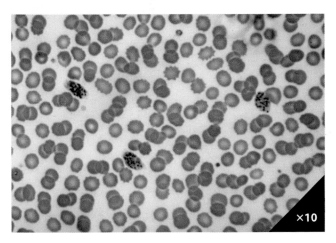

▲ **Fig. 9.74** Blood smear which shows three schizonts of *P. ovale*. The red blood cells are enlarged and an oval shape. Each schizont contains approximately eighteen merozoites.

Malaria as a lethal epidemic disease

Case 9.12

In 1980, the elders in a remote village in the high mountains of Papua New Guinea (PNG) decided they would like to be able to access the perceived benefits of being part of the development occurring elsewhere in PNG. So, a road was built to connect with the road system of the rest of the country (see Fig. 9.75).

There was a population of about 700 in the village and its surrounding area. The road allowed motor vehicles to reach the village, but an undesirable consequence of this was that along with the road came Anopheline mosquitoes infected with malaria parasites.

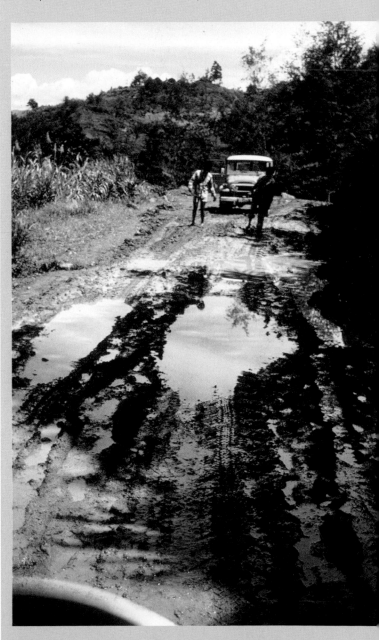

▲ **Fig. 9.75** In 1980, a village in the high mountains of Papua New Guinea became linked to the road system of the rest of the country.

In this part of the country, it rained heavily almost every day and the mosquitoes bred in the puddles of water along the unsealed road (shown in Fig. 9.76). The road came right to the doors of the village houses (see Fig. 9.77). In the vicinity of the houses, there were depressions in the ground made by the motor vehicles, the footprints of the people and the pigs that roam and forage in the village (see Fig. 9.78). These water-filled depressions became small puddles, where mosquitoes could breed. The collections of water were soon teeming with mosquito larvae.

Within a few weeks of the completion of the road, this community that was not immune to malaria developed an epidemic of *P. falciparum* malaria. A victim of the epidemic appears in Figure 9.79, overleaf. There were about 100 deaths before a health team was alerted and came to the rescue. The village elders then decided to allow the road to return to jungle (illustrated in Fig. 9.80, overleaf).

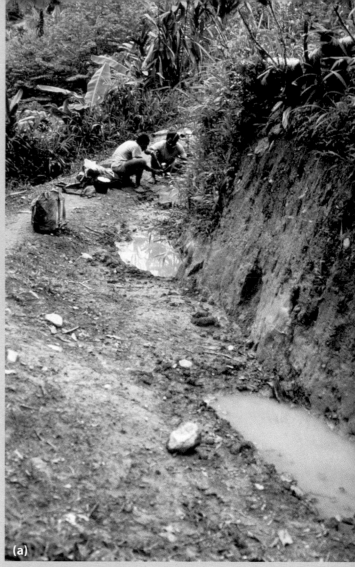
(a)

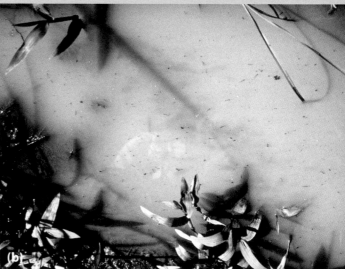
(b)

▲ **Fig. 9.76(a)** Motor vehicles made tracks in the road, which became filled with water. **(b)** Mosquitoes laid eggs in the water and the puddles were soon teeming with mosquito larvae.

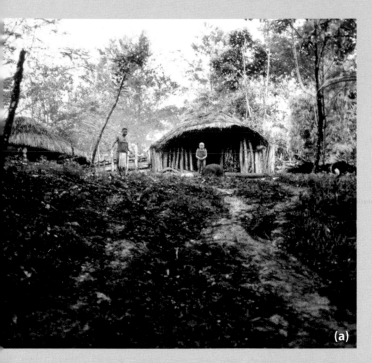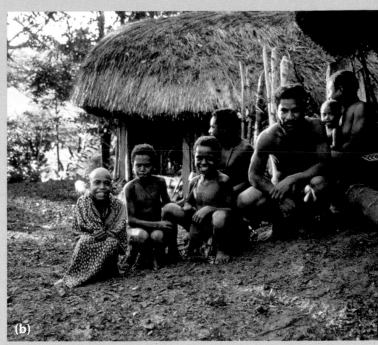

▲ **Fig. 9.77(a) and (b)** The road and the mosquitoes went right to the doors of the village houses.

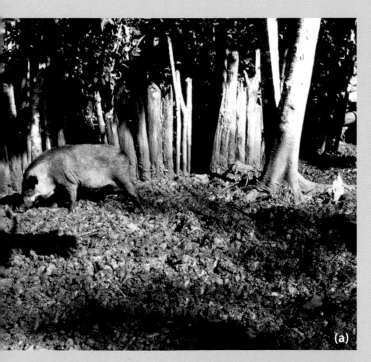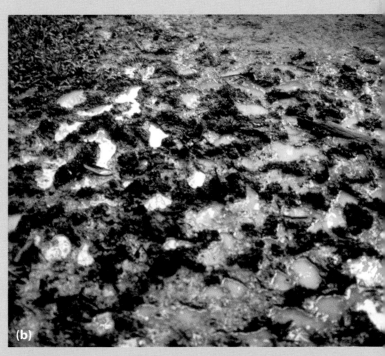

▲ **Fig. 9.78(a) and (b)** In the village, footprints of the people and the pigs created more puddles of water. These, too, became filled with mosquito larvae.

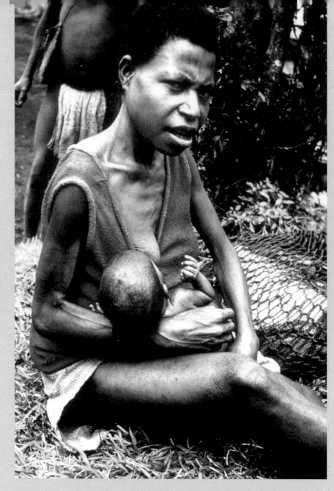

This episode underlines the killing power of epidemic malaria, and why it is such an important global disease.
Malaria can be confusing and sometimes difficult to diagnose because it presents in many different clinical manifestations. On the other hand, as illustrated by Case 9.13, the treating doctor may be tricked by another disease that mimics malaria in its clinical presentation.

▲ **Fig. 9.79** This emaciated woman died of malaria the day after this photograph was taken. Her child died, too, because it was frail and there was no one to care for it.

▼ **Fig. 9.80(a) and (b)** Village elders decided to allow the jungle to grow over the road, but the damage was already done.

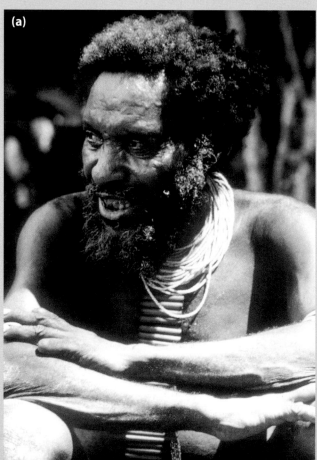

(a)

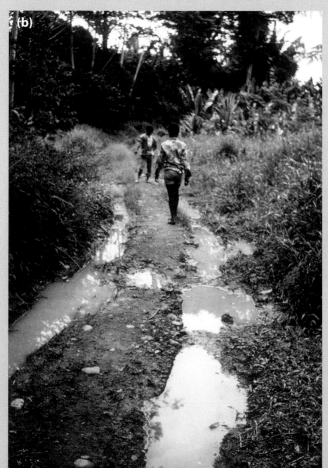

(b)

Case 9.13

A 21-year-old Australian woman returned to Brisbane from a holiday in a neighboring country where malaria is endemic. She presented with intermittent fever that appeared to have a cyclical pattern, heavy sweating and splenomegaly.

The first diagnosis to be considered was malaria. The peripheral blood film (see Fig. 9.81), however, showed a very high white cell count at 140 000 per cubic mm and numerous blast cells with the features of acute myeloblastic leukemia. There were no malaria parasites seen.

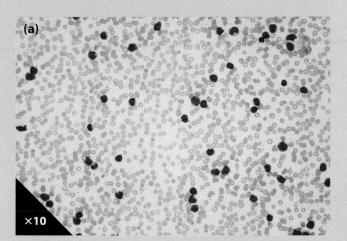 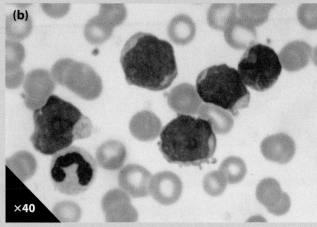

▲ **Fig. 9.81(a) and (b)** Views of the blood film from a 21-year-old woman recently returned from a holiday in a malaria endemic country, who presented with symptoms suggestive of malaria. It shows an elevated white cell count with a high percentage of blast cells consistent with a diagnosis of acute myeloblastic leukemia.

Malaria control and prospects for the twenty-first century

By the beginning of the twentieth century quite a lot was known about malaria. The causative organism had been identified. It had been shown that the parasite was transmitted from person to person by mosquitoes of the genus Anopheles. The breeding habits of these mosquitoes had been studied, and their numbers could be reduced by destroying their breeding grounds by drainage of swampy areas and areas of stagnant water.

In the middle of the twentieth century, insecticides (such as dichloro-diphenyl-trichloro-ethane (DDT)) were developed and shown to be effective in killing the adult mosquitoes and controlling the larval forms by spraying the insecticide on the waters of the breeding areas.

Biological control of mosquito larvae was attempted.

New chemotherapeutic agents were introduced to treat malaria. These were highly effective in killing the parasites in humans. By taking small doses of these drugs prophylactically, infection could be prevented.

From the late 1960s, this situation began to change. Mosquitoes became resistant to DDT. The complications of spraying with insecticide became apparent. The malarial parasites began to develop resistance to the chemotherapeutic agents. Governments were not able to spend the necessary amounts of money required to maintain malaria control programs.

At the beginning of the twentieth century, there was great optimism that malaria could be eradicated from the world. Certainly, there was a short time in evolutionary history when humans were able to live and work in malarial areas without succumbing to the disease. At the end of the twentieth century, the dream of malaria eradication remained unattained.

In the twenty-first century, new measures will need to be developed to control mosquito breeding. New drugs will need to be found. Much research has been centered on the attempt to develop a vaccine for malaria. The effectiveness of the various types of vaccine will need to be tested in the twenty-first century.

The twentieth century has been an exciting time for those involved in the understanding and treatment of malaria in all its aspects. The twenty-first century promises to be equally challenging and exciting.

Toxoplasmosis

Toxoplasmosis is a disease caused by the protozoan parasite *Toxoplasma gondii* (shown in Fig. 9.82), which occurs world-wide. Cats were thought to be the definitive hosts and they show no signs of infection (see Life cycle 9.5).

The organisms are present in the small intestine, where the oocysts are formed. These are excreted in feces and contaminate the environment, where they are ingested by a wide range of warm-blooded animals, including humans (see Fig. 9.83).

In these hosts, oocysts are found in tissues. It used to be thought that the main source of infection for humans was the ingestion of oocysts passed in the feces of domestic cats, but studies reported in 2000 showed that a wide range of mammalian hosts carried oocysts of toxoplasmosis. Eating raw or undercooked game meat may also lead to infection.

Toxoplasmosis

Domestic cats are reservoir hosts. They pass oocysts in their feces. Oocysts contaminate the environment, e.g. sand pits where children play and children become infected by hand-to-mouth contamination.

Some marsupials are also reservoir hosts, e.g. eating undercooked kangaroo meat in Australia has caused infections.

▲ **Life cycle 9.5** Toxoplasmosis.

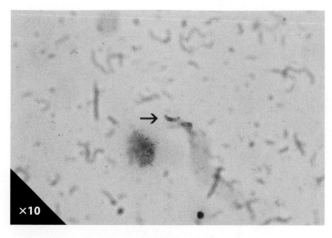

×10

▲ **Fig. 9.82** Individual crescentic toxoplasma organisms grown in culture in peritoneal fluid of a laboratory mouse. Tissue culture and polymerase chain reaction (PCR) tests can also be used in diagnosis.

▼ **Fig. 9.83** Young boy playing in a sand pit. Cats like to defecate in these sand pits and children may be infected with toxoplasma cysts by hand-to-mouth contamination.

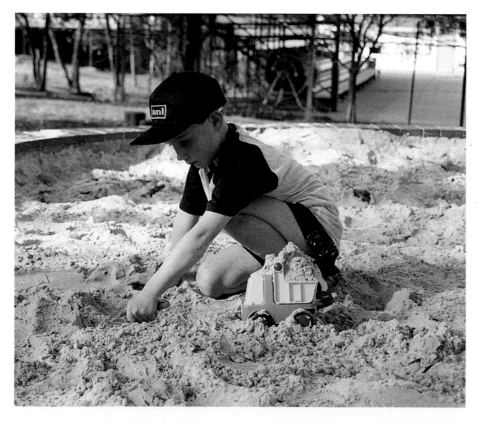

Clinicopathologic entities in toxoplasmosis

A number of clinicopathologic entities are recognized in toxoplasmosis, namely lymphadenopathy, neonatal toxoplasmosis, neonatal encephalitis and toxoplasmosis in immune-suppressed patients.

Lymphadenopathy

The most common presentation is with lymphadenopathy, particularly cervical lymphadenopathy. This may be an isolated finding or may be associated with a febrile illness. The lymph node is excised for diagnosis and to exclude more serious pathology. The histologic appearances in lymph nodes are illustrated in Figure 9.84.

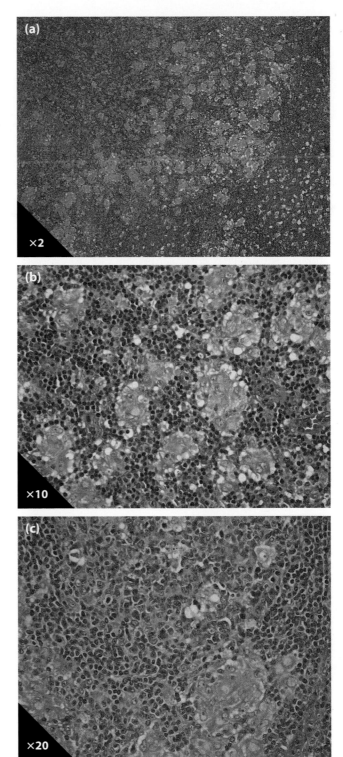

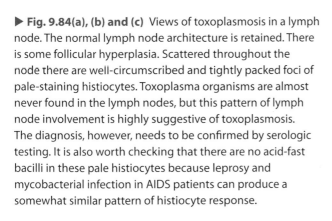

▶ **Fig. 9.84(a), (b) and (c)** Views of toxoplasmosis in a lymph node. The normal lymph node architecture is retained. There is some follicular hyperplasia. Scattered throughout the node there are well-circumscribed and tightly packed foci of pale-staining histiocytes. Toxoplasma organisms are almost never found in the lymph nodes, but this pattern of lymph node involvement is highly suggestive of toxoplasmosis. The diagnosis, however, needs to be confirmed by serologic testing. It is also worth checking that there are no acid-fast bacilli in these pale histiocytes because leprosy and mycobacterial infection in AIDS patients can produce a somewhat similar pattern of histiocyte response.

Neonatal toxoplasmosis

The most serious infection with toxoplasma occurs when a pregnant woman becomes infected. The organism crosses the placenta and infects the fetus. The baby may then be born with chorioretinitis and/or encephalitis. This results in considerable morbidity and, often, mortality.

A small outbreak of neonatal toxoplasmosis in Brisbane, Australia, was traced to some gourmet kangaroo meat that the mothers of the infected infants had eaten at the same restaurant. The kangaroo is one of the many Australian native animals that harbor toxoplasma organisms (see Fig. 9.85).

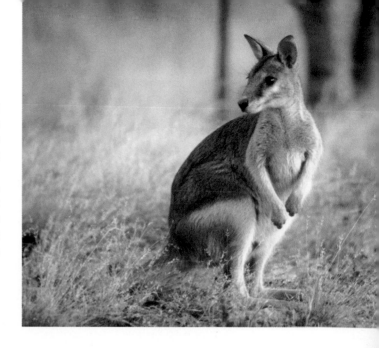

▶ **Fig. 9.85** Kangaroo. One of the many Australian native animals that harbor toxoplasma organisms.

Case 9.14

A 1-year-old female died from encephalitis and chorioretinitis. The clinical and pathologic features of this case are illustrated in Figures 9.86–9.90.

▼ **Fig. 9.86** Ophthalmoscopic appearance of a 1-year-old female, who had congenital toxoplasmosis. There is a black area lateral to the optic disc. This is consistent with an area of necrosis and calcification.

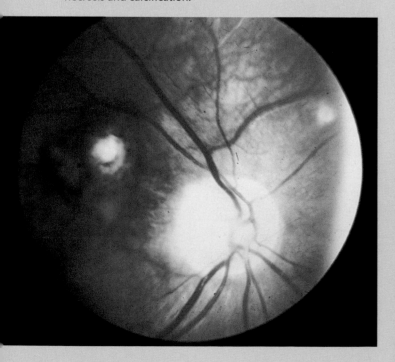

▼ **Fig. 9.87** Post-mortem examination of the eye showed the macroscopic appearance of chorioretinitis. The area of necrosis and calcification corresponds with that seen through the ophthalmoscope.

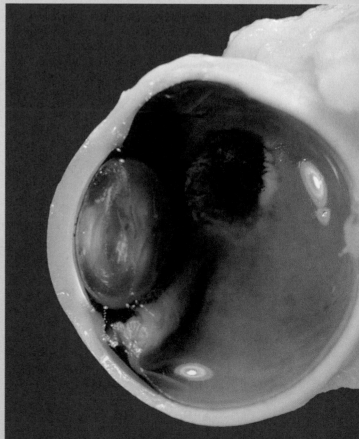

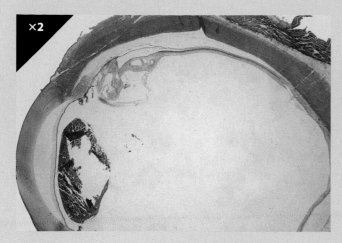

▲ **Fig. 9.88** View of a section of the child's eye. Towards the top right of the section, there is a gap in the retina.

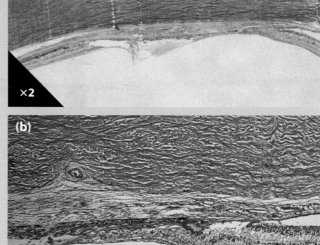

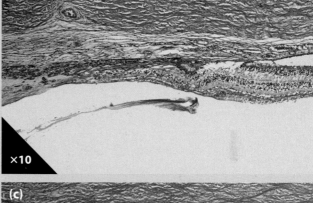

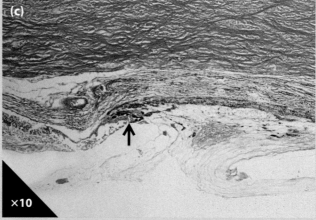

▶ **Fig. 9.89(a), (b) and (c)** Gap in the retina demonstrated more clearly at higher magnification. Adjacent to the area of retinal necrosis, the retina shows marked edema. The area of retinal necrosis shows the presence of a moderate amount of calcification (*see arrow*).

▶ **Fig. 9.90** Higher magnification view of the edge of the necrotic retina shows a focus of chronic inflammation with a probable cyst in the middle.

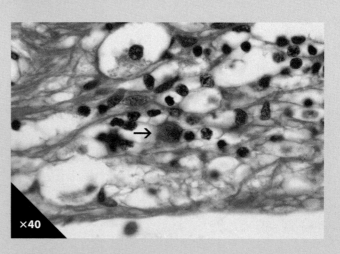

Neonatal encephalitis

Case 9.15

A 7-week-old female was referred for investigation of hydrocephalus. A magnetic resonance imaging (MRI) scan showed the hydrocephalus and there was some calcification in the right eye (see Fig. 9.91). This was suggestive of the presence of toxoplasmosis. Soon after referral, the child died.

Examination of the brain at post mortem confirmed the hydrocephalus. The cortex was very thin and the brain cut with a gritty sensation suggesting the presence of calcification in the hemispheres.

The gross appearances in the brain are illustrated in Figures 9.92 and 9.93.

The microscopic changes are illustrated in Figures 9.94–9.97, continued overleaf. The right eye showed changes similar to those demonstrated in Case 9.14 (see pages 328 and 329).

▶ **Fig. 9.91** MRI scan of the brain in a 7-week-old female showed hydrocephalus and some calcification in the right eye. These features are suggestive of toxoplasmosis.

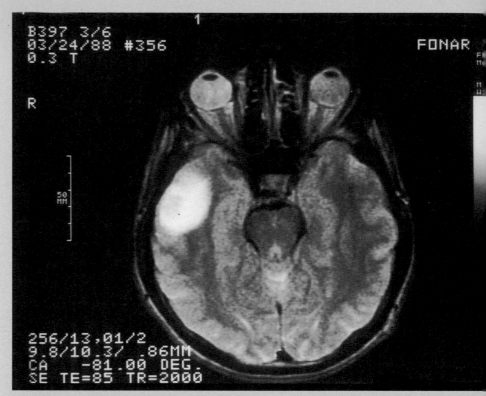

▶ **Fig. 9.92** Surface of the brain showed areas of depression, which corresponded with areas of cortical necrosis when the brain was sliced.

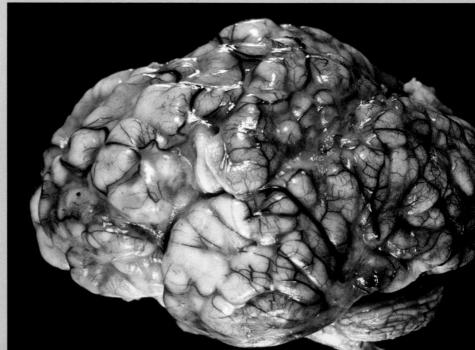

► **Fig. 9.93(a) and (b)** Slices through the brain showed gross hydrocephalus with marked thinning of the cerebral cortex in some areas. As the brain was being cut, there was a slightly gritty sensation, which corresponded with calcification in the thinned cortex. Calcification lining the dilated ventricles can often be seen in X-rays of children with neonatal toxoplasma encephalitis.

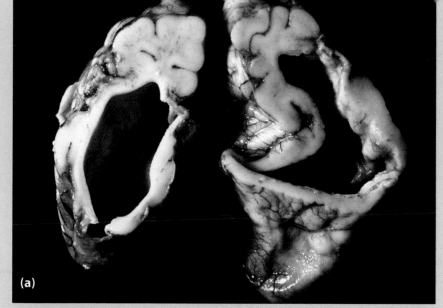

(a)

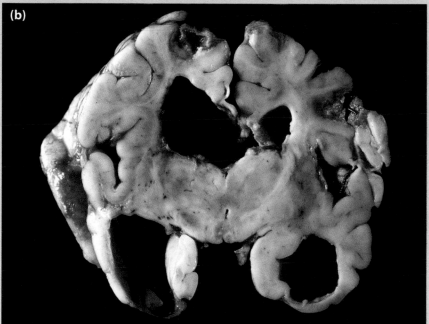

(b)

▼ **Fig. 9.94** View of a slice of the whole brain of a neonate who died of toxoplasmosis. There is generalized hydrocephalus with dilatation of the complete ventricular system. The mid brain portion of the brain (*see arrows*) shows calcification, hemorrhage, necrosis and inflammation. (The brain is stained with a von Kossa stain that stains calcium black.)

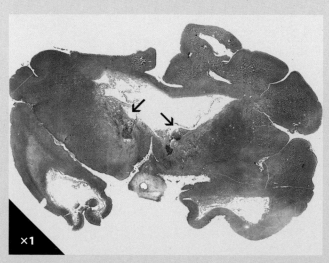

×1

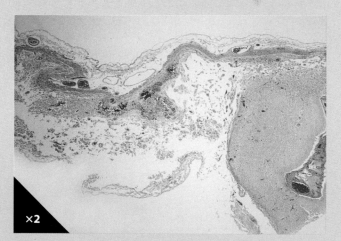

×2

▲ **Fig. 9.95** View through a thin area of the cerebral cortex of the brain examined in Figure 9.94. The brain substance has been almost completely lost and there is a large amount of calcification in the remaining cortical tissue. This is associated with a mild chronic inflammatory cell infiltration.

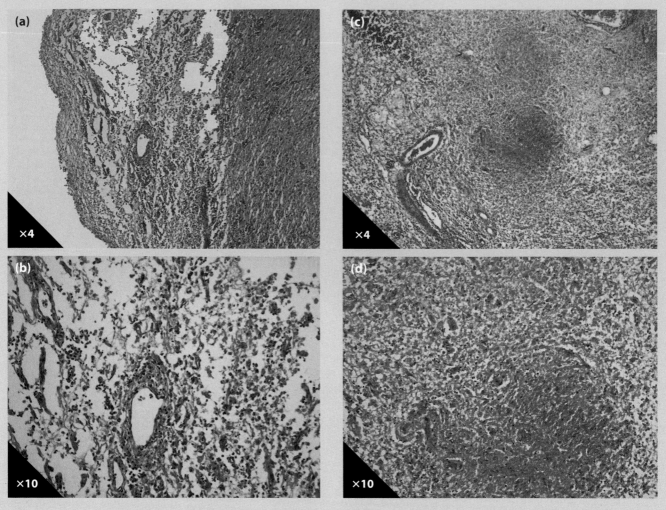

▲ **Fig. 9.96(a), (b), (c) and (d)** Views of the areas of hemorrhage and necrosis of the brain.

▶ **Fig. 9.97** View of the mononuclear inflammatory cell reaction associated with the areas of hemorrhage and necrosis. Occasional cysts of toxoplasma can be found in these areas (*see arrow*).

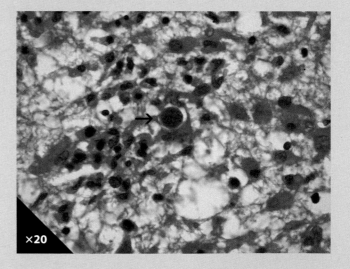

Toxoplasmosis in immune-suppressed patients

Toxoplasma encephalitis and toxoplasma myocarditis (see Fig. 9.98) are well-recognized opportunistic infections in immune-suppressed patients, particularly in relation to AIDS and chemotherapy for cancer. The toxoplasma encephalitis has the usual appearance of an encephalitis from any cause, that is focal areas of necrosis of cerebral tissue associated with a mononuclear inflammatory cell infiltrate. Toxoplasma cysts are found in the brain (indicated in Fig 9.97).

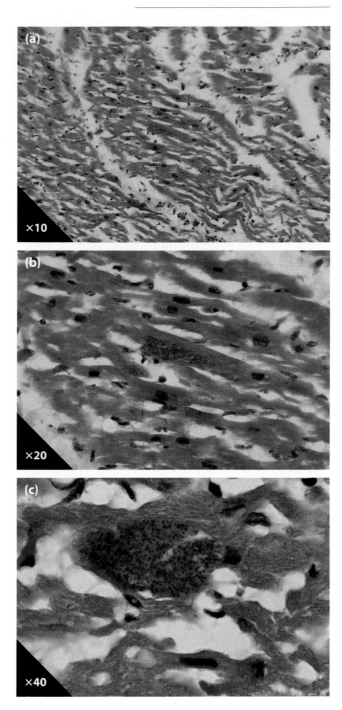

▲ **Fig. 9.98(a), (b) and (c)** Views of the heart of a middle-aged male who died from AIDS. The toxoplasma cyst is expanding the myocardial muscle fiber. In this case, there is no inflammatory reaction associated with the cyst.

Amebiasis

Amebiasis is an infection with the protozoan parasite *Entameba histolytica*. The human is the only host (see Life cycle 9.6). Cysts are passed in the feces. These contaminate fingers and/or food. The ingested cysts germinate in the small intestine to release trophozoites, which invade the mucosal surface of the colon causing blood-stained diarrhea—amebic dysentery. The organism occurs in every country of the world, particularly in communities in which sanitation is poor.

Amebic dysentery

Amebic dysentery presents as diarrhea with mucus and blood in the stool. The diagnosis is made by identifying trophozoites

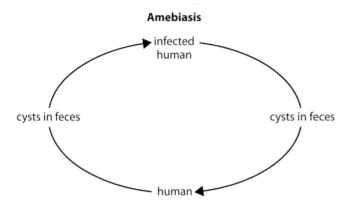

Amebiasis

Trophozoites invade tissues and produce cysts in the gut.

▲ **Life cycle 9.6** Amebiasis.

of *E. histolytica* in the diarrheal stool. The traditional method for doing this is by the examination of freshly passed feces. A blood-stained area of feces should be selected and mixed with warm saline on a warmed glass slide. It is then examined on a warm microscope stage. The slowly motile trophozoites can be seen. Pseudopods project from the organism and the cytoplasm flows into them.

The problems with this method of diagnosis are that the feces must be kept warm from the time it is passed; the examination must be done on a warmed microscope stage; and the microscopist must be experienced in identifying the organism. Even in a sophisticated laboratory, it is not easy to have all of these things available 'at call'.

A more practical method of diagnosis is by a histopathologic examination of tissue biopsied from a colonic ulcer. The tissue and exudate from the surface of the ulcer should be placed in a biopsy specimen jar containing 10 per cent formalin. It is always important to collect as much exudate as possible because this is where the amebas will be found. A routine hematoxylin and eosin (H&E) stain is perfectly adequate for identifying amebas.

E. histolytica trophozoites are slightly larger than macrophages and their nuclei have a centrally placed karyosome, with uniformly distributed peripheral chromatin. Ingested red blood cells are present in their cytoplasm. In an examination of feces, it is important to distinguish pathogenic *E. histolytica* from nonpathogenic amebas such as *E. dispar*—which is identical in appearance but does not show erythrophagocytosis. The two Entamebas can be distinguished on an enzyme-linked immune sorbent assay (ELISA) test.

Case 9.16

A 25-year-old female returned to Brisbane, Australia, after a month-long holiday in Nepal. She developed a blood-stained diarrhea (see Figs 9.99 and 9.100), which she allowed to continue for about 12 months before she sought medical assistance.

The reason this patient allowed her diarrhea to continue for 12 months without seeking medical advice was that she was living an 'alternative lifestyle' and she thought it beneficial for her body that she should be 'purging it' in this manner.

She was thin but not emaciated and she was afebrile. She had no other medical complaints apart from the diarrhea. Sigmoidoscopy showed the presence of mucosal ulcers with normal mucosa between the ulcers (see Fig. 9.101).

Rectal biopsy showed normal noninflamed mucosa; but in the purulent exudate on the mucosal surface, there were many trophozoites of *E. histolytica* (illustrated in Figs 9.102 and 9.103, overleaf).

She was treated with metronidazole. The diarrhea ceased by day 4 of treatment and she was feeling well and starting to put on weight by day 10.

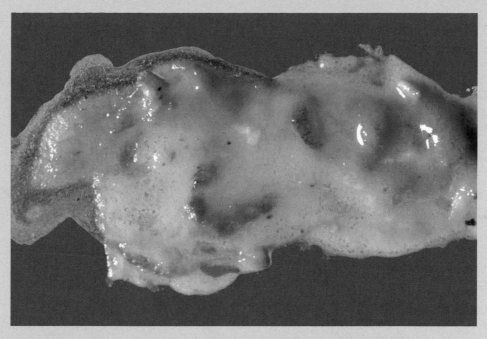

▲ **Fig. 9.99** Sample of blood-stained feces from a 25-year-old female who complained of blood-stained diarrhea.

▼ **Fig. 9.100** The feces had become dry by the time the photograph had been taken, so it was scraped off the slide and processed as for a cell block. An ameba has been fixed in the process of sending out a pseudopod in its ameboid movement. When they are fresh, the amebas move sluggishly like this.

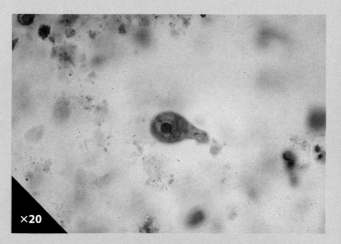

×20

▼ **Fig. 9.101** Sigmoidoscopy view shows some pale ulcers with normal red mucosa between them.

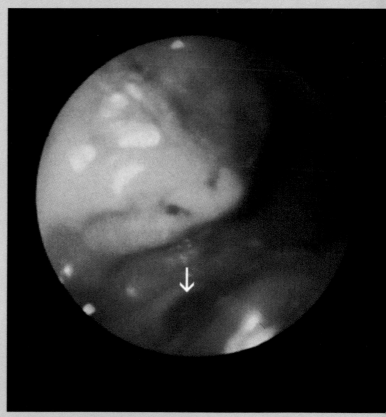

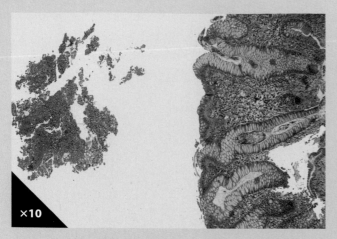

×10

▲ **Fig. 9.102** Rectal biopsy shows a noninflamed rectal mucosa with purulent exudate on the surface.

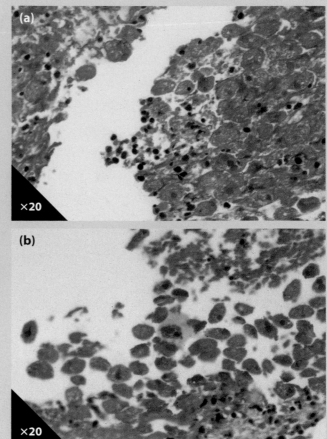

(a)

×20

(b)

×20

▶ **Fig. 9.103(a) and (b)** Views of the purulent exudate show numerous trophozoites of *E. histolytica*. The nuclei of the organisms can be seen and the cytoplasm is filled with red blood cells.

Acute amebic colitis

Figure 9.104 shows a fixed specimen of a portion of the colon from an elderly woman who died in a terminal-care facility from acute amebic colitis during a small epidemic of amebic dysentery among the inmates. It shows the characteristic appearance of amebic ulcers. The ulcers are undermined, and the intervening mucosa is relatively unaffected. The ulcers in amebic colitis can be viewed in life and biopsied via a colonoscope.

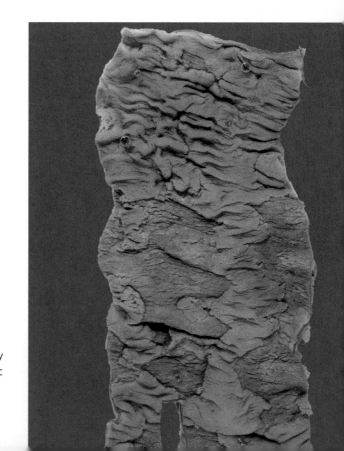

▶ **Fig. 9.104** Fixed specimen of a portion of the colon from an elderly woman who died from acute amebic colitis. It shows the characteristic appearance of amebic ulcers in the colon.

Ameboma

It is well known that *E. histolytica* can cause inflammatory masses that mimic the symptomatology of large bowel malignancies. When this occurs, the most common sites are the rectum and the cecum. The lesions are called amebomas.

The surgical dictum (especially in tropical countries) is that one should not operate on bowel cancer without having a histologic diagnosis first.

Case 9.17

A male, aged 34 years, from Papua New Guinea, who was working in Australia, developed lower abdominal pain and vomiting, with a palpable mass in the right iliac fossa.

A diagnosis of obstructing neoplasm was made and a right hemicolectomy was performed. As this was an emergency situation, no colonoscopy was done.

The pathology of the surgical specimen is illustrated in Figures 9.105–9.109, continued overleaf.

This case illustrates the problem confronted by doctors who are presented with a disease with which they are not familiar in a visitor from another country or in a recently returned traveler.

It is important for doctors to be aware of the country of origin and the travel history of every patient they see, so that they will consider alternative diagnostic possibilities apart from those of diseases with which they are more familiar.

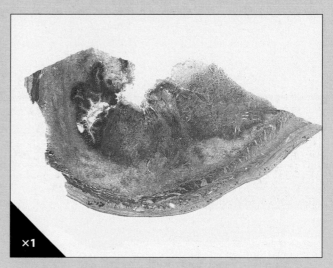

▼ **Fig. 9.105** Ameboma of the cecum. The walls of the cecum and the terminal ileum are thickened by fibrosis. The mucosa is thickened and ulcerated.

▲ **Fig. 9.106** Microscopic section of the cecum shows the thickening by fibrosis more clearly. The mucosa is stained blue and the wall is stained pink.

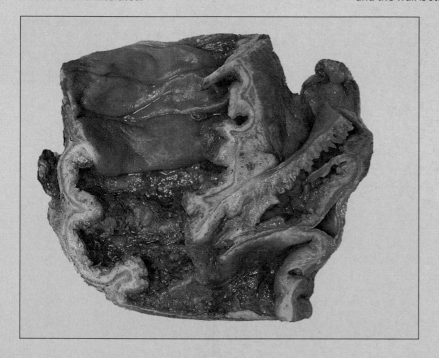

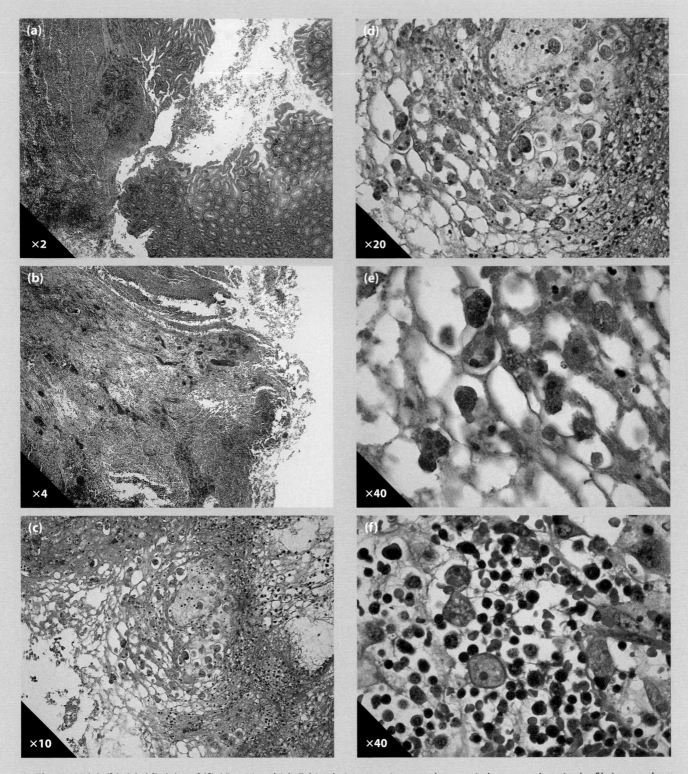

▲ **Fig. 9.107(a), (b), (c), (d), (e) and (f)** Views in which *E. histolytica* organisms can be seen in large numbers in the fibrinopurulent exudate lining the ulcerated mucosal surface of the bowel. They are slightly larger than histiocytes. Note the somewhat eccentric nuclei and the ingested red blood cells.

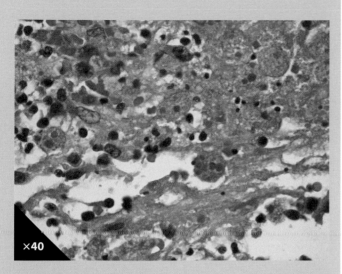

▲ **Fig. 9.108** As the organisms invade the bowel wall, they cause tissue necrosis.

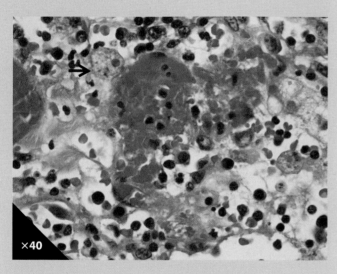

▲ **Fig. 9.109** Organisms enter damaged blood vessels and they are then carried throughout the body, causing abscesses in other organs—particularly the liver. (The *arrow* identifies an organism that is about to enter a damaged blood vessel.)

A doctor in Brisbane, Australia, had a narrow escape from an unnecessary colectomy some 30 years ago. He developed a blood-stained diarrhea towards the end of a holiday in Europe. As soon as he arrived home in Brisbane, he went to consult one of his surgical colleagues.

'Yes,' said the surgeon, 'I agree that you have a rectal carcinoma. I will send a biopsy to the pathologist and arrange the theatre for first thing tomorrow morning.'

The following morning, the colectomy was about to be performed. Premedication had been given when the pathologist telephoned with new information. 'There are amebas present. It must be an ameboma.'

The operation was abandoned, and treatment with metronidazole was begun.

It is impressive how quickly E. histolytica *infections respond to therapy. The patient's diarrhea stopped within a few days and no mass could be palpated in the rectum after day 3 of treatment.*

The incident was recalled at the time of this Brisbane doctor's eightieth birthday celebration in 2007.

Amebic liver abscess

Liver abscesses may be unilocular or multiloculated. They occur most commonly in the right lobe of the liver. The abscess can be localized by radiological imaging. Needle aspiration produces brown-colored pus. Microscopic examination of this pus is unhelpful because the viable organisms are present only in the advancing edge of the abscess. Even when the edge of the abscess has been biopsied, only rarely can organisms be found.

Abscesses may rupture into the pericardium with fatal consequences as illustrated in Case 9.18, overleaf.

Liver abscesses are usually treated by anti-amebic drugs alone, but sometimes additional drainage through a fine catheter is required for complete resolution. If open surgical drainage is undertaken as a primary treatment, the mortality is increased.

Case 9.18

A 49-year-old male was referred to Brisbane, Australia, from Papua New Guinea for treatment of what was diagnosed there as acute amebic dysentery and liver abscess.

Unfortunately, the surgeon decided to perform an open drainage of the abscess, and during the night following the surgery the abscess ruptured into the pericardium causing a cardiac tamponade and the patient died.

Post-mortem examination revealed the presence of multiple ulcers throughout his colon. These were most concentrated in the cecal region.

The liver showed a multiloculated abscess in the right lobe and the pericardial effusion was confirmed (illustrated in Figs 9.110 and 9.111).

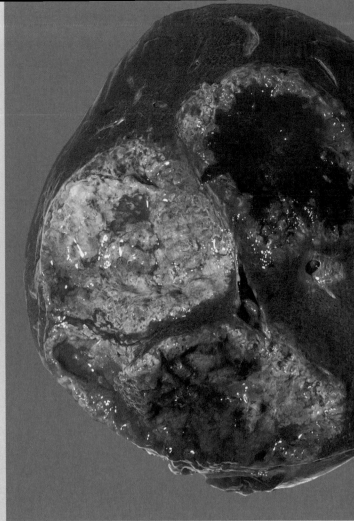

▲ **Fig. 9.110** Multiloculated amebic abscess in the right lobe of the liver.

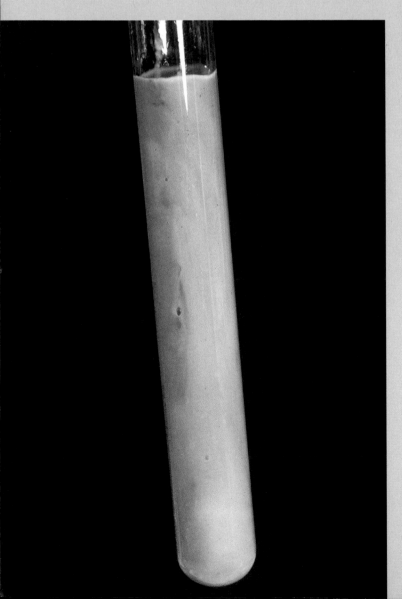

◀ **Fig. 9.111** Tube of brown pus (sometimes called anchovy sauce pus) from the liver abscess.

Cutaneous amebiasis

The *E. histolytica* parasite may invade the skin and produce an epithelial hyperplasia that closely resembles the appearance of squamous cell carcinoma. This invasion occurs under two circumstances, involving the abdominal wall and the anogenital region.

Abdominal wall

- The parasite invades the skin of the abdomen. This invasion can occur in either of two ways:

  - as a fistula from an ameboma of the gut (nearly always in the ileo cecal region)
  - as a fistula that forms following surgical removal of an ameboma that is wrongly considered to be a carcinoma. An example of this is illustrated in Case 9.19.

Anogenital region

- The parasite invades the skin of the anogenital region.
- This invasion follows contamination of the affected area by diarrheal feces or by sexual intercourse. Illustrative examples of this are demonstrated here.

Case 9.19

A 32-year-old female presented with symptoms of bowel obstruction. Investigations revealed what was thought to be a carcinoma of the cecum.

A right hemicolectomy was performed. There was some delay in dispatching the surgical specimen for reporting on the histology. When the specimen was finally reported a few weeks later, an inflammatory mass was found and amebas were present in the purulent exudate.

The patient was recalled. By this time, she had two fistulae—one from the drain from the surgical excision and the other from the paramedian surgical incision wound (shown in Fig. 9.112).

A biopsy from the edge of one of the sinuses showed the features of cutaneous amebiasis.

She was given a course of emetine hydrochloride (the now old-fashioned antiamebic drug), and the sinuses ceased to drain within a few days. They healed without further incident.

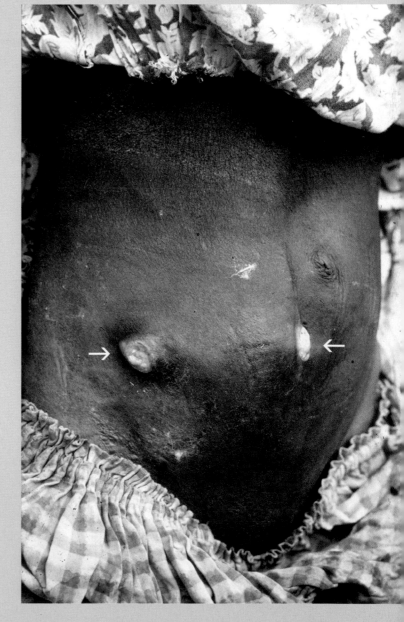

▶ **Fig. 9.112** This 32-year-old female developed fistulae following a right hemicolectomy for a misdiagnosis of carcinoma of the cecum. The correct diagnosis in retrospect was an ameboma of the cecum.

Perianal lesions

In 1962, the pathology laboratory in Port Moresby, Papua New Guinea, received a number of specimens from different doctors who had drawn a diagram of a patient in lithotomy position (see Fig. 9.113), with a perianal lesion (see Fig. 9.114), which they queried as an anal carcinoma which they biopsied. One doctor excised the whole lesion (see Fig. 9.115).

Sections of the lesions showed the microscopic appearances of cutaneous amebiasis (see Figs 9.116 and 9.117). The normal skin merged into the lesion, which consisted in an area of epitheliomatous hyperplasia. This appearance made many pathologists make a diagnosis of squamous cell carcinoma when similar sections were shown as problem cases at educational meetings during subsequent years—but if one looks along the surface of the thickened epidermis, there are 'cracks' in the epidermis. These areas are lined by purulent exudate in which there are numerous trophozoites of E. histolytica. In some places, the organisms can be seen eroding into the epidermis.

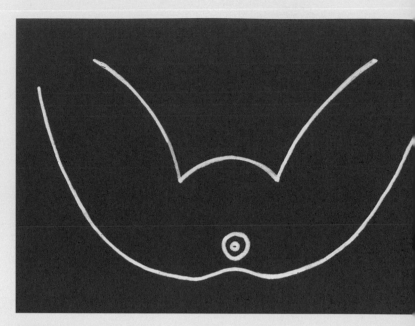

▲ **Fig. 9.113** Diagram of a patient in lithotomy position with a query carcinoma of the anus.

◀ **Fig. 9.114** Patient with the lesion depicted in the diagram in Figure 9.113.

▼ **Fig. 9.115** This perianal lesion was excised with a clinical diagnosis of carcinoma.

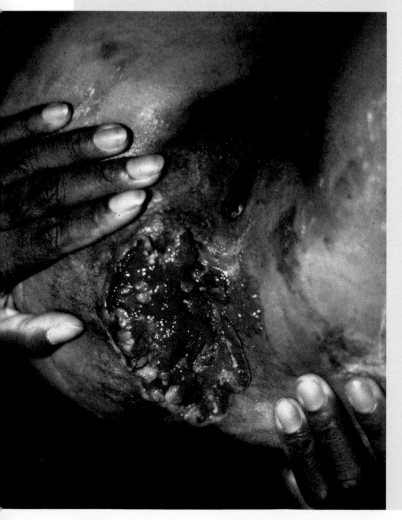

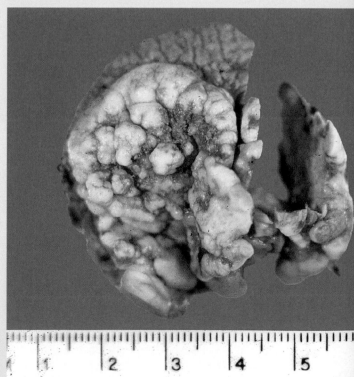

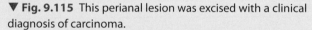

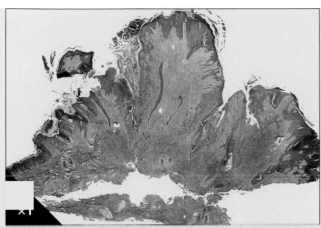

◀ **Fig. 9.116** View of the biopsy from the excised lesion of Figure 9.115. It shows the characteristic appearances of cutaneous amebiasis. The normal skin merges into the lesion, which consists in an area of epitheliomatous hyperplasia.

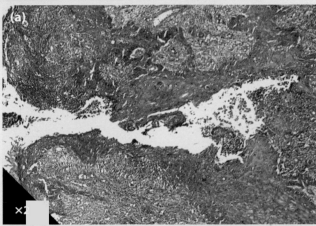

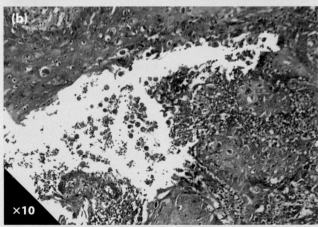

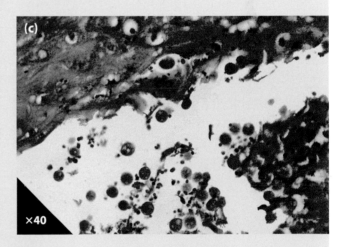

◀ ▼ **Fig. 9.117(a), (b) and (c)** If one looks along the surface of the thickened epidermis, there are 'cracks' in the epidermis. These areas are lined by purulent exudate in which there are numerous trophozoites of *E. histolytica*. The organisms can be seen invading the superficial layer of the stratum corneum. There is a moderately heavy inflammatory reaction in the dermis, but no organisms can be seen there.

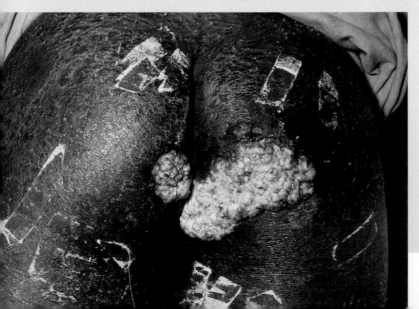

Unlike other organisms that are found in the inflammatory reaction in the dermis, E. histolytica *are present in the exudate on the surface. In this respect, they are similar to the organisms of syphilis (which also occur in the surface exudate of the skin lesions).*

An occasional case of cutaneous amebiasis was encountered in which the lesions were not directly associated with the anus (see Fig. 9.118).

◀ **Fig. 9.118** Biopsy of these lesions on the buttocks showed the appearances of cutaneous amebiasis.

Genital lesions

Biopsies from a number of cases involving the groins and external genitalia of females were received in the pathology department in Port Moresby, Papua New Guinea (see Figs 9.119–9.121).

An even greater number of cases involving the prepuce and glans penis were received, sufficient to create a reproducibly recognizable syndrome of 'amebic balanitis' (see Figs 9.122–9.124, continued overleaf).

It was soon realized that this was an important type of sexually transmitted infection (STI) in Papua New Guinea at that time. Figures 9.119–9.123 illustrate this condition.

Donovanosis (granuloma inguinale) was already recognized as being a very common cause of STI in Papua New Guinea. The clinical appearances of these lesions are very similar to those of cutaneous amebiasis.

With knowledge of the local pattern of disease, it became a rule of thumb for surgeons and medical students that any hypertrophic lesion in the anogenital region should be considered as being donovanosis, amebiasis, and then as a very last possibility, carcinoma.

At the time of Independence for PNG in 1975, many doctors left, and others who had no knowledge of the local disease patterns had to re-learn many of the lessons that had already been learned. So, a few cases of amebic balanitis were treated by amputation with a clinical diagnosis of carcinoma (Fig. 9.124, overleaf).

Cases of sexually transmitted cutaneous amebiasis occurred in some of the homosexual communities in the United States soon after AIDS was recognized in the early 1980s.

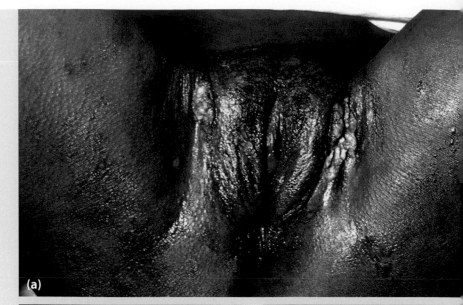

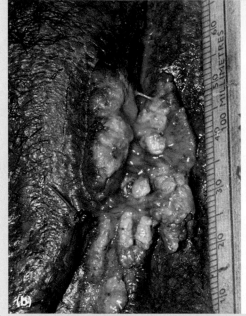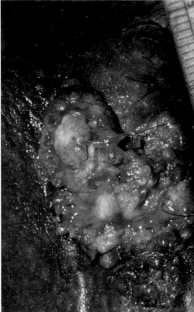

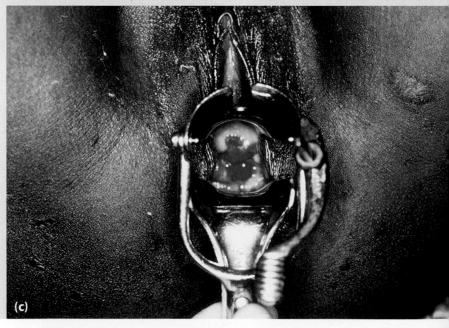

▶ **Fig. 9.119(a), (b) and (c)** Female aged 40 years. She had hypertrophic and ulcerated lesions in both groins. Vaginitis and cervicitis were present as well. Amebas were identified in smears from all the skin lesions and from the cervix. Biopsy showed cutaneous amebiasis.

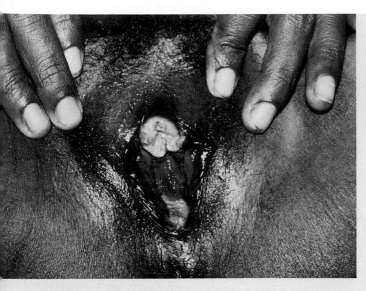

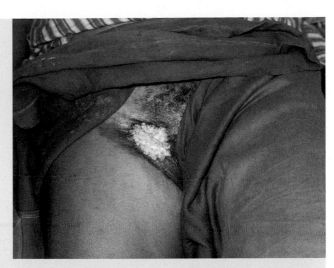

▲ **Fig. 9.121** Woman with a cutaneous amebiasis lesion in the right groin.

▲ **Fig. 9.120** Lesion of the clitoris. The clinical diagnosis was carcinoma of the clitoris, but the biopsy showed cutaneous amebiasis.

▼ **Fig. 9.122** Amebic balanitis. At first, there is swelling of the prepuce. This may lead to urinary obstruction, which is relieved when the amebas burrow right through the prepuce and form a fistula through which the glans penis can protrude. The glans can be seen on the left (B) and the prepuce on the right (A).

▼ **Fig. 9.123** Four days after starting treatment the lesion shown in Figure 9.122 had healed well.

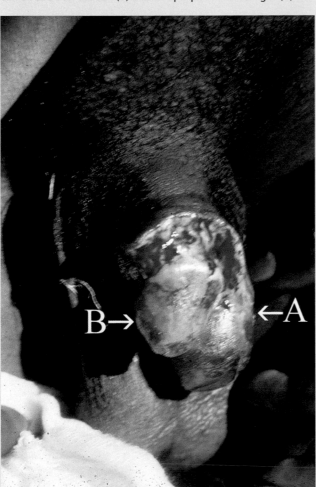

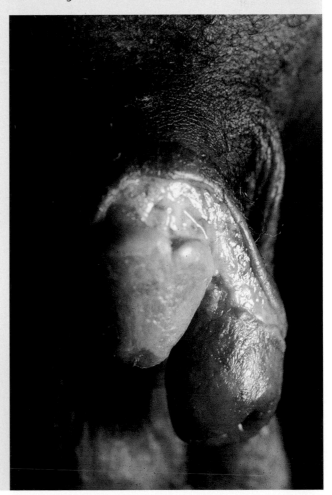

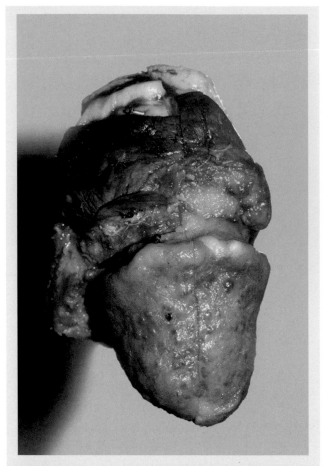

▲ **Fig. 9.124** Amebic balanitis treated by amputation because of a clinical misdiagnosis of carcinoma in 1980.

Perpetuation of the *E. histolytica*

Amebiasis is perpetuated by patients recovering from an acute attack of dysentery who pass organisms in the form of cysts in the feces. The cysts contaminate fingers or food and are ingested, and the cycle is continued.

The cyst of *E. histolytica* needs to be distinguished from other cysts that may be found in feces. The cyst of the non-pathogenic Entameba *E. dispar* is identical, while *Entameba coli* is larger and has eight nuclei. The trophozoite form of *E. dispar* does not show erythrophagocytosis, which is a feature of the trophozoite of *E. histolytica.*

Cysts of *E. histolytica* and *E. coli* are illustrated in Figures 9.125 and 9.126.

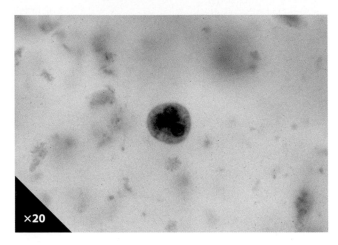

▲ **Fig. 9.125** The *E. histolytica* cyst is fairly small, 10–20 microns in diameter. It contains four nuclei, each with a well-defined central karyosome. This cyst needs to be distinguished from the cysts of non-pathogenic *Entameba*. *E. dispar* is identical, while *Entameba coli* is larger and has eight nuclei.

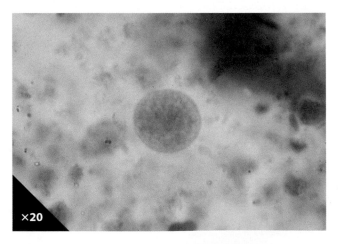

▲ **Fig. 9.126** *Entameba coli* cyst photographed at the same magnification as the *E. histolytica*. It is larger and has 8 nuclei.

Free-living amebas

Free-living amebas are organisms that are normally found in the environment and are normally nonpathogenic. Two of them will be demonstrated here:

- *Naegleria fowleri*, which causes meningitis, and
- *Acanthameba*, which is frequently found in people who wear contact lenses, and which occasionally causes meningitis in immunocompromised people.

Naegleria fowleri

N. fowleri is a small ameba which causes meningitis that is frequently fulminating, with death occurring within 1–2 weeks of the onset of the infection. Cases have been reported from many parts of the world.

The infected patients have usually been swimming in freshwater lakes or swimming pools. They present with an acute onset of fever and the symptoms and signs of meningitis. The cerebrospinal fluid (CSF) contains large numbers of inflammatory cells. Sometimes, motile amebas can be seen on the counting chamber during a CSF examination.

At post mortem, there is a variable opacity of the meninges, and cut slices of the brain show focal areas of hemorrhage and necrosis. The small amebas are present in the subarachnoid space and in the Virchow Robin spaces surrounding the blood vessels that penetrate into the brain (shown in Figs 9.127 and 9.128). The olfactory bulb is often destroyed. It is thought that the organisms enter the brain through the cribriform plates and directly invade the olfactory nerves.

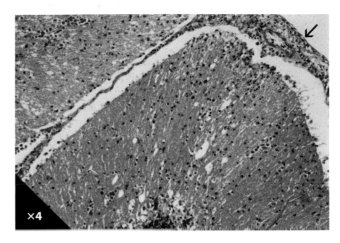

▲ **Fig. 9.127** *N. fowleri.* View of a meningitis with lymphocytes and amebas in the subarachnoid space (*see arrow*).

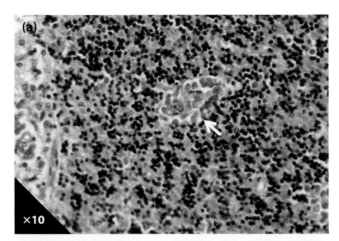

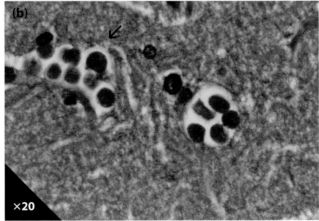

▲ **Fig. 9.128(a) and (b)** The small amebas can be seen in the perivascular space (the Virchow Robin space) within the brain.

Balantidiasis

Balantidiasis is an infection caused by the protozoan organism *Balantidium coli* (see Figs 9.134 and 9.135). This organism occurs in many parts of the world and it is a rare cause of diarrhea in humans. The organism lives in the intestine of many animals, and humans are infected by ingesting cysts in food or water.

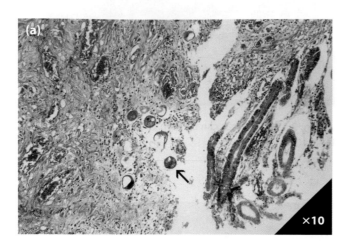
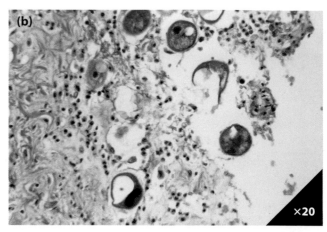

▲ **Fig. 9.134(a) and (b)** Views of an ulcer in the colon. *Balantidium coli* organisms can be seen in the base of the ulcer. These are large organisms approximately 50 microns in diameter. They are round, have a large nucleus and vacuolated cytoplasm. In freshly passed feces, the organisms are motile and the cilia are easily seen on the surface of the organism.

▶ **Fig. 9.135** View of formalin fixed feces from diarrheal stools. The tiny cilia can be seen on the surface of the organism adjacent to the macro nucleus.

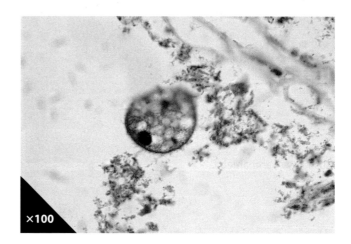

Giardiasis

The protozoan parasite *Giardia lamblia* occurs in most parts of the world. Infection is probably acquired by drinking water contaminated with Giardia cysts.

It causes diarrhea by infection of the small intestine, particularly the duodenum. Quite often, this diarrhea is severe and intractable. The patient often loses weight and sometimes has frank malabsorption.

The diagnosis is made either by finding the organisms in a small bowel biopsy or by finding motile flagellated organisms in fluid aspirated from the duodenum, or in diarrheal feces (illustrated in Figs 9.136–9.139, continued overleaf).

The organisms form cysts and these may be found in feces (see Fig. 9.140, overleaf).

Molecular biological tests, ELISA and PCR are also available for diagnostic testing.

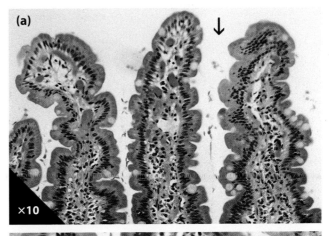

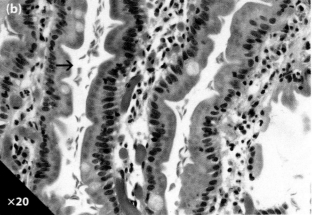

▲ **Fig. 9.137(a) and (b)** Large numbers of Giardia organisms can be seen in the surface mucus and in the recesses between adjacent villi.

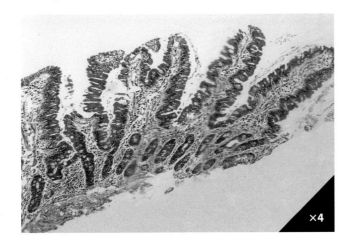

▲ **Fig. 9.136** Small intestinal biopsy from a patient with giardiasis. The small bowel is morphologically normal. The villi are of normal length. There is no inflammation.

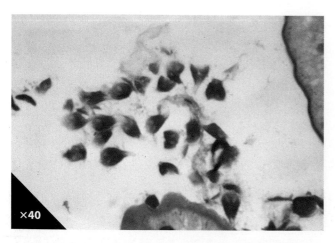

▲ **Fig. 9.138** View showing the trophozoites at different angles. The pear-shape of the organism is best seen in the front face view and then the two nuclei are visible, resembling a pair of eyes. The flagellum is at the pointed end of the parasite.

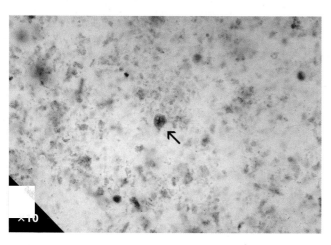

▲ **Fig. 9.139** Motile trophozoite of Giardia from a wet preparation of duodenal aspirate.

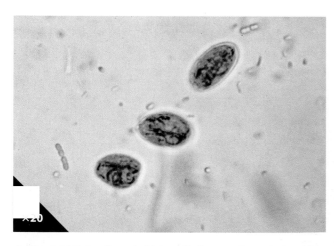

▲ **Fig. 9.140** Small, oval, thick-walled cysts of *Giardia lamblia* in a sample of feces.

Trichomoniasis

Trichomonas vaginalis is a flagellated protozoan parasite. It infects the vagina causing acute inflammation and the symptoms of acute vaginitis. The motile organism can be seen in a wet preparation in which a drop of the purulent exudate is placed on a microscope slide and covered by a cover slip. It may also be identified in a Papanicolaou smear from the cervix (see Fig. 9.141).

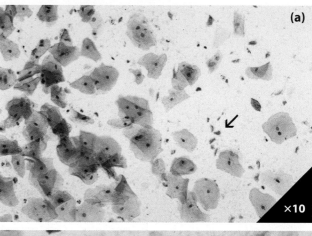

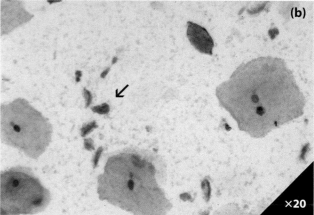

▲ **Fig. 9.141(a) and (b)** Papanicolaou smear from the cervix. Trichomonas organisms can be seen.

Cryptosporidium

Cryptosporidium is a protozoan parasite which is a not uncommon cause of diarrhea. It affects immunocompetent people but is more severe in those who have immune suppression from whatever cause. Localized epidemics have occurred as a result of contamination of drinking water or the water in public swimming pools.

The diagnosis is made by demonstrating the oocysts of the parasite in feces. This can be done by using a wet mount, a modified Ziehl Neelsen (ZN) stain or by immuno fluorescent microscopy (see Fig. 9.142).

Cysts may also be seen in histologic sections of small bowel biopsies (illustrated in Figs 9.143 and 9.144).

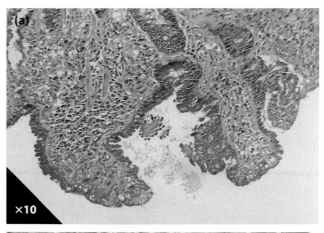

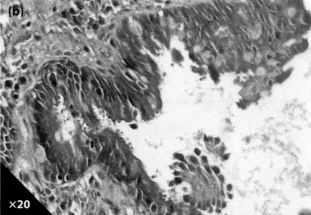

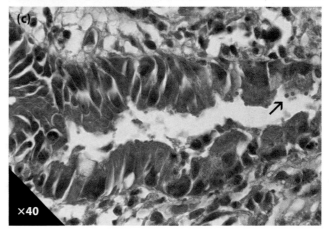

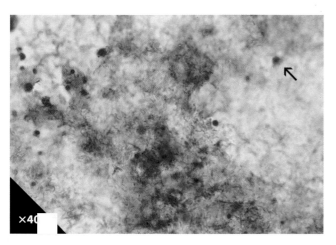

▲ **Fig. 9.142** Oocysts of Cryptosporidium in a smear of feces from a patient with diarrhea.

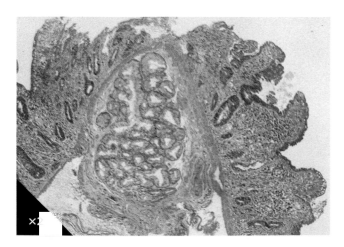

▲ **Fig. 9.143** Small intestinal biopsy showing partial atrophy with shortening of the villi.

▲ **Fig. 9.144(a), (b) and (c)** Views of oocysts of Cryptosporidium, which appear as tiny blue 'dots' attached to the surface of small intestinal mucosal epithelial cells.

Microsporidium

Microsporidium infection is caused by a species of protozoan parasite of the order Microsporidia. It is an obligate intracellular spore-forming protozoan. The commonest species encountered is *Enterocytozoon bieneusi*.

This organism is responsible for about one-third of the diarrhea that occurs in HIV-positive AIDS patients. First recognized in 1985, it has been identified in AIDS patients in most parts of the world.

The diagnosis is made by finding spores of the microsporidium in feces. These stain with a modified Trichrome stain. They measure 1–2.5 microns in diameter. They are slightly smaller than the oocysts of cryptosporidiosis, and more difficult to find (see Fig. 9.145). They can also be seen (although with some difficulty) in duodenal biopsies.

Since these organisms are virtually impossible to see in routine sections, it is recommended that a Warthin Starry stain be added to the routine battery of stains that should be used to identify the various organisms that may cause opportunistic infection in AIDS patients (see Figs 9.146, 9.147 and 9.148).

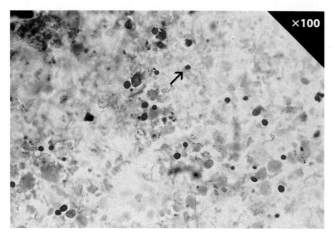

▲ **Fig. 9.145** Spores of *Enterocytozoon bieneusi* in diarrheal feces of an AIDS patient. The feces sample was concentrated and stained with a modified Trichrome stain.

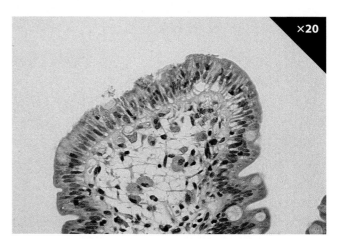

▲ **Fig. 9.147** At this magnification, it is not possible to see spores in the cytoplasm of surface epithelial cells.

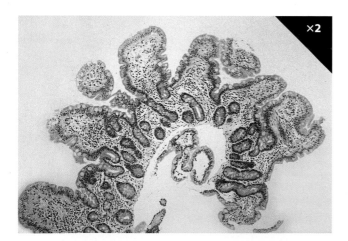

▲ **Fig. 9.146** Routine H&E stained section of a duodenal biopsy from an AIDS patient viewed at low magnification. The biopsy shows the changes of acute duodenitis, with some shortening of villi and a mild increase in inflammatory cells, mainly mononuclear inflammatory cells in the lamina propria.

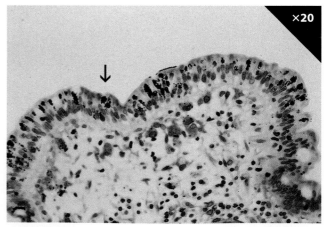

▲ **Fig. 9.148** The organisms are much more easily seen in a Warthin Starry stained section, examined at the same magnification.

Acknowledgments

- Fig. 9.1 Courtesy of Kathy Bevin, Brisbane, Australia.
- Figs 9.2 and 9.3 Courtesy of the Armed Forces Institute of Pathology (AFIP), Washington, USA.
- Fig. 9.4 Courtesy of Jaime Rios Dalenz, La Paz, Bolivia.
- Fig. 9.5 Courtesy of Samuel de Oliveira, Sao Paulo, Brazil.
- Fig. 9.6 Courtesy of Marcello Franco, Sao Paulo, Brazil.
- Fig. 9.7 Courtesy of David Tan, Kuala Lumpur, Malaysia.
- Figs 9.8–9.10 Courtesy of Graeme Beardmore, Brisbane, Australia.
- Fig. 9.11 Courtesy of Tony Allworth and Dominic Wood, Brisbane, Australia.
- Fig. 9.12 Courtesy of Paul Hofman, Nice, France.
- Fig. 9.13 Courtesy of Victor Harrison, London, England.
- Fig. 9.14 Courtesy of Geoffrey Crawford, Brisbane, Australia.
- Fig. 9.15 Courtesy of Sandeep Sen, Patna, India.
- Fig. 9.19 Courtesy of Michel Huerre and the Librarian, Institut Pasteur, Paris, France.
- Fig. 9.20 Leitz monocular microscope kindly loaned to the author by Bob Butterworth, Wild-Leitz, Brisbane, Australia.
- Fig. 9.22 Courtesy of David Perel, Brisbane, Australia.
- Figs 10.25 and 10.26 Photographed with permission of the Curator of the Museum of Medical History, Pavia, Italy.
- Fig. 9.31 Courtesy of James and Peggy McCartney, Adelaide, Australia.
- Fig. 9.32 Photographed with permission of Keith Macadam and the librarian, London School of Tropical Medicine, London, England.
- Figs 9.34 and 9.35 Photographs made possible by the collaboration of A.K. Hatti, Director of the School of Tropical Medicine, Calcutta, India.
- Figs 9.36 and 9.37 Photographed with the collaborative assistance of A.K. Banerjee, Calcutta, India.
- Fig. 9.38 Photographed with permission of Florabel Mullick, Director, Armed Forces Institute of Pathology (AFIP), Washington, USA.
- Fig. 9.40 Photographed by Robin Cooke, with permission of Dan Connor, Armed Forces Institute of Pathology (AFIP), Washington, USA.
- Fig. 9.41 Courtesy of Charles Hasyler, Papua New Guinea.
- Fig. 9.48 Courtesy of Leonard Champness, Papua New Guinea and Geelong, Australia.
- Fig. 9.50 From Cooke, R.A. and Stewart, B., *Colour Atlas of Anatomical Pathology*, third edn, Churchill Livingstone, Edinburgh, 2004.
- Figs 9.53 and 9.54 Courtesy of Drs A.K. Banerjee and Chaterjee, Calcutta, India. Photographed by Robin Cooke.
- Figs 9.57–9.74 Blood smears. Courtesy of the scientific staff of the Royal Brisbane Hospital Haematology Department. Photographed by Robin Cooke.
- Figs 9.75–9.80 Courtesy of Peter Sharp, Papua New Guinea and Alice Springs, Australia.
- Fig. 9.82 Courtesy of David Tan, Kuala Lumpur, Malaysia.
- Fig. 9.86 Courtesy of Paul Spiro, Brisbane, Australia.
- Figs 9.105–9.109 Courtesy of David Williams, Townsville, Australia.
- Fig. 9.118 Courtesy of Maurice Cave, Papua New Guinea and Rockhampton, Australia.
- Fig. 9.119 Courtesy of Roger Rodrigue, Papua New Guinea and Melbourne, Australia.
- Fig. 9.120 Courtesy of Stan Reid, Papua New Guinea and Perth, Australia.
- Fig. 9.121 Courtesy of Ian Welch, Papua New Guinea and Brisbane, Australia.
- Fig. 9.124 Courtesy of Prasantha Murthy, Papua New Guinea and Griffith, Australia.
- Fig. 9.128 Courtesy of Renata Kalnins, Melbourne, Australia.
- Fig. 9.130 Courtesy of Tony Tannenberg, Brisbane, Australia.
- Figs 9.131 and 9.132 Courtesy of Roy Axelsen, Brisbane, Australia. Photographed by Robin Cooke.
- Fig. 9.133 Courtesy of Jenny Robson, Brisbane, Australia.
- Fig. 9.135 Courtesy of David Tan, Kuala Lumpur, Malaysia.
- Figs 9.145–9.148 case information on microsporidium infection in AIDS patients. Courtesy of Andrew Field, Director of Anatomical Pathology, St Vincent's Hospital, Sydney, Australia. Photographed by Robin Cooke.

10

Parasitic infections
Nematodes, trematodes and cestodes

Nematodes

Nematodes are round worms. Some of the more important ones that infect humans will be considered in this section.

Bancroftian and Malayan filariasis

Filariasis is a disease caused by infection with the filarial worms *Wuchereria bancrofti* and *Wuchereria (Brugia) malayi*. The adult worms live in the sinusoids of lymph nodes, particularly in the inguinal region (see Life cycle 10.1).

The two species of filarial worm can be identified by minor morphological differences in the adult worms and in the microfilariae.

- *W. bancrofti* is found in most parts of the tropical world.
- *B. malayi* is confined to India, South-East Asia and mainland China.

Both species of worm produce similar clinicopatholgic manifestations. The female worms produce microfilariae, which are found in the peripheral blood. These microfilariae are covered by a sheath and they demonstrate nocturnal periodicity (that is, they are present in larger numbers in the peripheral blood during the night than during the daytime).

The microfilariae are transmitted by a variety of mosquito species.

Filariasis (*Wuchereria* and *Brugia* species)

An infected human harbors adult worm in lymphatics; and microfilariae in the blood.

↓

Many species of mosquito bite infected humans and transmit microfilariae to uninfected humans.

▲ **Life cycle 10.1** Filariasis—*Wuchereria* and *Brugia* species.

These references support the content of chapters 9 and 10:

Binford, C.H. and Connor, D.H., *Pathology of Tropical and Extraordinary Diseases*, vols I and II, Armed Forces Institute of Pathology (AFIP), Washington, DC, 1976.

Kean, B.H., Mott, K.E. and Russell, A.J., *Tropical Medicine and Parasitology Classic Investigations*, vols I and II, Cornell University Press, New York, 1978.

The adult worms of *W. bancrofti* were first identified in 1876 by Joseph Bancroft (see Fig. 10.1) in Brisbane, Australia, in chylous hydrocoele fluid. Bancroft associated them with the microfilariae found in 1866 by Otto Wucherer (1820–1873) in Bahia, Brazil, in the urine of three patients with chyluria. In the 10 years between these two discoveries, microfilariae were found in blood and their association with elephantiasis of legs and scrotum was confirmed.

The adult worms are 50–100 mm in length and quite thin (shown in Fig. 10.2). They are usually found in matted coils in the lymphatic vessels, particularly in inguinal lymph nodes, but sometimes elsewhere, for example in the region of the epitrochlear lymph node at the elbow. The females give birth to microfilariae, which then circulate in the peripheral blood.

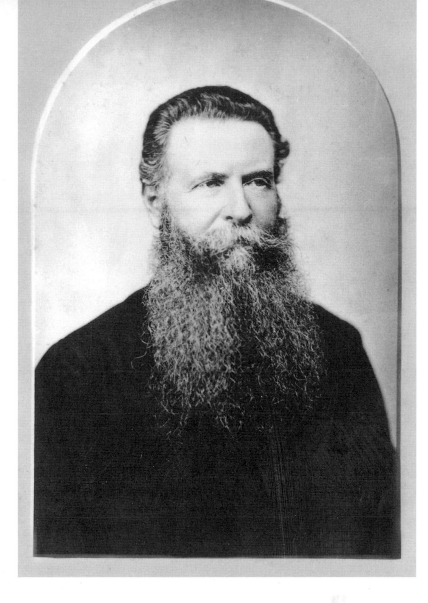

▶ **Fig. 10.1** Joseph Bancroft (1836–1894), who found in chylous hydrocoele fluid the adult filarial worm that came to be called *Wuchereria bancrofti*.

▼ **Fig. 10.2** Matted mass of adult filarial worms.

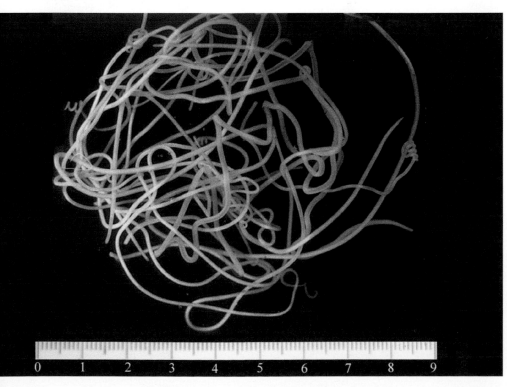

Identification of the microfilariae

The microfilariae are more numerous at night than during the daytime, so to be sure of seeing them, the blood sample is best taken during the night. Their motility is seen to advantage in a wet preparation, in which a drop of blood is placed on a microscope slide and covered by a cover slip. The motile microfilariae can be easily seen with a low-power objective of the microscope. They wriggle through the red blood cells with their sheath draped around them.

In stained peripheral blood smears, the microfilariae are most easily seen in the tail of the film when the film is examined with a low-power objective (illustrated in Figs 10.3–10.8).

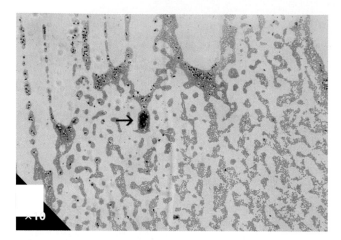

▲ **Fig. 10.3** Microfilaria in the tail of a peripheral blood smear.

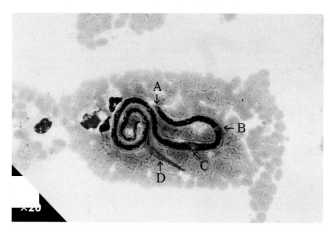

▲ **Fig. 10.4** *W. bancrofti* microfilaria cephalic space (A), nerve ring (B), excretory pore (C), sheath (D).

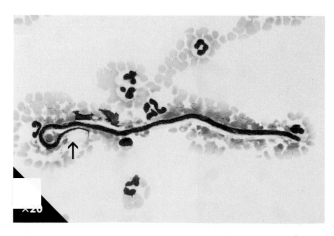

▲ **Fig. 10.5** *W. bancrofti* microfilaria. The nuclei extend right to the tip of the tail.

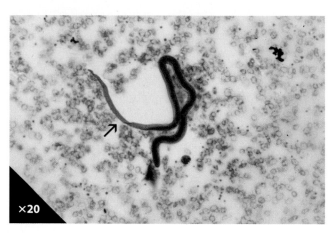

▲ **Fig. 10.6** *W. bancrofti* microfilaria. The sheath is nicely shown.

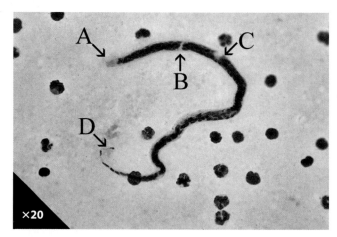

▲ **Fig. 10.7** *B. malayi* microfilaria cephalic space (A), nerve ring (B), excretory pore (C), two discrete nuclei at the tip of the tail (D).

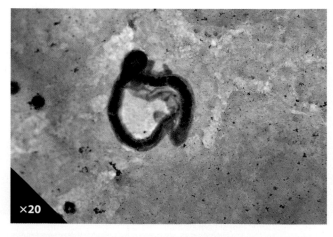

▲ **Fig. 10.8** *B. malayi* microfilaria. The sheath is nicely shown.

Clinical features of filariasis

The filarial worms, like other parasites, can live for many years in their human host without producing any clinical manifestations. When symptoms are present they are fever, lymphadenitis and swelling, particularly of legs, testis or spermatic cord (see Fig. 10.9). This is associated with a peripheral blood eosinophilia. At a later stage, the inguinal lymph nodes may become markedly enlarged.

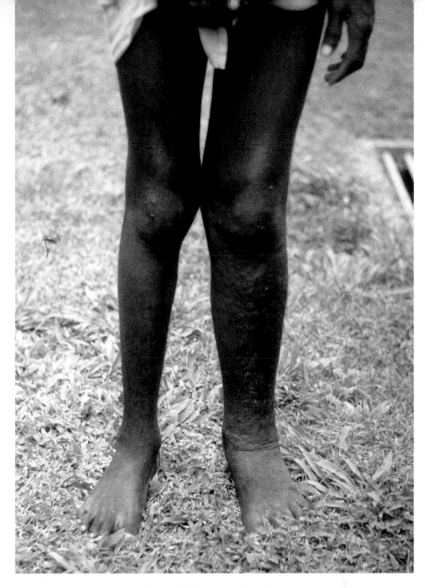

▲ **Fig. 10.9** Young male whose left leg is swollen from acute filariasis.

Case 10.1

A young adult male in Papua New Guinea (PNG) presented with markedly enlarged inguinal lymph nodes (see Fig. 10.10, overleaf). A fairly large piece was excised from the matted mass of lymph nodes. This showed the appearances of filarial lymphadenopathy, as illustrated in Figures 10.11–10.14, continued overleaf.

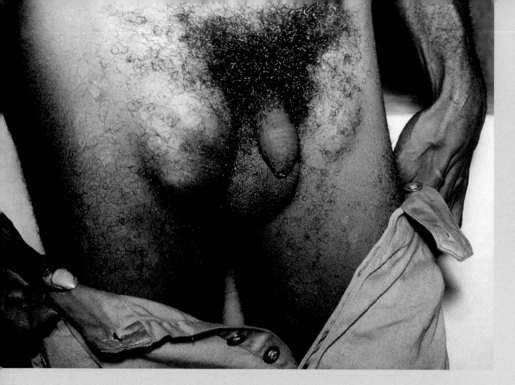

◀ **Fig. 10.10** Young adult male with markedly enlarged inguinal lymph nodes that on biopsy were shown to contain adult filarial worms.

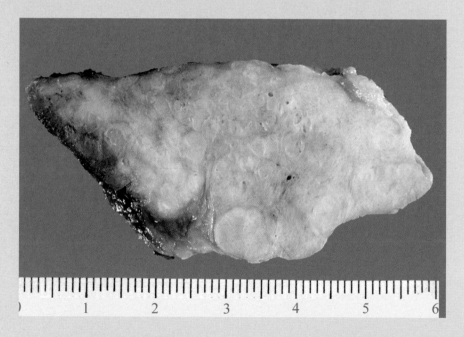

◀ **Fig. 10.11** Macroscopic appearance of an enlarged inguinal lymph node resulting from the presence of adult filarial worms. Note the presence of marked distortion of the architecture by fibrosis. (The enlarged lymph nodes may show no macroscopic abnormality, but more often there is marked fibrosis and distortion of the normal morphology of the lymph node.)

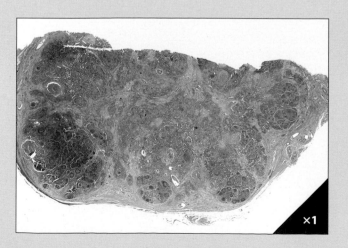

◀ **Fig. 10.12** Low magnification view of the section taken from the lymph node. It shows the marked distortion of the normal lymph node architecture with the blue staining lymphoid tissue separated by broad bands of pink-staining fibrous tissue. The lymphatic sinusoids can be seen to be considerably dilated.

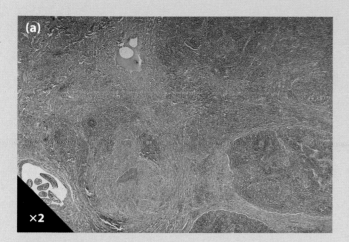
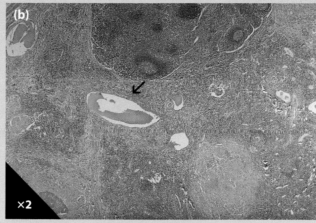

▲ **Fig. 10.13(a)** In the bottom left corner, adult filarial worms can be seen in one of these dilated lymphatics. **(b)** The dilated lymphatics (*indicated by the arrow*) can be more easily seen.

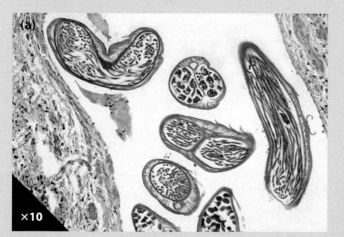
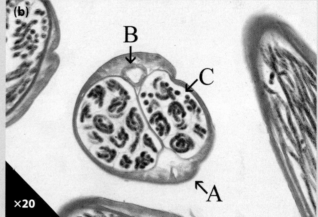

▲ **Fig. 10.14(a)** Adult female worms can be seen cut in cross section. **(b)** High magnification view of a transverse section of an adult female worm—the cuticle is staining pink (A), alimentary canal (B), bi-lobed uterus that contains microfilariae (C).

Appearances of filarial lymphadenopathy seen in another case are illustrated in Figure 10.15.

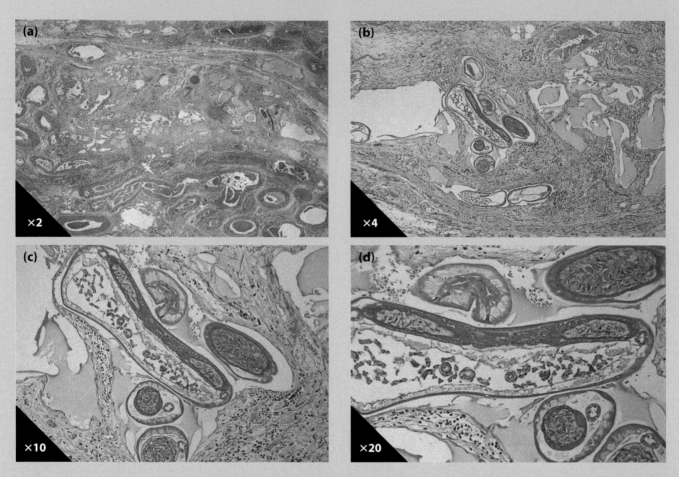

▲ **Fig. 10.15(a), (b), (c) and (d)** Section from an inguinal lymph node. It shows dilated lymphatics and many filarial worms. Some of the worms have died and an eosinophil proliferation has been induced by this.

Case 10.2

A 23-year-old man, who had been working in Papua New Guinea, was admitted to a hospital in Brisbane with a hard tumor in the epididymis of his left testis.

A clinical diagnosis of testicular tumor was made and an orchidectomy was performed. Histologic examination showed the presence of a granulomatous reaction to a degenerating filarial worm (see Fig. 10.16).

A later stage of the process is calcification (see Fig. 10.17).

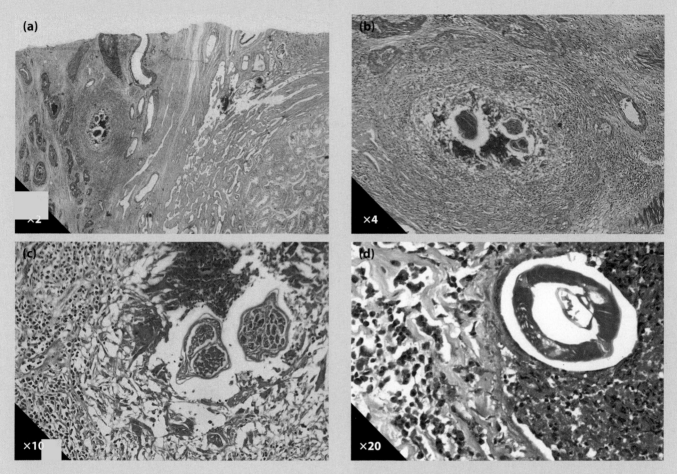

▲ **Fig. 10.16(a), (b), (c) and (d)** Seminiferous tubules of the testis can be seen on the right of **(a)**. In the epididymis on the left, there is a granulomatous reaction around partially degenerate adult filarial worms. In the higher magnification views, the brisk eosinophil reaction to the degenerate parasite can be seen. Sometimes in cases such as this, the degenerate worm is not seen in the first sections taken, nor in the first levels examined. If the clinical information suggests the possibility of filariasis, the pathologist should cut deeper sections through the paraffin block in an attempt to find filarial worms.

▶ **Fig. 10.17** Section taken from an epididymal tumor from another patient. In this case, the dead worms have become calcified.

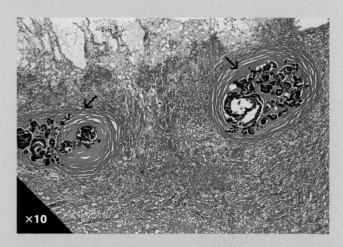

Occasionally, rupture of obstructed lymphatics within the bladder wall can cause chyluria (as shown in Fig. 10.18). Microfilariae circulate through the peripheral blood. They usually do not cause any reaction in the organs which they traverse. As a result, microfilariae may be found incidentally in histologic preparations of various organs (see Figs 10.19 and 10.20). Occasionally, a worm can be found in the eye (shown in Fig. 10.21).

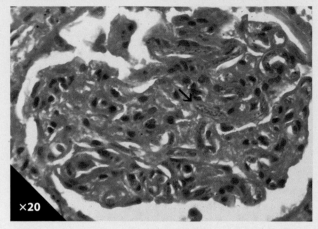

▲ **Fig. 10.19** Microfilariae in a capillary within a renal glomerulus.

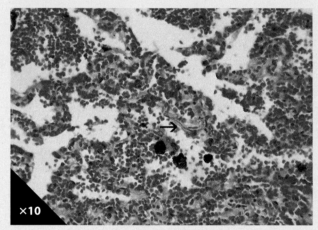

▲ **Fig. 10.20** Microfilariae in a capillary in the alveolar wall of the lung.

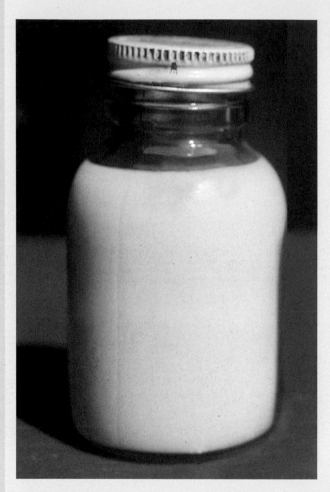

▲ **Fig. 10.18** Sample of urine showing chyluria. Occasionally, rupture of obstructed lymphatics within the bladder wall results in a leakage of chyle into the urine and passage of a milky urine. Otto Wucherer found microfilariae in chyluria specimens and Joseph Bancroft found adult worms in chylous hydrocoele fluid.

▶ **Fig. 10.21** Adult filarial worms are found occasionally in an aberrant situation, for example an adult worm is present in the anterior chamber of the eye of this patient. The patient will notice the worm intermittently in the eye because it leaves the anterior chamber and burrows back into the eye tissue. It can be removed surgically, but patience is often needed until the worm actually appears again in the anterior chamber. Surgery must then be done 'at once' in order to 'catch' the worm.

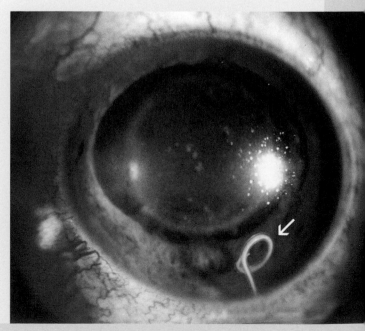

In heavily endemic areas, a small number of patients with longstanding infection develop the condition of elephantiasis. This phenomenon has been a medical curiosity of tropical regions. The parts of the body most often affected by elephantiasis are the legs, the scrotum, the vulva and breasts in women (see Figs 10.22–10.25).

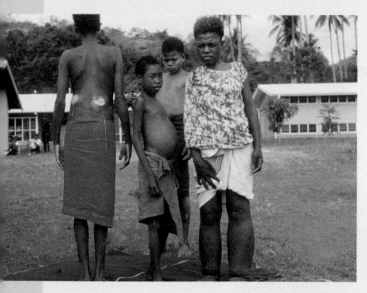

▲ **Fig. 10.22** Patients with different medical conditions. The woman on the right has filarial elephantiasis of both legs. The boy in the middle has splenomegaly from malaria.

▼ **Fig. 10.23** Elephantiasis of the left leg.

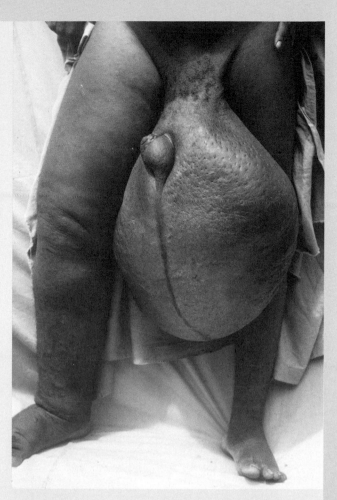

▲ **Fig. 10.24** Elephantiasis of the right leg and scrotum.

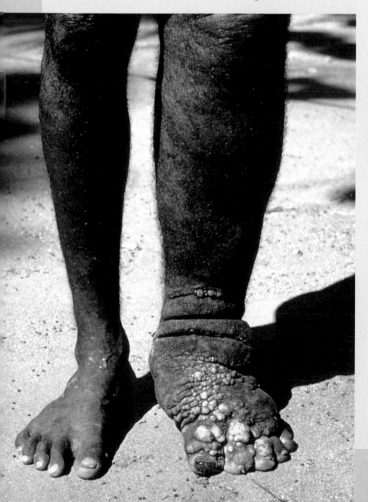

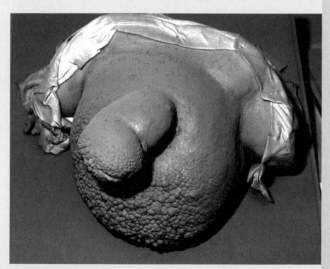

▲ **Fig. 10.25** Wax model from the early 1900s, showing elephantiasis of the scrotum in a man from north Africa.

Onchocerciasis

Onchocerciasis is caused by the filarial worm *Onchocerca volvulus*, which occurs in central Africa and Central and South America. The infection is transmitted from one person to another by a biting black fly (*Simulium*), which lives in the vegetation beside fast-flowing streams and rivers (see Life cycle 10.2).

The adult worms live in the dermis and subcutaneous tissue, where they cause subcutaneous nodules. Microfilariae are found in the dermis and subcutaneous tissue.

The main clinical effects of onchocerciasis are caused by the migrating microfilariae. They cause severe itching, and when they invade the eye they cause keratitis, which may lead on to blindness (depicted in Fig. 10.26).

The diagnosis is confirmed either by finding microfilariae in a sample of fluid extracted from a skin snip, or when a histopathologic examination is made of a subcutaneous lump.

Filariasis (*Onchocerca* species)

Infected humans (adult worms and microfilariae in connective tissue and the dermis of the skin).

↓

Flies of the *Simulium* species transmit microfilariae to uninfected humans.

▲ **Life cycle 10.2** Filariasis—*Onchocerca* species.

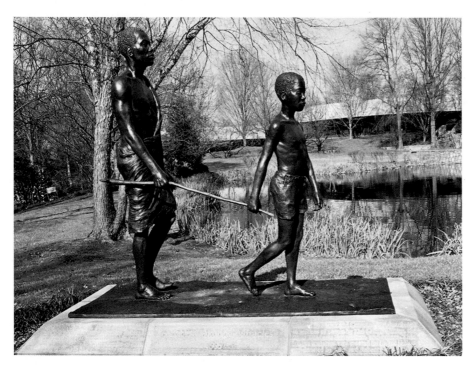

▲ **Fig. 10.26** Bronze sculpture in the grounds of the Jimmy Carter memorial in Atlanta, Georgia, USA. It depicts a young boy leading an old man blinded by onchocerciasis. The tragedy used to be that the boy ultimately would be blind, too. The Jimmy Carter foundation funds research to control onchocerciasis.

Case 10.3

An Australian male, aged 30 years, had been working in Nigeria for some years. While there, he developed a subcutaneous lump over his right hip. When he returned to Brisbane, he had the lump excised. Adult worms and microfilariae were seen in the fibrous nodule, as illustrated in Figures 10.27 and 10.28.

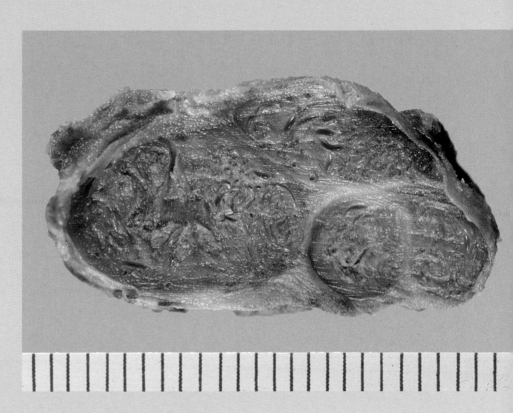

▶ **Fig. 10.27** Cut surface of a subcutaneous lump removed from the right hip region of an Australian male, aged 30 years, who had been working in Nigeria.

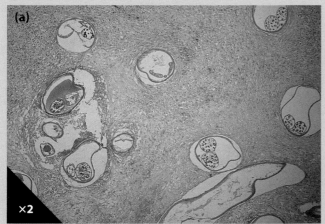

(a) ×2

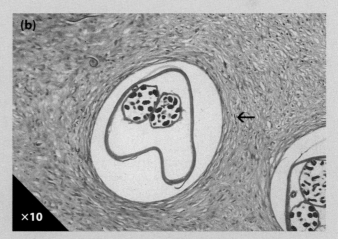

(b) ×10

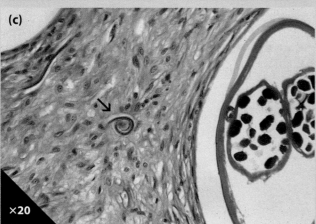

(c) ×20

◀ ▲ **Fig. 10.28(a), (b) and (c)** Microscopic section shows a fibrotic nodule through which there are many adult Onchocerca worms cut in transverse section. The morphology of these worms is similar to that of *W. bancrofti*, but the distinctions are that the adult worms are found in a subcutaneous nodule and not in a lymph node, and the microfilariae (*indicated by the arrow*) are nonsheathed and they are present in the dermis.

Dirofilariasis

Dirofilariasis is an infection with the filarial worm *Dirofilaria immitis*—the dog heartworm. The adult worms form tangled masses in the right ventricle of the hearts of dogs (see Life cycle 10.3). Untreated, this condition results in death of the animal.

Microfilariae circulate in the blood and are transmitted to other animals, and incidentally to humans by a wide variety of mosquito species.

In humans, the worms develop in the right ventricle of the heart and then die before reaching maturity. The dead worms may then become lodged in a small pulmonary artery. Here, they cause thrombosis and an area of infarction of the lung.

The lesions are usually asymptomatic and come to notice only when a chest X-ray for some other reason shows the appearance of a 'coin' lesion. This is removed surgically to exclude a diagnosis of lung tumor.

The correct diagnosis is made by finding the degenerate worm in the center of the infarcted lung tissue.

Dirofilariasis

Dog—adult worm in the heart and microfilariae in the blood.

↓

A number of different species of mosquito transmit microfilariae to humans.

▲ **Life cycle 10.3** Dirofilariasis.

Case 10.4

A female, aged 62 years, was shown to have a 'coin lesion' in the mid zone of the right lung (see Fig. 10.29). This was treated by partial lobectomy. The lesion was shown to be a small area of infarction. In the center of the lesion, a partially necrotic filarial worm was found.

The pathologic changes are illustrated in Figures 10.30–10.33, continued overleaf. A diagnosis of dirofilariasis was made.

▶ **Fig. 10.29** Chest X-ray of a female aged 62 years. There is a rounded, well-circumscribed, mid zone opacity in the right lung. This was treated by partial lobectomy.

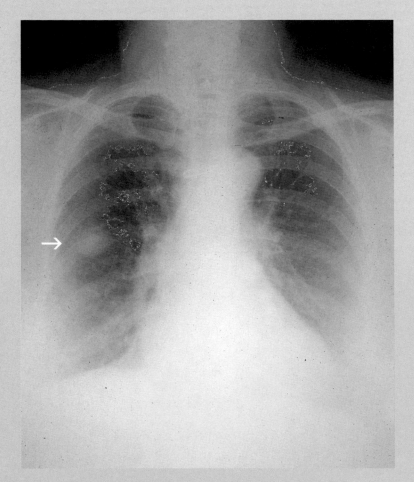

▶ **Fig. 10.30** The lung specimen has been sliced in two. The abnormal area consists of a well-circumscribed, homogeneous, firm, white tumor.

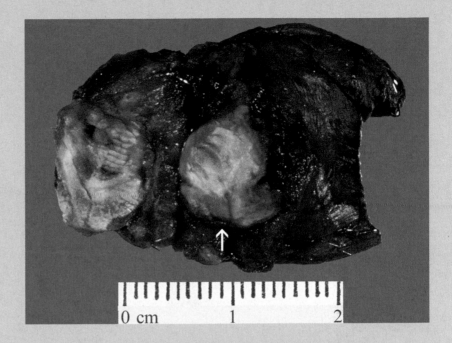

▶ **Fig. 10.31** Microscopic section of this tumor shows that it is an area of necrosis (infarction).

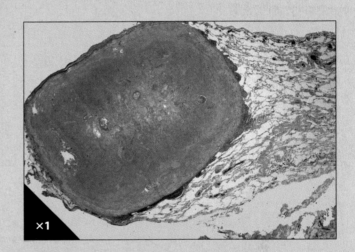

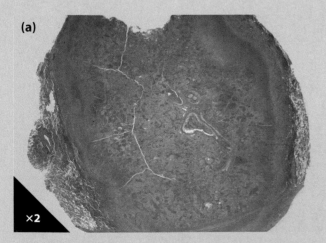

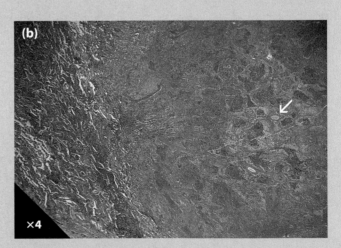

▲ **Fig. 10.32(a) and (b)** The area of necrosis is surrounded by a rim of fibrous tissue, in which there is a chronic inflammatory cell reaction. In the center of the necrotic area, there is a degenerate filarial worm.

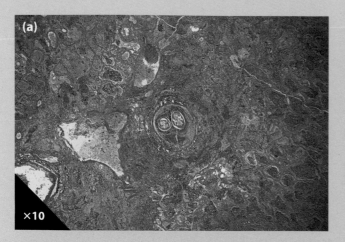

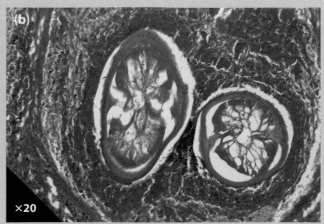

▲ **Fig. 10.33(a) and (b)** The morphology of the worm is shown more clearly at higher magnification.

Trichinosis

Trichinosis occurs when larvae of the nematode *Trichinella spiralis* invade the peripheral muscles of humans.

The adult worms are present in the intestines of pigs, bears and humans (see Life cycle 10.4).

As a result of strict meat inspection laws, the disease is not as widespread as it used to be, and it has become almost confined to hunters of bears or of wild pigs. In Canada, it is estimated that 25 per cent of bears harbor adult *T. spiralis* worms in their intestines (see Fig. 10.34).

Occasionally, infected meat may be mixed with hamburger meat. This practice has resulted in a few minor epidemics of trichinosis.

Once the infected meat is swallowed, the larvae develop into adults in the intestine. The new generation of larvae are passed into the bloodstream and then settle in peripheral muscles. Symptoms include diarrhea, nausea, myalgia and periorbital edema. Patients with myalgia due to trichinosis usually have a marked eosinophilia.

The diagnosis is confirmed by muscle biopsy. Serologic tests may be helpful with antibodies peaking in the second or third month post infection.

Trichinella

Pigs and other animals, e.g. bears, with adult worms in the gut.

↓

Larvae settle in the muscle.

↓

Humans become infected by eating undercooked meat.

▲ **Life cycle 10.4** Trichinella.

▶ **Fig. 10.34** Licensed hunter with the Canadian bear he had shot. It is estimated that 25 per cent of these bears harbor adult *T. spiralis* worms in their intestines.

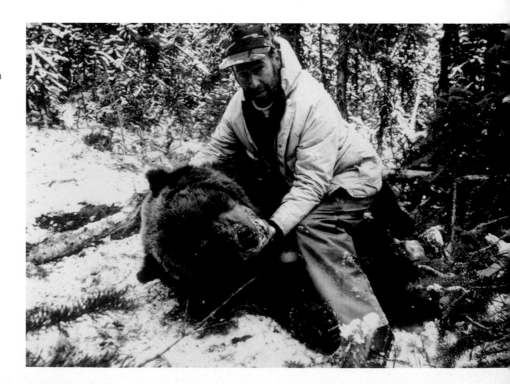

Case 10.5

A young man presented to a hospital in Vancouver, Canada, complaining of generalized myalgia. As part of his investigations, he had a muscle biopsy. This showed the presence of larvae of *T. spiralis* (see Fig. 10.35),

Further history revealed that he had recently eaten hamburger meat at an eatery in an outer suburb of Vancouver. Epidemiologic investigations revealed that a number of other people who had eaten at the same place around that time had similar symptoms. The proprietor was found to have mixed some bear meat he had acquired with the ordinary meat.

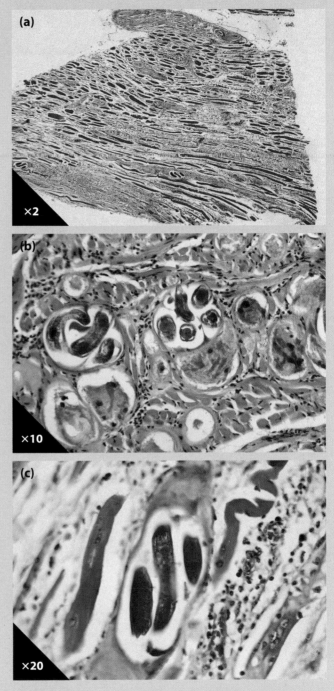

▲ **Fig. 10.35(a), (b) and (c)** Muscle biopsy from a young man who presented with myalgia to a hospital in Vancouver, Canada. Larvae of *T. spiralis* can be seen. There is some fibrosis and chronic inflammation together with a few eosinophils.

Cutaneous larva migrans

Cutaneous larva migrans is a condition caused by penetration of the skin by the infective larvae of dog and cat hookworms. It occurs particularly in children because they are most likely to be playing in soil or sand contaminated by the feces of dogs and cats.

Case 10.6

A male, aged 5 years, presented with an intensely itchy area on his left leg (see Fig. 10.36). It had developed over the previous few days and it appeared to be progressing. It had the appearance of a serpiginous track on the skin surface.

A small biopsy was taken from what appeared to be the advancing end of the track. The biopsy showed an inflammatory reaction that included many eosinophils (see Fig. 10.37, overleaf). No larvae could be seen. The boy was treated with thiabendazole (the recommended drug at the time) and the rash subsided.

▶ **Fig. 10.36(a) and (b)** Cutaneous larva migrans. An itchy rash consisting of serpiginous tracks on the left leg of a male 5 years of age. It had been developing for the previous few days.

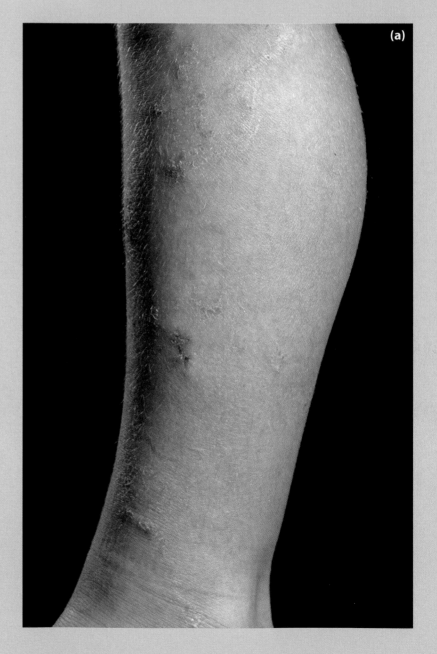

(a)

The track in the skin is made by the movement of the larva through the upper dermis. It is usually not possible to find the larva in a skin biopsy because it is in the skin in advance of the obvious rash on the skin surface. All one sees is the reaction caused by its passage.

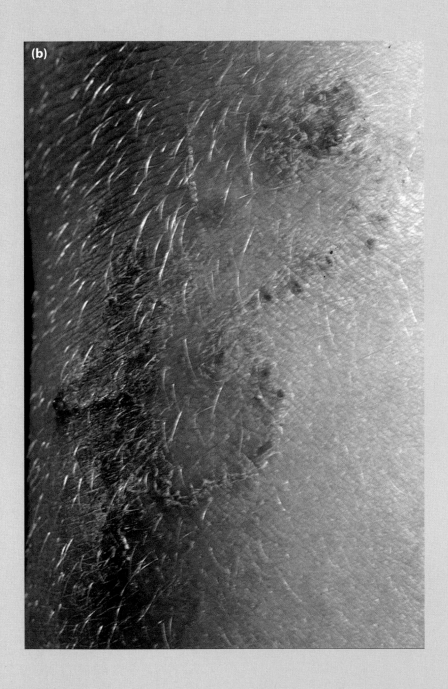

▼ **Fig. 10.37(a), (b) and (c)** Cutaneous larva migrans. Views of a skin biopsy from the advancing end of one of the serpiginous tracks. It shows the typical microscopic features of allergic dermatitis, consistent with an insect bite. The changes being— spongiosis at the dermo epidermal junction, and perivascular inflammatory cell infiltration that extends throughout the dermis and into the subcutaneous tissue. The predominant inflammatory cell is the eosinophil. No larvae were found.

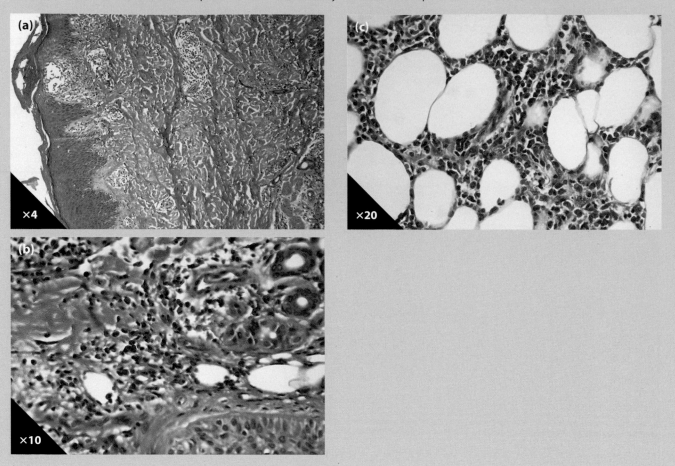

Visceral larva migrans

Visceral larva migrans occurs as a result of penetration of the viscera of humans by the larvae of *Toxocara canis* and *Toxocara cati* that occur commonly in the intestines of dogs and cats.

Case 10.7

A child with fever and eosinophilia had a diagnostic liver biopsy. A granuloma was found, in which a transverse section of a nematode larva consistent with *T. canis* was identified (see Fig. 10.38).

Serologic tests are now available for diagnosis but they were not available when this case was received into the pathology department of the hospital.

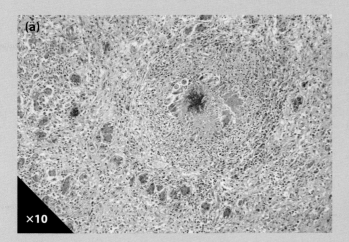
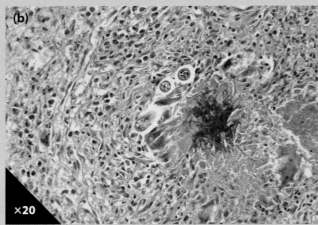

▲ **Fig. 10.38(a) and (b)** Views of a granuloma in a liver biopsy, showing a granuloma containing a transverse section of a larva consistent with *T. canis*.

Angiostrongyloidiasis

Angiostrongyloidiasis is a condition in which the nematode *Angiostrongylus cantonensis* invades the spinal cord causing eosinophilic meningitis, and the brain causing encephalitis. Human infections with this organism have been reported in Indonesia, Thailand, Vietnam, the Philippines, Australia and a number of islands in the Pacific Ocean.

The rat is the main host with the worm being found in the lungs, hence the name 'rat lung worm' (see Life cycle 10.5).

The intermediate hosts are slugs or snails. Humans become infected by accidentally eating infected slugs or snails or the mucus these animals leave on fresh vegetables in vegetable gardens.

Angiostrongylus

Adult worms in rats.

↓

Larvae passed in feces are ingested by snails.

↓

Snails are eaten by rats.

Humans are infected by eating snails which may be on green vegetables.

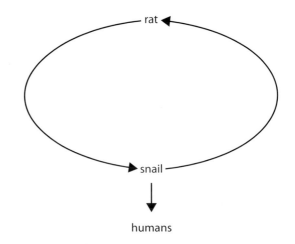

▲ **Life cycle 10.5** Angiostrongylus.

Case 10.8

A 12-month-old male presented at a children's hospital in Brisbane with a history of being unwell for 2 days. He was lethargic and would not move his legs. He was afebrile, hypertensive and had a rash on the thighs. There were no objective signs of joint or nerve damage.

Over the next few days, the lassitude increased and he became areflexic. On the sixth day of admission, he developed a temperature. Cerebrospinal fluid examination revealed 300 cells/cubic mm. Most of these cells were eosinophils. The rest were mononuclear cells.

The next day, a small worm was seen in his retina (see Fig. 10.39). This was sucked out and identified as an angiostrongylus worm.

A diagnosis of eosinophilic meningitis due to *A. cantonensis* was made.

Mental deterioration progressed and death occurred 3 weeks after admission. In the days before death, respiratory difficulties were encountered and some non-diagnostic opacities were seen on chest X-ray.

Post-mortem examination revealed extensive hemorrhage and necrosis in the white matter of the brain. The grey matter was relatively spared. Many small worms were visible in the necrotic tissue.

The distal part of the spinal cord showed gross edema and extensive necrosis and hemorrhage of the neural tissue. Numerous adult worms were present in the necrotic tissue. The lungs showed a number of solid areas that had the appearance of infarcts.

The pathologic and parasitologic features are illustrated in Figures 10.40–10.57 (see pages 376–381).

▼ **Fig. 10.39** Angiostrongyloidiasis. Ophthalmoscopic view of a worm in the retina. The worm appears as a black filament (*indicated by the arrow*). In reality, it was moving.

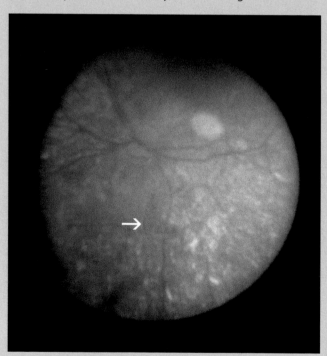

▼ **Fig. 10.40** Lumbar spinal cord and cauda equina. The dura has been opened to reveal the spinal cord. The distal half of the cord shows gross edema with necrosis and hemorrhage. Large numbers of small worms can be seen in the necrotic neural tissue.

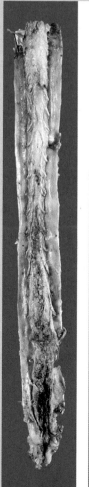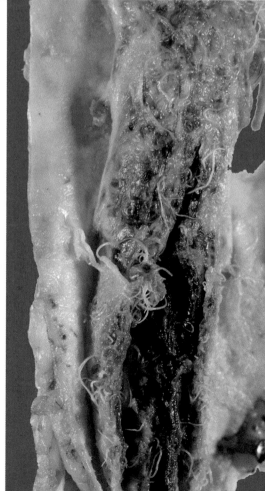

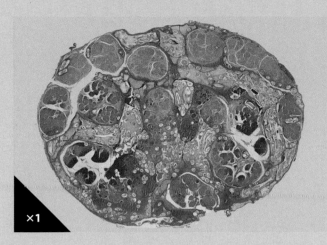

▲ **Fig. 10.41** Transverse section taken through the cauda equina. The hemorrhage and necrosis can be seen. The individual nerve bundles of the cauda are widely separated by the worms and the inflammatory response they have elicited.

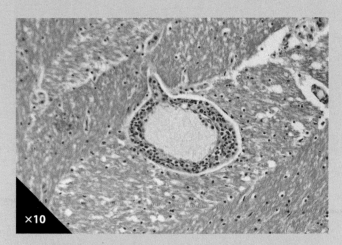

▲ **Fig. 10.44** At a higher magnification, the predominance of eosinophils in the inflammatory infiltration can be seen; hence the name 'eosinophilic meningitis' for this condition.

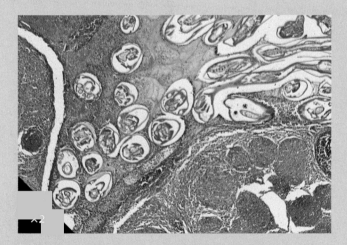

▲ **Fig. 10.42** The cauda equina showing partially degenerate worms.

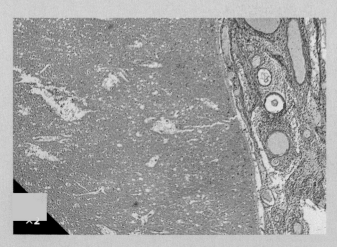

▲ **Fig. 10.43** Transverse section through the lumbar spinal cord showing the inflammatory infiltration in the subarachnoid space (*on the right*).

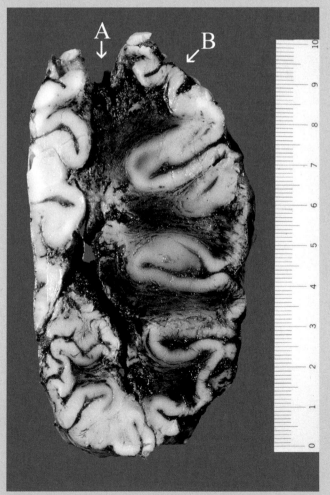

▲ **Fig. 10.45** Slice through one hemisphere of the brain. It shows extensive hemorrhage and necrosis in the white matter (A). The grey matter is relatively spared (B).

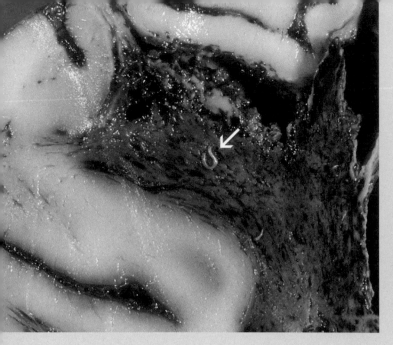

▲ **Fig. 10.46** Closer view of another area of the brain. The hemorrhage and necrosis in the white matter is more clearly visible and a worm can be seen in this tissue. The cortical grey matter is edematous and partially necrotic.

▲ **Fig. 10.47** View of the edge of the sulcus noted in Figure 10.46, which shows the necrosis of the white matter (encephalomalacea) and the worm noted macroscopically.

▼ **Fig. 10.48** Vertical slice through the left lung. It shows a wedge-shaped, firm area in the middle lobe, which has the appearance of a pulmonary infarct (*indicated by the arrow*).

▼ **Fig. 10.49(a) and (b)** These views show the infarction was caused by worms occluding the pulmonary artery.

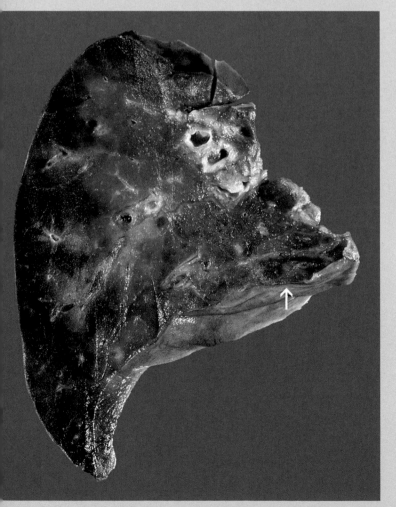

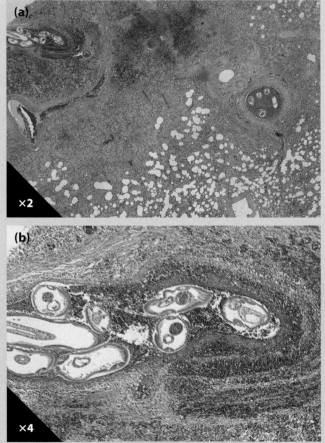

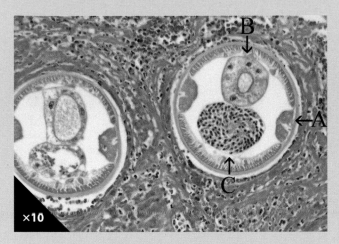

▲ **Fig. 10.50** Transverse section of a moderately well-preserved worm. It is the lower end of a male worm. The body wall and the two lateral chords (A) are seen. The internal structure consists of alimentary canal (B) and testis (C).

▼ **Fig. 10.51(a) and (b)** Degenerate worm that has elicited a brisk eosinophil reaction.

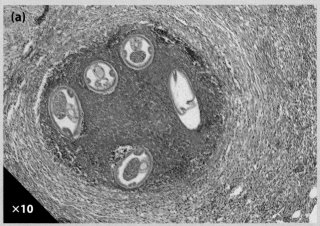

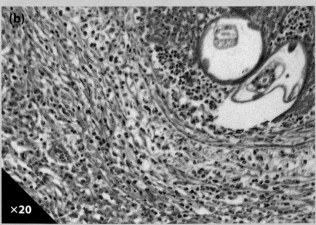

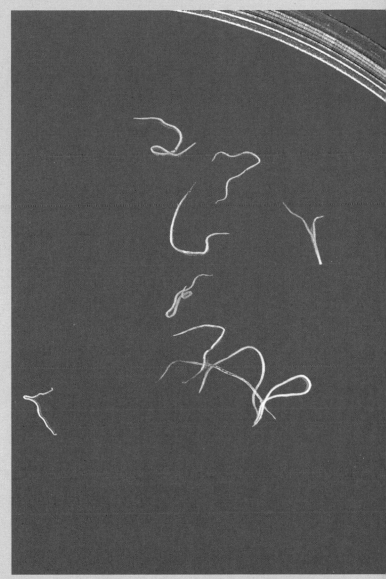

▲ **Fig. 10.52** Angiostrongylus worms were recovered from the formalin solution in which the spinal cord was fixed, and from the spinal cord itself. The worms each measured about 10–12 mm in length. Single worms were then placed in mounting medium on a microscope slide in order to examine their morphology in greater detail.

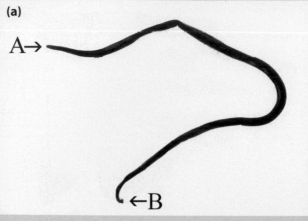

(a)

A→

←B

(b)

←B

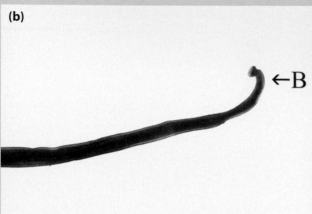

(c)

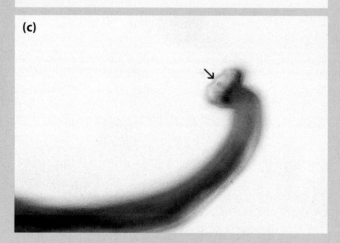

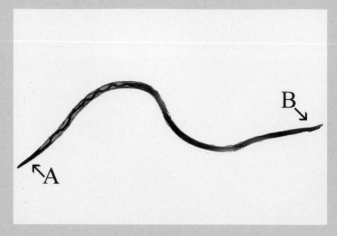

B↘

↖A

▲ **Fig. 10.54** Angiostrongylus female worm. Head (A). Tail (B).

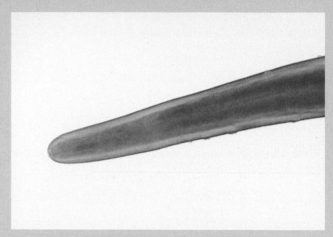

▲ **Fig. 10.55** Angiostrongylus. Head end of the female worm showing the esophagus.

▲ **Fig. 10.53** Angiostrongylus male worm. **(a) and (b)** Note the pointed head (anterior) end (A) and the slightly curved tail (posterior) end (B). The tail end has a copulatory bursa. **(c)** One of the two copulatory spicules in the bursa.

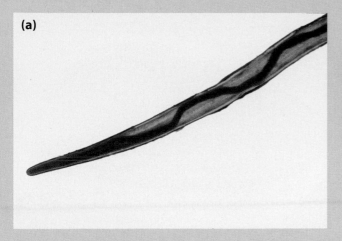
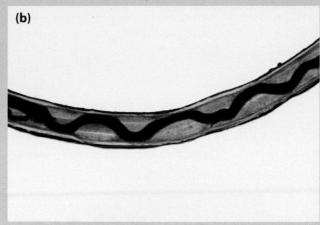

▲ **Fig. 10.56(a) and (b)** Angiostrongylus. Within the female worm, the uterus coils around the intestine.

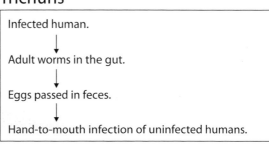

▶ **Fig. 10.57** Angiostrongylus. Tail end of the female worm.

Trichuriasis

Trichuriasis is caused by hand-to-mouth infection with the nematode *Trichuris trichiura* (the whipworm) (see Life cycle 10.6).

The thin anterior end of the worm becomes attached to the mucosa of the cecum or colon. The worm occurs in all parts of the world and is one of the most common parasitic infections of humans. Infection with *T. trichiura* is usually asymptomatic.

The eggs are found during a routine examination of feces. The eggs have a characteristic oval shape, with a plug in each end. They measure approximately 50 × 20 microns and they are a light brown color (shown in Fig. 10.58, overleaf). The adult worms are 30–40 mm in length. The males have a tightly curled tail, and the female has a pointed tail.

Trichuris

Infected human.
↓
Adult worms in the gut.
↓
Eggs passed in feces.
↓
Hand-to-mouth infection of uninfected humans.

▲ **Life cycle 10.6** Trichuris.

The pathology of some worms found during routine pathologic practice in Papua New Guinea are illustrated in Figures 10.59–10.63.

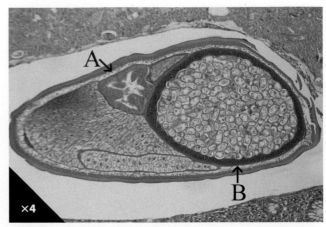

▲ **Fig. 10.60** *T. trichiura*. Section through the body of the worm. Alimentary canal (A). Uterus containing eggs (B).

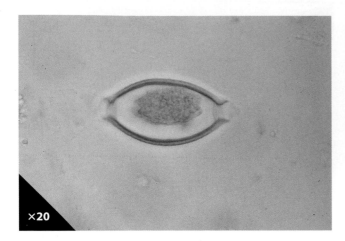

▲ **Fig. 10.58** *T. trichiura*. Trichuris egg in a sample of feces. The light brown, oval egg has a plug at each end.

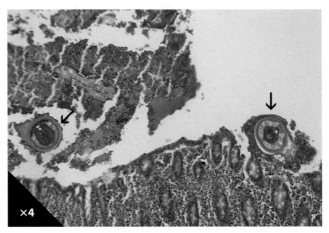

▲ **Fig. 10.61** *T. trichiura*. Two segments of the head end of the worm embedded in the muscosal epithelium.

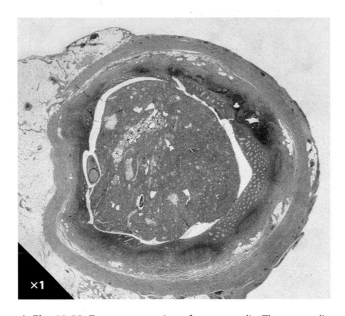

▲ **Fig. 10.59** Transverse section of an appendix. The appendix is not inflamed but transverse sections of a worm can be seen in the lumen. There are two components to the worm: a larger component and two smaller components. They correspond to a transverse section through the body and head respectively of a Trichuris worm.

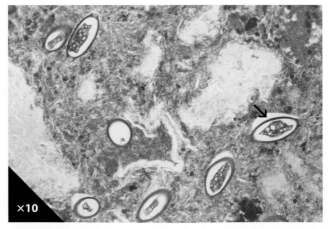

▲ **Fig. 10.62** Feces in the lumen of an appendix with some Trichuris eggs.

▶ **Fig. 10.63** In another area of the section shown in Figure 10.62, eggs of *Ascaris lumbricoides* can be seen as well (*indicated by the arrow*)—so there was a mixed infection (which is quite common in areas of high parasitic endemicity).

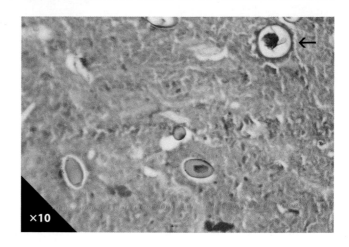

Case 10.9

A 12-year-old male from a tropical country was admitted to a sophisticated children's teaching hospital in a nontropical country. The boy was complaining of severe melena. As part of the diagnostic work-up, an isotope scan was performed (see Fig. 10.64). This indicated that the major bleeding was occurring in the region of the cecum.

A clinical diagnosis of angiodysplasia was made. The cecum was examined with a pediatric endoscope through a small incision made in the cecum. The bleeding area was identified (see Fig. 10.65, overleaf) and the abnormal area of cecum was excised.

When the bowel was opened and the blood cleared away, there were numerous *T. Trichuris* worms attached to the mucosa. It was then clear that what is usually a trivial and common parasitic infection had been overinvestigated and overtreated. The surgical pathology involved is illustrated in Figures 10.66–10.71, overleaf.

It is extremely unusual for T. trichiura *infection to produce clinical symptoms. This case illustrates how* T. trichiura *can cause clinical symptoms and how in a sophisticated medical environment an incorrect diagnosis can be made.*

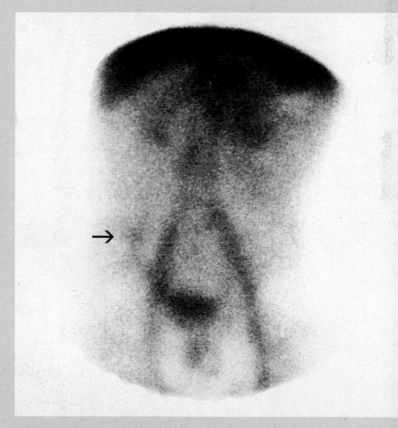

▲ **Fig. 10.64** Isotope scan showed a bleeding site in the region of the cecum.

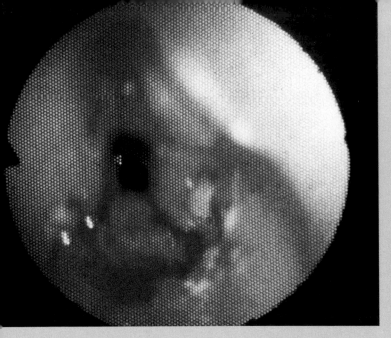

▲ **Fig. 10.65** Bleeding area in the cecum, viewed through a pediatric endoscope.

▼ **Fig. 10.66** Piece of the cecum showed the presence of one of the many worms that were attached to the mucosal epithelium.

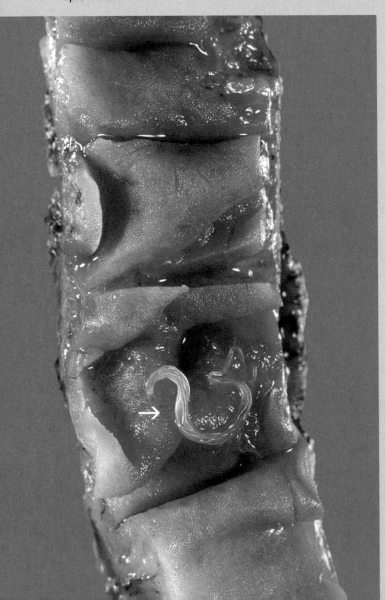

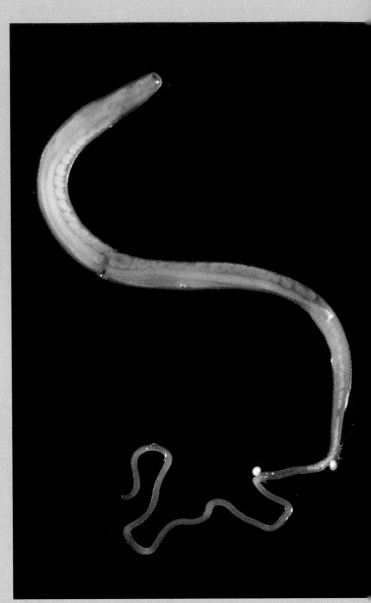

▲ **Fig. 10.67** One of the worms removed from the specimen. It shows the characteristic appearance of an adult *T. trichiura* worm. The head end is thin, and the body and tail are much thicker. This appearance has led to the name 'whipworm' for this parasite.

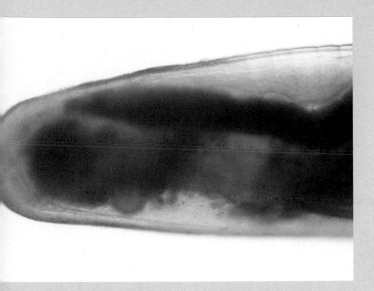

▲ **Fig. 10.68** Tail of a female Trichuris worm.

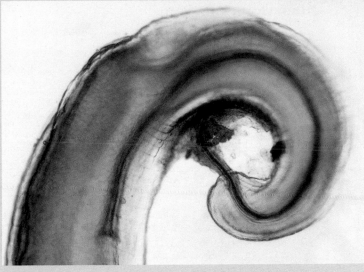

▲ **Fig. 10.69** Hooked tail of a male Trichuris worm, showing the retractile spicule.

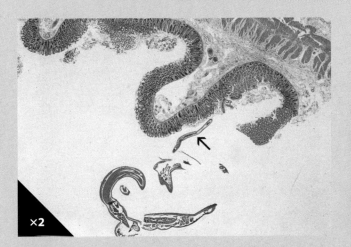

×2

▲ **Fig. 10.70** View of a Trichuris worm with its head end embedded in the mucosa of the cecum.

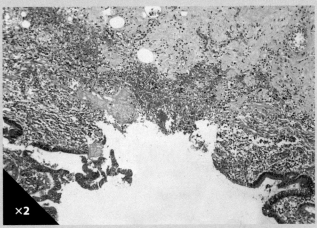

×2

▲ **Fig. 10.71** View of one of the many mucosal ulcers in the cecum caused by the Trichuris worms. Presumably, the bleeding was coming from these ulcers.

Hookworm infection

The two species of hookworm—*Ancylostoma* and *Necator*—that are found in humans can be distinguished by specialist parasitologists, but both species produce the same pathology. The organism is found in almost all parts of the world.

There is no intermediate host. Eggs are passed in the feces of humans. Infective larvae (filariform larvae) hatch from the eggs and then invade unprotected skin of humans who may be sitting or walking in the contaminated area (see Life cycle 10.7).

The adult worms become attached to the mucosa of the duodenum. They cause blood loss, resulting from the ulceration of the mucosa as the organisms attach themselves to the mucosal epithelium. In the majority of cases, infection is asymptomatic but the commonest presentation is with symptoms of iron deficiency anemia.

The pathologic and parasitologic features of hookworm infection are demonstrated in Figures 10.72–10.79, continued overleaf.

Hookworms

Infected human.

↓

Adult worm in the gut.

↓

Eggs passed in feces.

↓

Motile larvae develop in soil.

↓

Larvae penetrate the skin (usually through the feet of uninfected humans).

▲ **Life cycle 10.7** Hookworms.

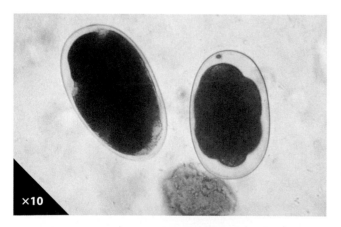

▲ **Fig. 10.72** Hookworm eggs in a sample of feces. The eggs are fairly large (60 × 40 microns), being easily visible with a ×10 objective of the microscope. The developing larvae can be seen through the transparent 'egg shell'. It is important to know how fresh the feces sample is—because about 24 hours after the feces has been passed, the hookworm larvae hatch and become motile. Morphologically, they resemble the larvae of *S. stercoralis*. So, the feces should be examined as soon as possible after it has been passed.

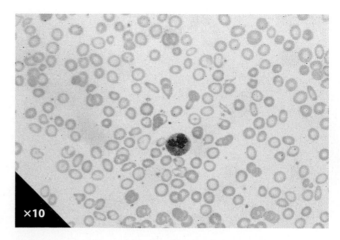

▲ **Fig. 10.73** Peripheral blood smear showing the features of an iron deficiency anemia—hypochromic, microcytic red blood cells. There is an eosinophil in the field, representing the fact that the iron deficiency anemia of hookworm infection is usually associated with an eosinophilia.

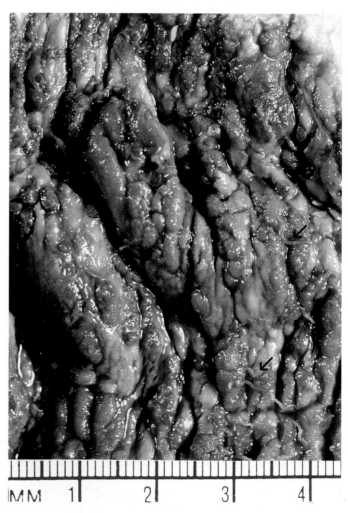

▲ **Fig. 10.74** Piece of small intestine from a child from Papua New Guinea suffering from Pig Bel (*Enteritis Necroticans*) caused by the exotoxin of *Clostridium perfringens*. An incidental finding is the presence of numerous small, white, thread-like worms attached to the mucosa (*indicated by the arrows*). These are adult hookworms (see also Fig. 10.94).

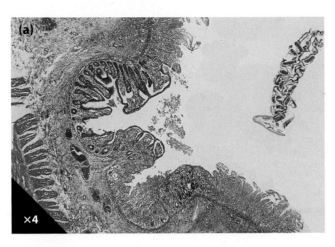

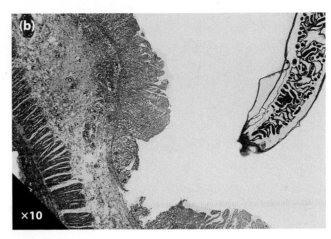

▲ **Fig. 10.75(a) and (b)** Views of a hookworm attached to an ulcer of the mucosal surface of the duodenum.

▶ **Fig. 10.76** Adult hookworms are about 10 mm long. The head end (anterior end) (A) is turned backwards at an acute angle, with the appearance of a hook, which gives the worm its name. The tail end of the female is pointed (B). The worm pictured here is a female.

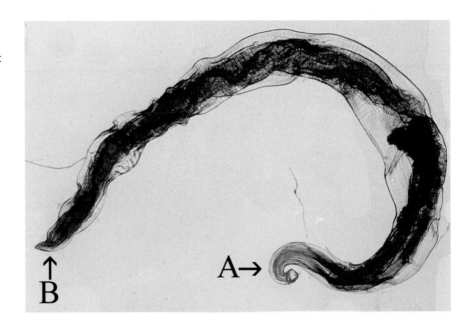

▶ **Fig. 10.77** The head end of the hookworm shows the 'teeth' by which the worm attaches itself to the mucosa. The esophagus can be seen through the cuticle.

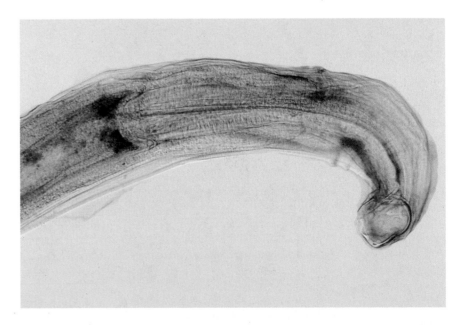

▶ **Fig. 10.78** Male hookworm—recognized by the appearance of the copulatory bursa at the tail end.

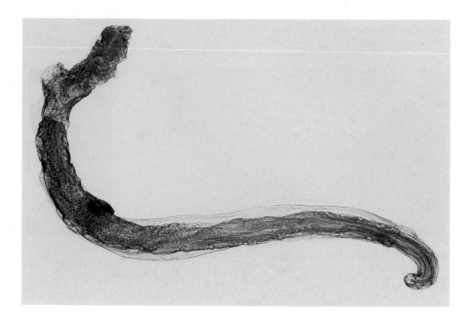

▶ **Fig. 10.79** Male hookworm—close-up view of the copulatory bursa (not shown in Fig. 10.78).

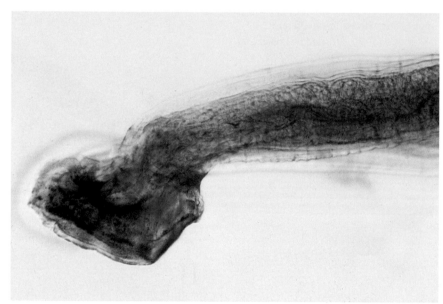

Strongyloidiasis

Strongyloidiasis is an infection with the nematode *Strongyloides stercoralis*. The motile larvae are passed in feces and become infective larvae in the soil, penetrating the skin of humans (see Life cycle 10.8).

It occurs worldwide and is a cause of diarrhea, particularly in malnourished children and in people who are immune suppressed.

The adult worms live in the small intestine. Motile, noninfective rhabditiform larvae are passed in the feces and transform into infective filariform larvae, which then penetrate the skin of the next host.

The diagnosis is made by finding motile larvae in freshly passed feces or by finding adult females or larvae in small intestinal biopsies. Serologic tests are also available for diagnosis.

Strongyloides

Infected human.

↓

Adult worm in the gut.

↓

Motile larvae passed in feces.

↓

In the soil they become infective larvae that penetrate the skin of uninfected humans.

▲ **Life cycle 10.8** Strongyloides.

Case 10.10

A 15-month-old, severely malnourished child died of pneumonia and meningitis. Post-mortem examination revealed a heavy infection with *S. stercoralis* parasites in the small intestine. This was considered to be so severe as to have contributed to the death of the child. This is an example of the so-called hyperinfection with a parasite (see Figs 10.80–10.84).

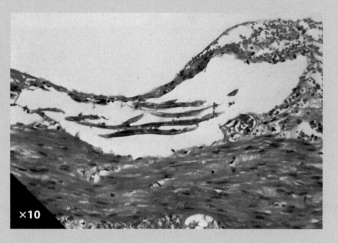

▲ **Fig. 10.82** Longitudinal section shows the presence of larvae in the base of an ulcer.

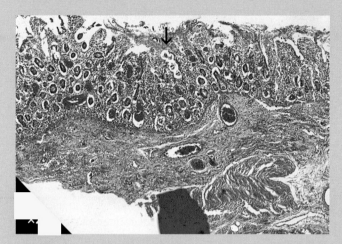

▲ **Fig. 10.80** Section of the duodenum. An adult female *S. stercoralis* can be seen in one of the crypts.

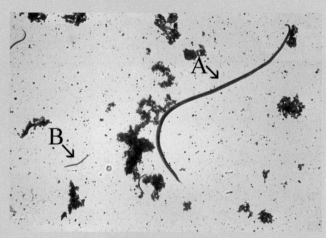

▲ **Fig. 10.83** Microscopic preparation made from feces taken from the duodenum shows an adult female worm (A) and a number of larvae (B).

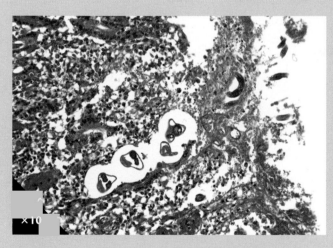

▲ **Fig. 10.81** At a higher magnification, the transverse sections of the female worm show the presence of an alimentary canal and a bi-lobed uterus within the cuticle of the worm.

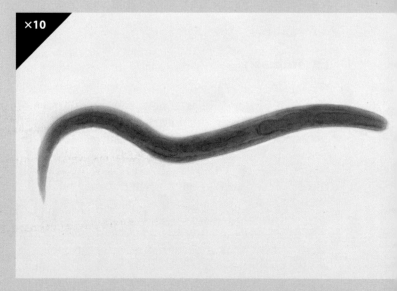

▲ **Fig. 10.84** *S. stercoralis* larva in a feces sample. It was motile in the fresh preparation.

To detect the presence of motile larvae, rather than doing a simple microscopic examination on feces, a more accurate test is to inoculate a concentrated specimen of feces onto an agar plate and to incubate it for 2 days. The parasites make tracks through the agar: all stages of the parasite can be seen on the plate (see Figs 10.85 and 10.86).

Serologic tests also are available for diagnosis.

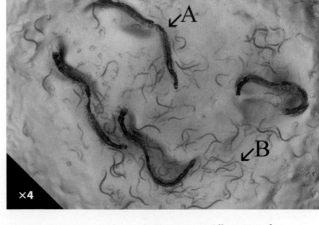

▲ **Fig. 10.86** All stages of *S. stercoralis* parasites, adults (A) and larvae (B) can be seen in the agar.

▼ **Fig. 10.85(a) and (b)** *(Left)* Concentrated specimen of feces inoculated onto an agar plate and incubated for 2 days. *(Right)* 'Tracks' made by the developing *S. stercoralis* parasites can be seen in the agar.

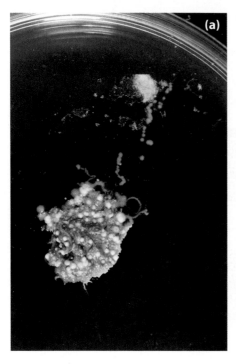

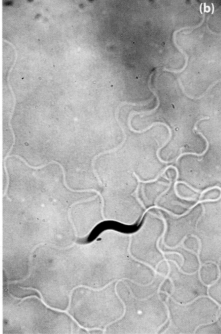

▶ **Fig. 10.87** Longitudinal section of an appendix. The lumen is filled with small Enterobius worms.

Enterobiasis

Enterobiasis is an infection by the nematode *Enterobius vermicularis* (pinworm). The worm is found in most countries of the world. Children are more often affected than adults. Transmission is by feces to hand-to-mouth contamination (see Life cycle 10.9).

The adult worms live in the colon. Male worms die after copulation and so they are not often found. The female migrates to the anus and deposits eggs on the perianal and perineal skin. This produces localized itching.

Enterobius worms are most frequently observed as incidental findings in appendectomy specimens. It is debatable whether the presence of worms in the appendix contribute to the symptomatology that results in appendectomy. Figures 10.87–10.91, continued overleaf, illustrate a case of Enterobius worms in an appendectomy specimen.

Enterobius eggs can be found in feces and sometimes in Pap smears, as illustrated in Figures 10.92 and 10.93, overleaf.

Enterobius

Infected human. Adult worms in the gut.

↓

Eggs passed in feces.

↓

Hand-to-mouth infection of uninfected humans.

▲ **Life cycle 10.9** Enterobius.

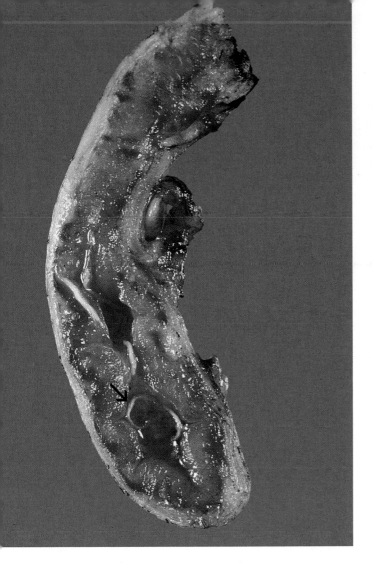

▼ Fig. 10.88 Microscopic view of a longitudinal section through the appendix, showing the Enterobius worms mainly cut in longitudinal section.

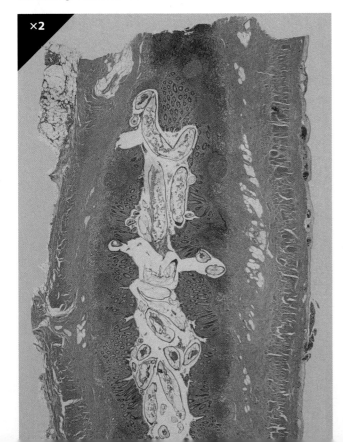

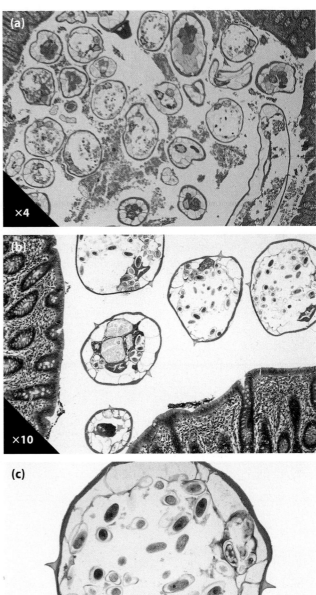

▲ Fig. 10.89(a) and (b) Views of female Enterobius worms cut in transverse section. **(c)** Lateral alae on the surface of the cuticle and eggs in the uterus are well seen.

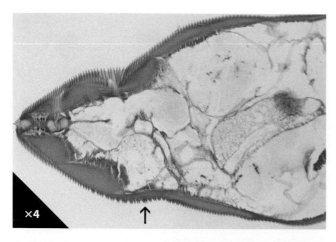

▲ **Fig. 10.90** Longitudinal section of the head end of a female Enterobius worm showing the lateral alae along the length of its cuticular covering.

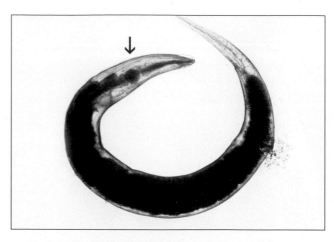

▲ **Fig. 10.91** Female Enterobius worm removed from the appendix. It measured 10 mm in length. The esophagus leads from the mouth to the prominent esophageal bulb (*indicated by the arrow*). The remainder of the worm is composed of uterus filled with eggs. The worm has a pointed tail.

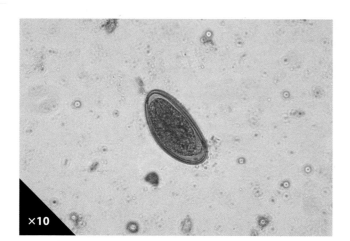

▲ **Fig. 10.92** Enterobius egg in a sample of feces. Eggs can be seen in feces or in a cellophane tape preparation from the perineum. They measure approximately 20 × 40 microns. They have a transparent capsule and they are flattened on one side.

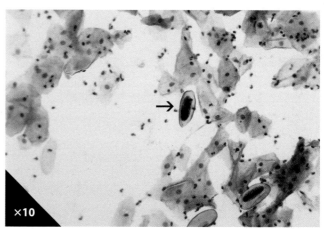

▲ **Fig. 10.93** Enterobius eggs sometimes can be seen as incidental findings in Papanicolaou smears from the cervix, as shown here.

Ascariasis

Ascariasis is caused by the nematode *Ascaris lumbricoides*. Adult worms live in the small intestine of humans. They vary in size from about 150 to 300 mm. Eggs are passed in the feces. The larval stage has a complicated life cycle, which includes passage through the lung (see Life cycle 10.10).

This parasite occurs in most parts of the tropical world and it is one of the most common parasites of humans. In endemic areas, in spite of a high infection rate, pathology caused by the worms is quite uncommon.

Worms are sometimes passed in feces, sometimes vomited or coughed up, and eggs are found in a high proportion of feces examined in any laboratory in any tropical country (see Figs 10.94–10.98, continued overleaf).

Serious pathology occurs in a heavy infestation, when worms become matted together and produce intestinal obstruction—usually in the region of the terminal ileum. This complication is frequently seen soon after commencement of antihelminthic drug therapy.

Worms sometimes migrate into the common bile duct, where they cause biliary colic.

Ascaris

> Humans and pigs with adult worms in the gut.
>
> ↓
>
> Eggs passed in feces.
>
> ↓
>
> Hand-to-mouth infection of uninfected humans.
> - Larvae develop in the small intestine and enter the bloodstream.
> - They pass through the lungs sometimes causing eosinophilic pneumonitis.
> - Larvae are then coughed up and swallowed.
> - When they next enter the small intestine they develop into adults.

▲ **Life cycle 10.10** Ascaris.

▶ **Fig. 10.94** Opened small intestine of a male, aged 6 years, from Papua New Guinea. The child had the condition called Pig Bel (*Enteritis Necroticans*), which is caused by the exotoxin of *Clostridium perfringens*. The adult Ascaris worms in the intestine were incidental findings. Of interest is the added presence of an adult hookworm towards the top left end of the specimen. This underlines the fact that ascaris and hookworm infections are very common in communities in tropical countries.

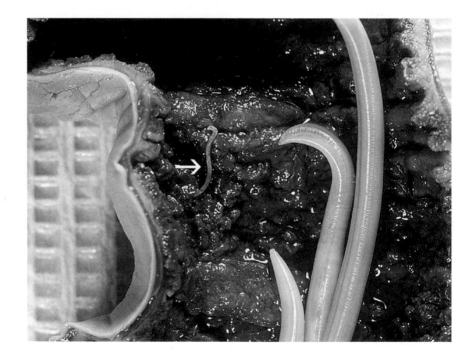

▶ **Fig. 10.95** Male Ascaris worm. The male has a tightly coiled tail.

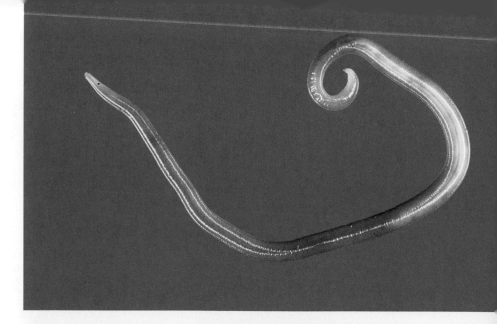

▶ **Fig. 10.96** Female Ascaris worm. The females have a pointed tail. Females reach a length of 350 mm. Males are somewhat smaller at 150–300 mm.

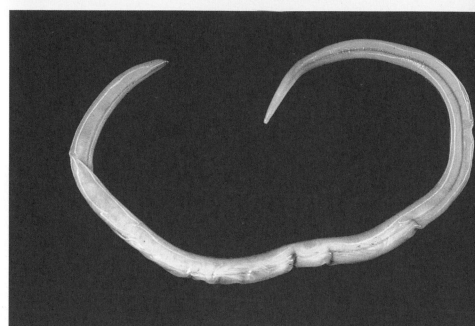

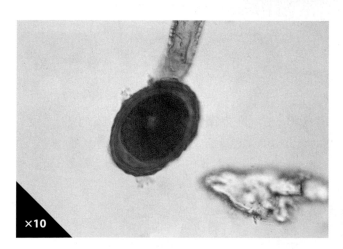

▲ **Fig. 10.97** Microscopic preparation of feces shows the characteristic brownish-colored Ascaris egg. The eggs measure approximately 50 × 40 microns. They are oval, with a thick shell: the shell may be smooth—but more frequently (as in this case), they have a bosselated surface. Fertile eggs may lose their outer bosselated layer.

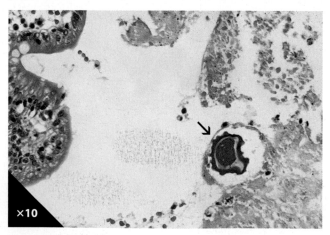

▲ **Fig. 10.98** Ascaris egg in the lumen of a tissue section of small intestine. The microscopic section was stained with routine hematoxylin and eosin (H&E) stain.

Case 10.11

A 41-year-old male Chinese seaman, whose ship was visiting the port of Brisbane in Australia, presented with a history of intermittent right upper abdominal pain for about 6 months.

A computed tomography (CT) scan of the upper abdomen showed dilatation of intrahepatic bile ducts (see Fig. 10.99). Endoscopy was performed and radio-opaque dye was injected in a retrograde manner into the common bile duct.

The X-ray showed marked dilatation of the common bile duct. There was a longitudinal filling defect within the duct (see Fig. 10.100).

The endoscopist noticed the tail of an Ascaris worm protruding through the ampulla of Vater. He clamped this and extracted the worm (see Fig. 10.101). This resulted in relief of the patient's symptoms. The patient was given follow-up drug treatment for his ascaris infection.

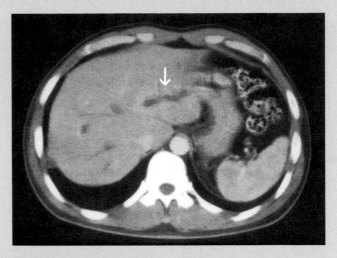

▲ **Fig. 10.99** CT scan of the upper abdomen showed dilatation of intrahepatic bile ducts.

▼ **Fig. 10.100** X-ray performed under endoscopic guidance showed marked dilatation of the common bile duct. There was a longitudinal filling defect within the duct.

▼ **Fig. 10.101** An Ascaris worm protruding from the ampulla of Vater was noticed by the endoscopist, who clamped it and removed it.

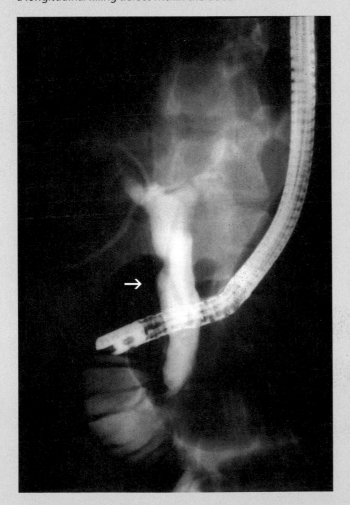

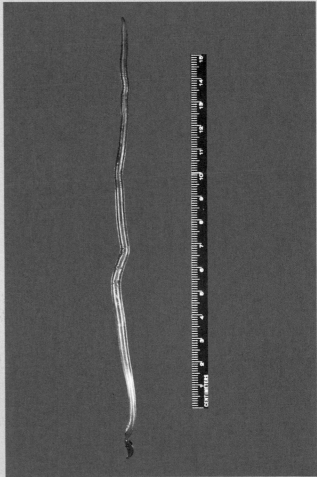

Trematodes

Schistosomiasis

Historical overview

The adult Schistosoma worms were first identified in Egypt in 1851, by Theodore Bilharz (1825–1862), who was a graduate of Freiburg University, Germany. The disease is sometimes called Bilharzia after him.

The life cycle through the snail host was identified in Egypt in 1914 by a team of scientists commissioned by the British Army to investigate this subject. The team leader was Robert Lieper (1881–1969), Director of the Division of Medical Zoology at the London School of Tropical Medicine.

The disease caused by S. japonicum *was elucidated by a number of Japanese workers. Perhaps the first account was in 1847 by Daijiro Fujii. He described a disease that was very common among the workers in the rice fields near Kata Mountain (Katayama), situated about 55 miles (85.5 km) north-west of Tokyo. From his description, it appears that sufferers died from portal hypertension and liver failure.*

In 1888, Tokuho Majima described the macroscopic and microscopic post-mortem appearances of cirrhosis and portal hypertension in a patient with Katayama disease. He drew the parasitic eggs that he found in the sections of liver. In retrospect, they resemble those of S. japonicum.

Fujiro Katsurada (1867–1946) trained at Tokyo University, Japan, and the University of Freiburg, Germany, and then became the Professor of Medicine at the Okayama Medical College.

In 1904, Katsurada published a definitive article on Katayama disease, which was prevalent in a number of widely separated prefectures throughout Japan. He identified the adult worm and its egg, and showed that it was the cause of Katayama disease by identifying the parasite in post-mortem tissue from patients who died from the disease. He pointed out that it was related to the parasite described by Bilharz but was distinctly different. He named the parasite Schistosoma japonicum.

Nowadays, the term 'Katayama fever' is used for the systemic illness that occurs early in the infection.

There are three different species of schistosomes—*Schistosoma haematobium, Schistosoma mansoni* and *Schistosoma japonicum.*

Infection occurs throughout the Middle East and Africa, South-East Asia and in South America.

- *S. haematobium* and *S. mansoni* are the causative species in Africa and South America.
- *S. japonicum* is the species in South-East Asia.

The intermediate host is a freshwater snail. For *S. haematobium* and *S. mansoni*, humans appear to be the definitive host. *S. japonicum* may be found in wild and domestic animals, as well as in humans (see Life cycle 10.11(a) and (b)). This

Schistosomes—other than *S. japonicum*

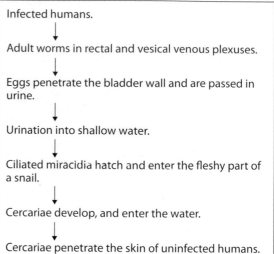

Infected humans.
↓
Adult worms in rectal and vesical venous plexuses.
↓
Eggs penetrate the bladder wall and are passed in urine.
↓
Urination into shallow water.
↓
Ciliated miracidia hatch and enter the fleshy part of a snail.
↓
Cercariae develop, and enter the water.
↓
Cercariae penetrate the skin of uninfected humans.

▲ **Life cycle 10.11(a)** Schistosomes other than *S. japonicum.*

Schistosomes—*S. japonicum*

Adult worms in rectal and vesical venous plexuses of infected humans and some reservoir animals.
↓
Eggs passed in feces. If feces are passed into water, ciliated miracidia emerge from the eggs and enter a snail.
↓
Cercariae develop and enter the water.
↓
Cercariae penetrate the skin of uninfected humans.

▲ **Life cycle 10.11(b)** *S. japonicum.*

extra reservoir host adds to the problems of disease control for this species.

The adult worms live in the blood vessels around the bladder and rectum. Eggs are passed in urine or feces.

- The egg of *S. haematobium* has a terminal spine (shown in Figs 10.102, 10.103 and 10.104).
- The egg of *S. mansoni* has a lateral spine (see Fig. 10.105).
- The egg of *S. japonicum* has a tiny and almost invisible spine on its outer shell.

The infective larva in the form of a miracidium quickly hatches and enters the flesh of the hump of a freshwater snail. Here, it develops into a fork-tailed form called a cercaria. The cercaria leaves the snail and swims in the shallow water of freshwater lakes and irrigation canals.

It penetrates the skin of humans wading in the shallow water. It then develops into an adult worm, which repeats the cycle.

The time taken between penetration of the skin to development of symptoms (the pre-patent period) is between 2 and 4 weeks.

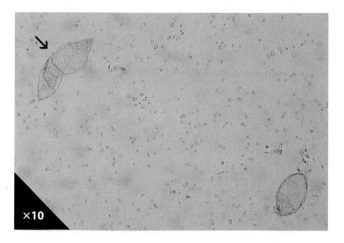

▲ **Fig. 10.102** Microurine showing the presence of red blood cells and a number of eggs with terminal spines (*S. haematobium*). Miracidia were hatching from some of the eggs (*see arrow*).

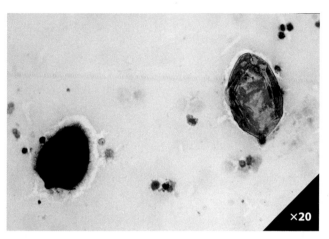

▲ **Fig. 10.104** Papanicolaou stain of a dried smear preparation made from the urine. It shows the eggs of *S. haematobium* with terminal spines (but not as clearly as in Fig. 10.103).

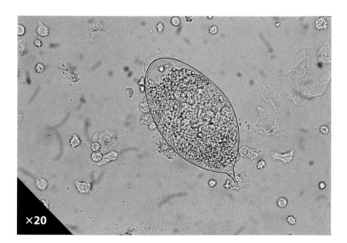

▲ **Fig. 10.103** An egg with a terminal spine consistent with a diagnosis of *S. haematobium*.

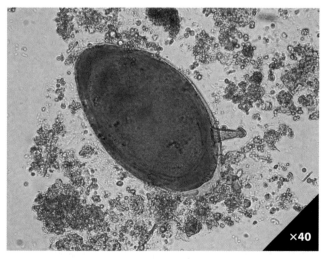

▲ **Fig. 10.105** Feces preparation with an egg of *S. mansoni* with a lateral spine.

Clinical manifestations of schistosomiasis

Case 10.12

A 20-year-old female presented with weight loss, recurrent attacks of colicky abdominal pain, and diarrhea with blood and mucus in the feces. About 4 weeks previously, she had returned from a holiday in southern Africa, which included a visit to Lake Malawi in Malawi (see Fig. 10.106).

Feces examination revealed no parasites, and no pathogenic organisms were cultured. The white cell count was not elevated, but 20 per cent of the leukocytes were eosinophils.

About a week later, she began to pass blood in her urine (see Fig. 10.107).

Microscopic examination of the urine showed the presence of *S. haematobium* eggs with a terminal spine (shown earlier in Figs 10.102, 10.103 and 10.104 on page 397).

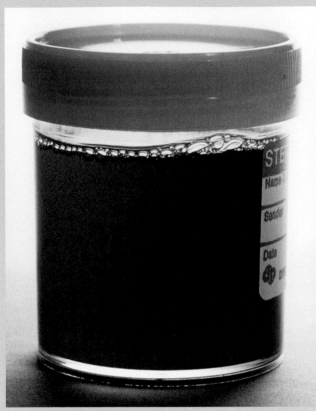

▲ **Fig. 10.107** About 5 weeks after returning from the tour, the young woman developed hematuria.

▼ **Fig. 10.106** A 20-year-old female and her companions on a small, sandy beach on the edge of Lake Malawi. She said that there were some snails on the sand and some of her companions were crunching them with their bare feet. (This would have shortened the life cycle by saving the cercariae the trouble of swimming in the water in search of a human host.)

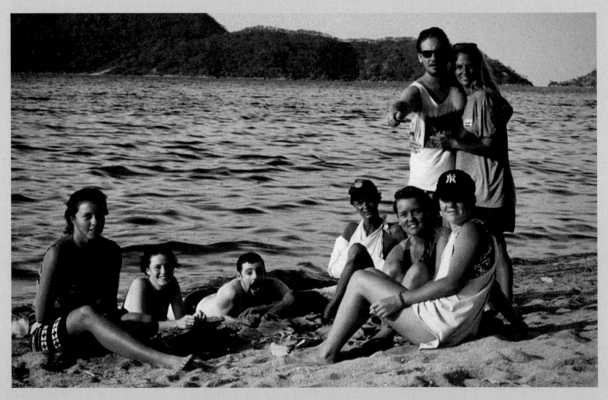

While the urine was being examined under the microscope, some of the eggs started moving. The egg shell was shed and a motile miracidium emerged—that is, hatched. It was covered with cilia, which were beating rapidly (illustrated in Fig. 10.108). It moved with a somewhat undulating movement. Figure 10.109 shows a cercaria, the form of the parasite that emerges from the hump of the snail. This is infective to humans.

The patient was treated with praziquantel. The symptoms gradually subsided and the eggs in the urine decreased in number. By 6 weeks, no further eggs were demonstrated in the urine.

An indirect hemagglutination test on the serum was positive for schistosome infection.

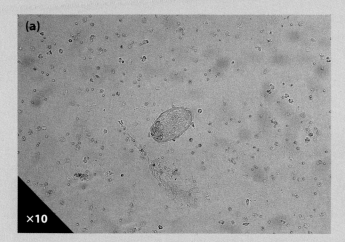
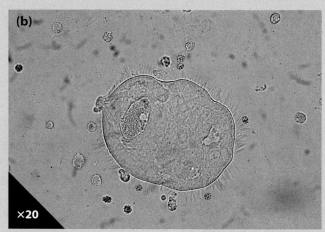

▲ **Fig. 10.108(a) and (b)** View of a miracidium covered with rapidly beating cilia.

▶ **Fig. 10.109** Cercaria with forked tail, released from the snail host. This is the stage of the parasite after the miracidium and the life form that penetrates the skin of humans.

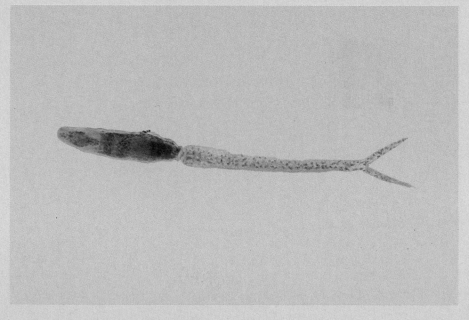

Case 10.13

A young man, who was a member of the tour group to Lake Malawi mentioned in Case 10.12, developed paraplegia. This was shown to be due to transverse myelitis of the cervical spinal cord, caused by a schistosome infection. He recovered almost full function over a period of 2 years.

Case 10.14

Another member of the tour group to Lake Malawi, mentioned in Case 10.12, see pages 398–399, returned to the United States and wrote to each of the people who had accompanied him on his tour to Lake Malawi. He developed an acute febrile illness, which was not malaria.

When he began to have epileptic fits, a space-occupying lesion was found in the brain. Biopsy showed the presence of schistosome eggs. He recovered after treatment, but he was warning all his traveling companions to have themselves tested for schistosomiasis.

Case 10.15

A team of Australian footballers visited Lake Kariba, in central Africa, as part of an African tour a few weeks after the patient from Case 10.12, see pages 398–399, had recovered. A brother of the patient brought this to the attention of her treating doctor, and a group of laboratory staff visited the team at one of their evening training sessions in Brisbane.

Blood was taken for serologic tests and urine for micro-urine tests. Of the team, 59 per cent returned positive serology tests for schistosomiasis. They were advised to seek medical attention if they developed symptoms.

Case 10.16

A number of other travelers who had visited Lake Malawi were seen in Brisbane for treatment within a few months of Case 10.12, see pages 398–399, being encountered. They all developed an acute flu-like illness with fever, abdominal pains and severe sweating in the evenings (Katayama fever).

Some of them had positive serology for schistosomiasis, while others had schistosome eggs in the urine.

The young woman in Case 10.12, see pages 398–399, said that her tour group had been informed by a leading travel guide book that in Lake Malawi there was no schistosomiasis. (Sometimes this disease is called Bilharzia.)

She had some doubts about this claim when she accompanied a friend from the group who attended the local hospital for treatment of a broken arm. The hospital had a ward labeled 'Bilharzia Ward'.

Dr Jenny Robson and the author wrote to the editors of the travel guide and informed them about the incorrect statement. The information was corrected in the next edition.

Pathology of schistosomiasis

The cercaria stage of the parasite penetrates the skin of humans as they wade in the shallow water of lakes and canals. It then develops into an adult worm that settles in the perirectal and perivesical veins. There the males and females copulate. The female lays eggs, which penetrate the adjacent tissue and cause damage that elicits a chronic inflammatory reaction by the host. Many eosinophils are found in the inflammatory infiltrate (see Figs 10.110–10.115, continued overleaf).

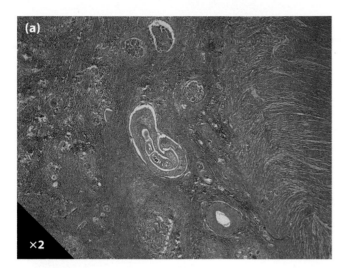

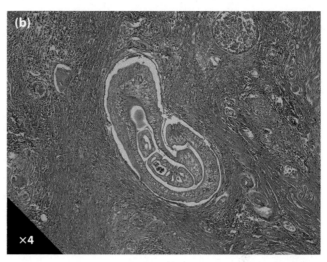

▲ **Fig. 10.110(a) and (b)** Views of adult schistosome worms in the pararectal tissues. The male worm is wider than the female and it encloses the female in what is called its gynecophoric canal.

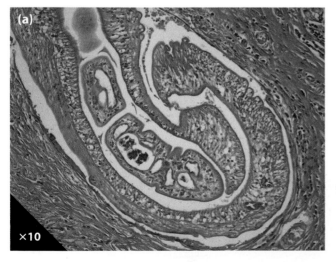

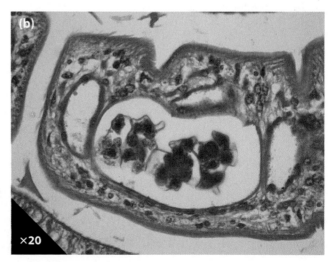

▲ **Fig. 10.111(a) and (b)** Views of the testes of adult schistosome worms.

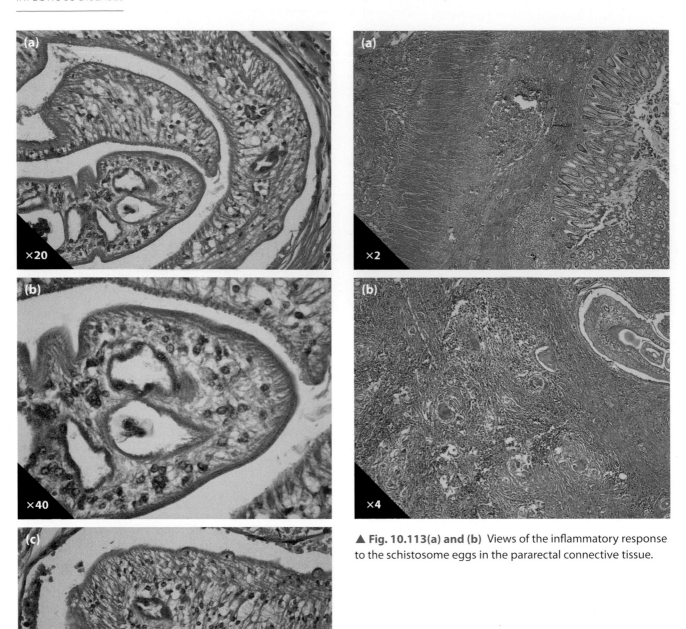

▲ **Fig. 10.113(a) and (b)** Views of the inflammatory response to the schistosome eggs in the pararectal connective tissue.

▲ **Fig. 10.112(a), (b) and (c)** Adult schistosome worms. Alimentary canal. Views of the lateral spaces.

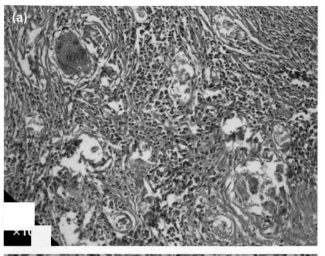

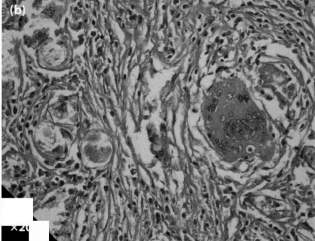

▲ **Fig. 10.114(a) and (b)** Magnified views of the inflammatory response shown in Figure 10.113.

Some eggs pass into the bloodstream and are carried to various sites, including appendix and cervix. In the liver, they cause periportal fibrosis and cirrhosis with the complications of this (see Figs 10.116–10.119, continued overleaf).

Eggs of *S. japonicum* in particular invade the lungs causing granulomas there as well (see Fig. 10.120, overleaf).

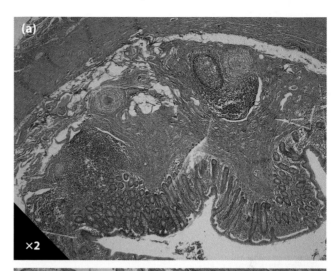

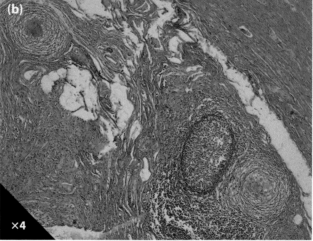

▲ **Fig. 10.116(a) and (b)** Views of an appendix with granulomas in its wall.

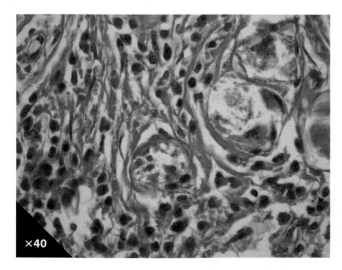

▲ **Fig. 10.115** Degenerate schistosome egg becoming calcified. There is a brisk eosinophil response to this.

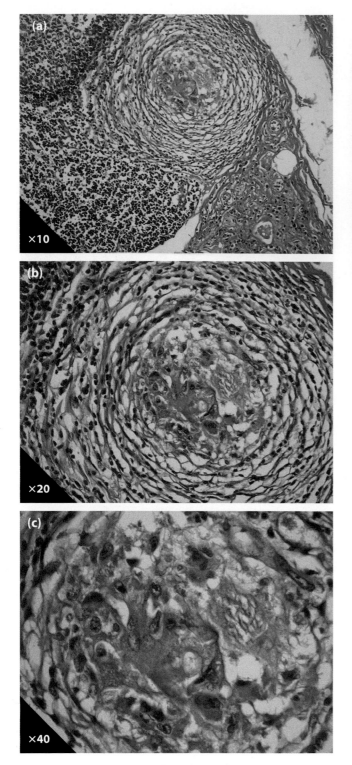

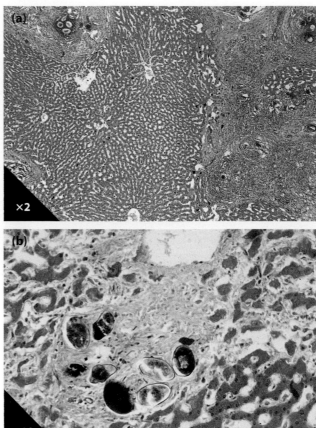

▲ **Fig. 10.118(a) and (b)** Portal tract area of a liver. There is marked periportal fibrosis and cirrhosis. Schistosome eggs are present in the portal tract. Liver involvement with portal hypertension is a common complication of schistosomiasis. This section came from the liver of an Australian serving in the Australian armed forces in north Africa in the 1940s who had not been outside Australia since then.

▲ **Fig. 10.117(a), (b) and (c)** Higher magnification view of a granuloma in the appendix.

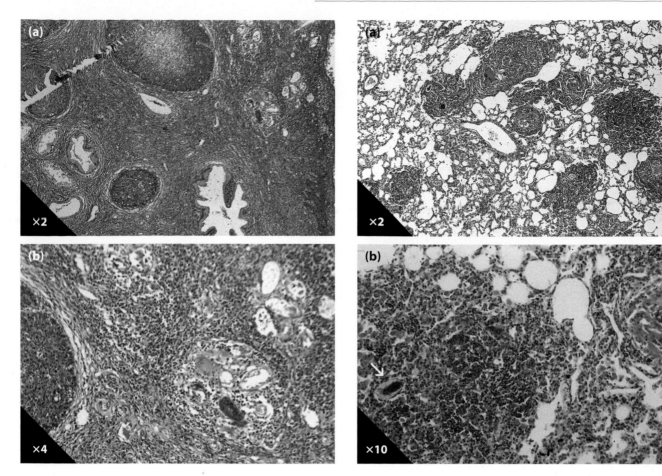

▲ **Fig. 10.119(a) and (b)** Biopsy of the cervix. It shows a squamous cell carcinoma. Longstanding schistosomiasis is thought to be a cause of cancer of the cervix and bladder.

▲ **Fig. 10.120(a) and (b)** Lung from a Chinese seaman, who died while his ship was visiting the port of Brisbane, Australia. It shows multiple granulomas, which contain schistosome ova. The species cannot be determined from H&E stained sections of tissue, but it was assumed that this infection could have been caused by *S. japonicum*.

Case 10.17

A 40-year-old male immigrant from South Africa presented with hematuria. An endoscopic examination of the bladder showed redness of the bladder mucosa. A red nodule on its surface was biopsied (shown in Fig. 10.121).

A diagnosis of schistosomiasis was made and the patient was given appropriate drug treatment.

Longstanding schistosomal infection of the bladder causes chronic inflammation and calcification. The bladder wall is thickened and the ureteric orifices become obstructed, causing hydronephrosis.

This condition in turn results in repeated urinary tract infections, as seen in two other patients illustrated in Figures 10.122 and 10.123.

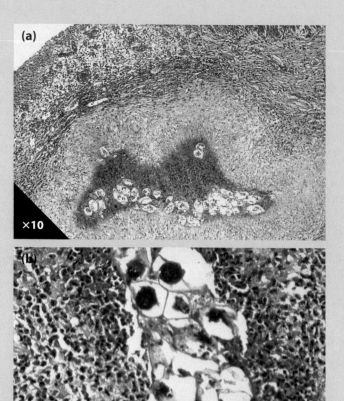

(a)

×10

(b)

×20

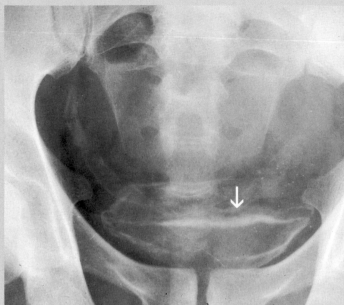

▲ **Fig. 10.122** X-ray from a young adult patient from Ghana shows a contracted, heavily calcified bladder resulting from chronic schistosomiasis.

▲ **Fig. 10.121(a) and (b)** An endoscopic biopsy of a red, nodular projection on the bladder mucosa of a male, 40 years old, who presented with hematuria. It shows an acute granulomatous reaction around schistosome eggs in the lamina propria. The overlying mucosa is ulcerated in some places and the blood vessels are dilated. The eggs are surrounded by large numbers of eosinophils.

▼ **Fig. 10.123** Serial X-rays taken over a period of a few hours, after an intravenous pyelogram in a young adult male from Egypt. The early film (*left*) shows a right hydroureter. As time passes, a dilated, left urinary system comes into view (*right*). That is, there is delayed filling of the hydroureters.

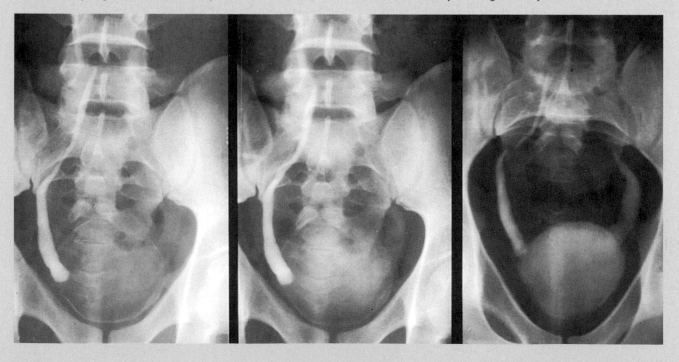

Case 10.18

A 43-year-old male was admitted to hospital for investigation of pain in his right loin. This was thought to be due to renal colic caused by renal calculi.

As part of the urologic investigation, endoscopy of the bladder was performed and it revealed the presence of a small, red nodule, which was biopsied. The biopsy was almost normal, but there were a few schistosome ova present and there was a very mild eosinophil response to them (see Fig. 10.124).

The patient had no symptoms referable to the bladder. He had lived in Australia for 25 years, after leaving Mauritius, an island off the east coast of Africa. During this time, he had had no symptoms of urinary tract disease and he had not left Australia—where schistosomiasis does not occur.

He was given antischistosome treatment on the basis of this finding. (Unfortunately, he was lost to follow up.)

In this case, the question is: is this a real disease that requires treatment, or are the schistosome eggs just passengers?

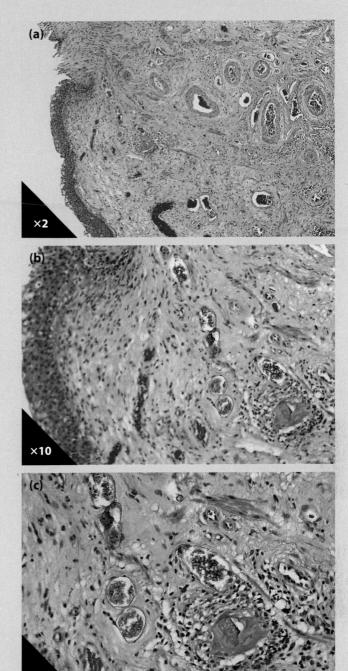

▲ **Fig. 10.124(a), (b) and (c)** Bladder biopsy that is almost normal except for the presence of a few schistosome ova. There is a mild eosinophil reaction associated with the ova.

Case 10.19

A 23-year-old Filipino woman, married to an Australian, developed obstructed labor that resulted from cephalo pelvic dysproportion (see Fig. 10.125). The baby was delivered by Caesarean section. During this procedure, the obstetrician biopsied some brown plaques that he saw on the serosal surface of the small intestine.

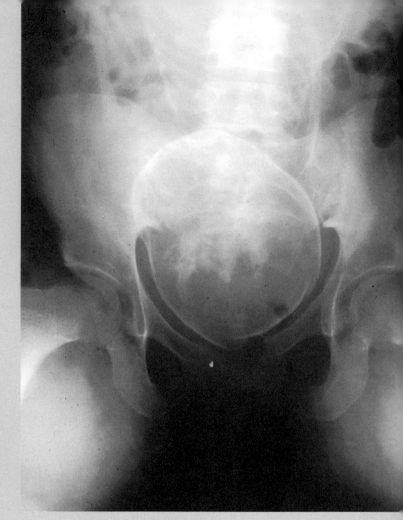

▶ **Fig. 10.125** X-ray of the pelvis of a 23-year-old Filipino woman, who had obstructed labor from cephalo pelvic dysproportion.

Microscopic examination of the plaques showed the presence of degenerate schistosome eggs associated with fibrosis (shown in Fig. 10.126).

The patient was given a course of antischistosome drug therapy. (But again—as in Case 10.18 on page 407—is this really active disease that needs treatment?)

Does the presence of a parasite mean that the patient has active disease that needs treatment?
This question may arise in many infectious diseases. In the absence of clinical disease caused by the identified infectious agent, how does one decide its importance to the patient?

The author is of the view that Case 10.18 on page 407 and Case 10.19 both illustrate the fact that most parasites live in a commensal relationship with humans and do not necessarily cause symptoms of disease.

Probably, neither patient needed treatment. The patient in Case 10.18 must have had the eggs lying dormant in the bladder for at least 25 years and the patient in Case 10.19 had degenerate and, therefore, nonviable eggs.

When patients present in a country where the parasitic disease in question does not occur, they are likely to be treated as though they have a disease. It is very likely that in a country where parasitic diseases are prevalent, they would not have had active treatment.

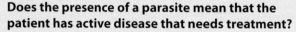

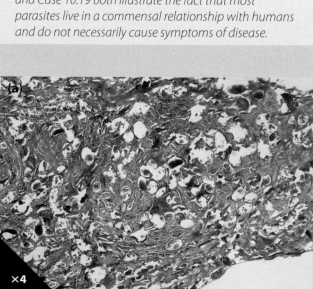

×4

×20

▲ **Fig. 10.126(a) and (b)** Brown plaque found on the surface of the small bowel at the time of Caesarean section. It shows numerous degenerate schistosome eggs surrounded by an area of fibrosis.

Clonorchiasis

Sometimes called the Chinese liver fluke, *Clonorchis sinensis* is a trematode which inhabits the biliary system of humans. It is found in China and its neighboring countries.

In Cambodia, Vietnam and Thailand, another species of liver fluke occurs—*Opisthorchis*. This species is so similar to the *C. sinensis* in morphology and behavior that there seems to be no practical reason for separating them for purposes of discussing their clinicopatholgic features.

Humans acquire the infection by eating uncooked or undercooked freshwater fish infected with the metacercaria stage of the parasite (see Life cycle 10.12). Mature flukes hatch in the duodenum and migrate to the bile ducts throughout the liver.

Even heavy infestations may not cause clinical symptoms. When symptoms do occur, they are those of biliary obstruction, jaundice and cholangitis. Some patients with longstanding infestation develop bile duct carcinoma of the liver.

Liver flukes (Clonorchis and others)

Infected humans.

↓

Eggs passed in feces.

↓

Ciliated miracidium hatch and enter a snail.

↓

Cercariae develop in the snail.

↓

Cercariae leave the snail and enter fish.

↓

Uninfected humans eat uncooked or undercooked fish.

▲ **Life cycle 10.12** Liver flukes.

Case 10.20

A middle-aged Korean seaman died from a myocardial infarction while his ship was visiting the port of Brisbane, Australia. A coronial post mortem was performed. An incidental finding was that the bile ducts of the liver were filled with liver flukes with the morphology of *C. sinensis* (shown in Figs 10.127 and 10.128, continued overleaf).

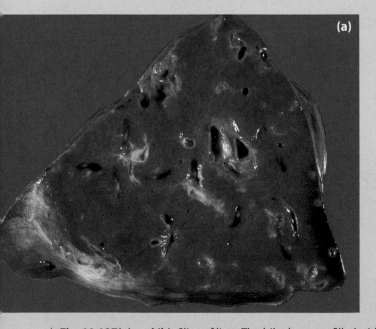
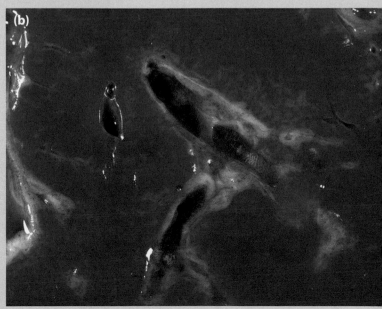

▲ **Fig. 10.127(a) and (b)** Slice of liver. The bile ducts are filled with liver flukes consistent with *C. sinensis*.

▶ **Fig. 10.128(a), (b) and (c)**
C. sinensis. Liver flukes removed from the bile ducts seen at low, medium and high magnification. Each one is approximately 20 mm in length. The internal structure is easily seen even in the unstained state. Oral sucker (mouth) (A). Esophagus (B)—which divides into two ceca (gut) (C) that extend the whole length of the body. Uterus (D). Seminal receptacle (E). Vas deferens (F). Testes (G). The ovary is at the lower end of the uterus near the seminal receptacle (not visible here).

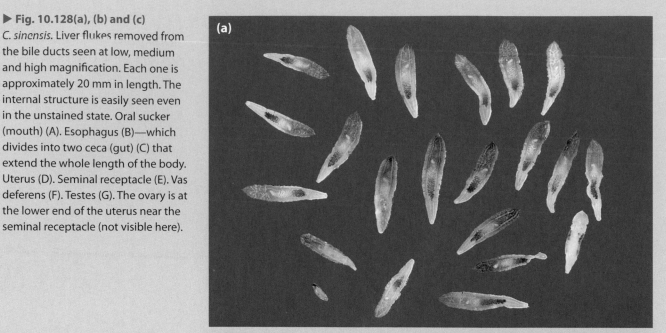

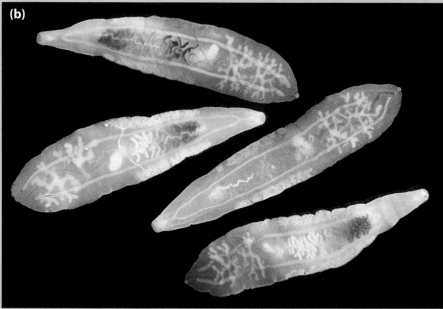

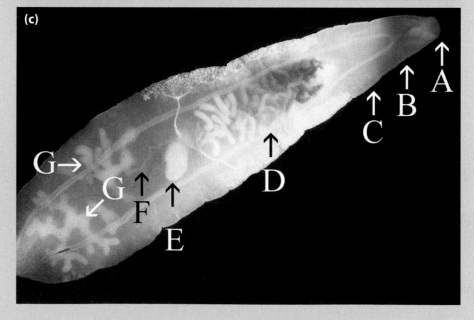

Further pathologic and parasitologic aspects of clonorchiasis are illustrated in Figures 10.129–10.136, continued overleaf.

(a)

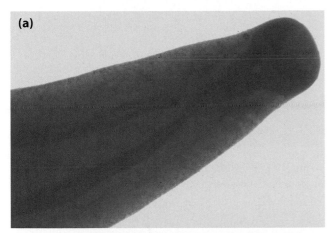

(b)

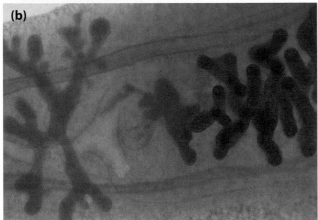

▲ **Fig. 10.129(a) and (b)** Stained *C. sinensis* fluke. The head is in **(a)**. The ovary can be seen in **(b)**, between the uterus on the right and the testes on the left.

▼ **Fig. 10.130** Two eggs of *C. sinensis* obtained by duodenal aspirate. They are small (about 30 × 10 microns). They have an operculum at one end.

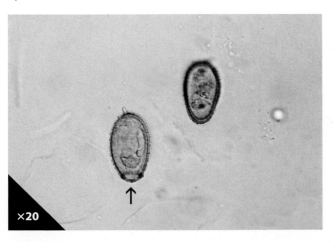

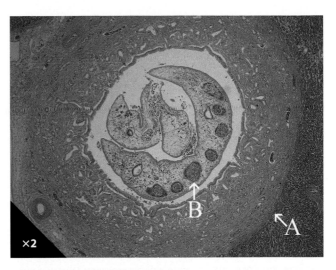

▲ **Fig. 10.131** Transverse section of a *C. sinensis* fluke in a bile duct in the liver. The epithelium of the bile duct is thickened and there is some periductal fibrosis (A). Testes can be seen at this magnification (B).

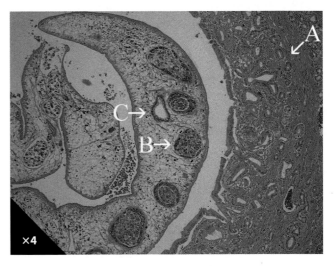

▲ **Fig. 10.132** Seen at higher magnification—thickened epithelium and periductal fibrosis (A), testes (B) and cecum (C).

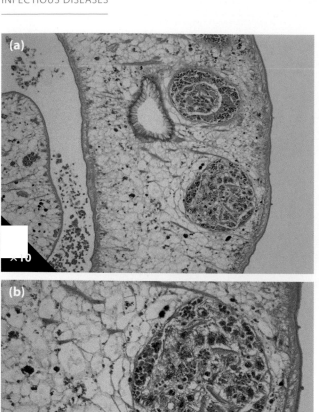

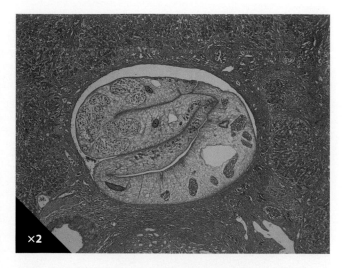

▲ **Fig. 10.134** Another *C. sinensis* fluke—cut through the anterior half, showing the uterus filled with eggs.

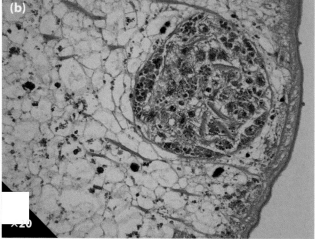

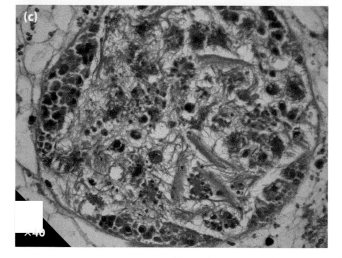

▲ **Fig. 10.133(a), (b) and (c)** Views of the testes.

▼ ▶ **Fig. 10.135(a), (b) and (c)** Three views of the uterus filled with eggs.

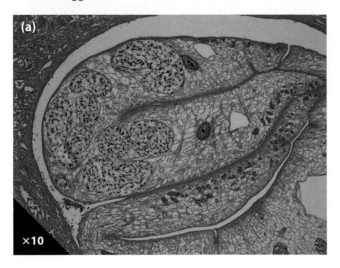

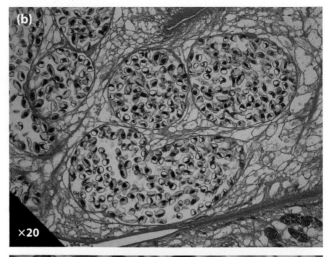

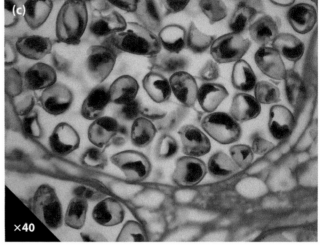

Liver cancer is a well-recognized complication of liver fluke infestation. The tumor is usually a cholangiocarcinoma.

▼ **Fig. 10.136** Specimen of liver showing a carcinoma filling the right lobe. The bile ducts were filled with *C. sinensis* flukes. Some flukes are collected in the inserted capsule.

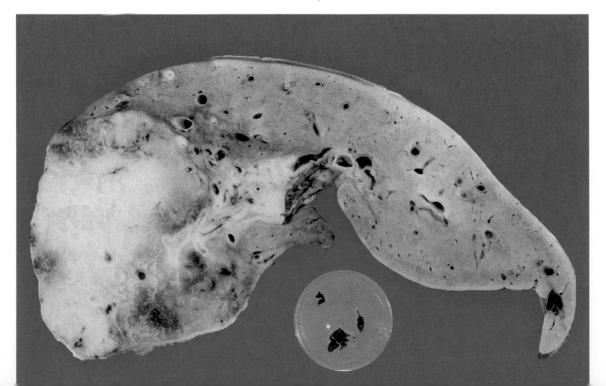

Paragonimiasis

Paragonimiasis is an infection by the trematode *Paragonimus westermani*—the oriental lung fluke. It is found in China, South-East Asia and some parts of South America.

It is transmitted by eating undercooked crabs or crayfish.

The adult fluke develops in the small intestine and then burrows through the intestinal wall to the abdominal cavity and then into the thorax, where it invades the lung. Flukes are found in bronchi or bronchioles, where they cause pneumonia and hemoptysis (see Figs 10.137 and 10.138).

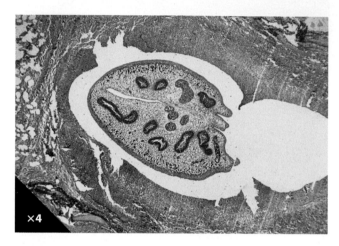

▲ **Fig. 10.137** Lung section from a male adult who died in Hong Kong SAR. A fluke in a distended bronchiole has a morphology consistent with *P. westermani*. The bronchiolar epithelium has been destroyed and pneumonia is present.

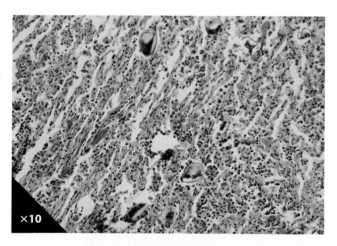

▲ **Fig. 10.138** Brown, thick-shelled eggs in the adjacent lung tissue.

Cestodes

Echinococcosis/hydatid disease

Echinococcosis occurs when humans are infected with the larval stage of the dog tapeworm *Echinococcus granulosus*.

Hydatid disease is prevalent in sheep-raising countries throughout the world. In sheep-raising communities, there is a close working relationship between sheep, dogs and humans (see Fig. 10.139).

The adult tapeworm lives in the gut of the sheep dogs (see Fig. 10.140). Eggs contaminate the environment. Following this contamination, humans and sheep become infected and develop the larval stage of the parasite—hydatid cyst.

Farmers kill some sheep for meat, and the offal is fed to the dogs. Liver in particular contains hydatid cysts and when the dog eats the cysts, the cycle is continued (see Life cycle 10.13).

Echinococcus granulosus

Sheep dogs with adult worms in their gut.

↓

Eggs passed in feces contaminate the environment.

↓

Eggs are eaten by sheep and humans.

↓

The larval stage of the parasite (hydatid cyst) develops in sheep and in humans.

↓

Sheep are butchered by sheep farmers for domestic meat consumption and the offal (liver, lungs, kidneys) are fed to sheep dogs.

↓

Sheep dogs develop adult worms.

Note: The life cycle of *Echinococcus multilocularis* is much as above, but the definitive host is the fox.

▲ **Life cycle 10.13** *Echinococcus granulosus*.

▼ **Fig. 10.139** Shearing time on a sheep station in the far west of Queensland, Australia. This shows the close association between the sheep farmer, the sheep dog helping to move the sheep, and the sheep.

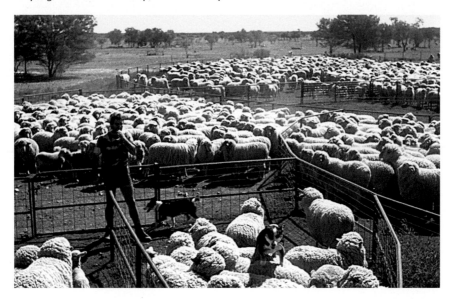

▼ **Fig. 10.140** Two dog tapeworms—*E. granulosus*. They are small worms, about 5 mm long. They have a head (scolex) with suckers and hooklets (A), and one mature and one gravid segment. In the gravid segment, the uterus is filled with eggs. The genital pore (B) opens laterally in the middle of the gravid segment.

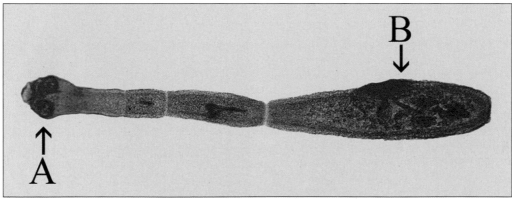

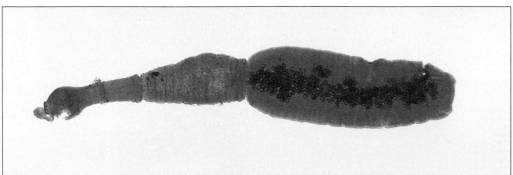

Pathology

Hydatid cysts slowly enlarge and, ultimately, they cause symptoms resulting from pressure effects. The liver is the most common organ to be involved, but hydatid cysts may occur in any organ. The cysts can be demonstrated by a number of different imaging techniques.

The treatment protocol is to begin with appropriate drug therapy aimed at killing the germinal epithelium. This is followed by surgical removal of the cyst.

There is usually a plane of separation between the laminated membrane of the cyst and the adjacent tissue. When a cyst is being removed, it is important to be very careful not to spill any of the contents of the cyst into the adjacent tissues, so as to minimize the risk of regrowth occurring.

The incidence of hydatid disease is greatly reduced by regular treatment of the sheep dogs with antihelminthics —the so-called 'deworming of the dogs'.

Case 10.21

A 40-year-old male sheep farmer had experienced a dragging pain in the right upper quadrant of his abdomen for some months. One day, in frustration, he punched himself firmly over the offending area. This induced an acute anaphylactic reaction (presumably caused by rupture of the hydatid cyst in his liver) and he was rushed to hospital for treatment.

An ultrasound examination revealed a space-occupying lesion in the left lobe of his liver and a diagnosis of probable hydatid cyst was made (see Fig. 10.141).

This diagnosis was confirmed at operation and the cyst was removed. The surgical pathology of this cyst is illustrated in Figures 10.142–10.147, continued overleaf. The patient's recovery was uneventful.

▼ **Fig. 10.141** An ultrasound examination showed a space-occupying lesion in the left lobe of the liver.

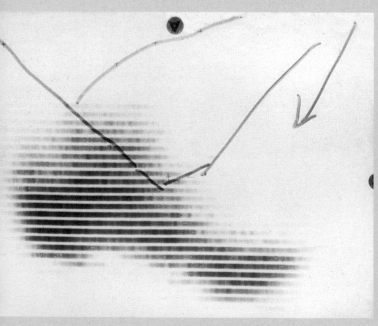

▼ **Fig. 10.142** The hydatid cyst being removed. Its firm, white, laminated membrane separated easily from the adjacent liver. The abdomen was carefully packed to prevent contamination of the peritoneal cavity.

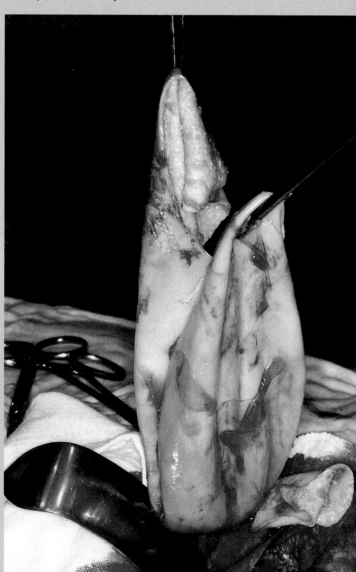

▶ **Fig. 10.143** View of the inner lining of the hydatid cyst. Multiple small nodules can be seen on its surface.

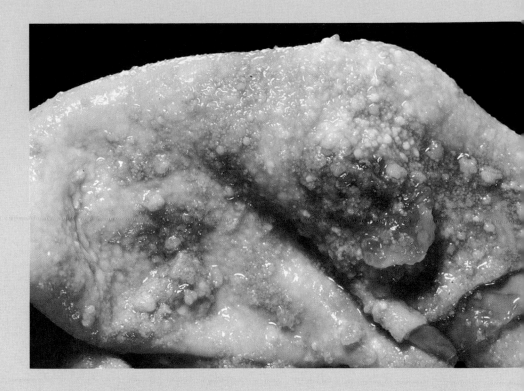

▶ **Fig. 10.144** View of laminated membrane (A). Germinal epithelium (B). Developing daughter cysts (C).

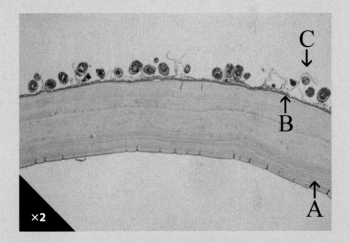

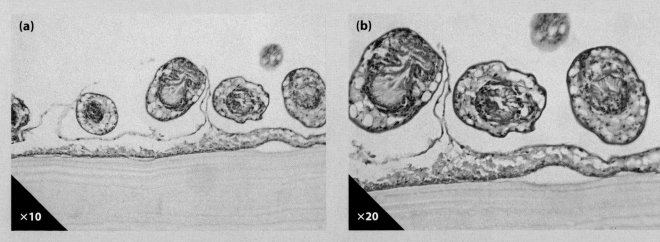

▲ **Fig. 10.145(a) and (b)** Higher magnifications of the laminated membrane, the germinal epithelium and the daughter cysts that develop from it.

► **Fig. 10.146** Well-formed daughter cyst with a developing head (scolex) within it.

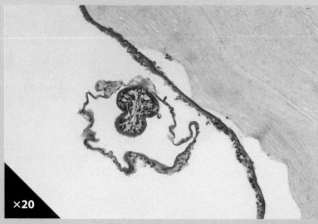

×20

► **Fig. 10.147(a) and (b)** The fluid within the cyst contains hooklets and heads of future worms, together with an amount of debris. This fluid is called 'hydatid sand'. When the fluid is centrifuged, the heads and hooklets can be seen in the unstained preparation. The second image of each pair is photographed under dark ground illumination, which enhances the appearance of the heads and hooklets.

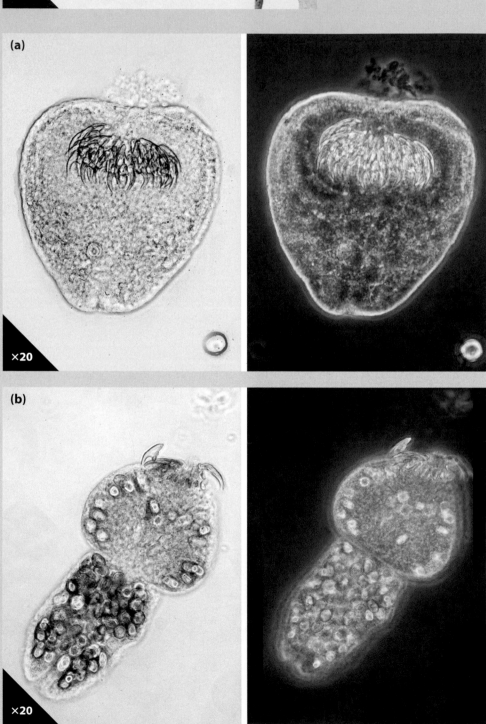

(a)

×20

(b)

×20

Case 10.22

A 53-year-old sheep farmer had an asymptomatic hydatid cyst in his liver at post-mortem examination. The cyst is shown in Figure 10.148.

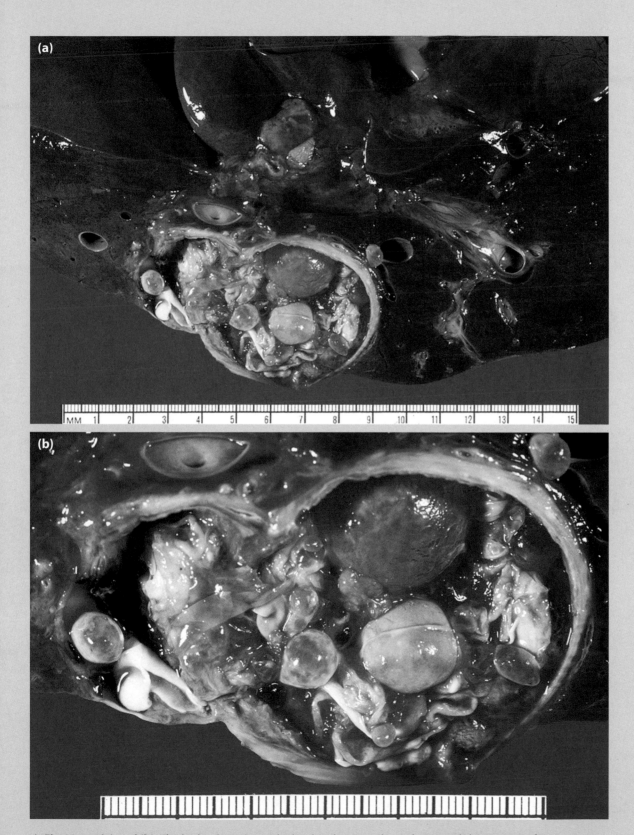

▲ **Fig 10.148(a) and (b)** The hydatid cyst has a thick, white laminated membrane and shows signs of expansion into the adjacent liver tissue. It contains multiple, thin-walled daughter cysts.

Case 10.23

A 40-year-old female had a partial hepatectomy to remove a calcified hydatid cyst.
The pathologic features of this are illustrated in Figure 10.149.

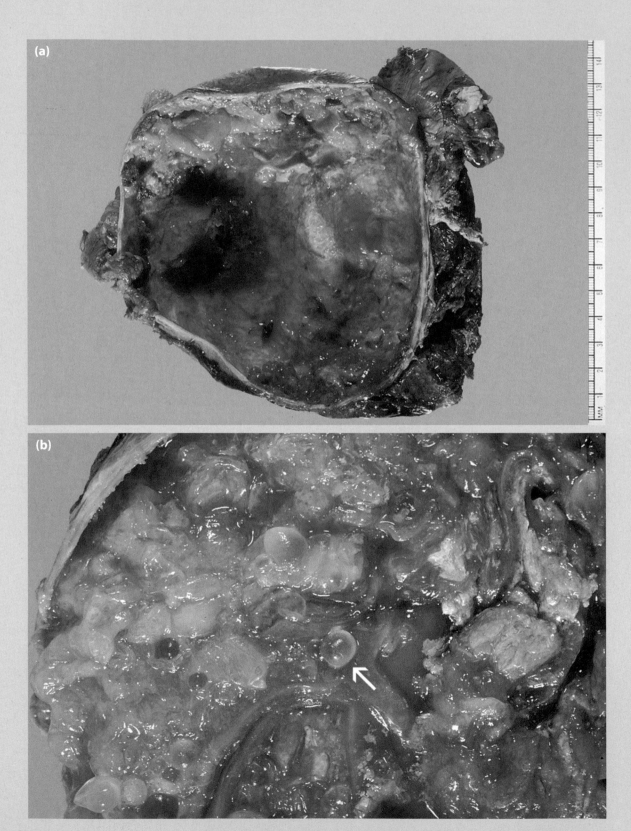

▲ **Fig. 10.149(a) and (b)** Partial hepatectomy to remove a calcified hydatid cyst. The cyst is well circumscribed; its wall is calcified; and some daughter cysts can be seen growing from its inner lining.

Case 10.24

A 10-year-old male was found to have eosinophilia on a routine blood count. A chest X-ray showed a space-occupying lesion in the lower lobe of his right lung (see Fig. 10.150). A provisional diagnosis of hydatid cyst was made and he was given a course of drug therapy.

A lobectomy was performed to remove the cyst. The surgical pathology is illustrated in Figures 10.151, 10.152 and 10.153, continued overleaf.

The child had not been exposed to a farm environment and neither had he had any known contact with dogs.*

Sometimes, it is not possible to identify the source of the infection, as was the case in this patient.

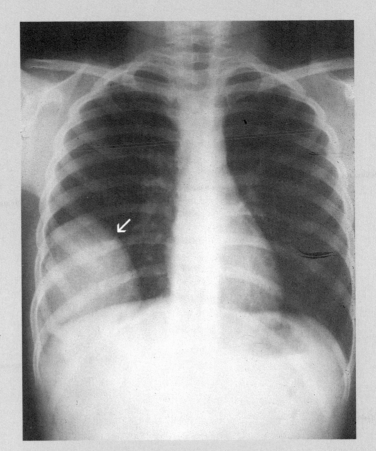

▶ **Fig. 10.150** Chest X-ray in a 10-year-old male showed a space-occupying lesion in the lower lobe of his right lung.

▶ **Fig. 10.151(a) and (b)** Lobectomy specimen showing the presence of a hydatid cyst. The laminated membrane has pulled away from the area of inflammatory reaction in the adjacent lung.

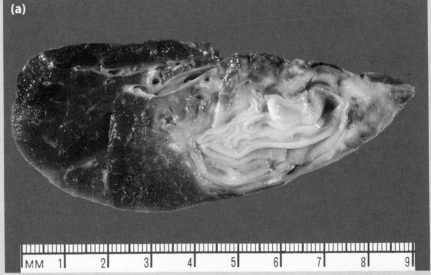

(a)

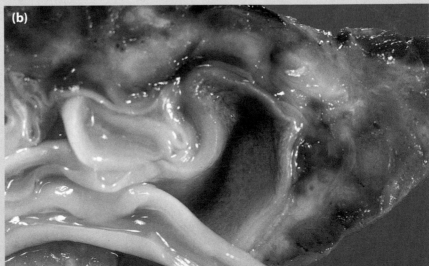

(b)

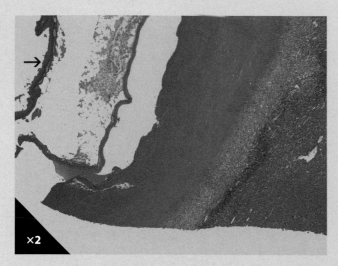

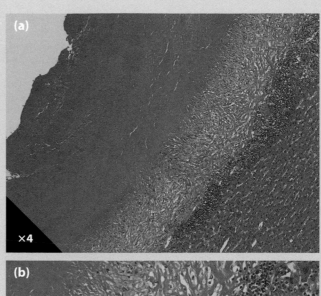

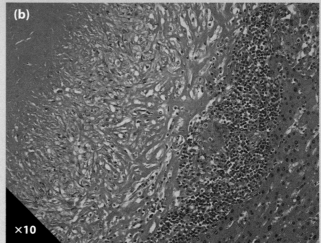

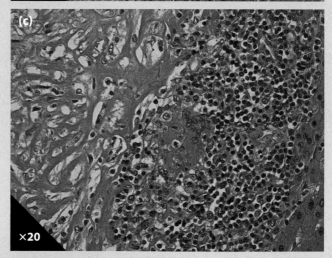

▲ **Fig. 10.152** View of the edge of the hydatid cyst. A piece of laminated membrane can be seen adherent to the adjacent lung. Often, the laminated membrane is the only microscopic indication of the presence of a hydatid cyst. It can then be diagnostic.

▲ **Fig. 10.153(a), (b) and (c)** Views of the chronic inflammatory reaction to the presence of the cyst in the lung. The lung further away from the cyst was normal.

Case 10.25

A female, aged 56 years, who lived in one of the main sheep-raising areas of Australia complained of a painful hip and a limp.

X-ray showed the presence of a cyst in the neck of the right femur (see Fig. 10.154). This was aspirated, and laminated membrane and scolices were demonstrated.

An X-ray of the humerus from another patient showing multiple hydatid cysts is illustrated in Figure 10.155.

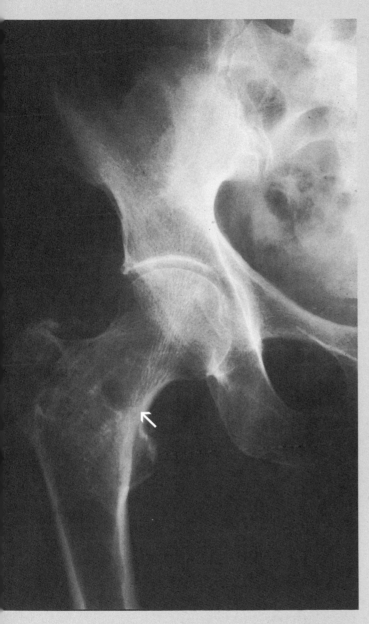

▲ **Fig. 10.154** X-ray showing a cystic lesion in the head of the right femur. Aspiration confirmed a diagnosis of hydatid cyst.

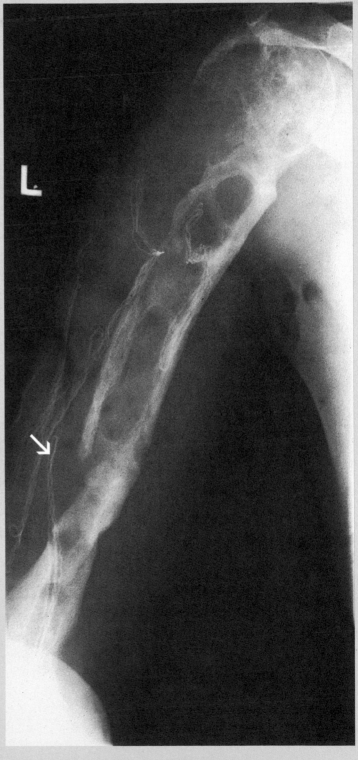

▲ **Fig. 10.155** X-ray showing a pathological fracture through one of multiple hydatid cysts in a right humerus.

Case 10.26

A male sheep farmer, aged 48 years, was admitted for amputation of his right femur because of a pathologic fracture caused by involvement of the bone by hydatid cyst. The daughter cysts were escaping from the marrow cavity and invading the thigh muscles (see Fig. 10.156).

▶ **Fig. 10.156(a) and (b)** Amputated femur showing a pathologic fracture at its distal end. The fracture has been caused by the replacement of the marrow cavity by an expanding hydatid cyst (A). The daughter cysts have extended through the fracture into the adjacent muscle (B).

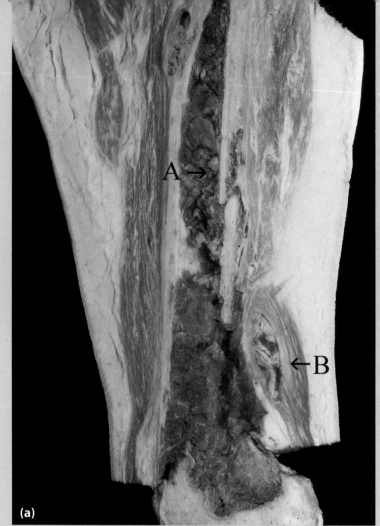

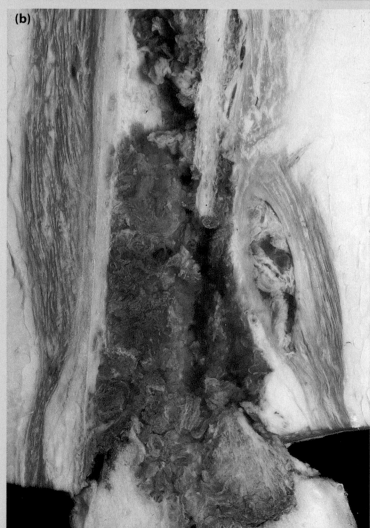

Case 10.27

A male, aged 10 years, presented with pain in the left loin. A palpable lump could be felt in the left upper quadrant of his abdomen.

Imaging revealed the presence of hydronephrosis and a space-occupying lesion in the left kidney. A nephrectomy was performed. The pathology of this is illustrated in Figure 10.157.

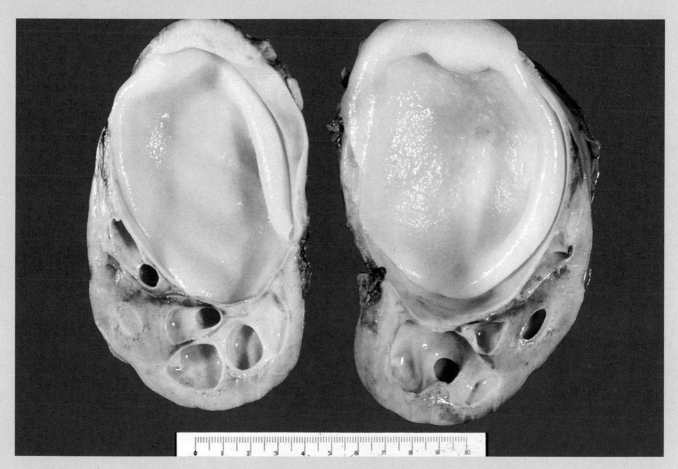

▲ **Fig. 10.157** The kidney has been sliced open to reveal that a hydatid cyst was the cause of the pathology. It has caused pressure on the calyceal system, which shows marked hydronephrosis. There is no evidence of infection. The white, laminated membrane is separating from the kidney substance.

Case 10.28

An 8-year-old male presented with the symptoms and signs of an intracerebral space-occupying lesion. An air encephalogram showed the presence of a large cystic lesion in the left frontal lobe (see Fig. 10.158). A left frontal lobectomy was performed.

The boy presented again 2 years later with a recurrence of symptoms. His condition deteriorated and he died soon after admission to the hospital.

Post-mortem examination revealed the presence of gross hydrocephalus, caused by a hydatid cyst that developed first in the region of the third ventricle (see Fig. 10.159).

A number of transparent daughter cysts were floating freely in the cerebrospinal fluid of the dilated ventricles (see Fig. 10.160).

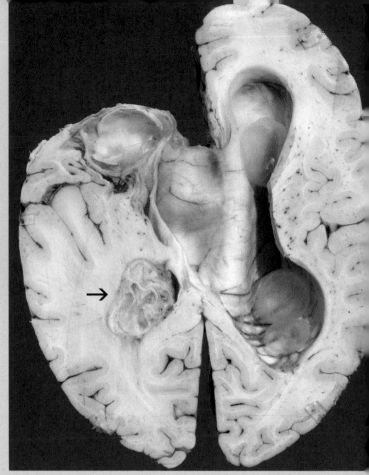

▲ **Fig. 10.159** Brain at post mortem 2 years after first presentation. It shows the absence of the left frontal lobe (which had been removed surgically as primary treatment of the presenting lesion) and gross hydrocephalus. A collapsed hydatid cyst can be seen in the posterior horn of the left lateral ventricle.

▼ **Fig. 10.158** An air encephalogram shows a large cystic lesion in the left frontal lobe and gross hydrocephalus.

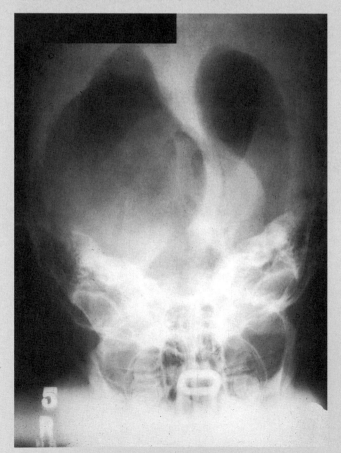

▼ **Fig. 10.160** Transparent daughter cyst floating freely in a dilated lateral ventricle.

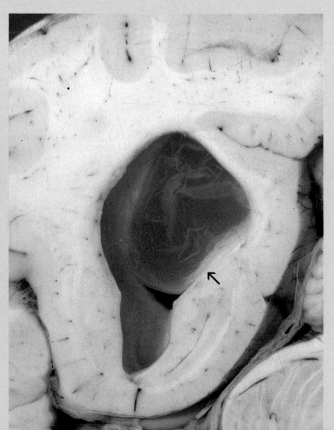

Echinococcus multilocularis

Echinococcus multilocularis is a second species of Echino-coccus. It is only found in certain areas of the world. The German pathologist Rudolph Virchow (1821–1902), from Berlin, is credited with being the first, in 1855, to identify this type of hydatid cyst.

It is called 'multilocularis' because the hydatid cyst contains numerous locules. The cyst is usually collapsed and degenerate when seen in surgical and post-mortem specimens. Low-magnification examination shows the collapsed laminated membranes that give it the multi-loculated appearance (see Fig. 10.161). The membranes are surrounded by the inflammatory reaction of the host organ.

This condition is demonstrated in Figures 10.162–10.165, continued overleaf.

The adult worm is similar to the *E. granulosus*, but is often slightly smaller. The worm is found in the alimentary canals of foxes, cats and various rodents. Infection occurs when another host ingests eggs passed in feces. Humans become infected when they accidentally enter the cycle by ingesting eggs (refer to Life cycle 10.13 on page 415).

In 1936, *E. multilocularis* was introduced into Hokkaido, the most northern of the larger islands of Japan, by foxes from Russia. In spite of active control measures, about 10 cases each year are still seen in the Hokkaido University Hospital.

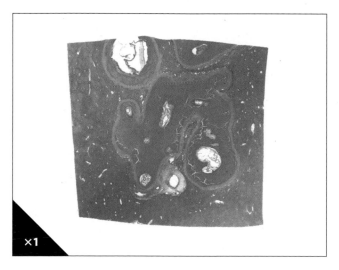

▲ **Fig. 10.161** Section of liver showing a collapsed hydatid cyst. It is degenerate, no viable germinal membrane can be seen and it has a multiloculated appearance.

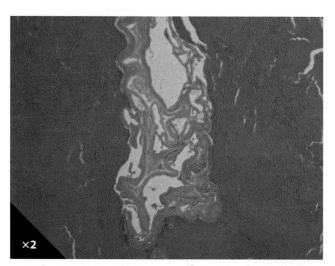

▲ **Fig. 10.162** An iridescent laminated membrane (from the section of liver shown in Fig. 10.161) can be seen but there is no viable germinal layer.

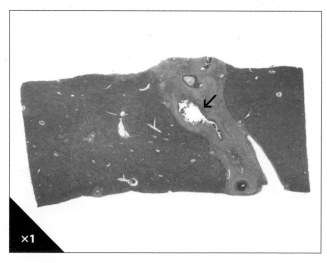

▲ **Fig. 10.163** Section of liver showing a collapsed hydatid cyst. There is marked periportal fibrosis and viable germinal membrane can be seen. Only a minority of these cysts show the presence of viable germinal membrane.

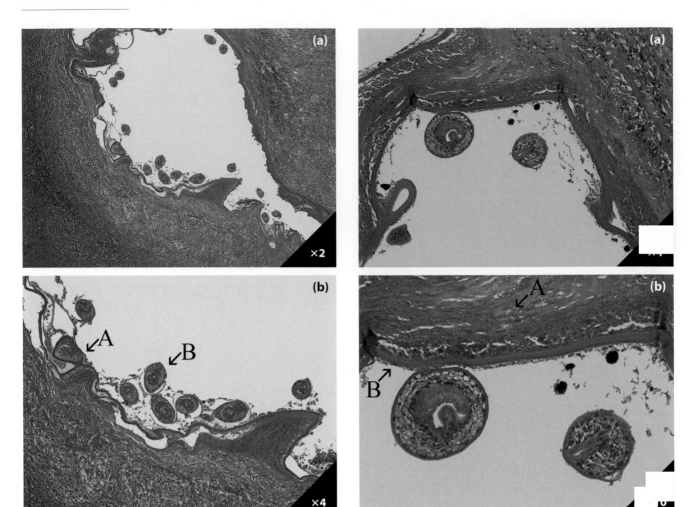

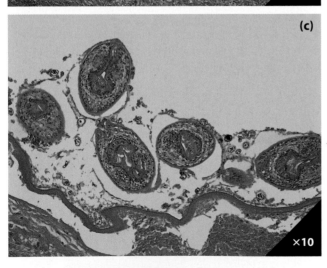

▲ **Fig. 10.164(a), (b) and (c)** Views of germinal membrane and 'developing daughter cysts' (B). The chronic inflammatory reaction of the host adjacent to the cyst can be seen.

▲ **Fig. 10.165(a) and (b)** At higher magnification the laminated membrane and the germinal layer (B) and the chronic inflammatory reaction of the host adjacent to the cyst (A) can be seen.

A cautionary tale

Not everything that at first sight appears to be parasitic disease is in fact caused by a parasite.

One of the most common situations in this regard occurs when a child about 12 months of age 'vomits' or 'regurgitates' a number of white cysts, which are up to about 10 mm in diameter (see Fig. 10.166). The mother is alarmed and wonders what this is. The doctor she consults telephones the laboratory to enquire whether they could be hydatid cysts.

The clinical history and the appearance of these cysts is quite characteristic. The cysts are all about the same size (10 mm), a white color and slightly sticky. When examined microscopically, the walls of the cysts are amorphous and without structure (see Figs 10.167, overleaf).

This appearance is due to the action of gastric juices on various forms of baby food fruit gel (shown in Fig. 10.168, overleaf). The doctor and the mother can be assured that this is not a parasitic infection. The offending material is gel cysts and they are of no consequence at all.

▼ **Fig. 10.166** Transparent cysts 'vomited' or 'regurgitated' by a 1-year-old child.

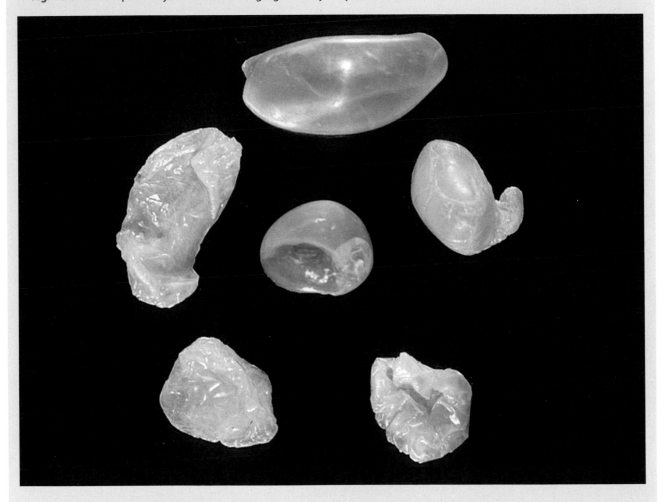

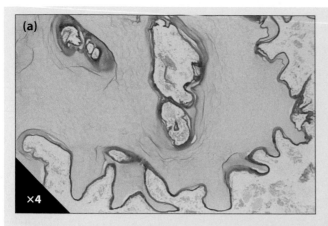
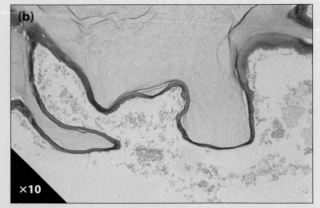

▲ Fig. 10.167(a) and (b) The cysts have an amorphous appearance in histologic sections. The diagnosis is gel cysts.

▶ Fig. 10.168 Fruit gel baby food. The action of gastric acid on this substance creates the gel cysts that may be regurgitated by young children.

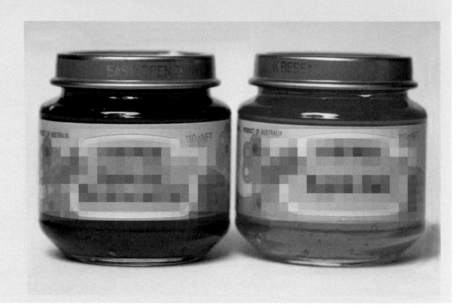

Sparganosis

Sparganosis is a condition in which a larva of a pseudophyllean tapeworm enters through the human skin and produces a subcutaneous inflammatory mass.

Adult tapeworms are mostly of the species *Spirometra mansonoides*, found in the intestines of dogs, cats and other animals. It occurs in most countries of the world. In Australia, most of the cases have manifested in farmers, farm workers or professional pig shooters. The exact life cycle of the parasite is not yet known.

Case 10.29

A 28-year-old male farmhand presented with a lump on his back. He said that it was moving slowly. It was excised and sent for histologic examination (see Figs 10.169 and 10.170).

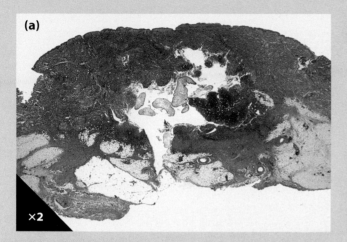

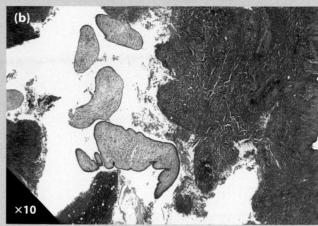

▲ **Fig. 10.169(a) and (b)** Section shows an abscess with a cross section of a 'worm' in the center.

▶ **Fig. 10.170** High-magnification view of the 'worm', which has the morphological features of a sparganum. It has a well-defined integument, no internal organs, and no scolices. The surface shows the presence of microvilli (A). On the inner surface of the integument, there is a line of well-defined tegumental cells. Within the body of the sparganum, there are a number of small muscle fibers (B). In the center, there is a small focus of calcification (which is a fairly common finding in this parasite).

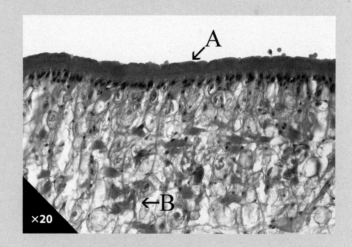

Case 10.30

An 81-year-old retired farmer had a lump on his left thigh. It was annoying him, so he had it excised. Histologic examination showed the presence of a sparganum (see Figs 10.171 and 10.172).

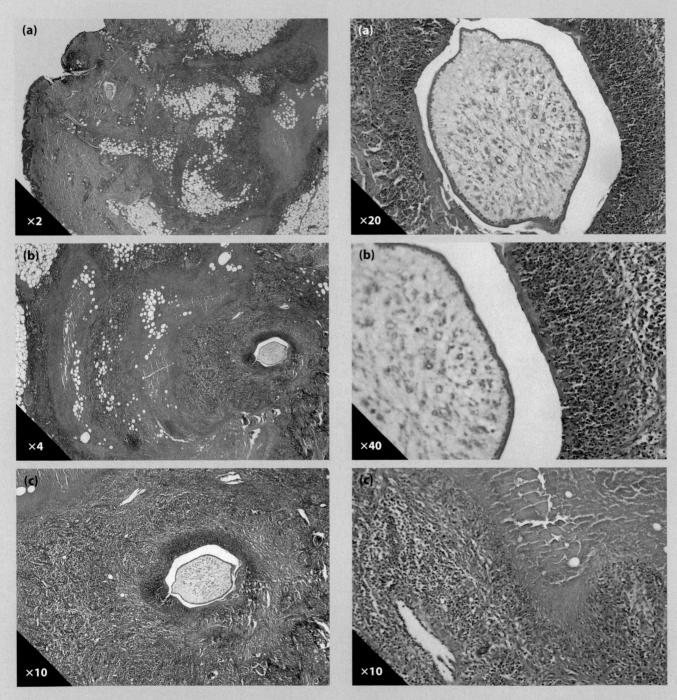

▲ **Fig. 10.171(a), (b) and (c)** Section shows a subcutaneous lesion with the appearance of an abscess. In the center of the abscess, there is a degenerate 'worm'.

▲ **Fig. 10.172(a), (b) and (c)** The worm has the features of a sparganum that is surrounded by a chronic inflammatory cell reaction. Small numbers of eosinophils are present in the inflammatory reaction.

Pig meat and sparganosis infection

In rural areas of Australia, wild pigs are numerous. They are regarded as a pest because they cause severe damage to the environment. Rural dwellers, especially males of all ages, often shoot the pigs for sport. Both of the men in Cases 10.29 and 10.30 (see pages 431–432) almost certainly acquired their sparganosis infections in this way.

In recent years, wild pig meat has become a gourmet dish in various countries. It is particularly sought after in Germany. Following the Chernobyl nuclear power reactor disaster in 1986, there was a demand for uncontaminated Australian wild 'boar' or pig meat. This resulted in a flurry of activity by professional pig shooters.

Professional pig shooters work during the wintertime and at night when it is cold. During the summertime, the meat would deteriorate before it could be frozen. The pig shooters have hunting dogs, which hold a shot pig until the shooter comes to make the final kill if it was not killed with the first shot. These dogs wear protective aprons to prevent injury from the pig tusks (see Fig. 10.173).

Soon after the pigs are shot, they are hung by one leg on the back of the shooters' truck and then disemboweled (see Figs 10.174 and 10.175, continued overleaf). At daylight, the pigs are transferred to a refrigerated truck, which holds approximately 500 pigs. These trucks then transport the carcasses to the nearest meat-processing plant.

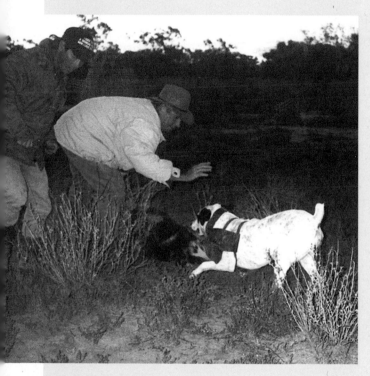

▲ **Fig. 10.173** Professional pig shooters employ dogs—protected with leather 'aprons'—to hold shot pigs that are not killed cleanly by the first shot, to prevent the pigs from getting away before they are finally killed.

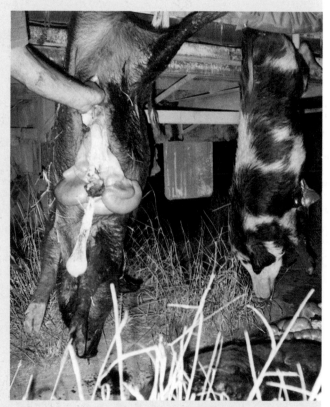

▲ **Fig. 10.174** The shot pigs are attached to the shooters' truck by one leg.

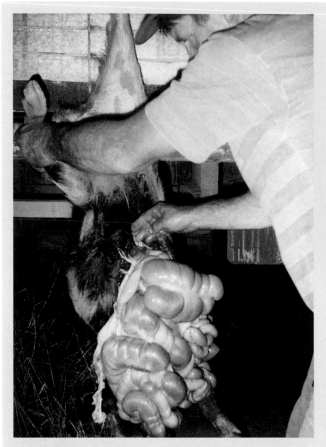

▲ **Fig. 10.175** The pigs are disemboweled. It is easy to see how infection from contaminated muscle can occur during this butchering process.

The butchered pig meat is inspected before being packaged. A small percentage of the carcasses contain sparganum larvae. The larvae are easily seen under the fascia covering the meat (shown in Figs 10.176 and 10.177). When the fascia is incised, the sparganum is liberated. It unfolds and is quite actively motile (see Figs 10.176, 10.177 and 10.178). Infected meat is condemned and discarded.

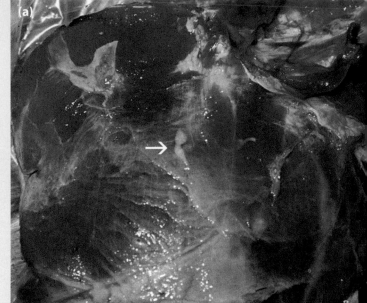

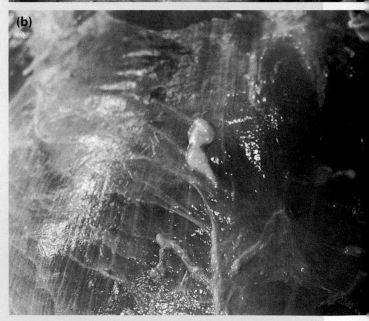

▲ **Fig. 10.176(a) and (b)** A white sparganum can be seen under the fascia in this pig meat that has been butchered and prepared for sale. The pig meat will have to be destroyed because it is infected.

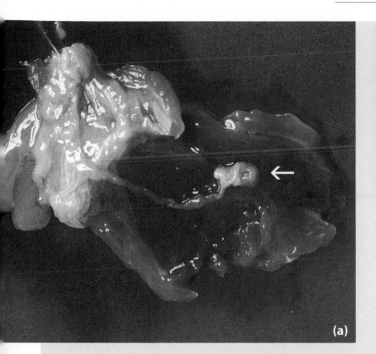

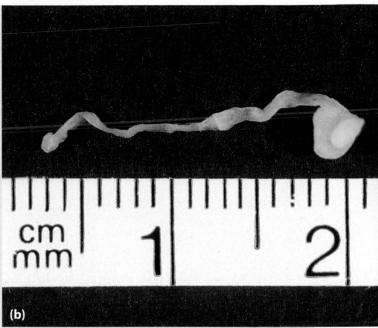

▲ **Fig. 10.177(a)** Piece of pig meat with a sparganum easily visible was selected for study and photography. **(b)** The sparganum was removed. It was sticky and motile, measuring approximately 20 mm in length. The thick end is the head.

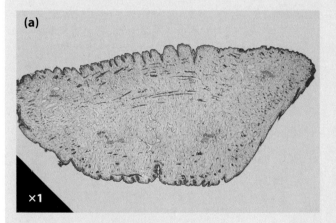

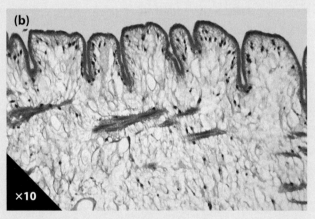

▲ **Fig. 10.178(a) and (b)** Transverse histologic section from the sparganum itself. It resembles exactly the appearance of the 'worm' found in the human cases.

Sparganosis is an uncommon infection. Pig shooters are much more likely to acquire brucellosis from the pigs, and this infection is quite commonly encountered in pig shooters in Australia.

Spargana are quite frequently found in frogs (see Fig. 10.179). In some parts of the world, infections of the eye and skin are treated with 'poultices' that consist of gutted frogs that are applied to the affected part of the body. Cases of sparganosis occur following this practice.

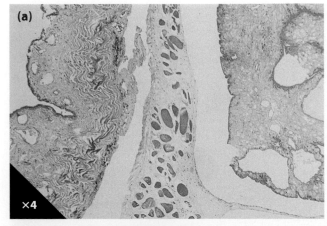

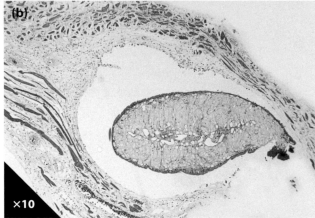

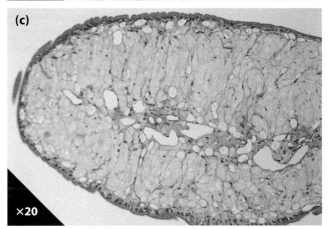

▲ **Fig. 10.179(a), (b) and (c)** Views of a section taken from the leg muscle of a common green tree frog found in one of the parks in the city of Brisbane, Australia. Naked eye inspection of the leg muscles showed the presence of numerous motile 'worms' within the muscle. The microscopic sections confirm that these are sparganum larvae. When frog poultices are used, it is not difficult to envisage direct transfer from frog to humans.

Cysticercosis

Cysticercosis is a condition in which the larval stage of *Taenia solium*—the pork tapeworm—becomes lodged in one or more organs of the human body. Humans are the definitive host of *T. solium* (see Life cycle 10.14(a) and (b)).

The adult tapeworm lives in the small intestine of humans. The tapeworm is flat and white and made up of multiple, contractile segments called proglottids (see Fig. 10.180).

The *T. solium* tapeworm begins its life cycle as the cysticercus, which is a white, thin-walled, transparent cyst—approximately 10 mm in diameter. Within this cyst, there is a small, white nodule approximately 1 mm in diameter. This is the head of a new tapeworm.

When the cysticercus is ingested, the wall of the cyst is digested, and the head is released and grows into an adult tapeworm. Parasitologic features of the *T. solium* tapeworm are illustrated in Figures 10.181–10.187, continued overleaf.

The tapeworm itself causes few or no symptoms. However, patients may notice the presence of flat, white, motile fragments of soft tissue (gravid proglottids) in their feces. Cysticerci, too, may cause no symptoms unless they involve vital structures in the body (such as the brain and the heart).

Taenia solium

Humans and pigs with adult worms in the gut.
↓
Eggs passed in feces.
↓
Infection is acquired from the contaminated environment.

▲ **Life cycle 10.14(a)** *Taenia solium.*

Cysticercosis

Pig with adult *T. solium* in the intestine.
↓
Eggs hatch in the intestine and the resulting oncospheres are carried in the blood to where they develop into cysticerci in muscle and other organs.
↓
Humans eat infected, undercooked pig meat and the scolices in the cysticerci develop into an adult tapeworm in the small intestine.
↓
Humans who already harbor an adult worm in their own intestine may get cysticercosis from ingesting eggs or gravid proglottids passed in their feces by hand-to-mouth infection—autoinfection.

▲ **Life cycle 10.14(b)** Cysticercosis.

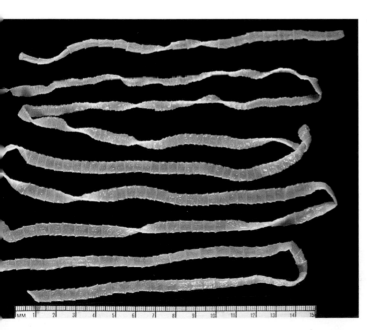

▲ **Fig. 10.180** An almost complete *T. solium* tapeworm, which was passed after the patient had been given treatment to expel the worm. The head end (*top*) is thinner than the distal end, which contains the gravid proglottids filled with eggs. (The head of this worm is missing.)

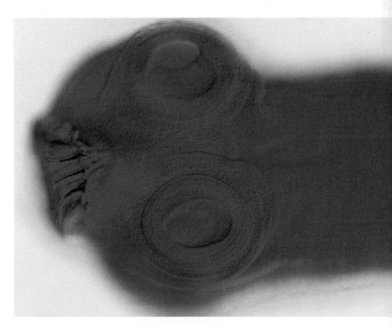

▲ **Fig. 10.181** Close view of a fresh scolex (head) of a *T. solium*. There is a row of hooklets above the part of the scolex, which bears the four suckers.

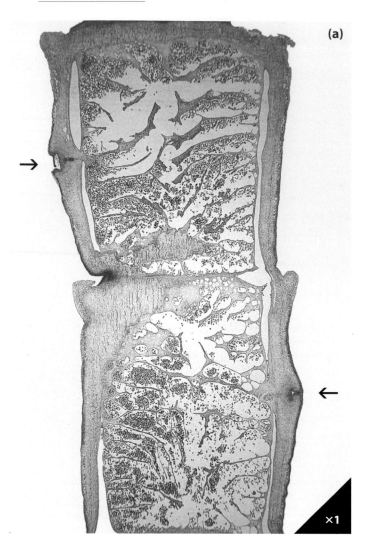

(a)

×1

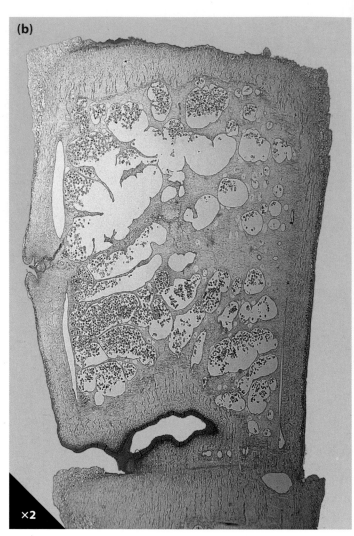

(b)

×2

▲ **Fig. 10.182(a) and (b)** Longitudinal section through two of the gravid proglottids. Genital pores open on alternate sides of succeeding proglottids.

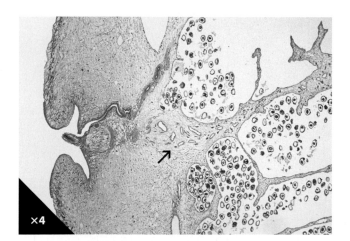

×4

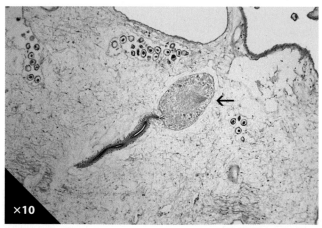

×10

▲ **Fig. 10.183** View of the genital pore shows the vagina opening superiorly as a well-defined tube. The vas deferens is a smaller tube and is somewhat twisted, as shown by the presence of large numbers of transverse sections leading away from the genital pore (*indicated by the arrow*). The testes consist of multiple small, rounded structures in the connective tissue septum between the branches of the uterus (*towards right*).

▲ **Fig 10.184** The oviduct can be seen leading from the ovary, which is situated at the proximal end of the proglottid.

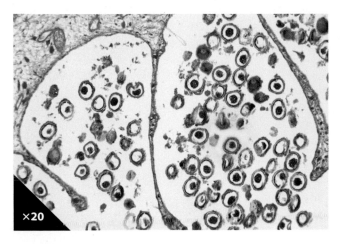

▲ **Fig. 10.185** High-magnification view of the multibranched uterus filled with eggs.

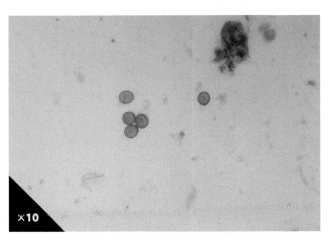

▲ **Fig. 10.186** Taenia eggs in feces.

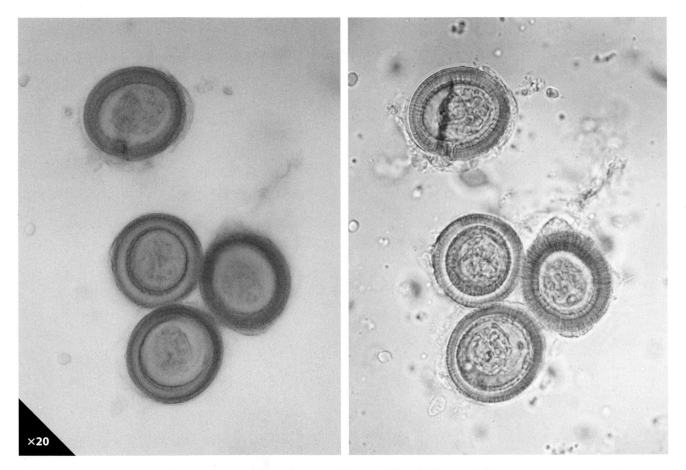

▲ **Fig. 10.187** At high magnification, Taenia eggs are brown and round, with a thick capsule. They measure approximately 36 microns in diameter. Under diffracted light (*right*) radial striations can be seen in the capsule of the egg. Eggs from all species of tapeworm are morphologically identical.

Case 10.31

A 30-year-old female Australian tourist agent visited Nepal on a familiarization tour (see Figs 10.188 and 10.189).

Some months after returning to Australia, she developed two subcutaneous lumps: one in the left breast and the other just below the breast. These lumps were excised (see Figs 10.190 and 10.191). Each one measured approximately 10 mm in diameter.

Examination revealed them to be cysticerci (see Figs 10.192–10.199 on pages 442–444). Presumably, this patient had eaten undercooked and infected pig meat during her tour.

An X-ray of the lower limb of another patient, illustrated in Figure 10.200 on page 444, shows the presence of multiple calcified bodies in the calf muscle: this is a result of past cysticercosis.

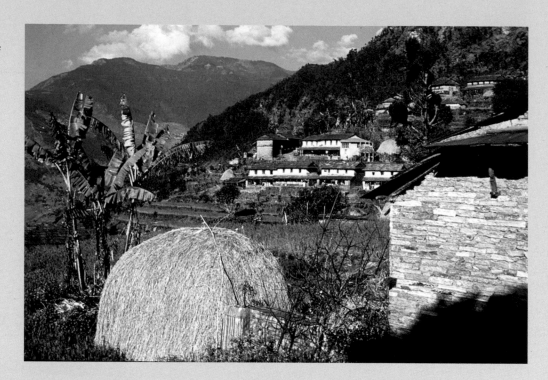

▶ **Fig. 10.188** Trekking in the high mountains of Nepal.

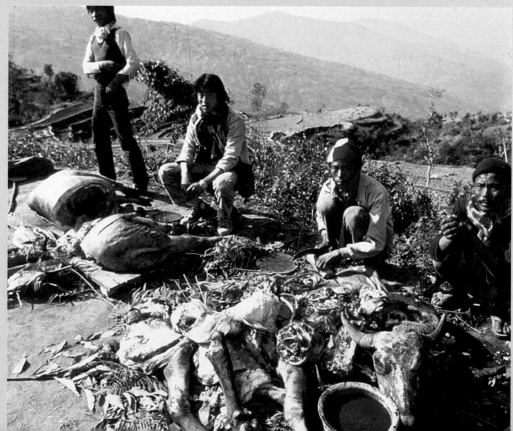

▶ **Fig. 10.189** Local people selling meat by the side of a trekking path in the high mountains of Nepal. Some of the meat was pig meat.

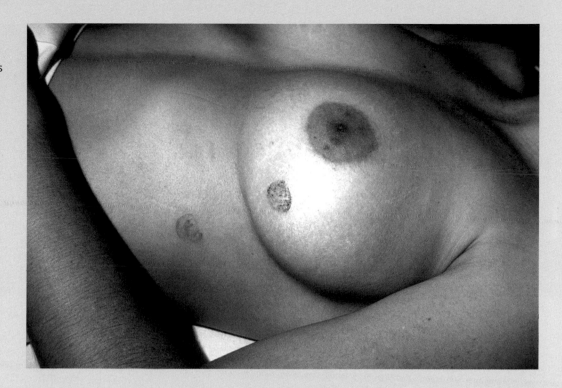

▶ **Fig. 10.190** This 30-year-old female has two subcutaneous lumps: one in the left breast and the other just below the breast.

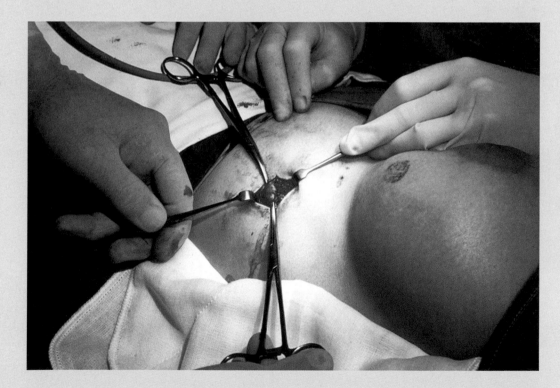

▶ **Fig. 10.191** Both lumps were excised. Each one was approximately 10 mm in diameter.

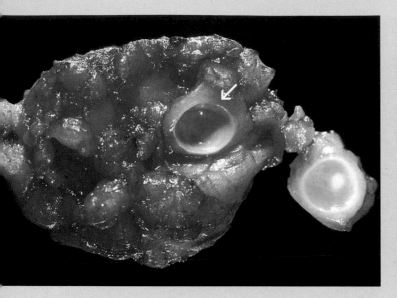

▲ **Fig. 10.192** One of the lumps is illustrated. The lesion was approximately 10 mm in diameter, and it was removed with some surrounding adipose tissue. It consists of a cyst. The piece on the right contains a small, white nodule. That on the left consists of an empty cyst cavity.

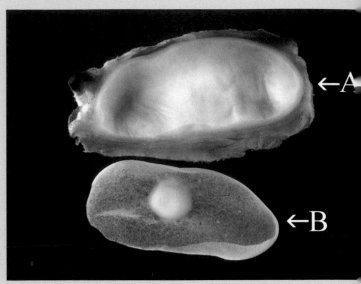

▲ **Fig. 10.194** Close view of the specimen shows the cyst wall (A)—which is the body's response to the presence of the parasite; and the cysticercus, which has a thin white wall and contains a tiny white spot (B)—the head of a new tapeworm.

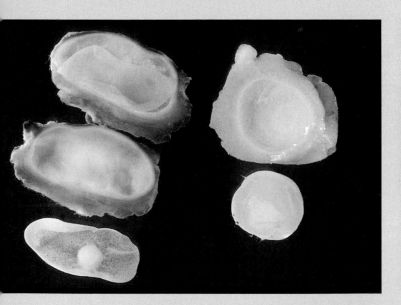

▲ **Fig. 10.193** When the cysts were cut across, a thin-walled, transparent structure floated out from the cyst. It separated easily from the cyst cavity, which was firm and did not collapse.

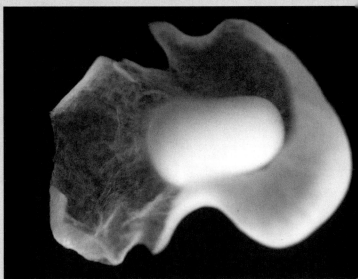

▲ **Fig. 10.195** Closer view of the specimen shows the structure of the cysticercus.

▼ ▶ Fig. 10.196(a), (b) and (c) Views of the head of the embryo tapeworm from the cysticercus. The hooklets in the scolex are well seen in **(c)**.

(a)

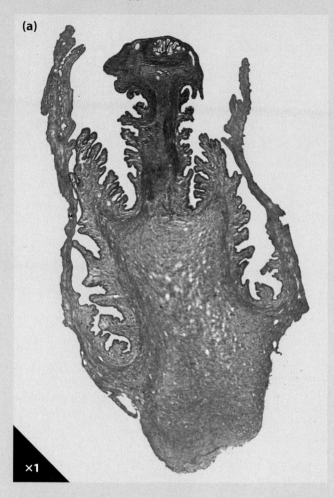

×1

(b)

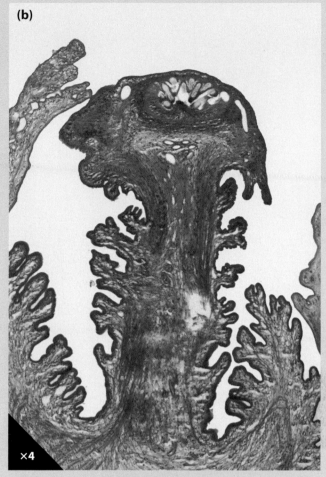

×4

(c)

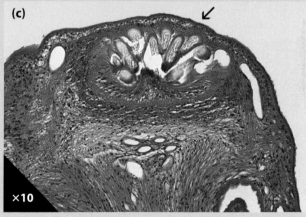

×10

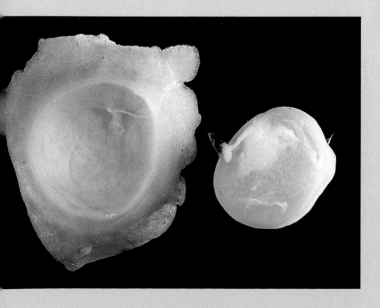

◀ Fig. 10.197 This is the second specimen to discuss a technical problem that arises when the specimen is being processed for histologic examination. Sometimes, a prosector allows the white membrane, that is the contents of the cyst, to disappear down the sink and then takes the section from the other half. When this happens, only the body's reaction to the parasite is seen in the section. A positive diagnosis cannot be made because no diagnostic part of the parasite has been included in the section. The correct procedure is to section not only the cyst wall, but also the cysticercus itself.

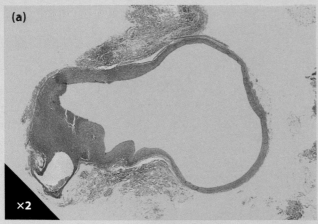

(a)

×2

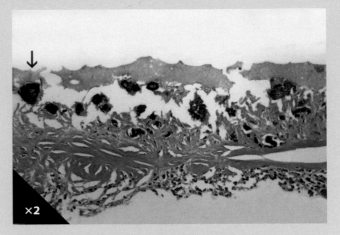

×2

▲ **Fig. 10.199** As the cyst ages, its wall becomes calcified. Foci of calcification can be seen in the wall of this cyst. Ultimately, the whole cyst degenerates and calcified bodies develop that are visible on X-ray.

(b)

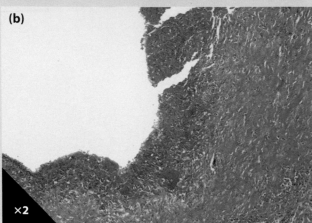

×2

(c)

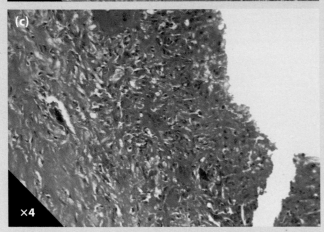

×4

▲ **Fig. 10.198(a)** Section from the left portion of the specimen from Figure 10.197 on page 443 shows the cyst wall. **(b) and (c)** Views of the cyst wall show a chronic inflammatory reaction only. There is no cysticercus in the section and the specimen is not diagnostic.

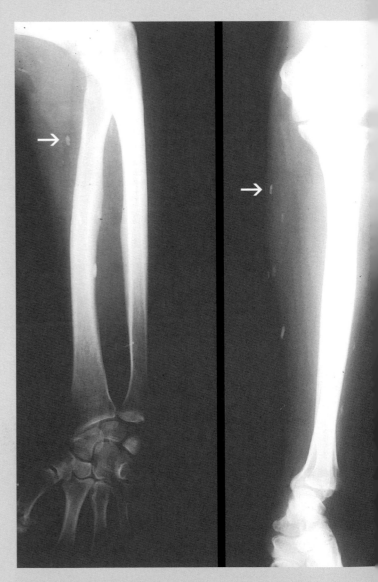

▲ **Fig. 10.200** X-ray of the lower limb of a 45-year-old male migrant from Greece living in Australia shows the presence of multiple calcified bodies in the calf muscle. This is a result of past cysticercosis.

Case 10.32

A 29-year-old Thai postgraduate student of agriculture presented at the student clinic of a university in Brisbane, Australia. He had multiple, soft, subcutaneous lumps: each approximately 10–15 mm in diameter on the right upper arm and chest (see Fig. 10.201).

Excision of one of these showed the typical appearance of cysticercosis (as demonstrated in Case 10.31, see pages 440–444).

He was given appropriate drug therapy and returned home to Thailand at completion of his postgraduate study. He wrote a few years later to say that he had developed some more similar lumps and that he was beginning to have headaches.

▼ **Fig. 10.201(a) and (b)** A 29-year-old male postgraduate student from Thailand presented with multiple soft subcutaneous lumps. Excision of one of these showed the typical appearance of cysticercosis.

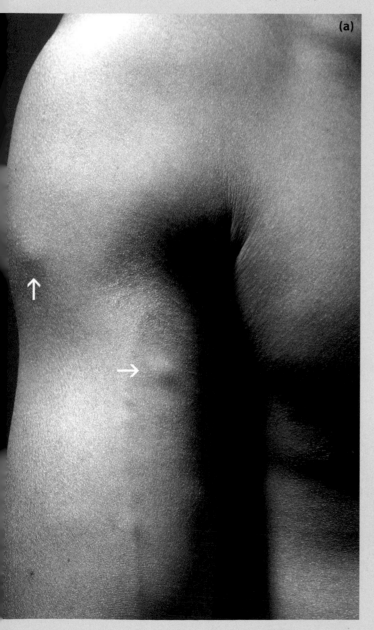 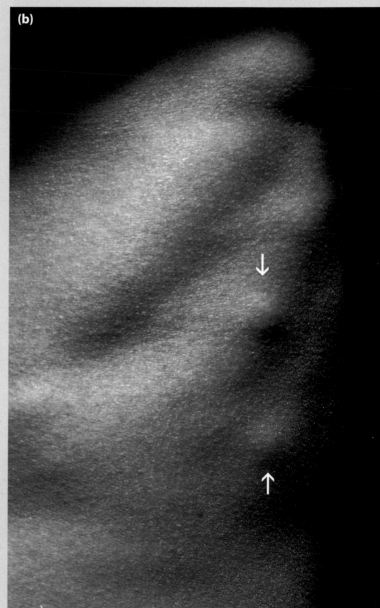

Case 10.33

A 72-year-old Pakistani immigrant to Australia died of a myocardial infarction. Post-mortem examination was performed at a teaching hospital in Brisbane. As an incidental finding, two transparent cysticerci were found under the leptomeninges (see Fig. 10.202). Other cysticerci were demonstrated deeper in the brain when it was examined in more detail (see Fig. 10.203).

Microscopic section of one of these cysticerci showed the presence of an embryo head of a tapeworm and a marked gliotic reaction around the parasite (see Fig. 10.204(a)). A section of another cysticercus showed no tissue reaction to the parasite (see Fig. 10.204(b)).

Figures 10.205 and 10.206, overleaf, show a CT scan and a gross specimen of very severe cysticercosis of the brain.

Cysticerci can be found in almost every organ in the body. Figure 10.207, overleaf, shows cysticerci in the eye and Figure 10.208, overleaf, shows them in skeletal muscle.

▶ **Fig. 10.202(a) and (b)** Unfixed brain of a male, aged 72 years, who had a number of cysticerci in the brain. He did not have any symptoms that could be related to the parasitic infection. Sometimes, however, symptoms of epilepsy occur in cases of cerebral cysticercosis.

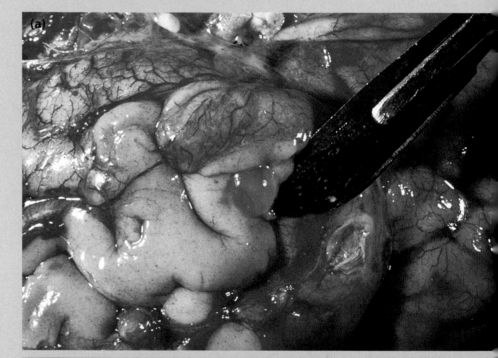

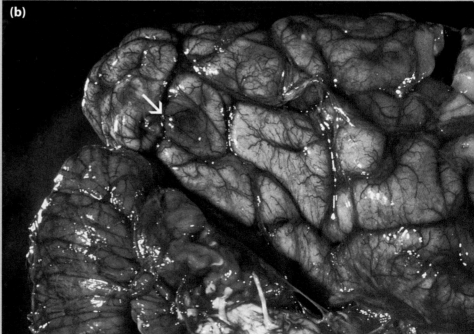

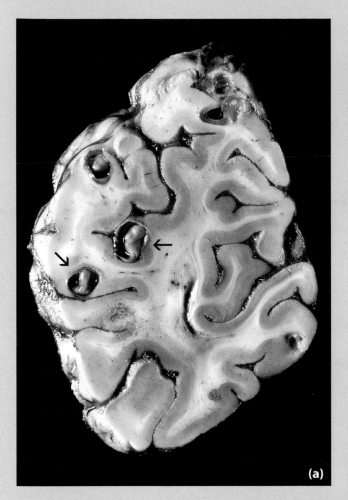

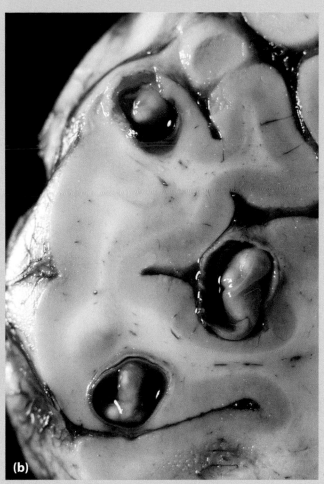

▲ **Fig. 10.203(a) and (b)** Slices of the fixed brain of the patient shown in Figure 10.202. Multiple cysticerci can be seen.

▼ **Fig. 10.204(a)** One of the cysticerci in the brain had a gliotic reaction around it.

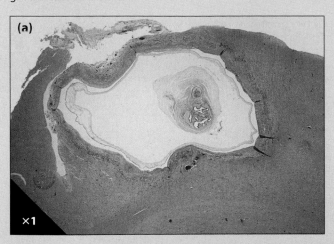

▶ **Fig. 10.204(b)** Another cysticercus in which there is no reaction around the parasite.

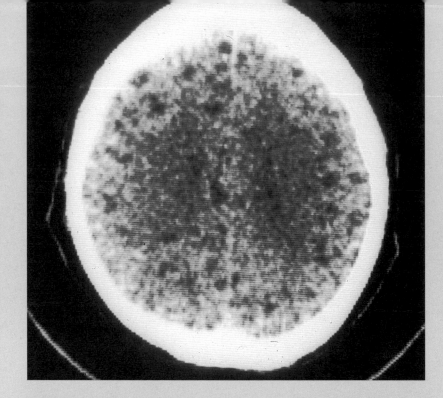

▶ **Fig. 10.205** CT scan of a 40-year-old female from Shandong, China. It shows a heavy infestation with cysticerci.

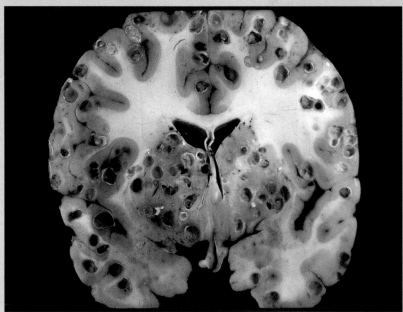

▶ **Fig. 10.206** Brain of a patient from West Irian, Indonesia, that shows a very heavy infestation with cysticerci similar to that seen in the CT scan. The patient had epilepsy during life.

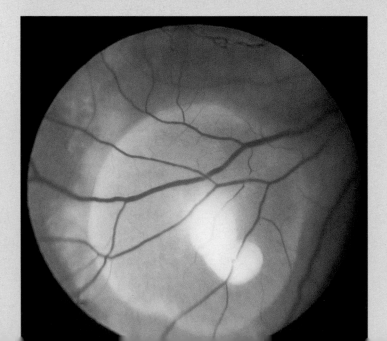

▶ **Fig. 10.207** Ophthalmoscopic view of a cysticercus present in the retina of the eye of an Indian patient from Chennai, India.

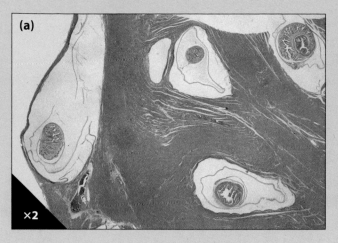 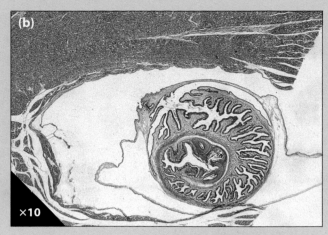

▲ **Fig. 10.208(a) and (b)** Views of cysticerci in skeletal muscle. There is no tissue reaction to the presence of the parasite.

Acknowledgments

- Fig. 10.1 Courtesy of John Pearn, Brisbane, Australia.
- Figs 10.7–10.8 Courtesy of David Tan, Kuala Lumpur, Malaysia.
- Fig. 10.9 Courtesy of Leonard Champness, Papua New Guinea and Geelong, Australia.
- Fig. 10.10 Courtesy of Walter Wood, Papua New Guinea and Brisbane, Australia. Photographed by Robin Cooke.
- Fig. 10.18 Courtesy of Leonard Champness, Papua New Guinea and Geelong, Australia.
- Figs 10.19–10.20 Courtesy of Ian Wilkey, Papua New Guinea and Brisbane, Australia.
- Fig. 10.21 Courtesy of J. Biswas, Mumbai, India.
- Figs 10.22–10.23 Courtesy of Leonard Champness, Papua New Guinea and Geelong, Australia.
- Fig. 10.24 Courtesy of Ian Reid, Papua New Guinea and Sydney, Australia.
- Fig. 10.25 Courtesy of Vincenzo Eusebi, Bologna, Italy.
- Fig. 10.30 Courtesy of Belinda Clarke and Tony Riley, Brisbane, Australia.
- Fig. 10.34 Courtesy of the hunter pictured in the photograph.
- Fig. 10.35 Courtesy of David Hardwick, Vancouver, Canada.
- Figs 10.36–10.37 Courtesy of Mike Powell, Brisbane, Australia. Photographed by Robin Cooke.
- Fig. 10.39 Courtesy of Chris Burke, Brisbane, Australia.
- Figs 10.40–10.57 case report on angiostrongyloidiasis. Courtesy of David Slaughter and Megan Turner, Brisbane, Australia. Parasitologic diagnosis of the worm removed from the eye was made by Paul Prociv, Brisbane, Australia. Photographed by Robin Cooke.
- Figs 10.64–10.65 Courtesy of the surgeon.
- Figs 10.80–10.84 Courtesy of Geoffrey Strutton, Brisbane, Australia.
- Figs 10.85–10.86 Courtesy of Jenny Robson, Brisbane, Australia.
- Figs 10.99–10.101 Courtesy of Mike Ward, Brisbane, Australia.
- Fig. 10.105 Courtesy of Jenny Robson, Brisbane, Australia. Jenny Robson also provided assistance with histories in Cases 10.13–10.16.
- Fig. 10.106 Courtesy of the patient, with the permission of her companions.
- Fig. 10.109 Courtesy of Lis Sedlak-Weinstein, Gold Coast, Australia.
- Fig. 10.116 section of granuloma in the wall of the appendix. Courtesy of Prasantha Murthy of Zambia, Papua New Guinea and Griffith, Australia. Photographed by Robin Cooke.
- Fig. 10.119 Courtesy of Pauline Close, Cape Town, South Africa.
- Fig. 10.120 Courtesy of John Tonge, Brisbane, Australia.
- Figs 10.122–10.123 Courtesy of Hiram Badderley, Egypt, Ghana, Bristol and Brisbane, Australia.
- Fig. 10.127(b) From Cooke, R.A. and Stewart, B., *Colour Atlas of Anatomical Pathology*, third edn, Churchill Livingstone, Edinburgh, 2004.
- Fig. 10.129 Courtesy of Lis Sedlak-Weinstein, Gold Coast, Australia.
- Figs 10.131–10.135 Case courtesy of Lloyd McGuire, Hong Kong, China, and Brisbane, Australia.
- Fig. 10.136 specimen of liver. Courtesy of Laurence Hou, Hong Kong, China, and John Kerr, Brisbane, Australia.
- Fig. 10.137 Courtesy of Dorothea Sandars, Brisbane, Australia.
- Fig. 10.139 Courtesy of Lorraine Pegler, Raymore Station, Quilpie, Australia.
- Fig. 10.142 Courtesy of Ron Aitken, Brisbane, Australia.

- Fig. 10.148b From Cooke, R.A. and Stewart, B., *Colour Atlas of Anatomical Pathology*, third edn, Churchill Livingstone, Edinburgh, 2004.
- Fig. 10.151 Courtesy of Ken Donald, Brisbane, Australia.
- Fig. 10.154 Courtesy of Arthur Beresford, Armidale, Australia.
- Fig. 10.155 Courtesy of John Earwaker, Brisbane, Australia.
- Fig 10.156 Courtesy of John Kerr, Brisbane, Australia.
- Figs 10.161–10.165 case information and histologic sections of *E. multilocularis*. Courtesy of Tomoo Itoh, Hokkaido University Hospital, Sapporo, Japan. Photographed by Robin Cooke.
- Fig. 10.171 Courtesy of Kevin Whitehead, Brisbane, Australia.
- Figs 10.173–10.175 Courtesy of Lorraine Pegler, Raymore Station, Quilpie, Australia.
- Figs 10.177–10.178 Infected pig meat was made available for study and photography by John Welch, Brisbane, Australia.
- Fig. 10.181 Courtesy of Lis Sedlak-Weinstein, Gold Coast, Australia.
- Fig. 10.188–10.189 Courtesy of John Mayze, Brisbane, Australia.
- Figs 10.190–10.191 Courtesy of John Sullivan, Brisbane, Australia.
- Fig. 10.200 Courtesy of Paul Mowat, Brisbane, Australia.
- Figs 10.202–10.203 Courtesy of Jack Little, Brisbane, Australia.
- Fig. 10.205 Courtesy of Hiram Badderley, Brisbane, Australia.
- Fig. 10.206 Courtesy of the Armed Forces Institute of Pathology (AFIP), Washington, USA.
- Fig. 10.207 Courtesy of J. Biswas, Mumbai, India.

Pandemic diseases

An epidemic disease is one that spreads quickly through a community, has a high rate of infection, lasts for a relatively short period of time and then disappears. When such diseases affect populations in a number of different countries, they are called pandemic diseases.

Pandemic diseases cause such serious social upheaval that they are recorded by historians at the time they occur. This chapter considers the main historical pandemic diseases that have occurred in many countries during the past few centuries—plague, smallpox and influenza. The two more recent pandemic diseases human immunodeficiency virus (AIDS) and severe acute respiratory syndrome (SARS) will be considered in the next chapter on 'emerging viral infections'.*

Plague

Plague is caused by the organism *Yersinia* (formerly *Pasteurella*) *pestis* a nonmotile, Gram-negative cocco-bacillus that shows bipolar staining. It grows on most culture media, including blood agar.

The organism normally lives in rats and other rodents. It is spread from one animal to another by the bite of fleas. Humans are infected upon accidentally entering the cycle by being bitten by fleas carrying the organism.

During the 1300s, there were many outbreaks of plague in Europe. These outbreaks were catastrophic. After the first case appeared, the disease spread rapidly through the population. The clinical manifestations were dramatic—with rapid onset of a high fever, prostration and death within a few days. Only a few victims survived.

---

*These references support the content of this chapter:

Hampson, A.W. and Mackenzie, J.S. The influenza viruses. *Med J Aust* 185:S39–S43, 2006.

Searle, J., Bryant, S. and Forgan-Smith, R. Clinico-pathological features in seven fatal cases of influenza A2/Hong Kong/68 pneumonia. *Med J Aust* 2:474–476, 1971.

Clinical manifestations

The organism caused subcutaneous hemorrhages that gave the skin a black color, hence the name 'Black Death' (see Fig. 11.1).

Axillary and inguinal lymph nodes became enlarged. Inguinal lymphadenopathy was particularly prominent. The swellings were called 'buboes' (shown in Fig. 11.2), Hence the name 'bubonic plague'.

Some patients developed pneumonia—pneumonic plague. This was almost universally fatal. Pneumonic plague seems to be the main manifestation of the occasional human cases that occur now as a result of infection from wild rodents and other animals. This is the situation for cases that occur in parts of the United States, like New Mexico, where the disease is endemic in prairie dogs. Humans become infected by fleas from infected animals that visit campsites in the desert to feed on scraps left by campers. This type of plague is sometimes called sylvatic plague.

▼ **Fig. 11.1** Moulage (wax model) by the Italian modeler Gaetano Zumbo (1656–1701), showing a group of people who died from the 'Black Death'. The skin is black from the hemorrhagic effect of the plague bacillus. It is interesting that Zumbo has shown a rat on the abdomen of one of his figures.

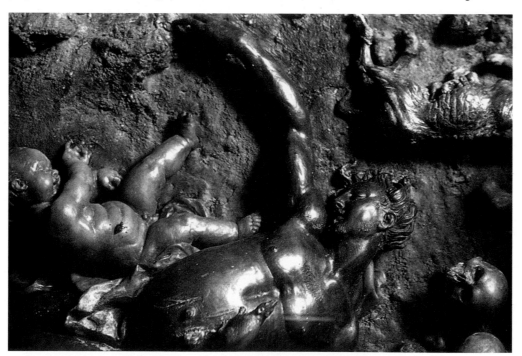

▼ **Fig. 11.2** Young Vietnamese woman has a left inguinal bubo. It was aspirated and plague bacilli were identified.

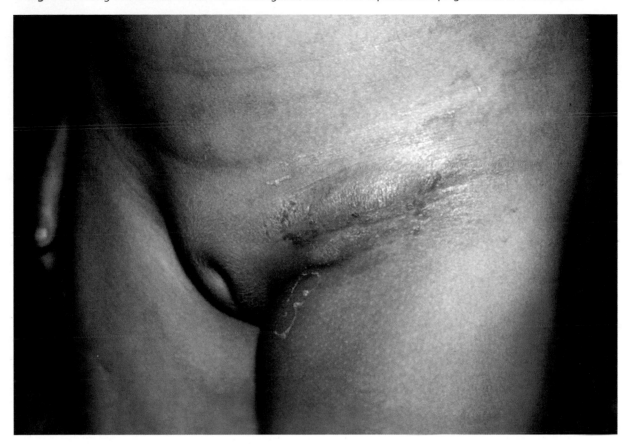

Case 11.1

In 1976, a 15-year-old male developed fever, headache and malaise the day after a family picnic in the countryside near Albuquerque, New Mexico. He had no clinical signs of disease until 4 days later, when he developed rectal bleeding with a prolonged prothrombin time. He was noted to have enlarged inguinal lymph nodes and pulmonary edema.

Aspiration of the lymph nodes yielded Gram-negative organisms identified as plague bacilli. He became progressively dyspneic and, in spite of antibiotic therapy, died on the fifth day of his illness.

Post mortem demonstrated the presence of pneumonia with numerous Gram-negative bacilli mixed with the purulent exudate (see Fig. 11.3). Inguinal lymph nodes showed hemorrhagic necrosis with numerous Gram-negative bacilli.

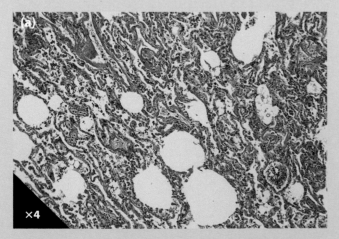
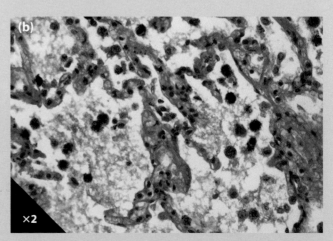

▲ **Fig. 11.3(a) and (b)** Sections of lung show plague pneumonia. Gram stain showed the presence of numerous Gram-negative bacilli.

Plague in the Middle Ages

It is not clear what the exact mortality was in the various outbreaks in Europe during the Middle Ages. Mortality seems to have varied from one outbreak to another. However, it was very high—in some places reaching 75 per cent of the population.

The high mortality rate changed the social order. For example, so many laborers died that the feudal system (the system of government based on an obligation of subjects to work for their king) was destroyed and laborers subsequently had much greater freedom to negotiate their terms of employment.

During the epidemics of the Middle Ages, doctors attending to patients with plague dressed in a black garb that covered them completely. They wore a beak-like mask, which had in its tip a cloth soaked in perfume to counteract the smell of death and disease. Even with these precautions, the doctors were not immune to the disease. Presumably, the rat fleas had no difficulty 'penetrating' these defences (see Figs 11.4 and 11.5).

▶ **Fig. 11.4** Model of a doctor in the Middle Ages dressed to attend to patients with plague.

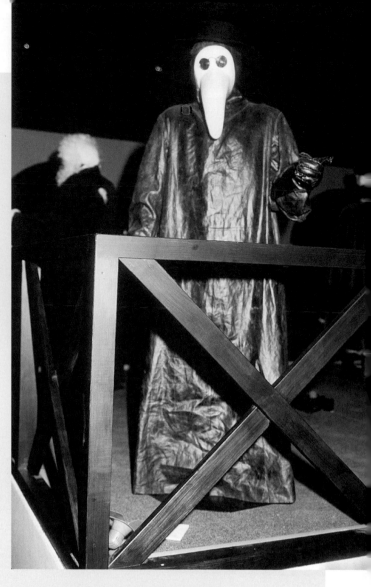

▼ **Fig. 11.5** Plague display in the Medical Museum in Lyon, France. The doctor is shown in his black gown. The pikes (spears) in the display next to him were used by city guards to keep strangers and visitors from entering the city during an epidemic of plague. This measure was aimed at preventing possibly infected people from bringing the 'contagion' into the city.

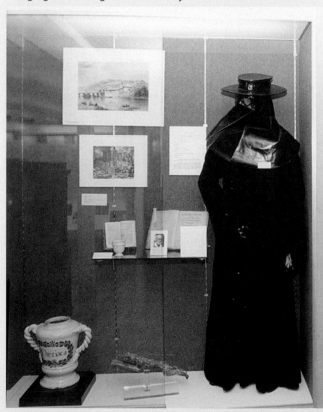

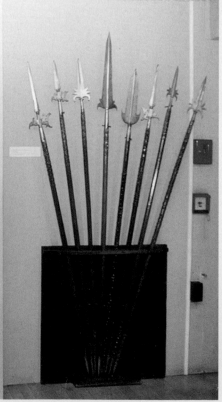

Plague epidemics in London and in Hong Kong

Two particularly dramatic epidemics are worth noting. The plague epidemic in London in the years 1664–1666 killed about 70 000 of a total population of about 460 000. It was controlled when a fire destroyed the city and its rats. These catastrophic events are commemorated by the Monument to the Great Fire of London, commonly known as 'The Monument' (see Figs 11.6, 11.7 and 11.8).

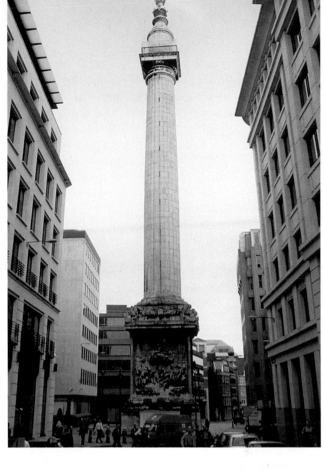

▶ **Fig. 11.6** The Monument in the City of London, at the junction of Monument Street and Fish Street, was erected to commemorate the Great Fire of 1666 and the Great Plague that preceded the fire.

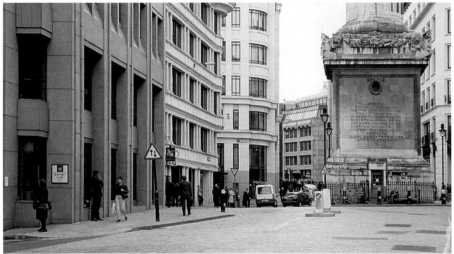

▶ **Fig. 11.7** Behind the Monument and to the left of it is the entrance to Pudding Lane, where the Great Fire is said to have started in a baker's shop.

▶ **Fig. 11.8** Plaque to commemorate the Great Fire.

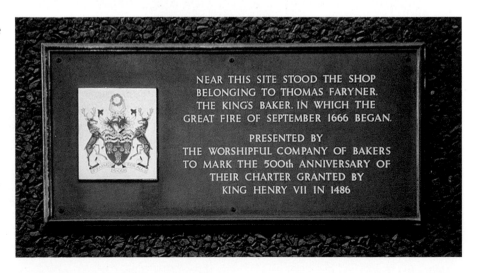

NEAR THIS SITE STOOD THE SHOP BELONGING TO THOMAS FARYNER. THE KING'S BAKER. IN WHICH THE GREAT FIRE OF SEPTEMBER 1666 BEGAN.

PRESENTED BY THE WORSHIPFUL COMPANY OF BAKERS TO MARK THE 500th ANNIVERSARY OF THEIR CHARTER GRANTED BY KING HENRY VII IN 1486

The second dramatic plague epidemic was an outbreak in Hong Kong SAR in 1894. This killed about 80 000 of an estimated population of 100 000. From Hong Kong, it spread to other parts of the world, subsequently killing some millions of people.

Apart from its severity, this outbreak was notable for the fact that the French microbiologist Alexandre Yersin (1863–1931), from the Pasteur Institute in Vietnam, identified the causative organism that now bears his name. He suggested that the disease was spread by the rat flea.

A few days after Yersin's identification of the organism, the leading Japanese microbiologist Shibasaburo Kitasato (1852–1931) reported identical findings. Soon after this, another Japanese scientist from the Hygiene Institute in Tokyo identified plague bacilli in fleas removed from an infected rat. This completed the understanding of the life cycle of the organism.

In the Middle Ages in Europe, the knowledge that infected people needed to be kept apart from healthy ones was applied to the construction of hospitals. Wards were constructed in such a way that they could be isolated from each other in times of epidemics. However, this principle of isolating infected patients did not necessarily apply to the conditions in individual wards where many patients shared a bed—sometimes with the sickest being placed nearest the edges of the bed (see Fig. 11.9).

What did ordinary people think about the cause of plague epidemics?

The powerful effect that plague had on the ordinary people, and what they thought about it can be seen in many of the cities and towns in Europe by the plague monuments constructed to commemorate the passing of the various epidemics.

The monuments were built to give thanks for the end of an epidemic. One of the most famous of these is the monument in the Graben in the center of Vienna, Austria (shown in Fig. 11.10).

Near Prague, in the Czech Republic, there is a church called 'The Bone Church'. It derives its name from the fact that during an epidemic of plague, there were so many deaths that there were not enough people to bury the dead. The bodies would normally have been buried in the cemetery attached to the church, but instead they were just left there unburied. When the epidemic was over, it was decided to decorate the church with the bones, rather than bury them in the conventional way (Fig. 11.11)

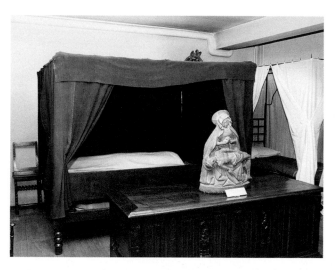

▲ **Fig. 11.9** Hospital bed from the Middle Ages in the Medical Museum in Lyon, France. Four patients were put in the bed with the sickest nearest the sides.

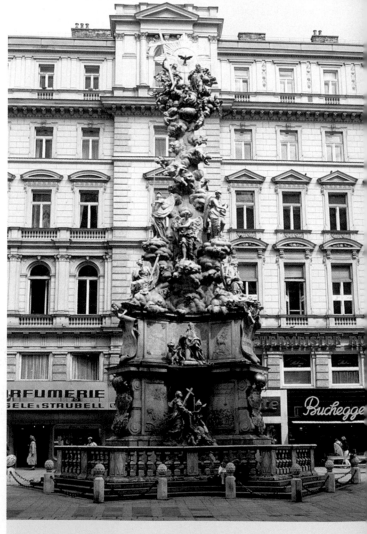

▲ **Fig. 11.10** Plague Monument in the Graben in the center of Vienna, Austria.

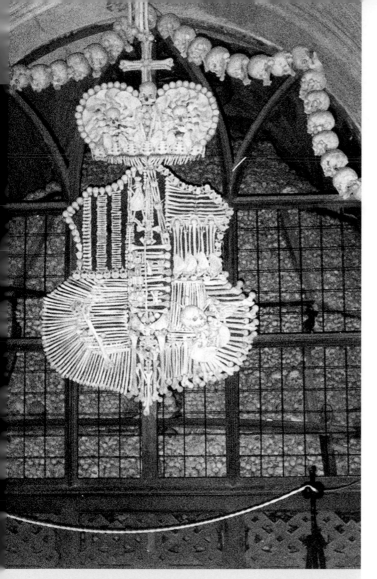

▲ **Fig. 11.11** Bones of plague victims decorating 'The Bone Church' near Prague, Czech Republic.

Could there be another epidemic of plague?

In many countries throughout the world, rubbish is placed for collection along the length of small streets in the cities (see Fig. 11.12). In older cities in Europe, for example in the older section of London, England, rubbish is also placed for collection outside buildings (see Fig. 11.13, overleaf). Before the introduction of proper sanitation practices in the early 1800s, rubbish was tossed into these narrow streets and removed mainly by rain. Rats bred under these conditions and this made it easy for foreign rats—bearing plague-infected fleas—to introduce plague into the local rats. This was at least partly responsible for the outbreaks of plague.

Today, if there is a breakdown of the orderly running of cities, for example by wars, earthquakes, tsunamis or industrial unrest, rubbish can accumulate and provide a fertile ground for the breeding of rats, and the spread of other infectious diseases as well.

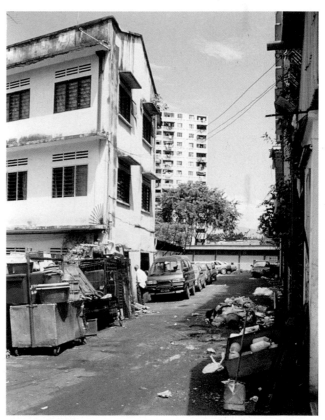

▲ **Fig. 11.12** Narrow street in a large city in South-East Asia, with garbage awaiting collection.

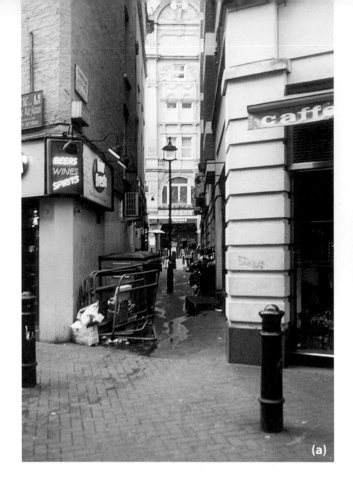

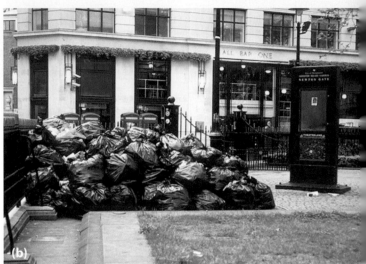

◀ ▼ **Fig. 11.13** Central London. **(a)** Laneway, Soho. **(b)** Leicester Square, early one Sunday morning before rubbish collection. It would only take a strike by garbage collectors for a few days (as actually happened in London some years ago) to recreate the conditions of the Middle Ages, with the risk of rats breeding and setting the stage for a potential recrudescence of plague and many other infectious diseases.

(a)

(b)

Smallpox

Smallpox is a disease caused by a virus that is highly infectious with a high rate of infection in a community that is not immune. It is spread by skin-to-skin contact. It causes severe illness and has a 50 per cent mortality rate.

Clinically, the patient presents with high fever and a vesicular rash that develops a few days after the onset of the fever. The rash consists of round, regular, deep-set vesicles that are mainly on the face and limbs—with relative sparing of the trunk (see Figs 11.14 and 11.15). The rash differs from that of chickenpox in that the vesicles are all about the same size, and are mainly on the face and limbs as against vesicles of varying size that are predominantly on the trunk.

In past centuries, it has been the cause of many serious epidemics. It is credited with causing the deaths of 40 million people during the eighteenth century.

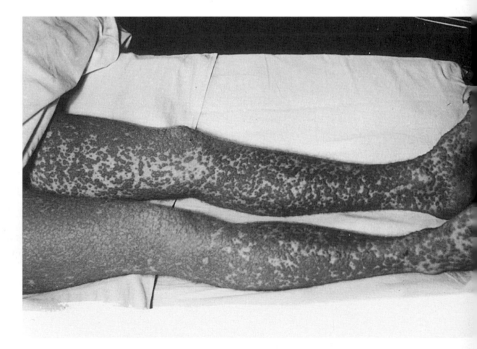

▲ **Fig. 11.14** African man, who died of smallpox in 1934. Note that the vesicles are large and close together, and they densely cover the legs. He had similar lesions on his face and arms.

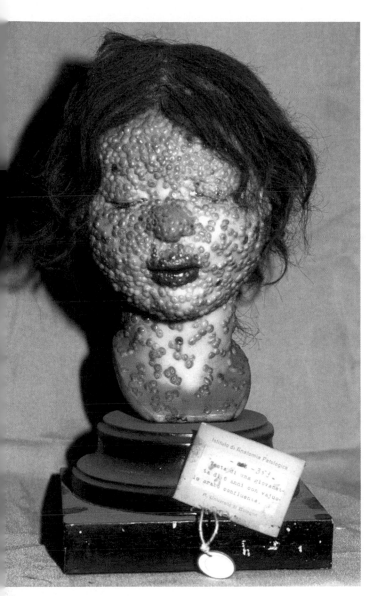

▲ **Fig. 11.15** Wax model of the face of a patient who had smallpox. Note the large vesicles covering the face. There are wax models of smallpox in many of the medical museums in Europe.

In 1977, it was claimed that this virus had been eradicated thanks to a vigorous worldwide campaign by the World Health Organization (WHO). With smallpox eradicated, it was argued that the remaining stocks of wild organism that were held in laboratories around the world should be destroyed, so that the organism would no longer be a danger to humanity.

An international meeting was held in 2003, at which it was decided not to destroy the remaining virus stocks because there was a real danger that it could be developed as a weapon of biological warfare or an agent of bioterrorism. If this happened, it would be important to have stocks from which vaccines could be manufactured quickly. So, supplies of the virus are now held in high security storage in a few designated infectious diseases laboratories in some countries.

History of smallpox vaccination

Edward Jenner (1749–1823), an English physician, introduced a successful method of prevention of infection by inoculating pus from cowpox through the skin—the process of vaccination. This caused a trivial illness and protected the person from smallpox.

Jenner's introduction of smallpox vaccination stemmed from an awareness that dairy farmers and other dairy workers became infected with cowpox (a trivial disease) and then did not contract smallpox.

In many countries, various forms of inoculation with pus from smallpox lesions had been attempted in order to prevent serious smallpox infection. One of the probable influences on Jenner was Lady Mary Montague, wife of the British ambassador to Turkey. She was impressed by the method used by Turkish women to prevent attacks of smallpox. They scratched the skin of normal people with a pin, dipped in pus from a smallpox lesion. This caused disease that was usually mild, but sometimes fatal. However, those who survived did not get smallpox later on. Lady Montague wrote to Jenner suggesting that he should try this in England.

In 1796, Jenner took pus from the cowpox lesions on the hand of a dairy maid, and inoculated this through scratches made on the skin of the 8-year-old son of one of his servants. Subsequently, the boy had a mild illness—with fever and a small pustular sore at the site of the inoculation—from which he soon recovered.

Six weeks later, Jenner did a similar inoculation on the boy, with pus from a case of smallpox. The boy remained well and did not get any infection following a further inoculation some months later. In fact, he lived into old age. This was the first documented successful use of vaccination to prevent a previously major killing disease.

Influenza

Influenza is a disease characterized by the sudden onset of fever over 100.4°F (38°C), headache, cough, generalized aches and muscle pain. It is transmitted by droplet infection. In the usual epidemics, symptoms last about a week and then recovery occurs. However, every few years, the infection is more virulent and there are some deaths either directly from influenza virus or from a bacterial superinfection.

In temperate climates, epidemics occur particularly during the winter months. In the tropics cases occur throughout the year. Some winter epidemics are more severe than others; and, occasionally and unpredictably, an epidemic spreads to many different countries—becoming a pandemic infection.

The most severe influenza pandemics in the twentieth century were the Spanish influenza (1918–1919), the Asian influenza (1957) and the Hong Kong influenza (1968–1969).

An interesting story of scientific sleuthing

In 2005, Dr Jeffrey Taubenberger and his research team at the Armed Forces Institute of Pathology (AFIP), Washington, reported[†] that they had identified the genetic code for the virus that caused the 'Spanish influenza'. This finding was assisted by samples from persons who had died of this disease in 1918.

In September 1918, thousands of US soldiers had died from this pandemic. Army pathologists had performed autopsies on many of them and had sent tissues to the AFIP for reporting. The tissue repository at the AFIP was searched by Dr Taubenberger and his team for this tissue. Over 120 cases were found on the files: 78 of these had lung tissue in paraffin blocks.

The team found fragments of the same viral RNA in two of these 78 cases. To be sure of these findings, it was necessary to examine frozen tissue so that they could determine that the viral RNA had not been denatured by the tissue processing.

The team reported their findings in *Science*, 1997, and 'wished' that they could get some frozen lung tissue from the 1918 epidemic.

A retired pathologist Johan V. Hultin read the 1997 paper and telephoned Dr Taubenberger to disclose that in 1951, as a graduate student, he had participated in the excavation of a gravesite in Brevig Mission (now Teller Mission), Alaska, where 85 per cent of the Inuit population of the Mission had died from Spanish influenza in 1918, and they had been interred in the Teller Mission graveyard in the permafrost. The objective of the 1951 excavation was to look for influenza virus in the lung tissue. By the methods available at that time, no virus was isolated, so the team went no further.

Dr Hultin offered to return to Teller Mission to find another sample of frozen lung tissue. So, in 1998, he did return and he obtained lung tissue from an Inuit woman who had died of Spanish influenza in 1918.

The researchers at the AFIP were able to confirm that the Inuit woman's lung tissue had viral RNA with the same genetic code as that of the two soldiers.

Influenza virus

There are three types of human influenza virus—types A, B and C. Serious disease is caused only by types A and B. The influenza A and B viruses have two major surface glycoprotein antigens:

- hemagglutinin—H, which is responsible for cell attachment, and
- neuraminidase—N, which assists with virus maturation and release.

These surface antigens continually undergo antigenic change—a phenomenon called 'antigenic drift'. This gives rise to subtypes of the viruses and explains why immunity gained from infection or vaccination to one subtype does not protect from infection with another subtype.

The disease was probably described by Hippocrates (460–377 BC), but since the virus was first isolated in 1933, it was found that winter epidemics were caused by influenza A. Anti-influenza vaccines were produced but it was soon realized that the virus quickly changed its antigenic composition. This showed in laboratory tests on the virus cultures, and by the fact that the vaccine prepared from a virus that caused one epidemic was not necessarily effective against the virus that caused the next epidemic.

This 'antigenic drift' is seen in Australia, where the influenza vaccine for the Australian winter is prepared from the influenza A virus causing influenza in the Northern Hemisphere winter. When it is administered in Australia, it is not always effective in preventing influenza because the infecting organism has changed its antigenic composition.

The major pandemic infections have been caused by newly formed subtypes of influenza A, developed by a process called 'antigenic shift' to which no-one has any immunity. The subtypes that caused the three major pandemics in the twentieth century are the Spanish influenza A/H1N1, the Asian influenza A/H2N2, and the Hong Kong influenza A/H3N2.

It has been established that the influenza viruses have evolved in an avian host, with migratory water birds being the major host for influenza A. Influenza B seems to have evolved into being a purely human pathogen.

---

†AFIP Letter, 163(3), 2005.

Some clinical and pathologic features of fatal influenza

Case histories of some deaths caused by Hong Kong influenza virus

In 1970 in Australia, there was a significant number of deaths, mainly from respiratory failure caused by Hong Kong influenza virus. The Australian cases followed those in the northern winter of 1969. Of the patients who died at a hospital in Brisbane, 13 had post-mortem examinations. Seven of these died from what on post-mortem examination was a primary influenza pneumonia. The other six showed changes of a superimposed bacterial pneumonia.

The average age of these 13 patients was 54.5 years and the average time from admission to death was 5.5 days.

The lungs were all more than twice normal weight and were firm and rubbery in consistency. Microscopically, the alveolar walls were thickened (see Figs 11.16 and 11.17). The alveoli were filled with oedema fluid and many were lined by hyaline membranes (shown in Fig. 11.18a and 11.18b, overleaf). The alveoli contained numerous alveolar lining cells that showed some dysplasia (see Fig. 11.18c, overleaf). In some areas, the alveolar lining cells showed squamous metaplasia. There was a variable chronic inflammatory cell infiltration present.

The Hong Kong influenza virus was isolated from the lungs of three of the pure influenza pneumonias and three of those who had superimposed bacterial pneumonia.

One case of myocarditis was encountered during the epidemic (see Figs 11.19 and 11.20).

Case 11.2

A male, aged 40 years, was admitted to a Brisbane hospital in 1970 with symptoms and signs of influenza. He had pneumonia and was extremely dyspnoeic. His condition deteriorated and he died 2 days after admission. Post mortem examination revealed heavy lungs which were firm and rubbery in consistency. Viral culture of lung tissue was positive for Hong Kong virus. The microscopic changes are shown in Figs 11.16–11.18, continued overleaf.

Note: During the influenza epidemic, a post mortem examination was performed on one child who died. This was a female aged 7 years. Her lungs showed similar changes to those seen in the adult cases, but viral culture of lung tissue was negative.

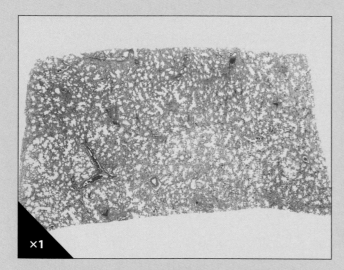

▲ **Fig. 11.16** View of a section of lung from a male, aged 40 years, who died following an attack of Hong Kong influenza, showing almost complete consolidation of this part of the lung.

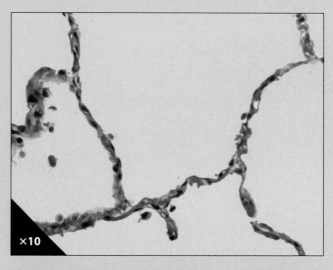

▲ **Fig. 11.17** View of an alveolar portion of a normal lung showing the thickness of the alveolar septae.

▼ ▶ **Fig. 11.18(a) and (b)** Views of the lung showing features of Hong Kong influenza pneumonia with thickened alveolar septae and the presence of hyaline membranes lining the alveoli. **(c)** Proliferation of alveolar lining cells some of which show moderate dysplasia.

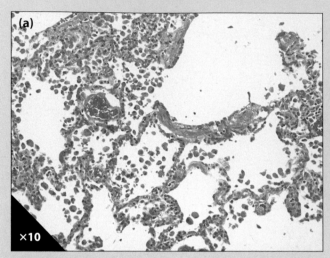

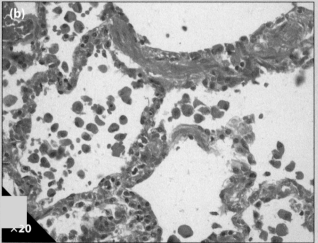

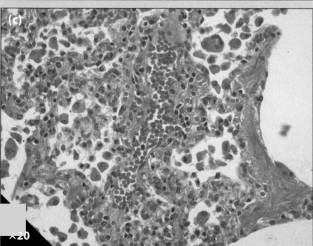

Case 11.3

A male, aged 31 years, was found dead in bed one morning after having had 'flu' for 2 days and complaining of chest pain and dyspnea. A coronial autopsy showed the lung changes of influenza, and the heart showed acute myocarditis.

The Hong Kong influenza virus was isolated from the lungs, which showed similar changes to those in Case 11.2. The changes in the heart are illustrated in Figs 11.19 and 11.20.

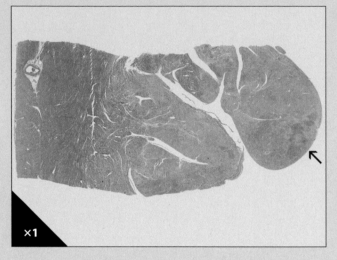

▲ **Fig. 11.19** View of a section taken from a hemorrhagic area in the myocardium of a male, aged 31 years, who was found dead at home after a 2-day history of dyspnea and chest pain. He had myocarditis caused by Hong Kong influenza.

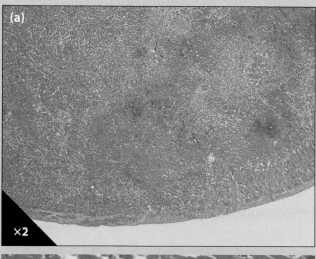

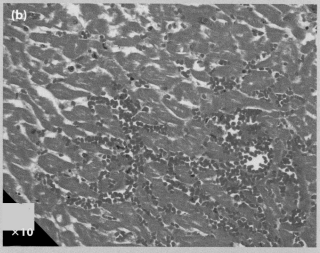

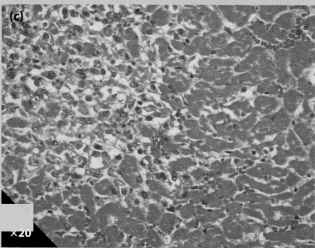

▲ **Fig. 11.20(a), (b) and (c)** Views of the myocardium showing the features of myocarditis—necrosis of myocardial muscle fibers, hemorrhage and an infiltration of mononuclear inflammatory cells.

Bird flu

Influenza A is primarily found in water birds, and the birds only rarely show evidence of disease. However, two subtypes in particular—H5 and H7—cross the species barrier and cause disease in domestic poultry and, sometimes, in humans.

In 1997, a new A/H5N1 subtype was isolated in Hong Kong SAR from an epidemic in domestic poultry. Since then, this virus has been isolated in sick or dead poultry in many countries in South-East Asia, with some reports from Africa and Europe as well. By 16 October 2006, the WHO reported 256 human cases from ten countries with 151 deaths. All of the human cases were associated with infected poultry or other birds. There has been no confirmed transmission from human to human. For a pandemic to occur, the virus will need to mutate to a form that is infective when passed from one human to another. The situation is being carefully monitored.

What of the future?

It is universally agreed that another pandemic similar to that of the Spanish influenza can and probably will occur. Whether it will be caused by the influenza A/H5N1, or some other subtype of the influenza A virus, or by one of the other 'emerging viral infections' cannot be predicted. Nor can the severity of such a pandemic be predicted. However, many countries have invested large sums of money in developing appropriate measures to identify early cases, to diagnose and treat them, and to contain any potential epidemic within their national borders. Global communication centers have also been established to ensure that the response to such a major pandemic will be properly coordinated.

Acknowledgments

- Fig. 11.1 Photographed with permission of the Curator, University of Bologna Museum, Bologna, Italy.
- Fig. 11.2 Courtesy of Geoffrey Bourke, Brisbane, Australia.
- Fig. 11.4 Photographed with permission at a display in Padua, Italy.
- Fig. 11.5 Photographed with permission of the Curator, Medical Museum, Lyon, France.
- Fig. 11.9 Photographed with permission of the Curator, Medical Museum, Lyon, France.
- Fig. 11.11 Courtesy of Justin Cooke, Brisbane, Australia.
- Fig. 11.14 Courtesy of James and Peggy McCartney, Adelaide, Australia.
- Fig. 11.15 Courtesy of Vincenzo Eusebi, Bologna, Italy.
- Fig. 11.18 Hong Kong influenza case information. Courtesy of Jeffrey Searle, Brisbane, Australia. Photographed by Robin Cooke.
- Fig. 11.20 case report on Hong Kong influenza. Courtesy of Ian Wilkey, Brisbane, Australia. Photographed by Robin Cooke.

Emerging viral infections

New pathogenic viruses are appearing all the time. There are many causes for this, for example as a result of genetic changes in existing viruses; as a result of animals being moved from their natural environment into close contact with humans; or as a result of humans moving into new environments, as occurs when forests are cleared for agriculture. The new viruses pose a challenge to all categories of health workers throughout the world because in a world where the movement of people is easier than it ever was, infectious diseases can spread with unprecedented speed.

Every time a virus of this type appears, people wonder whether it will be of similar severity to some of the serious historical pandemic diseases, particularly the influenza epidemic of 1918–19. Any new pandemic disease will not be strictly comparable with those of the past, because medical science now has better tools with which to combat them, and there are international management strategies in place that can deal with the global nature of the diseases.

In this chapter, the two most famous of recent pandemic diseases are considered: human immunodeficiency virus (AIDS) and severe acute respiratory syndrome (SARS).

- AIDS first appeared in 1981 and is still causing major problems in many countries.
- SARS first appeared in 2002 and disappeared by the end of 2004.

Two other infections are also discussed here: the monkeypox virus and the Hendra virus, because they give different perspectives to this topic.

- Monkeypox virus infection, discussed in Case 12.5 (see pages 477–478).
  In this case, the disease occurred as a result of moving an animal (a prairie dog) from its natural environment into a domestic environment with humans. The monkeypox virus is considered in the light of the epidemiology and problems in diagnosis and management.
- Hendra virus infection, discussed in Cases 12.6, 12.7 and 12.8 (see pages 481–488).
  Hendra virus caused a fatal disease in horses and then 'jumped the species barrier' to cause serious disease, and in some cases death, in the humans who were associated with them. The Hendra virus is considered from the standpoint of the difficulties in diagnosis and management of a new virus.

These considerations lead on to consider how humans are exploiting naturally occurring organisms, and newly emerging viruses to wage biological warfare, and how some nations, terrorist organisations and individuals may further exploit these organisms to engage in terrorist activities.

Human immunodeficiency virus (HIV)—the cause of AIDS

In 1981, physicians on both coasts of the United States reported clusters of homosexual men with unusual opportunistic infections and tumors, who had been previously healthy. Cases in Los Angeles had *Pneumocystis carinii* pneumonia (PCP), diarrhea and thrush, while those in New York and San Francisco presented with Kaposi sarcoma (KS) and PCP. Within 2 years of the original report, cases were identified in 15 US states, in Europe and in central Africa.

Epidemiologists defined the disease as having a long incubation period, with eventual destruction of the immune system (CD4 lymphocytes) and death in most cases. They determined that the syndrome consisted of an early phase of lymphadenopathy followed by a period of apparent latency, and, finally, immunosuppression complicated by various opportunistic infections and specific tumors (KS and B-cell lymphoma).

The etiologic agent is a retrovirus, human immunodeficiency virus (HIV). There are two subtypes—HIV1 and HIV2. (HIV2 is limited to West Africa.) HIV is called a retrovirus because its genetic material is RNA. This is converted into DNA by an enzyme, reverse transcriptase, that is present in the virus. This allows the HIV to enter the DNA of the host cell and take over its function. (The process in other viruses is that DNA is converted into RNA.)

HIV is transmitted by anal and vaginal sexual intercourse, by transfusion of blood or blood products, via transplacental or intrapartum exposure, and by the sharing of infected needles. Untreated, the mortality of AIDS is high. It has caused many deaths, particularly in tropical Africa. The World Health Organization predicts that by 2010, Asia will have the greatest number of AIDS cases.[*]

Serologic tests have been introduced for diagnosis, and antiretroviral agents are able to suppress virus replication, thus lowering morbidity and mortality. Effective treatment requires multiple drugs because both primary and secondary drug resistance is common.

Altered host response in HIV infection and in AIDS

A complex combination of alterations in host response occurs over the stages of HIV infection. The defects are seen in both acute and chronic phases of inflammation. If we understand the usual histologic reaction to infective agents in the immune competent host, as well as how the underlying deficiency can alter the histologically observable immune response, we can predict the most likely cause of a given reaction.

The normal host has several mechanisms to prevent and control infection. Nonspecific barriers (skin and mucosal surfaces) block entry of microorganisms into the host. If these fail, the body has an incremental defense system that evolves from a nonspecific 'innate' reaction to a highly specific 'adaptive' response.

Acute inflammation is primarily controlled by the 'innate' defense system and can function with humoral, cellular or combined immune deficiencies if the neutrophil count is adequate and there is active myelopoiesis.

Adaptive immunity allows the host to identify and remember specific pathogens through activity of B and T lymphocytes that express specific receptors. The cytokine profiles of CD4+ T helper lymphocytes define two separate arms of the response: Th-1 (cellular immunity) and Th-2 (humoral immunity).

Cytokine activity of Th-1 and Th-2 are both synergistic and antagonistic. Cell-mediated immunity (CMI) relies on the complex interaction of antigen presenting cells, T-cells, cytokines and other factors. The antigen presenting cells (APCs) (macrophages, Langerhans and dendritic cells) process and present antigen with MHC-II molecules to activate naïve T-cells. Th-1 cell cytokines activate macrophages, natural killer (NK) cells and other components of CMI.

Activated macrophages have enhanced intracellular killing and secrete cytokines responsible for many of the signs of infection. Tumor necrosis factor (TNF)-α induces fever, shock and inflammation, as well as induction of angiogenesis and deposition of extracellular matrix.

CD8 cytotoxic lymphocytes are another important component of cellular immunity. They are able to kill cells that present foreign peptides (viral infected or neoplastic cells) and help to control nonviral intracellular pathogens.

The Th-2 mediated component of adaptive immunity is primarily a B-cell response characterized by antibody (immunoglobulin) formation and activation of the classic complement pathway.

HIV-associated defects in immunity

Nonspecific barriers, such as skin and mucosae, are altered by the use of antibiotics (changes in normal microbiota), inflammation, drug reactions, malnutrition and the presence of intravenous lines or catheters. Complement function is impaired in late-stage AIDS. Neutrophil function is normal in early stages of HIV infection and can be protective in late-stage disease if recruitment is maintained.

Due to the effects of high viral loads, drug-induced bone marrow suppression or replacement of the bone marrow by tumor and infection, most patients have some level of neutropenia as well as neutrophil and natural killer (NK) cell dysfunction at multiple times during the course of the disease. Altered production and activity of monocytes and macrophages affects both innate and adaptive immunity. Dendritic/Langerhans cells demonstrate decreases in phagocytosis, chemotaxis and cytokine production, as well as poor antigen presentation. NK cells are unable to effectively recognize and kill target cells (malignant or infected cells).

---

*Statistics are available at UNAIDS.org.

In advanced stages of HIV infection, the marked disruption of lymphoid tissue and loss of follicular dendritic cells limits the host's ability to process antigen and mount specific responses to pathogens. Loss of cellular immunity is the hallmark of AIDS. Due to the loss of CD4+ T-cells and the subsequent defects in the protective action of lymphokines, macrophage and CD8+ killing and cytokine activity, the host is subject to overwhelming opportunistic infections.

There are qualitative and quantitative defects in CD4 cells due to HIV infection. The resulting indirect effects include loss of cytokine production, dysregulation of B-cell function, loss of CMI and 'holes' in the immunologic repertoire that may not be restored with the use of anti-retroviral therapy.

Most alterations in humoral immunity are related to B-cell hyperactivation and hypergammaglobulinemia infections associated with neutropenia and neutrophil dysfunction.

Infections associated with neutropenia and neutrophil dysfunction

- Bacteria: Enterobacteria, Pseudomonas, Enterococci, Streptococci.
- Fungi: Candidiasis, Aspergillosis.

Infections associated with defective cell-mediated immunity

- Bacteria: Mycobacteria, Listeria, Salmonella, Rhodococcus.
- Fungi: Pneumocystis, Histoplasmoses, Cryptococcus.
- Viruses: Herpes, CMV, Varicella, EBV.
- Protozoa: Toxoplasmosa, Cryptosporidia, Leishmania.

Viral-induced tumors

- EBV-related lymphomas (B-cell, CNS and Hodgkin).
- HPV-associated squamous neoplasms.
- Herpes hominis virus-8: Kaposi sarcoma, multicentric Castleman's.

Infections associated with IgG-deficiency

- *S. pneumoniae*, *H. influenzae*, other encapsulated organisms.
- *Pneumocystis carinii*, Giardia, Cryptosporidia.

Immune restoration syndrome

Following the initiation of highly active antiretroviral therapy (HAART), some patients develop exaggerated local and systemic inflammatory reactions. The immune restoration syndrome usually occurs within the first few months of initiating therapy and coincides with a rapid increase in CD4+ T lymphocytes and the resulting immune reconstitution. The reaction is thought to be due to increased hypersensitivity to the antigens. These paradoxical reactions have been reported most commonly in cases of tuberculosis

and mycobacterium avium complex (MAC) disease involving lymph nodes.[†]

Some presenting manifestations of HIV/AIDS

- Case 12.1 Lymphadenopathy
- Case 12.2 Opportunistic infection
- Case 12.3 A specific tumor

[†]There are no specific references on immuno restoration syndrome, but there are many reviews of immunology and pathology in normal and HIV-infected persons.

Case 12.1

A 45-year-old HIV-infected woman presented with parotid swelling, which had been increasing over the past several months. She also had generalized lymphadenopathy, but no other significant symptoms.

Her CD4 T-cell count was 212 cells/microliter. She was taking Trizivir (an antiretroviral agent). Biopsy of the left parotid gland was performed (see Figs 12.1, 12.2 and 12.3).

Diagnosis: Parotid lymphoepithelial lesion (HIV-associated sialadenopathy).

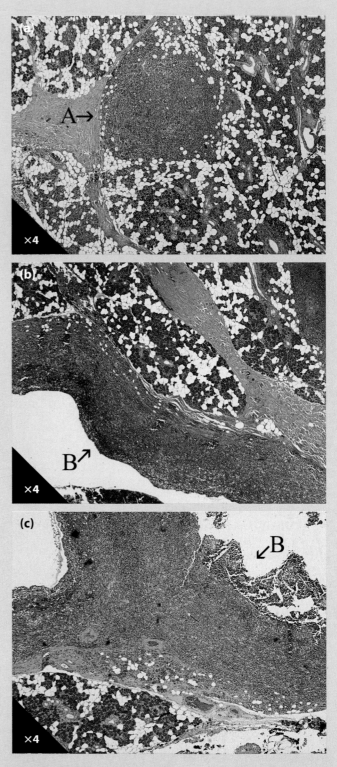

▲ **Fig. 12.1(a), (b) and (c)** Sections of parotid gland showing nodular (A) and cystic (B) lymphoid hyperplasia. The lymphoid tissue shows the characteristic changes of hyperplasia described in lymphoid tissue in other areas of the body.

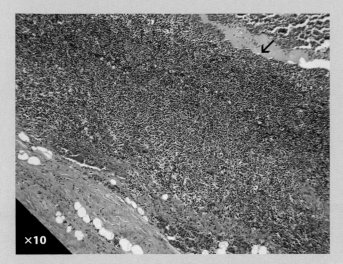

▲ **Fig. 12.2** The cysts are lined by epithelial cells.

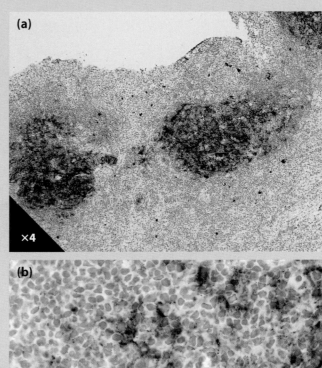

▲ **Fig. 12.3(a) and (b)** HIV p24 (gag) antigen is positive in the follicular dendritic network and individual cells within the lymphoid tissue.

Case 12.1 discussion

Persistent generalized lymphadenopathy (PGL), one of the earliest manifestations of HIV infection, is defined by the Centers for Disease Control (CDCs) as 'palpable lymphadenopathy of more than 1 centimeter that involves more than two extrainguinal sites, and has persisted for more than 3 months'.

Three types or stages have been described, but they actually represent a constellation of changes that may occur along a spectrum from florid hyperplasia to marked atrophy. In the early stages of HIV-infection, often prior to the onset of any other symptoms, the hyperplastic changes predominate. There are large, geographic follicles that have varying amounts of cytolysis, focal hemorrhage and tingible body macrophages. Mantle zone lymphocytes may invade the follicle or may be moderately to markedly decreased

in number Monocytoid B-cell hyperplasia, vascular proliferation, intrafollicular plasmacytosis, erythrophagocytosis and Warthin-Finkeldey type giant cells occur. Involutional and atrophic changes are found in more advanced stages of HIV infection.

A particular form of hyperplasia occurs in salivary gland associated lymphoid tissue, which is characterized by the formation of lymphoepithelial cysts in parotid or other glands. The lymphoepithelial lesion was described initially in 1958. It is reported frequently in association with HIV infection and often occurs early in the course of HIV disease. Bilateral parotid involvement is more common than unilateral disease. Although the lymphoepithelial lesion is benign, malignant transformation can occur, especially in patients with low CD4+ T-cell lymphocyte counts.

Case 12.2

A 10-year-old African boy had been severely ill in hospital for more than 2 months. HIV infection was diagnosed 12 months before. The presenting symptoms at that time included abdominal pain, cough and thrush. His CD4 T-cell count was 4 cells/microliter.

He was started on antiretroviral therapy and there was an increase in CD4 count to 153 cells/microliter over 6 months.

Clinically, he was thought to have tuberculosis and was started on antimycobacterial therapy, although all cultures were negative. He had a retroperitoneal mass from which a biopsy was taken (see Figs 12.4 and 12.5).

Diagnosis: Disseminated tuberculosis: Immuno restoration syndrome.

▶ **Fig. 12.4(a), (b) and (c)** Section of the retroperitoneal mass showed it to be a lymph node that contained necrotizing and suppurative granulomas.

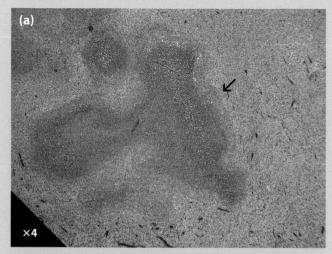

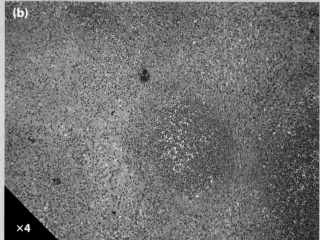

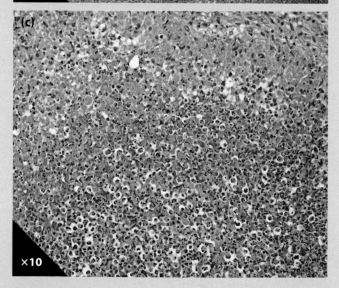

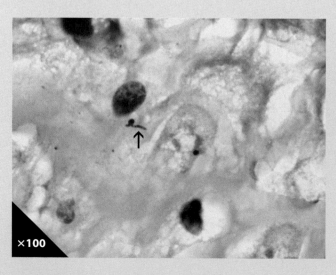

◀ **Fig. 12.5** Rare acid-fast bacilli (AFB) were present.

| 470 |

Case 12.2 discussion

Mycobacterium tuberculosis infection, either pulmonary or extrapulmonary, is an AIDS-defining disease. Persons with HIV infection are uniquely susceptible to both primary, reinfection and reactivation disease due to *M. tuberculosis*. This susceptibility is in part responsible for recent increases in the incidence of tuberculosis in countries where HIV infection has become established.

In the United States, the prevalence of co-infection is approximately 4 per cent, but in Africa and Asia the rate may be as high as 40–80 per cent.

Because *M. tuberculosis* is a virulent pathogen, it is often the earliest infection in the course of declining immunocompetence. Tuberculosis itself is immunosuppressive and causes a depression in blood CD4+ lymphocyte counts in both HIV-infected and noninfected persons.

The histologic patterns of tuberculosis reflect the integrity of the cellular immune response of the patient. There are three patterns of cellular immune response that correlate with the stage of HIV infection—granulomatous, hyporeactive and anergic.

Patients with relatively intact cellular immunity will have a typical granulomatous response with few organisms. As the CD4+ lymphocyte count drops, cellular immunity decreases and there is a loss of Langhans giant cells and a decrease in epithelioid macrophages. In this hyporeactive stage, there is poor intracellular killing of mycobacteria. The caseous centers enlarge and coalesce, and AFBs are numerous, both in the areas of necrosis and within macrophages. In the final stages of AIDS, there is pyohistiocytic response and myriads of AFB.

The immune restoration syndrome is associated with increases in CD4 counts and the resulting immune reconstitution. These paradoxical reactions have been reported in cases of tuberculosis and MAC disease and often involve the cervical or mesenteric lymph nodes. There is usually fever, swelling and, in the case of mesenteric adenopathy, abdominal pain and malabsorption.

Cultures can be negative. Histologic features include reactive lymphadenopathy, edema and granulomatous reactions, often with few or no AFB identified.[#]

#The section on immuno restoration syndrome is based on information from:

Lucas, S. and Nelson, A.M., Pathogenesis of tuberculosis in human immuno-deficiency virus-infected people. In *Tuberculosis: Pathogenesis, Protection and Control*, American Society for Microbiology, Washington, 503–513, 1994.

Case 12.3

A 55-year-old man presented with a previous diagnosis of oral and cutaneous Kaposi sarcoma. He now had anemia, rectal bleeding and a rectal mass. He had been on antiretroviral therapy for 12 months. The rectal mass was biopsied (illustrated in Figs 12.6–12.9, see pages 472–473).

Diagnosis: Kaposi sarcoma, human herpes hominis 8 (HHV8) infection.

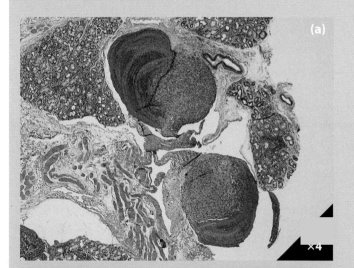
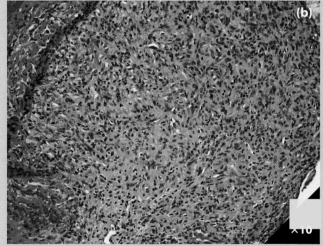

▲ **Fig. 12.6(a) and (b)** Sections of rectal mucosal biopsy show a nodular spindle-cell proliferation.

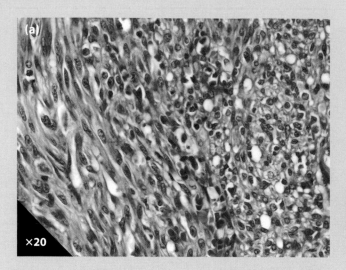
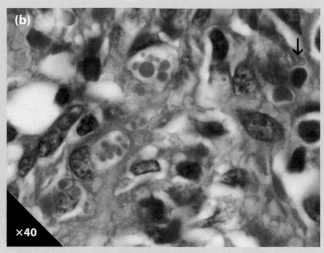

▲ **Fig. 12.7(a) and (b)** Vascular slits and intracytoplasmic hyaline globules.

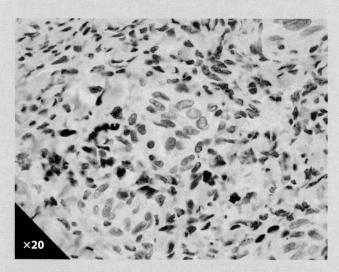

▲ **Fig. 12.8** Cells show positive staining with HHV8 antinuclear antigen.

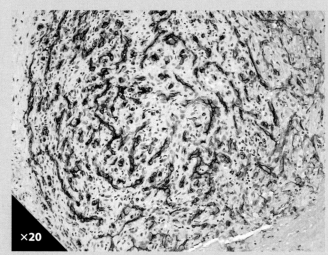

▲ **Fig. 12.9** Cells show positive staining with CD34.

Case 12.3 discussion

Kaposi sarcoma tumor cells are plump to elongated spindle cells arranged haphazardly. Mitosis, necrosis and nuclear pleomorphism are rare. The clefts or vascular slit-like spaces may contain red blood cells or hemosiderin.

PAS-positive intracytoplasmic hyaline globules can be found, but they are not pathognomonic. Plasma cells and coarse granules of hemosiderin are concentrated mostly at the periphery of the lesion.

The CD34 immunostain demonstrates the vascular origin of the spindle cells and lines the cleft-like spaces. The etiologic agent of KS is HHV8.

SARS

Severe acute respiratory syndrome (SARS), a life-threatening respiratory disease, was first recognized in Guangdong province, China in November, 2002. It quickly spread to many other countries. On 12 March 2003, the World Health Organization issued a global alert about the mysterious pneumonia. Within 2 weeks, a new coronavirus had been isolated from patients with SARS. It was named the SARS-associated coronavirus (SARS-CoV). Within a year, the outbreak had been controlled, and it subsided.

Clinically, the disease was characterized by the sudden onset of high fever and nonproductive cough, with dyspnea and rapidly progressive pneumonia. Lymphopenia of CD4 and CD8 T-cells was one of the earliest and most important findings in SARS patients. There were about 800 deaths, but only a relatively few post-mortem examinations were performed. One of the largest post-mortem series was reported from the Department of Pathology, Peking University Health Science C Department of Pathology, Peking University Health Science Center.

The typical morphological changes seen were:

- diffuse alveolar damage with hyaline membrane formation and pulmonary interstitial fibrosis, and
- generalized injury to the lymphoid tissue.

Seventy per cent of deaths were due to respiratory failure, and the lung was thought to be the portal of entry of the virus. However, other organs, especially the lymphoid organs, and gut and renal epithelium were also affected. Infection and destruction of the lymphocytes resulted in an acute immunodeficiency. Survival was determined by the absolute T-lymphocyte count.

SARS infection resulted in cases showing a spectrum of severity of symptoms, and only the severe cases demonstrated the typical pathologic changes described above. Typically children are especially vulnerable to viral diseases, but this is not the case with SARS. Physiological lymphoid hyperplasia of lymphoid tissue in childhood may account for the rare occurrence of SARS during the first decade of life.

Case 12.4

A 24-year-old psychotic male was found on the street, with fever and nonproductive cough. On admission, his body temperature was 103.0°F (39.2°C). Blood tests showed: WBC 4.8 × 10/L (neutrophils 83.3%, lymphocytes 12.4%), platelets 214 × 10/L and hemoglobin 5.4g/dL).

A chest X-ray demonstrated bilateral patchy infiltrates in the lower lobes (see Fig. 12.10). The patient was treated with antibiotics and ribavirin.

His symptoms improved from day 8 to day 11 post admission. On day 12, his temperature suddenly rose to 103.46°F (39.7°C) and watery diarrhea appeared 2 days later.

The chest X-ray showed progression of the patchy infiltrates and oxygen saturation dropped to 83 per cent from 85 per cent. Corticosteroids were administered, but lymphopenia persisted (0.7 × 10 /L on day 16). The ALT (28U.L) and AST (37U/L) were within normal limits.

He was maintained on mechanical ventilation for 5 days, but died of respiratory failure 20 days after admission.

Serologic testing identified SARS-CoV antibody just prior to his death. An autopsy was performed 24 hours after death.

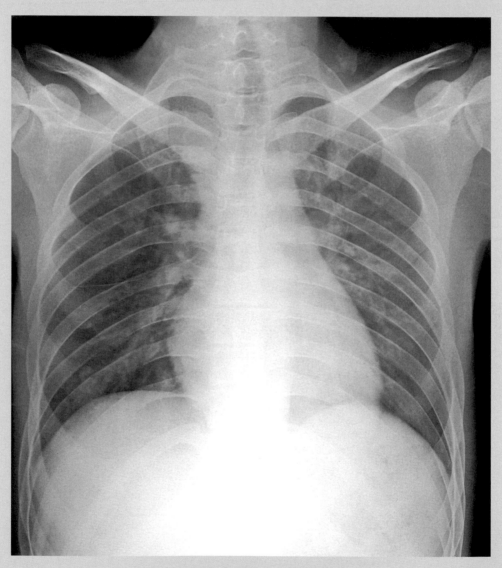

▲ **Fig. 12.10** Chest X-ray on day 12 of illness. It shows patchy infiltrates.

Morphological findings

Pathologic abnormalities were seen in the lungs, spleen, lymph nodes, liver and intestines. The lungs were heavy, firm, red and had the consistency of liver (see Fig. 12.11).

Microscopic examination showed diffuse alveolar damage with hyaline membrane formation, intra-alveolar edema, interstitial mononuclear inflammatory cell infiltration, and focal alveolar and interstitial fibrosis. There was an increase in macrophages both in number and in size. Multinucleated giant cells were present (see Figs 12.12 and 12.13, continued overleaf).

The spleen and lymph nodes were atrophic with loss of follicles (see Fig. 12.14, overleaf). There was atrophy of the mucosal lymphoid tissue, and pseudo-membranous enteritis was present in the ileum. Centri lobular necrosis was observed in the liver.

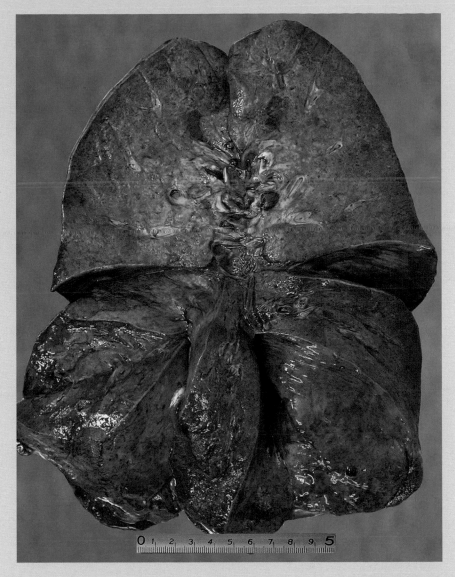

▲ **Fig. 12.11** Grossly, the lungs were heavy, firm and red, and had the consistency of liver.

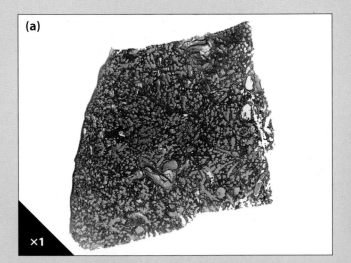

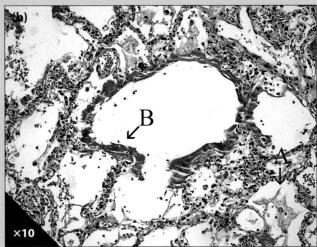

▲ **Fig. 12.12(a) and (b)** Microscopic views of the solid-looking lung section show intra-alveolar edema (A), hyaline membrane formation (B), and interstitial mononuclear inflammatory cell infiltration.

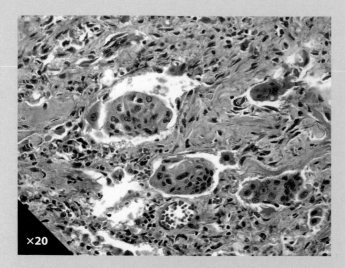

▲ **Fig. 12.13** Alveolar collapse, interstitial fibrosis and multinucleated giant cells.

In situ hybridization for SARS viral sequence detected positive signals in the cytoplasm of some epithelial cells of the trachea, bronchi, bronchioles, lungs, intestine, renal distal tubules and the central nervous system neurons (see Figs 12.15 and 12.16).

Some lymphocytes in the spleen, lymph nodes, mucosal-associated lymphoid tissue and pulmonary interstitial infiltrate were also positive (see Fig. 12.17).

Most importantly, SARS virus was also detected in the lymphocytes and monocytes of circulating blood. Coronavirus-like particles were observed in these cells by electron microscopy (shown in Fig. 12.18).

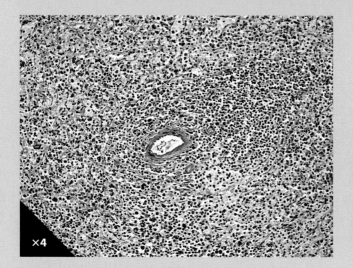

▲ **Fig. 12.14** Spleen shows atrophy with loss of follicles.

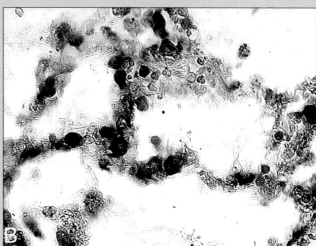

▲ **Fig. 12.15** In situ hybridization of SARS viral sequence detected positive signals in the cytoplasm of some epithelial cells of the lungs.

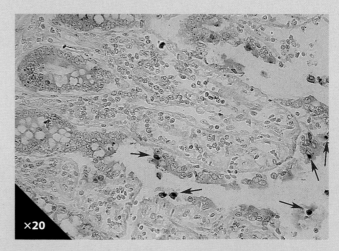

▲ **Fig. 12.16** In situ hybridization of SARS viral sequence detected positive signals in the cytoplasm of isolated mucosal epithelial cells of the small intestine.

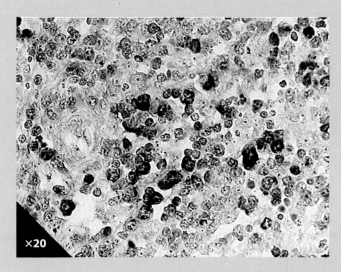

×20

▲ **Fig. 12.17** Lymphocytes in the spleen are positive for SARS viral sequence by in situ hybridization.

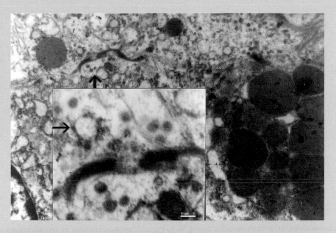

▲ **Fig. 12.18** Electron microscopy shows coronavirus-like particles in epithelial cells of the small intestine.

Monkeypox virus infection

Case 12.5

On 18 May 2003, in a city in the United States, a 30-year-old female, her 33-year-old husband and their 6-year-old daughter purchased two prairie dogs from a pet trade show. Both animals appeared healthy at the time of purchase but 3 days later, one of the animals appeared ill, displaying lethargy, wasting and anorexia. On 24 May that animal died. The following day, the second animal developed similar signs and died 2 days later. The family members had had extensive contact with the animals and, on 29 May, all three family members developed sore throat, fever, headache and fatigue.

The 30-year-old female had no prior medical history. She developed sore throat, headache, fever and malaise, and a small painless papule on her left cheek. Over the next 48 hours, the throat soreness and malaise worsened, and additional lesions developed, most prominent on the chest and arms.

On 2 June, she presented to a primary care physician, where she was noted to have a vesiculopustular rash with hemorrhagic manifestations, progressing in a uniform manner to include the entire body, most prominent on the trunk and including the palms and soles (see Fig. 12.19). Approximately 150 lesions were present.

▼ **Fig. 12.19** Monkeypox. Clinical appearance of one of the skin lesions.

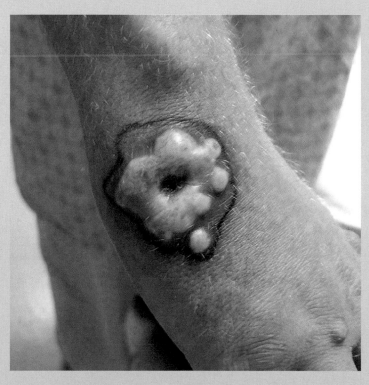

She was referred to a dermatologist, where a diagnosis of possible staphylococcal infection was made; no treatment was rendered at this time. That same evening, the patient experienced acute worsening of throat pain, as well as a sense of airway obstruction. She was seen in an emergency room, where she was given a bolus of prednisone, with subsequent improvement of shortness of breath.

On 4 June, the patient's daughter was hospitalized with recent onset seizures. The mother was now noted to have approximately 200 lesions, most prominent on the face, trunk, arms, legs, palms and soles. All lesions had a similar morphology, and no scabbing was noted.

By 7 June, several of the lesions began to scab, and the 30-year-old female patient experienced improvement of systemic symptoms. On 9 June, skin biopsies of several lesions were obtained. By 11 June, sloughing of scabs had begun, and the patient remained otherwise systemically well. By 16 June, all lesions had developed scabs, most of which had sloughed. The patient subsequently remained without systemic symptoms. She experienced extensive scarring over skin areas where the rash had been present.

Diagnosis: Monkeypox virus infection.

Human monkeypox—commentary

Human monkeypox was first identified in Zaire, now the Democratic Republic of Congo (DRC), in 1970, near the end of smallpox eradication efforts in Africa. Outbreaks of human illness have been documented in the DRC in recent years, involving over 450 suspected cases. Additional cases have been sporadically reported in other western and central African countries. Studies of the disease in Western countries and central Africa describe clinical characteristics similar to that of smallpox. The recent US outbreak represents the first time that human monkeypox has been identified outside Africa.

Clinicians initially evaluating patients included smallpox as a possible differential diagnosis. After accessing the CDC (Centers for Disease Control and Prevention) website and its information on the recently observed human monkeypox disease associated with prairie dog exposure, it was realized that the pustular rash lesions were more likely to be from the orthopoxvirus monkeypox.

Monkeypox virus is a double-stranded DNA virus of the genus Orthopoxvirus. It is genetically distinct from other orthopoxviruses, including variola virus (the cause of smallpox) and vaccinia virus (the virus used as smallpox vaccine). Descriptive studies conducted in Africa through 1986 have provided most of our understanding of the human disease and epidemiology.

Transmission is primarily by large droplets or direct contact. Compared with transmissibility of smallpox, transmission of monkeypox is inefficient. However, recent studies suggest that as the number of never-smallpox-vaccinated individuals increase, the number of secondary transmission events have also increased.

Following an incubation period of 7–19 days, clinical monkeypox is characterized by a prodrome of fever, headache and fatigue. Lymphadenopathy is common and may distinguish this infection from smallpox. While many patients in the outbreak in the United States had extensive lymphadenopathy, this feature was noted in only one of the patients. Generally, the rash evolves uniformly as macules, papules, vesicles and pustules, and then crusts over a period of 2–3 weeks. Lesions are most prominent on the head and extremities, and often involve the palms and soles.

Histopathologic features included variable degrees of ballooning, spongiosis, reticular degeneration, eosinophilic cytoplasmic granules, multinucleation, nuclear melding and hyperchromasia. Lesions were associated with abundant, mixed inflammatory cell infiltrates, often including eosinophils, at various levels of the dermis. The virus was distributed predominantly in the cytoplasm of epidermal keratinocytes, but also in dermal fibroblasts, endothelium and hair shaft epithelium (see Figs 12.20–12.23, continued overleaf).

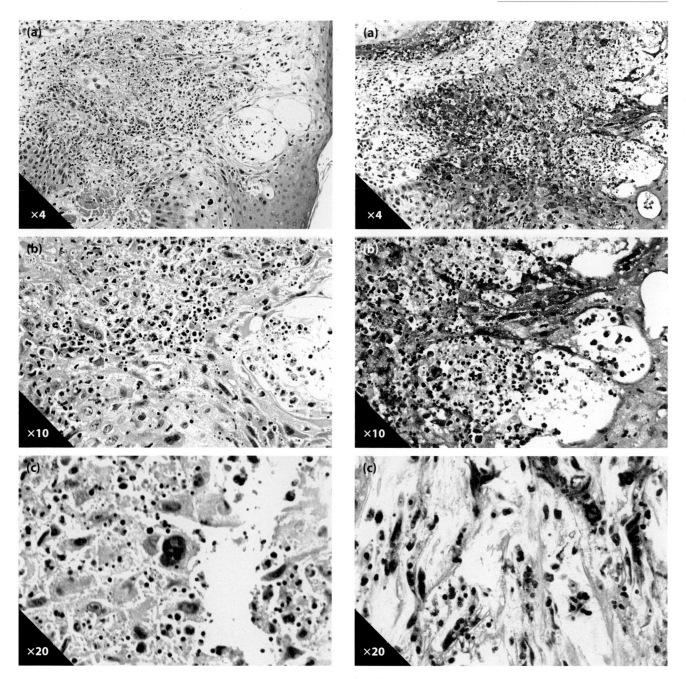

▲ **Fig. 12.20(a), (b) and (c)** Focal spongiosis and ballooning degeneration of epidermal keratinocytes with vesicle formation. The vesicles had extensive necrosis and karyorrhectic debris, accompanied by neutrophils. The dermis showed mixed perivascular inflammatory infiltrates.

▲ **Fig. 12.21(a), (b) and (c)** Immunohistochemical stains demonstrated abundant staining of orthopox viral antigens (the small red dots) within the cytoplasm of swollen keratinocytes and within the karyorrhectic debris in the vesicle.

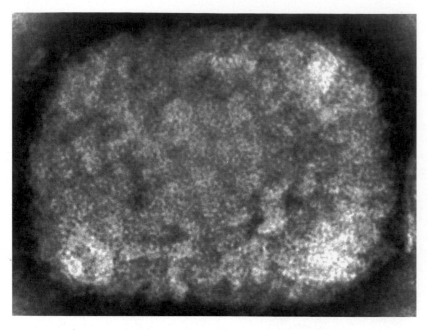

▲ Fig. 12.22 Negative stain electron microscopy of vesicular fluid.

A range of novel diagnostic methods—including PCR, serology and immuno-histochemistry—can be used to confirm various orthopoxvirus infections (including monkeypox). Antiorthopoxvirus IgM reactivity in CSF may be useful in diagnosing encephalitis due to orthopoxviruses.

Hendra virus outbreak

Human cases of Hendra virus

- Case 12.6 Pneumonia
- Case 12.7 Encephalitis

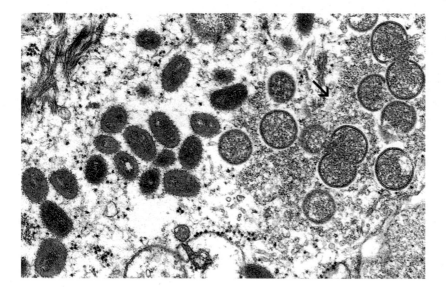

▲ Fig. 12.23 Thin section electron microscopy image of the skin biopsy showed pox virus particles.

Case 12.6

A 49-year-old male racehorse trainer presented in 1994 with an influenza-like illness 6 days after the death of a mare in his stables. He was a heavy smoker. Examination revealed fever and an increased respiratory rate. He was hypoxic and required oxygen therapy. Hemoglobin and white cell count were normal. He had severely deranged liver function tests.

A chest X-ray showed diffuse alveolar shadowing (see Fig. 12.24). Microscopy and culture of sputum, blood and bronchial washings did not reveal any organisms.

He was admitted to an intensive care unit and treated with a range of antibiotics. Despite this, he became febrile 32°F (up to 40°C), and his renal function deteriorated. Continuous dialysis was instituted. He developed an arterial thrombus in his right leg. This was treated with heparin and urokinase. He rapidly deteriorated and 7 days after admission, he developed cardiac irritability, which led to prolonged periods of asystole and then death.

Post-mortem examination was performed and the main pathology was found in the lungs, which were heavy, congested and showed multiple focal areas of hemorrhage and pneumonia. Hyaline membranes lined many of the alveolar spaces and there was proliferation of bronchial epithelial lining cells. Some of these cells contained viral inclusions (see Figs 12.25–12.28, overleaf).

Diagnosis: Pneumonia caused by the Hendra virus. (The diagnosis was made a considerable time after the death and after much laboratory and epidemiologic work had been done.) This diagnosis was confirmed by the identification of Hendra virus in the kidney (particularly) and other tissue obtained from the post mortem.

▼ Fig. 12.24 Chest X-ray showing increased shadowing in both lower lobes.

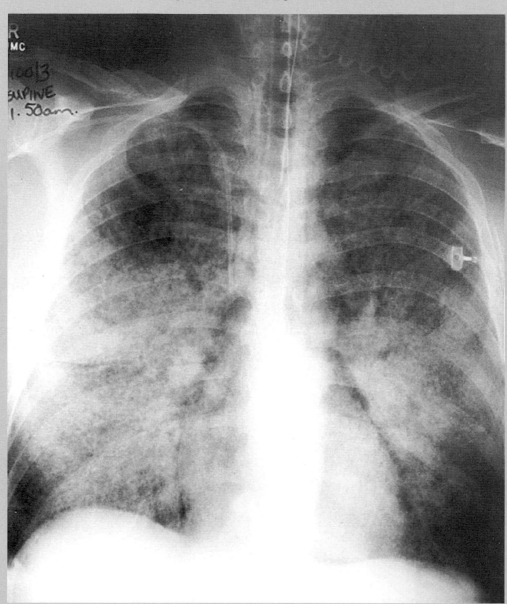

▶ **Fig. 12.25** Low-magnification view of lung showing focal areas of pneumonia.

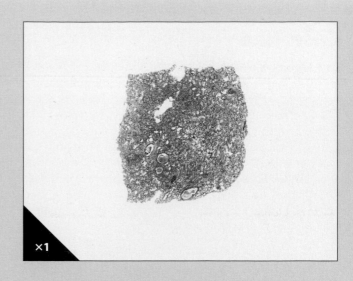

▼ **Fig. 12.26(a), (b) and (c)** Microscopic views of one of the areas of bronchopneumonia.

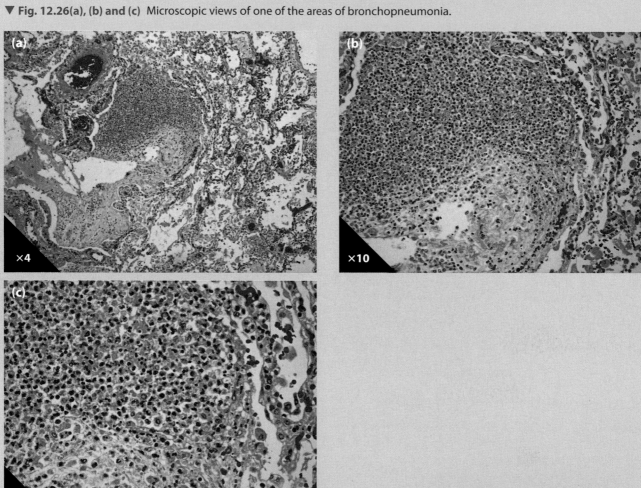

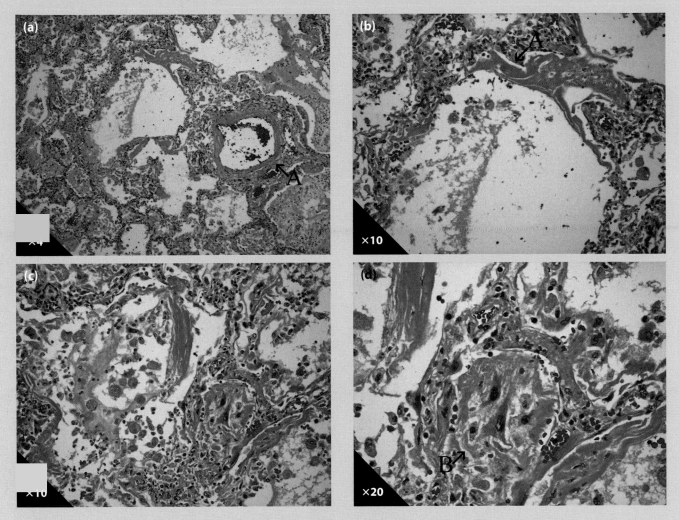

▲ **Fig. 12.27(a), (b), (c) and (d)** Hyaline membranes (A), and hyperplasia of bronchial epithelial lining cells (B).

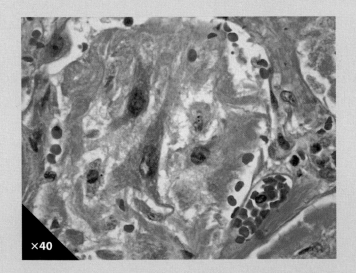

◀ **Fig. 12.28** Hyperplastic cells. Some contained viral inclusions—but not these particular cells.

Case 12.7

A 35-year-old male presented with a 12-day history of sore throat, headache, drowsiness, vomiting and neck stiffness. The clinical diagnosis was meningitis, for which no cause was found.

Oral antibiotic treatment was begun and a day or two later a lumbar puncture was performed and the CSF examination showed a total white cell count of 560/cubic mm with 82 per cent neutrophils, protein 1820 ng/L (150–450 ng/L) and glucose 4.7 mmol/L (2.5–4.5 mmol/L). Bacterial culture—no growth; no virus detected. The patient made a full recovery.

The patient was admitted to hospital 12 months later, with a 2-week history of irritable mood, low back pain and tonic-clonic seizures. Two days prior to admission, he had had three focal motor seizures involving the right arm.

MRI scans showed the appearances consistent with meningeal inflammation involving a number of cortical gyri and widespread cerebral necrosis (see Figs 12.29 and 12.30).

By day 7 of the hospital stay, he had developed a dense right hemiplegia, signs of brain stem involvement and coma. Fever developed during this week. He remained febrile and deeply unconscious until death 25 days after admission.

Examination of the brain at post mortem showed the features of viral meningitis and encephalitis which correlated with the appearances seen in the MRI scans (see Figs 12.31, 12.32 and 12.33, continued overleaf).

CSF from his second and fatal admission showed the presence of neutralizing antibodies to Hendra virus. Serum

▶ **Fig. 12.29** MRI (T1 weighted) linear serpiginous 'train track' areas of high signal consistent with meningeal inflammation involving a number of cortical gyri.

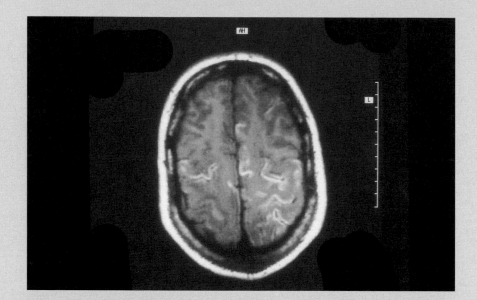

▶ **Fig. 12.30** MRI (T2 weighted) areas of high signal in both temporal lobes (A) and to a lesser extent the parietal and occipital lobes (B) (gray and white matter are involved). This is consistent with widespread cerebral necrosis. (Note that the mucosal lining of the frontal sinuses is outlined. This is not pathologic.)

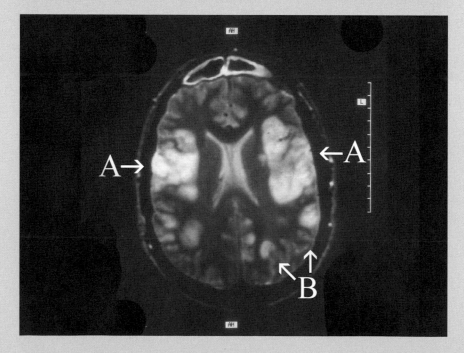

taken during the fatal illness showed a high titre of neutralizing antibodies to Hendra virus.

Immunohistochemistry carried out on brain tissue with rabbit antiserum for Hendra virus was positive.

Diagnosis: Encephalitis caused by the Hendra virus. (Diagnosis was made much more quickly than in Case 12.6 see pages 481–483.)

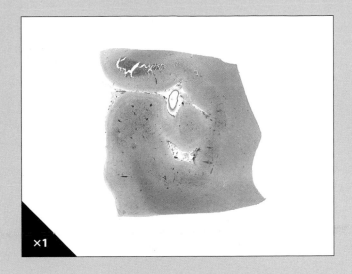

▶ **Fig. 12.31** View of a section of brain.

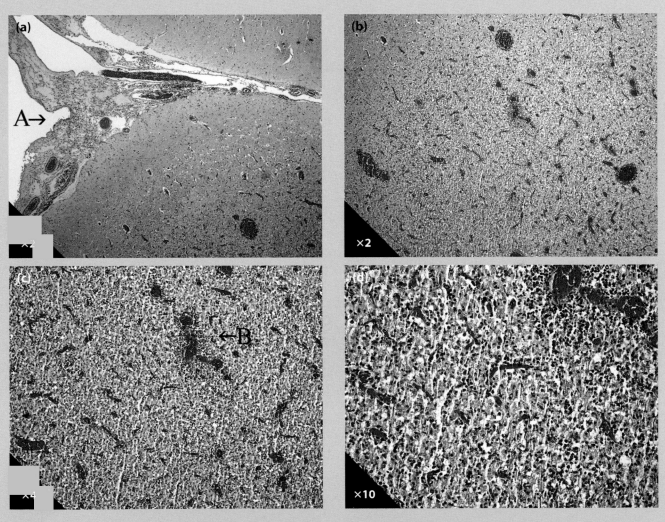

▲ **Fig. 12.32(a), (b), (c) and (d)** Low- medium- and high-magnification views of the brain showing an infiltration of mononuclear inflammatory cells in leptomeninges (A), and Virchow Robin space (B)—meningitis.

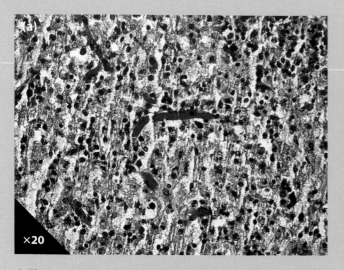 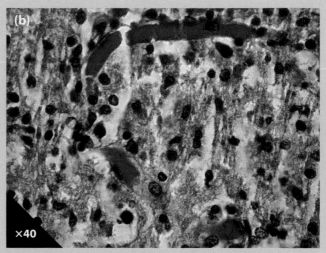

▲ **Fig. 12.33(a) and (b)** Cerebral cortex showing necrosis and chronic inflammation—encephalitis.

Equine cases of Hendra virus

Case 12.8

Two thoroughbred geldings were killed in extremis after a short, febrile illness. Six days later, 13 horses from the same suburban stable and one in an adjoining stable had been killed or died after developing acute severe respiratory disease, The incident was treated as an outbreak of exotic disease.

One horse had been dead for 12 hours or so but, allowing for the more advanced post-mortem decomposition in the latter animal, the pathologic changes in these horses were very similar.

At post mortem, there was evidence of severe recent self-trauma about limbs and head, and blood-tinged foam was present at the nostrils. The airways were almost completely filled with thick, fine, stable foam (edema fluid) ranging from white to blood-tinged (see Figs 12.34 and 12.35).

The lungs were not collapsed or consolidated in any part but were extremely heavy, variably congested according to gravitational influences, and showed patchy recent hemorrhages which ranged in size and severity throughout the lung parenchyma (see Figs 12.36 and 12.37, continued overleaf). The pleura was strikingly thickened by edema and there was excess thoracic and pericardial fluid. These accumulations were more pronounced in the longer-dead horse. There were a few accumulations of yellow edema fluid in loose areolar tissue in the dorsal retroperitoneum, thoracic inlet and between some muscle planes unrelated to areas of trauma.

There was recent blood-staining of ingesta in the proximal parts of the small bowel and in the distal colon, but no real evidence of enteritis.

Microscopic changes were present in the renal cortex (see Fig. 12.38, overleaf).

Hendra virus was isolated from post-mortem material.
Diagnosis: Equine Hendra virus infection.

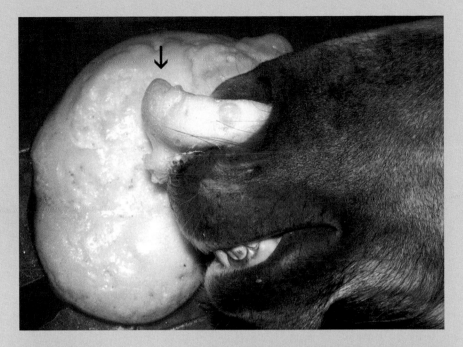

▶ **Fig. 12.34** Suffocatingly voluminous stable foam (edema fluid) issuing from the nose of a horse with severe acute pulmonary edema. This is a nonspecific finding, not restricted to cases of Hendra virus infection.

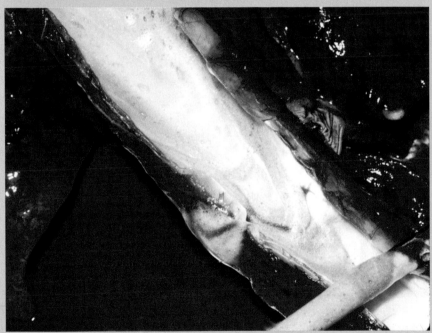

▶ **Fig. 12.35** Stable foam filling the trachea of a horse dead of severe acute pulmonary edema. Again, not pathognomonic in any sense of acute Hendra virus infection.

▶ **Fig. 12.36** Lung. Recent intraparenchymal hemorrhage in acute equine Hendra virus infection with no accompanying inflammation.

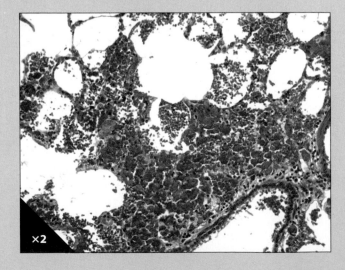

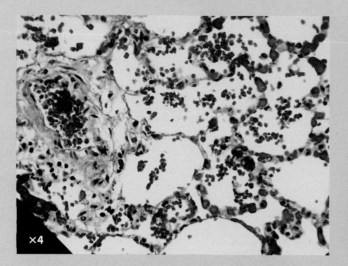

▲ **Fig. 12.37** Lung. Many endothelial cells are represented only by pyknotic nuclear fragments. This septal capillary destruction is probably responsible for the hemorrhage and edema.

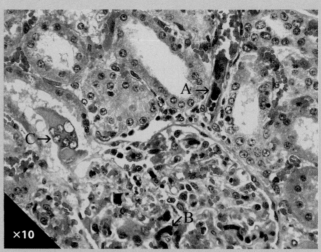

▲ **Fig. 12.38** Renal cortex showing syncytium formation in endothelial cells of an afferent arteriole (A), glomerular capillaries (B) and in epithelial cells (possibly parietal Bowman's capsular epithelium) sloughed into the origin of the proximal tubule (C).

Hendra virus—commentary

The Hendra virus outbreak occurred in 1994. The three presentations describe the clinical and pathologic features produced in humans and horses by the same previously unrecognized virus. It was given the name Hendra virus after the place where the first cases were found. Hendra is a suburb of Brisbane, Australia, where two major racetracks are located, and many racehorses are stabled in the area.

Extensive epidemiologic tests were carried out in relation to these cases. 296 contacts, including the veterinarian wife of the patient who died from encephalitis, were seronegative to the Hendra virus. Other veterinarians who performed autopsies on the horses also tested negative for serum antibodies against the Hendra virus. Those tested included spouses of the patients, people who worked closely with the infected horses, and healthcare workers at the hospitals where the patients were managed. 2000 thoroughbred racehorses were tested and 5000 specimens were examined from over 40 other animal and bird species. None of them was found to be positive.

In an attempt to identify a reservoir of the virus, fruit bats (*Pteropus* species) were tested for the presence of Hendra virus, and 9 per cent of them were found to be positive. Experimental studies demonstrated that the virus could be transmitted from bats to horses, and between horses.

From September 1998 to June 1999, an outbreak of a clinically similar disease caused by a closely related virus appeared in Malaysia and Singapore. This virus was called Nipah, after the town in northern Malaysia where the first case was diagnosed. The outbreak in Malaysia affected more than 250 patients with a case fatality of approximately 40 per cent. The symptoms were of a flu-like illness complicated by encephalitis. There was a strong history of contact with pigs.

About this time, the same virus caused a febrile, flu-like illness associated with either encephalitis or pneumonia in 11 abattoir workers in Singapore.

As for the Hendra virus, the Nipah virus was also found in fruit bats. The intermediate host was pigs, rather than horses, and experimental transmission was obtained between pigs.

Further studies have confirmed the identity of the Hendra and Nipah viruses. They are now classified as a separate genus (Henipavirus) of the subfamily Paramyxovirinia of the family Paramyxoviridia. (The morbilli virus that causes measles is also a genus within the same subfamily.)

Since these outbreaks of Hendra virus in 1994, and Nipah in 1998 and 1999, only a few further human cases have been reported.

Biological warfare/bioterrorism

A chemical or an organism that can quickly cause severe debilitating disease in an enemy would appeal to an attacker. However, the attacker must be able to protect themselves from the agent being used, or otherwise have an antidote or a protective vaccine. The number of chemicals and organisms that would be suitable for this sort of activity is probably somewhat limited, but it is a sad fact of life that there are governments, terrorist organizations and individuals thinking about a wide range of possibilities.

Anthrax has received considerable attention in recent years as a potential agent in biological warfare, and as a weapon for bioterrorism. In 1979, there was an accidental release of anthrax spores from a weapons research laboratory in the Ural Mountains in what was then the Soviet Union. About 60 people died. The clinical features of the cases were similar. Fever developed one day and drowsiness was followed by unconsciousness and death one or two days later.[‡]

Post-mortem examinations on 42 cases revealed a hemorrhagic, necrotizing pneumonia at the presumed site of entry of the inhaled organism, the presence of hemorrhagic necrosis of the thoracic lymph nodes and hemorrhagic mediastinitis, a hemorrhagic meningitis and multiple gastrointestinal submucosal hemorrhages.

Microscopically, the various sites of involvement showed hemorrhage, very little inflammation and numerous, large, Gram-positive bacilli—the pathologic hallmarks of *Bacillus anthracis* infection. The organism *B. anthracis* was cultured from 20 of the cases.

In the months following the terrorist attack on the twin towers of the World Trade Center in New York on September 11 in 2001, a number of US senators and others received mail containing a fine white powder that contained *B. anthracis* spores. Some infections were reported.

What of the future?

From the historical vignettes in this book, it can be seen that our present knowledge about infectious diseases has been acquired by the painstaking observations and experiments of workers in many different countries. Health workers throughout the world are united in a team that is engaged in protecting their fellow citizens from the ravages of these diseases. It is important for them to be able to diagnose and treat not only diseases that occur in their own environment, but also to know about diseases that occur elsewhere, because with the speed and ease of modern travel, people may acquire an infection in one country and then become sick by the time they reach another one. Timely diagnosis and treatment is important for the individual, but with potentially epidemic diseases, the whole community is depending on the health workers for protection.

Acknowledgments

- Figs 12.1–12.9 report on AIDS. Courtesy of Ann Marie Nelson, Chief, Division of AIDS Pathology, Armed Forces Institute of Pathology (AFIP), Washington, USA.
- Figs 12.10–12.18 report on SARS. Courtesy of Jiang Gu, Professor and Chair, Department of Pathology; and Dean, School of Basic Medical Sciences, Peking University, Beijing, China. (In association with staff member Xueying Shi.)
- Figs 12.19–12.23 report on monkeypox virus. Courtesy of Sherif R. Zaki, Chief, Infectious Disease Pathology Activity, Division of Viral and Rickettsial Diseases, National Center for Infectious Diseases, Centers for Disease Control and Prevention, Atlanta, USA.
- Figs 12.24–12.28 case report on Hendra virus. Courtesy of Anthony J. Ansford, pathologist, and Joseph G. McCormack, infectious diseases physician, Brisbane, Australia. Photographed by Robin Cooke.
- Figs 12.29–12.33 case report on Hendra virus. Courtesy of Ian Brown, pathologist, and John O'Sullivan, neurologist, Brisbane, Australia. Photographed by Robin Cooke.
- Figs 12.34–12.38 report on equine Hendra virus. Courtesy of Roger Kelly, veterinary pathologist, Brisbane, Australia.

---

‡Report of cases from the Ural Mountains was obtained from:

Abramova, F.A., Grinberg, L.M., Yampolskaya, O.V. and Walker, D.H. Pathology of inhalational anthrax in 42 cases from the Sverdlovsk outbreak of 1979. *Proc Natl Acad Sci USA* 90(6):2291–2294, 1993.